DIFFERENTIAL DIAGNOSIS OF
LYMPHOID DISORDERS

DIFFERENTIAL DIAGNOSIS OF LYMPHOID DISORDERS

TSIEH SUN, M.D.
Chief, Division of Clinical Pathology
Department of Laboratories
North Shore University Hospital—
Cornell University Medical College
Manhasset, New York
and
Professor of Clinical Pathology
Department of Pathology
Cornell University Medical College
New York, New York

MYRON SUSIN, M.D.
Attending Pathologist
Department of Laboratories
North Shore University Hospital—
Cornell University Medical College
Manhasset, New York
and
Clinical Associate Professor of Pathology
Department of Pathology
Cornell University Medical College
New York, New York

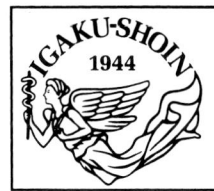

IGAKU-SHOIN   New York * Tokyo

Published and distributed by

IGAKU-SHOIN Medical Publishers, Inc.
One Madison Avenue, New York, New York 10010

IGAKU-SHOIN Ltd.,
5-24-3 Hongo, Bunkyo-ku, Tokyo 113-91.

Copyright © 1996 by IGAKU-SHOIN Medical Publishers, Inc.
All rights reserved. No part of this book may be translated or
reproduced in any form by print, photo-print, microfilm, or any
other means without written permission from the publisher.

Library of Congress Cataloging-in-Publication Data

Sun, Tsieh.
   Differential diagnosis of lymphoid disorders / Tsieh Sun and Myron Susin.
     p.   cm.
   Includes bibliographical references and index.
   1. Lymphomas—Diagnosis—Handbooks, manuals, etc. 2. Blood—
Diseases—Diagnosis—Handbooks, manuals, etc. 3. Diagnosis,
Differential—Handbooks, manuals, etc. I. Susin, Myron.
II. Title.
   [DNLM: 1. Lymphoma—diagnosis. 2. Diagnosis, Differential. QZ
350 S957d 1995]
RC280.L9S843   1995
616.99′242075—dc20
DNLM/DLC   95-19893
for Library of Congress   CIP

ISBN: 0-89640-289-4   (New York)
ISBN: 4-260-14289-5   (Tokyo)

Printed and bound in the U.S.A.

10 9 8 7 6 5 4 3 2 1

*To our wives Sue and Janet
for their constant support, patience, and understanding.*

ACKNOWLEDGMENT

We wish to acknowledge Drs. I. J. Su of the National Taiwan University, T. T. Kuo of Chang Gung College of Medicine and Technology, Taiwan, Anna-Luise Katzenstein of the State University of New York at Syracuse, and Harry Ioachim of Lenox Hill Hospital, New York, for providing us with histologic sections of unusual cases; the Armed Forces Institute of Pathology for providing photos of some rare diseases; our pathology colleagues at the North Shore University Hospital for sharing their cases with us; Dr. Saul Teichberg for providing electron-microscopic illustrations; the technologists in the flow cytometry, immunopathology, molecular genetics, and electron-microscopy laboratories for skillful technical assistance; the staff of our medical library for prompt interlibrary service; and last but not least, Lynn Bartholomew for impeccable secretarial assistance.

PREFACE

Hematopathology has always been a great challenge to the pathologist because of its complexity and the subtle differences between various entities. It is even more so in recent years owing to the explosion of new techniques in immunopathology, cytogenetics, and molecular biology and to the development of specific therapeutic regimens for hematologic neoplasms. Therefore, making a distinction between lymphoid hyperplasia and lymphoma is no longer sufficient; the knowledge of lymphoma subclassification is now demanded of the pathologist by clinical hematologists and oncologists, so that an effective treatment can be tailored. In fact, the expansion in the area of atypical lymphoproliferative disorders makes the distinction between a benign and a malignant condition no longer an easy task. The application of new techniques has created more disease entities. The Revised European-American Classification of Lymphoid Neoplasms (REAL classification), published in 1994, listed at least 10 new entities that have not been recognized in other classifications.

To meet this unprecedented challenge, many books on hematopathology have been published in the last few years. Some of them are highly authoritative and comprehensive, but these books are so voluminous that some of the readers may be overwhelmed.

Bearing this situation in mind, we are presenting a concise handbook aiming at the practicing pathologist for quick reference. Our emphasis is on the differential diagnosis of the new and relatively new lymphoma entities, including most of those listed in the REAL classification, but some old entities that require recognition in the differential diagnosis are also included. One of the common weaknesses in textbooks of hematopathology is the neglect of benign lesions; thus we have made a conscious effort to describe these lesions in detail. Although it is almost impossible to make a definitive morphologic diagnosis of some subclassified lymphomas, especially in the T-cell category, we have made serious attempts to guide the reader to reach a preliminary morphologic diagnosis by providing important morphologic criteria and abundant illustrations. In addition, up-to-date information on new diagnostic tools is furnished in each chapter and an overview of these new techniques is presented at the early part of the book so that the reader may have a basic understanding of the clinical application of the ancillary studies.

The goal of this book is not to replace but to complement those comprehensive textbooks of hematopathology. We hope that the readers may find this book helpful in their busy daily practice of pathology so that they would read a voluminous textbook only at their leisure.

CONTENTS

1. General introduction   1
2. Cell markers and classification of lymphoid neoplasms   3
3. Ancillary studies for lymphoid disorders   13
4. Reactive lymphoid hyperplasias   25
5. Differential diagnosis of granulomatous lymphadenitis   49
6. Differential diagnosis of storage histiocyte disorders   62
7. Hodgkin's disease vs. lymphomas with Reed–Sternberg-like cells   69
8. Differential diagnosis of Castleman's disease (angiofollicular hyperplasia)   82
9. Follicular lymphoma vs. follicular hyperplasia vs. mantle-cell lymphoma   90
10. Composite lymphoma vs. Richter's syndrome vs. mixed small- and large-cell lymphoma   102
11. Pseudolymphoma vs. lymphoma of mucosa-associated lymphoid tissue vs. T-cell-rich B-cell lymphoma   110
12. Hairy-cell leukemia vs. monocytoid B-cell lymphoma vs. splenic lymphoma with villous lymphocytes   120
13. Lymphoblastic lymphoma vs. Burkitt's lymphoma vs. acute lymphoblastic leukemia   132
14. Anaplastic large-cell Ki-1 lymphoma vs. Hodgkin's disease, metastatic carcinoma, and malignant histiocytosis   143
15. Thymoma vs. malignant lymphoma vs. Hodgkin's disease   150
16. Angioimmunoblastic lymphadenopathy vs. immunoblastic lymphadenopathy-like T-cell lymphoma   158
17. T-cell lymphoma vs. malignant and benign histiocytosis   164
18. True natural-killer-cell lymphoma vs. natural-killer-like T-cell lymphoma   175
19. Mycosis fungoides/Sézary syndrome vs. adult T-cell leukemia/lymphoma   181
20. Cutaneous lymphomas vs. carcinomas   190
21. Differential diagnosis of angiocentric immunoproliferative lesions   197
22. Lymphoplasmacytic lymphoma vs. plasmacytoma vs. plasmacytoid T-cell lymphoma (plasmacytoid monocytoid sarcoma)   204
23. Granulocytic sarcoma vs. large-cell lymphoma vs. true histiocytic lymphoma   215

Index   225

1
General Introduction

The lymphocyte is the major component of the human immune system and plays an important role in both the humoral and cellular arms of the immune system. Therefore, lymphoid reactions are among the most common phenomena, occurring frequently in a broad spectrum of benign conditions. These conditions are often so similar that they may not be easily distinguishable. Sometimes, they may even mimic malignant diseases. In patients with immune deregulation, for instance, the lymphoid cells that react to antigenic stimulation may appear atypical or malignant. In some cases, in fact, posttransplantation lymphoproliferative disorder can be distinguished from lymphoma only by withdrawal of immunosuppressive therapy to see if there is a resurgence of normal lymphocytes. In other conditions, lymphoid hyperplasia may terminate in lymphomas, such as in patients with the acquired immunodeficiency syndrome (AIDS).

In between reactive lymphoid disorders and lymphomas, a third category, designated *atypical lymphoproliferative disorders*, has emerged in recent years. These disorders, which include angiocentric immunoproliferative lesions, angioimmunoblastic lymphadenopathy, and systemic Castleman's disease, pose a great challenge to pathologists.

As can be expected, the most difficult task in the field of lymphoid disorders is to make an accurate diagnosis of lymphoma. Lymphomas are thought to be the result of a developmental arrest in various stages of lymphoid evolution, which differs in terms of T-cells, B-cells, and natural-killer (NK) cells. Lymphomas are also derived from different compartments of the lymph node or the spleen. For B-lymphocytes, lymphomas can originate from the follicular center, mantle zone, and marginal zone. The distinction of all these subtypes of lymphomas is often impossible without the help of modern technology.

To make this situation even more complicated is the fact that two different lymphomas can coexist side-by-side (e.g., composite lymphoma), and a low-grade lymphoma can transform into a high-grade lymphoma (e.g., Richter's syndrome). In fact, there is evidence to indicate that even low-grade B-cell lymphomas can transform into each other or become a hybrid form (e.g., hairy-cell leukemia/chronic lymphocytic leukemia). This close association of various tumor cells inevitably causes confusing histopathologic features, and a clearcut diagnosis under these conditions is not always achievable.

Furthermore, the lymphoid organs (lymph node, bone marrow, spleen, and thymus) are involved not only by lymphocytes but also granulocytes, histiocytes, thymic epithelial cells, and carcinoma cells, which may be associated with such conditions as granulocytic sarcoma, malignant histiocytosis, storage histiocyte disorders, thymoma, and metastatic carcinoma. These diseases are frequently confused with and need to be distinguished from lymphoid disorders.

All the conditions that are mentioned above are part of the intriguing problems that we must be concerned with in the diagnosis of lymphoid disorders. In many conditions, the differences between two entities are so subtle that a diagnosis represents only a subjective interpretation of an ambiguous condition. Fortunately, new technological advances have come to the rescue. The first B-cell marker, surface immunoglobulin, remains the most useful marker in distinguishing a benign from a malignant disease by identifying clonality in terms of light-chain restriction. The subsequent development of monoclonal antibodies and flow cytometry has greatly enhanced the fine-tuning capability of lymphocyte characterization: the cell lineage, developmental stage, immunologic function, activation status, and proliferative activity. On this basis, lymphomas are classified and subclassified. In the revised European–American Classification of Lymphoid Neoplasms, published in 1994, 23 lymphoid neoplasms are listed, 10 of which have never before been included in any other lymphoma classification.

The weakness of immunophenotyping such as the failure to identify the clonality of T-cell neoplasms is compensated by the development of genotyping. When gene rearrangement is equivocal, cytogenetic studies frequently help determine the malignant or benign nature of a lesion. The recent development of the polymerase chain reaction and *in situ* hybridization techniques have made these new techniques even more practical.

The subclassification of lymphomas has been followed by the development of new therapeutic regimens. This progress makes the accurate diagnosis and subclassification of lymphomas imperative since clinical hematologists and oncologists have begun to demand a precise diagnosis so that they can make their treatment more specific.

This book represents our effort in helping to solve the problems mentioned before through the discussion of morphologic features and laboratory techniques and their roles in establishing the diagnosis. Clinical manifestations are also included in individual chapters as these are essential in making a differential diagnosis. Bearing in mind that many pathologists may not have access to the latest technology, we have emphasized morphologic criteria and supplemented them with abundant illustrations to facilitate the recognition of characteristic diagnostic features. On the basis of the histopathologic features, the reader may achieve a preliminary diagnosis, and may accordingly request appropriate ancillary tests from a commercial laboratory of immunopathology and molecular biology.

Because of the intimate relationship between benign and malignant conditions in the field of lymphoid diseases, it is difficult to separate them in different sections of the text. However, a rough organization has been arranged to keep similar topics together. Chapter 2, for example, depicts the new concepts of lymphocyte evolution from the bone marrow to the parafollicular zone. This basic knowledge is important for the reader in order to understand how lymphomas are classified and why some tumors have similar phenotypes. Chapter 3 provides a basic understanding of the theory and techniques behind immunophenotyping and cytogenetic molecular analysis, so that the reader may develop some background knowledge of these techniques before encountering them in subsequent chapters. After the three introductory chapters (Chapters 1–3) are three chapters describing benign lymphoid disorders (Chapters 4–6). Because of the sheer number of entities associated with reactive lymphoid hyperplasia and granulomatous lymphadenitis, Chapters 4 and 5 are not divided into clinical features, pathology, and laboratory findings. The remaining chapters use the same format for easy search of information. Each chapter also singles out a few entities for an in-depth discussion, and for those newly recognized entities, they are described in particular detail.

Hodgkin's disease is discussed mainly in Chapter 7, but it is also included in the differential diagnosis in other chapters, such as in the chapter on Castleman's disease (Chapter 8). Chapters 9–13 are devoted to B-cell lymphomas. Chapters 13–21 include T-cell lymphomas, natural-killer-cell lymphomas, and histiocytic disorders. Chapter 22 discusses plasma-cell neoplasms; and Chapter 23, granulocytic sarcoma.

Since there is a plethora of publications dealing with lymphomas and atypical lymphoproliferative disorders, it is impossible to include an exhaustive list of references for each chapter, which is also not the style of a handbook. However, we have tried to include the most up-to-date and representative articles for the reader to refer to; in some chapters, it is as up-to-date as 1995. The availability of several comprehensive textbooks in recent years has helped us avoid any major omission in content. However, since this book is meant to be a quick reference text, the reader is encouraged to consult the following books listed in the bibliography for topics that are not covered in this book.

BIBLIOGRAPHY

1. Lennert K, Feller AC: *Histopathology of Non-Hodgkin's Lymphomas* (based on the updated Kiel classification), 2nd ed, Berlin, Springer-Verlag, 1992.
2. Swerdlow SH: *Biopsy Interpretation of Lymph Nodes*, New York, Raven Press, 1992.
3. Stansfeld AG, d'Ardenne AJ (eds): *Lymph Node Biopsy Interpretation*, Edinburg, Churchill Livingstone, 1992.
4. Knowles DM (ed): *Neoplastic Hematopathology*, Baltimore, Williams & Wilkins, 1992.
5. Lukes RJ, Collins RD: *Tumors of the Hematopoietic System, Atlas of Tumor Pathology*, 2nd series, Washington DC, Armed Forces Institute of Pathology, 1992.
6. Sun T: *Color Atlas/Text of Flow Cytometric Analysis of Hematologic Neoplasms*, New York, Igaku-Shoin, 1993.
7. Ioachim HL: *Lymph Node Pathology*, 2nd ed, Philadelphia, Lippincott, 1994.
8. Brunning RD, McKenna RW: *Tumors of the Bone Marrow, Atlas of Tumor Pathology*, 3rd series, Washington DC, Armed Forces Institute of Pathology, 1994.
9. Isaacson PG, Norton AJ: *Extranodal Lymphomas*, Edinburgh, Churchill Livingstone, 1994.
10. Jaffe ES: *Surgical Pathology of the Lymph Nodes and Related Organs*, 2nd ed, Philadelphia, Saunders, 1995.

2
Cell Markers and Classification of Lymphoid Neoplasms

Lymphocytes can be divided phenotypically into T-cell, B-cell, and natural-killer (NK) cell. While the ontogeny of T-cell and B-cell has been well established, that of natural-killer cell is still unclear.[1] In the embryonic stage, T-cell precursors are produced in the bone marrow, and migrate to the thymus, where the thymocytes pass through the subcapsular region to the cortex and finally medulla, becoming mature thymocytes (2–4). The earliest stage of thymocyte, also called *stage I thymocyte* or *prothymocyte*, is composed of about 13% of the entire thymocyte population (Table 2–1).[4] It expresses terminal deoxynucleotidyl transferase (TdT) in the nucleus; CD3 in the cytoplasm; and CD38, CD71, and the earliest T-cell surface marker, CD7, on the surface (Table 2–1). Some studies also indicated the presence of surface HLA-DR, CD34, and possibly CD2 at this stage.[2] Stage II thymocytes, also called *common thymocytes*, include subcapsular and cortical cells and represent approximately 75% of the total thymocyte population. In this stage, CD1, CD2, CD5, CD7, and CD8 are expressed. CD4 and CD8 are usually coexpressed, or only one of the two is expressed. Stage III thymocytes, also called *medullary* or *mature thymocytes*, consist of about 15% of the thymic-cell population. The mature thymocytes express additional surface CD3 as well as T-cell receptor protein and start to divide into CD4+, CD8− and CD4−, CD8+ subgroups. When the mature thymocytes enter into the peripheral circulation, they become postthymic or peripheral T-cells, which lose the CD38 marker.

The development of B-cells is confined to the bone marrow. In the B-cell progenitor stage, only HLA-DR, CD34, and TdT are expressed (Table 2–2). Additional antigens, CD10, CD19, CD20, and CD22 appear in the next stage, pre-pre-B-cell stage.[2-4] The pre-B-cell stage is characterized by the presence of cytoplasmic μ chain without accompanying light chain and the loss of CD34. In the immature B-cell stage, surface IgM as well as immunoglobulin light chains and CD21 start to appear. CD10 usually disappears at this stage, but it is frequently present on Burkitt's lymphoma cells, which are considered immature B-cells.[5] When B-cells become mature, IgD appears on the surface side by side with IgM. The mature B-cells are considered resting or "virgin" until becoming activated by their contact with antigens. As heavy-chain switching occurs on B-cell activation, the activated B-cells express surface IgA or IgG instead of IgM/IgD. CD21 disappears at this stage, but activation antigens, such as CD38 and CD71, and proliferation-associated antigen Ki-67 are frequently expressed. Activated B-cells finally develop into the terminal stage, plasma cell. Plasma cells synthesize cytoplasmic immunoglobulin and express surface CD38, PCA-1, and PC-1. Some activated B-cells may become memory B-cells, which have an immunophenotype similar to that of either a resting B-cell[4] or an activated B-cell.[6]

The circulating lymphocytes may migrate to the lymph nodes, the mucosal follicles, and other extranodal sites depending on their surface homing receptors for high endothelial venules in various tissues.[7] In the lymph node, lymphocytes travel from one compartment to another, undergoing further morphologic changes.

INTRANODAL DISTRIBUTION AND DEVELOPMENT OF LYMPHOCYTES

The lymph node contains four compartments: the cortex, paracortex, medullary cords, and sinuses (Fig. 2–1). The cortex is composed of lymphoid follicles. A primary follicle contains aggregates of resting or virgin B-cells.[6,8] After antigenic stimulation, resting B-lymphocytes become activated, leading to proliferation and blastic transformation. A germinal center is formed and is surrounded by a mantle zone (Fig. 2–2), which comprises the same resting B-cells (Fig. 2–3) as those in the primary follicles. The follicle with a germinal center is called a *secondary follicle*. The germinal center is subdivided into dark and light zones; the dark zone is composed primarily of noncleaved cells (centroblasts), and the light zone consists of cleaved cells (centrocytes) (Fig. 2–4–2–6). The centrocytes are the mature form of the proliferating centroblasts. Some of the activated B-cells (centrocytes) migrate to the medullary cords and differentiate into plasma cells. Other activated B-cells transform into memory B-cells, which move to the outer follicular mantle zone, known as the *marginal zone*.[11] The memory B-cells are protected from apoptosis by the normal

4 DIFFERENTIAL DIAGNOSIS OF LYMPHOID DISORDERS

TABLE 2.1
Immunophenotype of Different Developmental Stages of T-Lymphocytes

Stage I: prothymocyte	Stage II: Common thymocyte	Stage III: mature thymocyte	Postthymic T-lymphocyte
TdT	TdT	TdT	CD7
cCD3	cCD3	cCD3	CD2
HLA-DR	CD7	CD7	CD5
CD7	CD2	CD2	CD4 or CD8
CD2 (±)	CD38	CD38	CD3
CD34	CD5	CD5	TCR
CD38	CD1	CD4 or CD8	
CD71	CD4	CD3	
	CD8	TCR	

Abbreviations: TdT = terminal deoxynucleotyl transferase; cCD3 = cytoplasmic CD3; TCR = T-cell receptor (TCR α/β 95%, TCR γ/δ 5%).

bcl-2 gene, which is expressed on B-cells after activation; thus they can survive for a long time.[12,13]

In the lymph node, T-cells are normally present in the paracortical area (T-zone) (Fig. 2–7), but small numbers of T-cells are also present in the follicles. T-cells can also be activated, leading to blastic transformation and proliferation. Tingible-body macrophages are frequently seen in proliferating germinal centers representing phagocytosis of apoptotic cells.

TABLE 2.2
Immunophenotypes of Different Developmental Stages of B-Lymphocytes

Progenitor B-cell: TdT, HLA-DR, CD34
↓
Pre-pre-B-cell: TdT, HLA-DR, CD34, CD19, CD22, CD10, CD20
↓
Pre-B-cell: TdT, HLA-DR, CD19, CD22, CD10, CD20, cytoplasmic μ chain
↓
Immature B-cell: HLA-DR, CD19, CD22, CD20, CD21, surface IgM
↓
Mature B-cell: HLA-DR, CD19, CD22, CD20, CD21, surface IgM/IgD
↓
Activated B-cell: HLA-DR, CD19, CD22, CD20, surface IgA, or IgG
↓
Plasma cell: Cytoplasmic immunoglobulins, CD38, PCA-1, PC-1

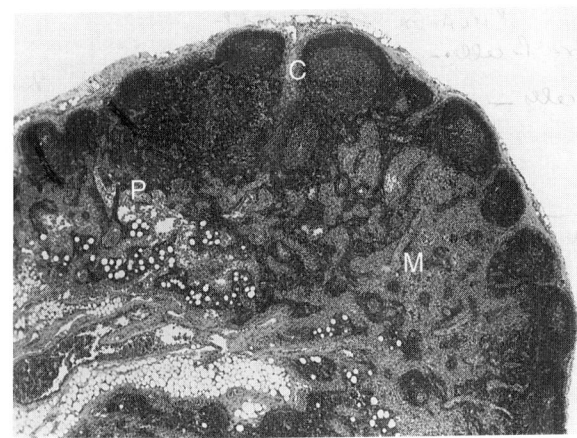

Fig. 2.1a. A normal lymph node showing the capsule, subcapsular sinus, the cortex (C) containing lymph follicles with germinal centers, the paracortex (P), and the medulla (M) including cords and sinuses. H&E (hematoxylin–eosin stain preparation) × 50.

The germinal centers also contain CD57+ natural-killer cells, which are sometimes used as a marker for collapsed follicles. However, demonstration of meshwork of follicular dendritic cells (dendritic reticulum cells) (Fig. 2–8) is especially useful in substantiating the diagnosis of B-cell lymphoma of follicular center origin, because these lymphomas usually intermingle with the dendritic meshwork even when they are located in the exranodal sites.[2] Similar to follicular dendritic cells, the interdigitating reticulum cells are also antigen-presenting cells, but they are located in paracortex and interact with T-lymphocytes.

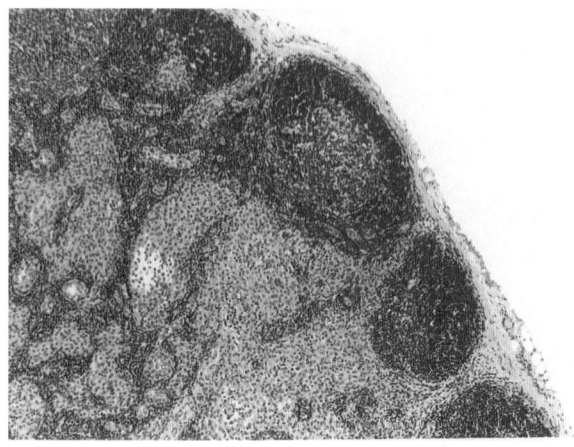

Fig. 2.1b. The cortex and paracortex of a normal lymph node. H&E, ×125.

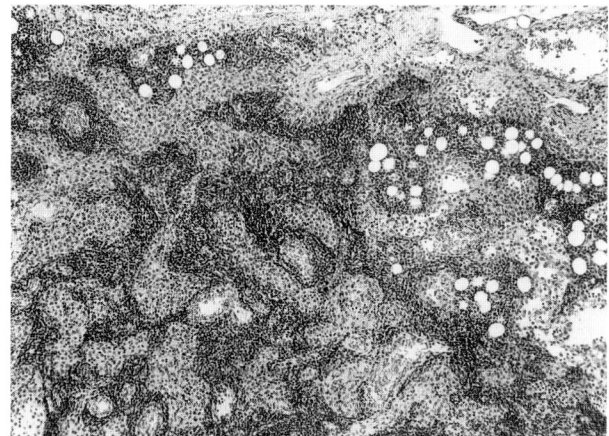

Fig. 2.1c. The medulla of a normal lymph node. H&E, ×125.

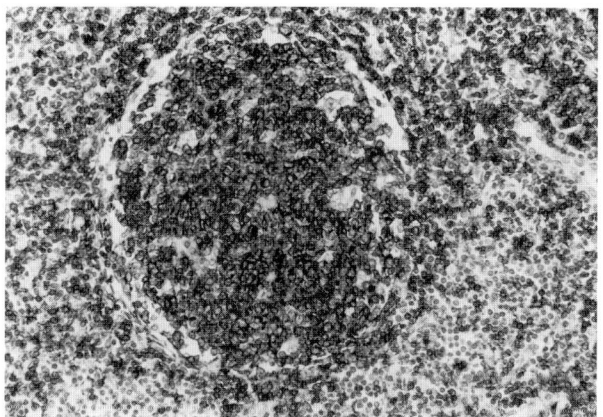

Fig. 2.3. A lymph follicle showing positive B-cell (CD20) staining of the cells in the germinal center and some cells in the mantle zone. Immunoperoxidase, ×250.

On the basis of current studies, the sequence of normal B-cell differentiation within the follicles is suggested as follows. In the mantle zone, small lymphocytes develop into intermediate lymphocyte and finally blastic lymphoid cells. The blasts then move into the germinal center and evolve through the stages of small noncleaved cell, large noncleaved cell, large cleaved cell, and small cleaved cell.[6]

The concept of intranodal B-cell differentiation has now expanded to cover the marginal zone and parafollicular zone (Fig. 2–9).[10] As mentioned before, when the activated B-cells transform into the memory B-cells, the latter migrate to the marginal zone and become marginal-zone cells. Under certain conditions, the marginal-zone cells move to the parafollicular, perisinusoidal area and become parafollicular B-cells. These cells have ovoid nuclei and relatively abundant, clear cytoplasm resembling monocytes and are thus called *monocytoid B-cells*. In lymphomas of mucosa-associated lymphoid tissue (MALT), the tumor cells are similar to monocytoid B-cells morphologically. Therefore, it is suggested that monocytoid B-cell lymphoma, lymphoma of MALT, and splenic marginal-zone lymphoma are all derived from the same origin:

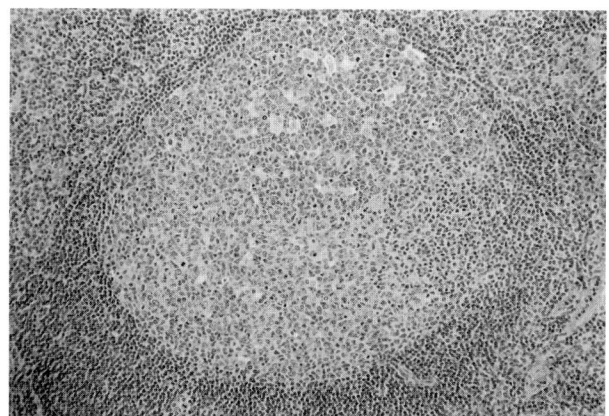

Fig. 2.2. A lymph follicle showing a germinal center surrounded by a mantle zone. The upper half of the germinal center is the dark zone consisting of noncleaved cells and some pale-stained macrophages. The lower half of the germinal center is the light zone consisting of cleaved cells. H&E, ×250.

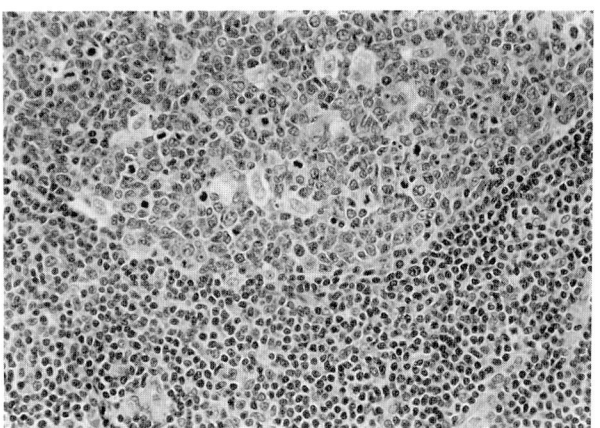

Fig. 2.4. A higher magnification showing the dark zone containing noncleaved cells and pale-stained macrophages; each is surrounded by a small space. Several mitotic figures are also present. Below the germinal center is the mantle zone. H&E, ×500.

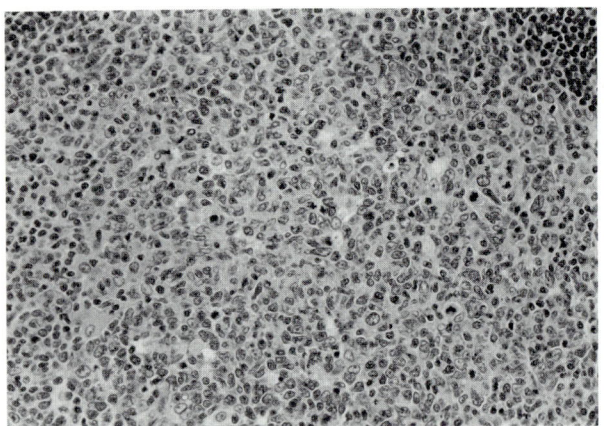

Fig. 2.5. A higher magnification showing the light zone which is composed of cleaved cells with many mitotic figures. H&E, ×500.

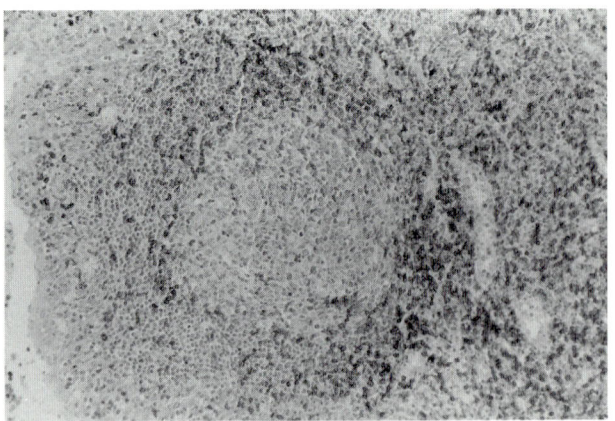

Fig. 2.7. A lymph node showing positive T-cell (CD45RO) staining of the cells in the interfollicular area and some cells in the mantle zone. Immunoperoxidase, ×125.

the marginal-zone B-cells.[10] Because of the morphologic similarity to monocytoid B-cell lymphoma, hairy-cell leukemia has also been included in this group of tumors.[14]

LYMPHOID ANTIGENS

Although cytologic morphology and tissue distribution are helpful guides to distinguish various types of lymphoid neoplasms, immunophenotyping is frequently needed for a precise diagnosis and classification of these tumors and for the distinction between benign and malignant conditions. The refinement of immunophenotyping has been achieved by the continuing discovery of large numbers of monoclonal antibodies that define the cell lineage, stage of development, and function of different cell types. The antigens to which monoclonal antibodies react can be divided into the following categories (Table 2–3).

1. *Lineage-associated antigens:* For lymphoid cells, there are three groups of antigens: the T-cells, B-cells, and natural-killer cells.[4,15] Among B-cell-associated antigens, CD19 and CD20 are most frequently tar-

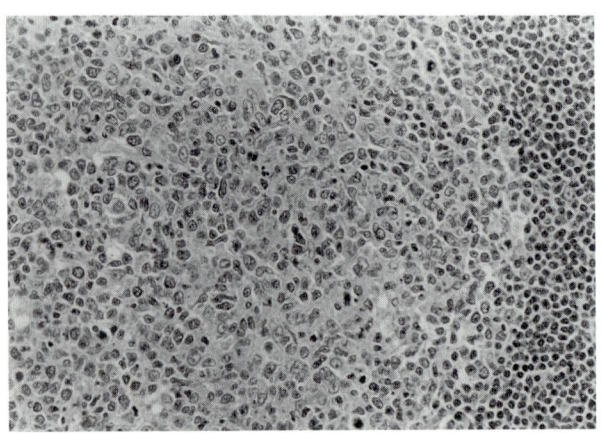

Fig. 2.6. Another view showing the light zone of germinal center, side-by-side with the mantle zone. H&E, ×500.

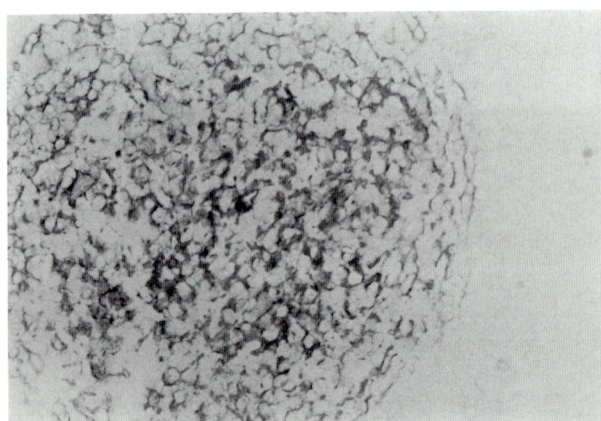

Fig. 2.8. A meshwork of follicular dendritic cells in the germinal center is demonstrated by CD21 (DRC-1) staining. Note the empty space at right representing the mantle zone with negative staining. Immunoperoxidase, ×500.

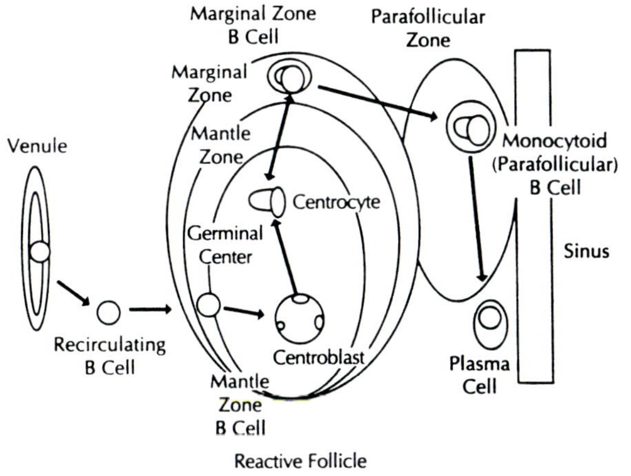

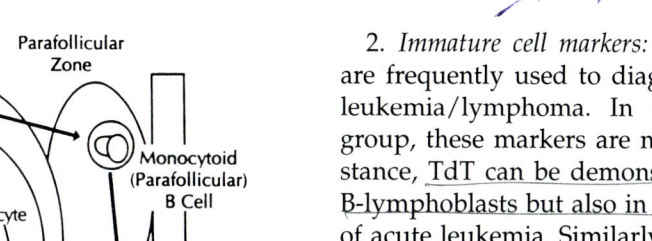

Fig. 2.9. Intranodal B-cell differentiation (maturation). (From Harris NL: *Arch Pathol Lab Med* 117: 771–775, 1993.)

geted. Other antibodies may help for subdivision of B-cell lymphomas and leukemias. For example, CD5, CD10, and CD23 are instrumental in distinguishing several low-grade B-cell lymphomas (small lymphocytic lymphoma, follicular lymphoma, and mantle-cell lymphoma).[16] Among T-cell-associated antigens, the pan-T-cell antigens, such as CD2, CD3, CD5, and CD7, are commonly targeted. However, T-cell subset analysis with CD4 and CD8 antibodies is frequently used in both benign and malignant conditions. For natural-killer cells, there are three specific antigens: CD16, CD56, and CD57.

TABLE 2.3
Categories of Surface and Nuclear Antigens

1. Lineage-associated antigens
   B-cell: CD19, CD20, CD21, CD22, CD23, CD24, CD32, PC-1
   T-cell: CD1, CD2, CD3, CD4, CD5, CD6, CD7, CD8, TCR
   NK-cell: CD16, CD56, CD57
2. Immature cell markers
   TdT, CD10, CD34
3. Activation antigens
   CD25, CD30, CD38, CD71, HLA-DR
4. Adhesion molecules
   CD11a/CD18 (LFA-1), CD56 (NCAM), CD54 (ICAM-1), CD102 (ICAM-2), CD106 (VCAM-1), CD31 (PECAM-1)
5. Proliferation-associated antigens
   Ki-67, PCNA

Abbreviations: TCR = T-cell receptor protein; PCNa = proliferating-cell nuclear antigen.

2. *Immature cell markers:* TdT and CD10 (CALLA) are frequently used to diagnose acute lymphoblastic leukemia/lymphoma. In contrast to the previous group, these markers are not lineage-specific. For instance, TdT can be demonstrated not only in T- and B-lymphoblasts but also in myeloblasts in some cases of acute leukemia. Similarly, CD10 can be detected in B- or T-cell lymphoblastic leukemias and demonstrated in follicular lymphoma. CD34 is found in both acute myeloblastic and lymphoblastic leukemias.

3. *Activation antigens:* These antigens appear on both T-cell and B-cell after activation, although they may also be demonstrated on cells in the resting stage. In lymphoma cases, the presence of a high percentage of activation-antigen-positive cells may indicate high aggressiveness of the tumor.[17] The most frequently used activation antigens are CD25 (IL-2 receptor), CD71 (transferrin receptor), and HLA-DR (a histocompatibility antigen). CD30 is also an activation antigen but is commonly used for the identification of Reed–Sternberg and Hodgkin's cells, as well as the ki-1 positive anaplastic large-cell lymphoma.

4. *Adhesion molecules:* Increasing numbers of adhesion molecules have been discovered in recent years. Their function is related mainly to lymphocyte homing by binding vascular surface proteins (addressins) of high endothelial venules.[18] The presence of the adhesion molecule LFA-1 (CD11a/CD18) in small lymphocytic lymphoma helps to distinguish it from chronic lymphocytic leukemia.[19] In addition, there are neural-cell adhesion molecules (NCAMs), CD56; intercellular adhesion molecules (ICAM-1 and ICAM-2), CD54 and CD102; vascular-cell adhesion molecule-1 (VCAM-1) CD106; and platelet-endothelial-cell adhesion molecule-1 (PECAM-1) CD31.

5. *Proliferation-associated antigens:* The commonly known proliferation-associated antigens include Ki-67 and proliferating-cell nuclear antigen (PCNA). Ki-67 is a nuclear antigen associated with proliferation and is expressed in all phases of the cell cycle except for the G_0 (resting) phase. PCNA, on the other hand, is present in low concentrations in G_1 and G_2–M phases, and in high concentration in S phase. Since these antigens are expressed only on the nuclei of proliferative cells, therefore, calculation of the percentage of Ki-67 or PCNA-positive cells may give a clue to the aggressiveness of the tumor.

Since the early 1980s, over 1000 monoclonal antibodies specific for leukocyte differentiation antigens have been developed. These antibodies are categorized into different functional groups, and those that

TABLE 2.4
Cell Specificity and Clinical Applications of Monoclonal Antibodies

Cluster designation	Monoclonal antibodies	Cell specificity	Clinical application
CD1a	Leu6, OKT6, T6	Thymocyte, Langerhans cells	T-ALL, T-lymphoma, histiocytosis X
CD2	Leu5, OKT11, T11	E-rosette receptor	T-ALL, T-CLL, T-lymphoma
CD3	Leu4, OKT3, T3	T-cell receptor complex	T-ALL, T-CLL, T-lymphoma
CD4	Leu3, OKT4, T4	Helper-inducer T-cell	Identification of T subset
CD5	Leu1, OKT1, T1	T-cell, B-cell from CLL	T-ALL, T-lymphoma, B-CLL
CD7	Leu9, OKT16, 3A1	T-cell, receptor for IgM-Fc	T-ALL, T-lymphoma
CD8	Leu2, OKT8, T8	Cytotoxic-suppressor T-cell	Identification of T subset
CD10	CALLA, OKBcALLa, J5	Immature B-cell and T-cell (rare)	ALL, B-lymphoma
CD11b	Leu15, OKM1, Mo1	Monocyte, granulocyte, NK-cell, T-suppressor cell	AML
CD11c	LeuM5, S-HCL3	Monocyte, B-cell from hairy-cell leukemia	AML, HCL
CD13	LeuM7, OKM13, My7	Monocyte, granulocyte	AML
CD14	LeuM3, OKM14, My4, Mo2	Monocyte, granulocyte	AML
CD15	LeuM1, My1	Monocyte, granulocyte, Reed–Sternberg cell	Hodgkin's disease
CD16	Leu11	NK cell, granulocyte, macrophage	NK-cell disorders
CD19	Leu12, OKpanB, B4	B-cell	B-ALL, B-CLL, B lymphoma
CD20	Leu16, B1	B-cell	B-ALL, B-CLL, B lymphoma
CD21	CR2, OKB7, B2	Follicular dendritic cell, B-cell, C3d receptor	B lymphoma
CD22	Leu14, OKB22, B3, S-HCL1	B-cell	B lymphoma, HCL
CD23	B6, Leu20	B-cell	B-CLL
CD25	IL-2, OKT26a, Tac	IL-2 receptor on T-cell (Tac antigen)	Hairy-cell leukemia, human T-cell leukemia
CD30	Ki-1, BerH2	Reed–Sternberg cell, T- or B-cell from lymphoma	Ki-1 anaplastic lymphoma, Hodgkin's disease
CD33	LeuM9, My9	Monocyte, granulocyte	AML
CD34	HPCA-1, My10	Precursors of hematopoietic cells	Acute leukemia
CD38	Leu17, OKT10, T10	Plasma cell, activated T- and B-cells	Multiple myeloma
CD41	J15	GPIIb/IIIa antigen on platelet and megakaryocyte	Megakaryocytic leukemia
CD42a & 42b	HPL14, AN51, 10P42	Platelet GPIX and GPIb	Megakaryocytic leukemia
CD43	MT-1, Leu22, L60	T-cell, some B-cells	T-lymphoma
CD45	HLe-1, LCA	All leukocytes	Lymphomas, leukemias
CD45RA	MT-2	T-cell, some B-cells	Follicular lymphoma
CD45RO	UCHL1	T subset, B subset, monocyte, granulocyte	T-lymphoma
CD56	Leu19, NKH-1	NK cell	NK-cell disorders
CD57	Leu7, HNK-1	NK cell, T subset	NK-cell disorders
CD61	10P61, VI-PL2	Platelet GPIIIa	Megakaryocytic leukemia
CD68	KP1	Monocyte, histiocyte	Monocytic and histiocytic neoplasms
CD71	Transferrin receptor, OKT9, T9	Activated T- and B-cells, macrophages, proliferating cells	Acute leukemias and lymphomas
CD74	LN2	B-cell, monocyte	B-lymphoma
CDw75	LN1	B-cell, T subset	B-lymphoma
CD103	HML-1, B-ly7	B-cell	HCL
	FMC7	B-cell	HCL, prolymphocytic leukemia
	HLA-DR	B-cell, activated T-cell, monocyte, granulocyte	B-cell neoplasms

TABLE 2.4 (Continued)

Cluster designation	Monoclonal antibodies	Cell specificity	Clinical application
	PCA-1	Plasma cell, monocyte (weak), granulocyte (weak)	Multiple myeloma
	RC-82.4	Erythroblast	Erythroleukemia
	Glycophorin	Erythroid series	Erythroleukemia
	TCR-1, βF-1, WT31	T-cell	T-lymphoma, T-leukemia
	TCR-δ1, TCS-1, antiδ	T-cell	T-lymphoma, T-leukemia

Abbreviations: ALL = acute lymphoblastic leukemia; AML = acute myelogenous leukemia; CLL = chronic lymphocytic leukemia; HCL = hairy-cell leukemia; NK = natural killer.

are reacting to the same antigenic epitope are assigned the same cluster designation (CD). In the 5th International Workshop on Leukocyte Differentiation Antigens held in Boston in 1993, the last cluster designation was CDw130.[20] These antibodies have been used mainly on fresh and appropriately frozen cells (Table 2–4). However, there is a group of newly developed antibodies that are reactive with antigens in fixed, paraffin-embedded sections (Table 2–5).[21] These antibodies are most helpful in morphologic correlation with immunophenotypes and in retrospective studies.

CLASSIFICATION OF LYMPHOMAS

Lymphomas are tumors of the immune system; therefore, their classification is expected to be complicated.[16,22] The rapid progress in the fields of immunology, cytogenetics, and molecular biology has greatly enhanced the understanding of lymphomas and facilitated their classification. The best known example is the changing concept of reticulum cell sarcoma to histiocytic sarcoma to large-cell lymphoma. Although true histiocytic lymphoma and reticulum-cell sarcoma do exist, they are rare tumors and most cases diagnosed as such in the early literature were probably large-cell lymphomas.

Modern classification of non-Hodgkin's lymphomas started with Rappaport.[23] His classification was based on the histologic pattern (nodular or diffuse), cytology (lymphocyte or histiocyte), and cell differentiation (well differentiated or poorly differentiated). Lukes and Collins' classification combined immunologic subtypes with morphology and proposed that immunologic phenotypes could be determined by morphologic features alone.[24] The Kiel classification proposed by Lennert and

TABLE 2.5
Monoclonal Antibodies Used in Paraffin-Embedded Sections

CD designation	Monoclonal antibody	Cell specificity	Major clinical application
CD3	CD3	T-cell	T-lymphoma
CD15	LeuM1	Myelomonocytes, Reed–Sternberg cells	Hodgkin's disease
CD20	L26	B-cell	B-lymphoma
CD30	BerH2	Reed–Sternberg cell, T- or B-cell	Hodgkin's disease, Ki-1 lymphoma
CD34	HPCA, My10	Lymphoid, myeloid	Lymphoblastic lymphoma
CD43	MT-1, Leu22, L60	T-cell, some B-cells	T-lymphoma
CD45	LCA	T- and B-cells	All lymphomas
CD45 RA	MT-2	T-cell, some B-cells	Follicular lymphoma
CD45 RO	UCHL-1	T-cell, some B-cells	Mainly T-lymphoma
CD68	KP-1	Monocyte, macrophage, mast cell	Histiocytic disorders
CD74	LN-2	B-cell	B-lymphoma
CDw75	LN-1	B-cell	B-lymphoma
	DBA-44	B-cell	Hairy-cell leukemia
	βF1	T-cell receptor α/β	T-lymphoma

associates is mainly morphologic with more cell types included.[25] The lesser known schemes include Dorfman, the British National Lymphoma Investigation, and WHO (U.N. World Health Organization) classifications. These six different schemes unavoidably caused some confusion among the pathologists; thus, the National Cancer Institute in the United States organized a team of experts to evaluate the available classifications and establish a "compromised" new scheme. As a result, a Working Formulation of non-Hodgkin's lymphomas for clinical use was proposed (Table 2–6).[26] The Working Formulation is relatively simple and yet incorporates all the major components from other schemes. Its major advantage is dividing the lymphomas into three prognostic groups that makes the Working Formulation clinically relevant.[16] It was promptly accepted and has been widely used, especially in North America. However, the Working Formulation does not identify individual disease entities and does not include many new entities, especially in the T-cell lymphoma category, that have appeared in recent years.[16,22] In addition, the new treatments used currently have changed the outlook of many diseases; thus the prognostic grouping may no longer be valid for some of the lymphomas. Therefore, some American hematologists and oncologists feel that the Working Formulation has outlived its usefulness.[16]

The Kiel classification was updated in 1992 (Table 2–7). It combines immunophenotypes with morphology, includes several new entities, and divides lymphomas into two prognostic groups. This new scheme has been widely used in Europe. The International Lymphoma Study Group, however, feels that the Kiel classification excludes primary extranodal lymphomas other than mycosis fungoides, does not include the morphologic subtypes of follicular lymphomas, and includes some morphologic subclassifications that may be difficult and poorly reproducible.[16]

Because of this situation, a revised European–American Classification of Lymphoid Neoplasms (REAL classification) has been proposed (Table 2–8).[16] This new scheme encompasses many new entities, covers both Hodgkin's disease and non-Hodgkin's lymphomas, and incorporates immunophenotypes and cytogenetics as the integral parts for diagnosis. For instance, the presence of a nodular pattern may be diagnosed as follicular (follicle center) lymphoma if CD10 is positive, or mantle-cell lymphoma if CD5 is positive, or lymphoma of the mucosa-associated lymphoid tis-

TABLE 2.6
A Working Formulation of Non-Hodgkin's Lymphoma for Clinical Usage

Low-grade
A. Malignant lymphoma, small lymphocytic
    Consistent with CLL
    Plasmacytoid
B. Malignant lymphoma, follicular, predominantly small-cleaved-cell
    Diffuse areas
    Sclerosis
C. Malignant lymphoma, follicular, mixed small-cleaved and large-cell
    Diffuse areas
    Sclerosis

Intermediate-grade
D. Malignant lymphoma, follicular, predominantly large-cell
    Diffuse areas
    Sclerosis
E. Malignant lymphoma, diffuse, small-cleaved-cell
    Sclerosis
F. Malignant lymphoma, diffuse, mixed small-/large-cell
    Sclerosis
    Epithelioid-cell component

G. Malignant lymphoma, diffuse, large-cell
    Cleaved-cell
    Noncleaved-cell
    Sclerosis

High-grade
H. Malignant lymphoma, large-cell, immunoblastic
    Plasmacytoid
    Clear-cell
    Polymorphous
    Epithelioid-cell component
I. Malignant lymphoma, lymphoblastic
    Convoluted-cell
    Nonconvoluted-cell
J. Malignant lymphoma, small noncleaved cell
    Burkitt's
    Follicular areas

Miscellaneous
    Composite
    Mycosis fungoides
    Histiocytic
    Extramedullary plasmacytoma
    Unclassifiable
    Other

sue if both CD5 and CD10 are negative. The anaplastic large-cell (CD30+) lymphoma in this scheme includes only the T-cell and null-cell type. When a CD30+ anaplastic lymphoma has a B-cell phenotype, it is classified under diffuse large-B-cell lymphoma. This new classification does not divide lymphoma into prognostic groups because the International Lymphoma Study Group believes that many lymphomas have a range of morphologic grades and clinical aggressiveness. This group also emphasizes that this scheme constitutes merely a framework for further study; some new entities may not prove to be real diseases, and some excluded entities may prove to be real diseases.

Throughout this book, we have used the Working Formulation as the basis of our classification of lymphomas. However, most of the new entities in the REAL classification are included for differential diagnosis, because we feel that these are items with which the general pathologist may not be familiar.

TABLE 2.7
Updated Kiel Classification of Non-Hodgkin's Lymphomas

B-cell	T-cell
Low-grade malignant lymphomas	
Lymphocytic	Lymphocytic
Chronic lymphocytic leukemia	Chronic lymphocytic leukemia
Prolymphocytic leukemia	Prolymphocytic leukemia
Hairy-cell leukemia	Small-cell, cerebriform Mycosis fungoides/ Sézary's syndrome
Lymphoplasmacytic/cytoid (immunocytoma)	Lymphoepithelioid (Lennert's lymphoma)
Plasmacytic	Angioimmunoblastic (AILD)
Centroblastic-centrocytic (follicular ± diffuse; diffuse)	T-zone lymphoma
Centrocytic (mantle-cell)	Pleomorphic, small cell (HTLV-1 ±)
Monocytoid, including marginal-zone cell	
High-grade malignant lymphoma	
Centroblastic	Pleomorphic, medium-sized and large cell (HTLV-1 ±)
Immunoblastic	Immunoblastic (HTLV-1 ±)
Burkitt's lymphoma	
Large-cell anaplastic (Ki-+)	Large-cell anaplastic (Ki-1 +)
Lymphoblastic	Lymphoblastic

Other rare types of lymphoma may be separately identified for T- and B-cell lymphomas, respectively.

TABLE 2.8
A Revised European–American Classification of Lymphoid Neoplasms

B-Cell Neoplasms
I. Precursor B-cell neoplasm: precursor B-lymphoblastic leukemia/lymphoma
II. Peripheral B-cell neoplasms
  1. B-cell chronic lymphocytic leukemia/ prolymphocytic leukemia/small lymphocytic lymphoma
  2. Lymphoplasmacytoid lymphoma/immunocytoma
  3. Mantle-cell lymphoma
  4. Follicle center lymphoma, follicular
    Provisional cytologic grades: I (small-cell), II (mixed small/large-cell), III (large-cell)
    Provisional subtype: diffuse, predominantly small-cell type
  5. Marginal-zone B-cell lymphoma
    Extranodal (MALT-type ± monocytoid B-cells)
    Provisional subtype: Nodal (± monocytoid B-cells)
  6. Provisional subentity: Splenic marginal zone lymphoma (± villous lymphocytes)
  7. Hairy-cell leukemia
  8. Plasmacytoma/plasma-cell myeloma
  9. Diffuse large B-cell lymphoma[a]
    Subtype: primary mediastinal (thymic) B-cell lymphoma
  10. Burkitt's lymphoma
  11. Provisional entity: high-grade B-cell lymphoma, Burkitt-like[a]

T-Cell and Putative NK-Cell Neoplasms
I. Precursor T-cell neoplasm: precursor T-lymphoblastic lymphoma/leukemia
II. Peripheral T-cell and NK-cell neoplasms
  1. T-cell chronic lymphocytic leukemia/ prolymphocytic leukemia
  2. Large granular lymphocyte leukemia (LGL)
    T-cell type
    NK-cell type
  3. Mycosis fungoides/Sézary syndrome
  4. Peripheral T-cell lymphomas, unspecified[a]
    Provisional cytologic categories: medium-sized cell, mixed medium/large-cell, large-cell, lymphoepithelioid-cell
    Provisional subtype: hepatosplenic γδ T-cell lymphoma
    Provisional subtype: subcutaneous panniculitic T-cell lymphoma
  5. Angioimmunoblastic T-cell lymphoma (AILD)
  6. Angiocentric lymphoma
  7. Intestinal T-cell lymphoma (± enteropathy-associated)
  8. Adult T-cell lymphoma/leukemia (ATL/L)

Continued

TABLE 2.8 (Continued)

9. Anaplastic large-cell lymphoma (ALCL), CD30[†], T- and null-cell types
10. Provisional entity: anaplastic large-cell lymphoma, Hodgkin's-like

Hodgkin's Disease
I. Lymphocyte predominance
II. Nodular sclerosis
III. Mixed cellularity
IV. Lymphocyte depletion
VI. Provisional entity: lymphocyte-rich classical HD

[a]These categories are thought likely to include more than one disease entity.

REFERENCES

1. Robertson MJ, Ritz J: Biology and clinical relevance of human natural killer cells. *Blood* 76:2421–2438, 1990.
2. Knowles DM, Chadburn A, Inghirami G: Immunophenotypic markers useful in the diagnosis and classification of hematopoietic neoplasms. In Knowles DM (ed): *Neoplastic Hematopathology*, Baltimore, Williams & Wilkins, 1992, pp 73–167.
3. Sun T: *Color Atlas/Text of Flow Cytometric Analysis of Hematologic Neoplasms*, New York, Igaku-Shoin, 1993; pp 18–25.
4. Stetler-Stevenson M, Medeirosi LJ, Jaffe ES: Immunophenotypic methods and findings in the diagnosis of lymphoproliferative diseases. In Jaffe ES (ed): *Surgical Pathology of the Lymph Nodes and Related Organs*, 2nd ed, Philadelphia, Saunders, 1995, pp 22–57.
5. Garcia CF, Weiss LM, Warnke RA: Small noncleaved cell lymphoma: An immunophenotypic study of 18 cases and comparison with large cell lymphoma. *Hum Pathol* 17:454–461, 1987.
6. Weisenburger DD, Chan WC: Lymphomas of follicles, mantle cell and follicle center cell lymphoma. *Am J Clin Pathol* 99:409–420, 1993.
7. Butcher E: Cellular and molecular mechanisms that direct leukocyte traffic. *Am J Pathol* 136:3–12, 1990.
8. Gloghini A, Carbone A: The nonlymphoid microenvironment of reactive follicles and lymphomas of follicular origin as defined by immunohistology on paraffin embedded tissues. *Hum Pathol* 24:67–76, 1993.
9. Lennert K, Feller AC: *Histopathology of Non-Hodgkin's Lymphoma*, 2nd ed, Berlin, Springer-Verlag, 1992, pp 29–39.
10. Harris NL: Low-grade B-cell lymphoma of mucosa-associated lymphoid tissue and monocytoid B-cell lymphoma. *Arch Pathol Lab Med* 117:771–775, 1993.
11. van den Oord J, de Wolf-Peeters C, Desmont V: The marginal zone in the human reactive lymph node. *Am J Clin Pathol* 86:475–479, 1985.
12. MacLennan I, Liu Y, Oldfield S, et al: The evolution of B-cell clones. *Curr Top Microbiol Immunol* 159:37–63, 1990.
13. Nunez G, Hockenberry D, McDonnell TJ, et al: Bcl-2 maintains B-cell memory. *Nature* 353:71–73, 1991.
14. Rosso R, Neiman RS, Paulli M, et al: Splenic marginal zone cell lymphoma: Report of an indolent variant without massive splenomegaly presumably representing an early phase of the disease. *Hum Pathol* 26:39–46, 1995.
15. Pirrucello SJ, Johnson DR: Reagents for flow cytometry: Monoclonal antibodies and hematopoietic cell antigens. In Keren DF, Hanson CA, Hurtubise PE (eds): *Flow Cytometry and Clinical Diagnosis*, Chicago, American Society of Clinical Pathologists, 1994, pp 56–91.
16. Harris NL, Jaffe ES, Stein H, et al: A revised European–American classification of lymphoid neoplasms: A proposal from the International Lymphoma Study Group. *Blood* 84:1361–1392, 1994.
17. Sun T, Brody J, Susin M, et al: Aggressive natural killer cell lymphoma/leukemia: A recently recognized clinicopathologic entity. *Am J Surg Pathol* 17:1289–1299, 1993.
18. Carlos TM, Harlan JM: Leukocyte-endothelial adhesion molecules. *Blood* 84:2068–2101, 1994.
19. Freedman AS, Nadler LM: Immunologic markers in non-Hodgkin's lymphoma. *Hematol/Oncol Clin N Am* 5:871–889, 1991.
20. Pinto A, Gattei V, Soligo O, et al: New molecules burst at the leukocyte surface: A comprehensive review based on the 5th International Workshop on Leukocyte Differentiation Antigens, Boston (USA), 3–7 November 1993, *Leukemia* 1994; 8:347–358.
21. Perkins SL, Kjeldsberg CR: Immunophenotyping of lymphomas and leukemias in paraffin-embedded tissues. *Am J Clin Pathol* 99:363–373, 1993.
22. Jaffe ES: An overview of the classification of non-Hodgkin's lymphoma. In Jaffe ES (ed): *Surgical Pathology of the Lymph Nodes and Related Organs*, 2nd ed, Philadelphia, Saunders, 1995, pp 193–204.
23. Rappaport H: *Tumors of the Hematopoietic System. Atlas of Tumor Pathology*, Armed Forces Institute of Pathology, 1966.
24. Lukes RJ, Collins RD: Immunological characterization of human malignant lymphomas. *Cancer* 34:1488–1503, 1974.
25. Lennert K, Feller AC: Histopathology of the non-Hodgkin's lymphomas (based on the updated Kiel classification), Berlin, Springer-Verlag, 1992, pp 13–28.
26. The non-Hodgkin's lymphoma pathologic classification project: National Cancer Institute sponsored study of classification of non-Hodgkin's lymphomas. *Cancer* 49:2112–2135, 1982.

3
Ancillary Studies for Lymphoid Disorders

The rapid development of hematopathology in terms of comprehension of pathogenesis and expansion of classification in lymphoid neoplasms is a direct result of the recent explosion in ancillary techniques for the study of lymphoid disorders. The first breakthrough was the subdivision of lymphocytes into T-cell and B-cell categories, which have become an integral part of new classifications of lymphoid neoplasms. The availability of monoclonal antibodies led to the discovery of the third lineage of lymphocytes, the natural-killer cells. Monoclonal antibodies may also characterize lymphocytes by determining their subsets (e.g., helper cells vs. suppressor cells) and developmental stages (e.g., thymic T-cell vs. postthymic T-cell). However, it is the development of flow cytometers with the multifluorochrome labeling technique that makes immunophenotyping a fine art. By analyzing multiple correlated surface markers on single cells, flow cytometry can further characterize and subclassify lymphoid tumors by their subtle differences.

However, some phenotypes may not be expressed on the cell surface, surface immunoglobulin of the same tumor may switch from time to time, and some coexistent or recurrent tumors may show different phenotypes although they are genetically derived from the same origin. Furthermore, the correlation and mechanism of a low-grade lymphoma transforming to a high-grade neoplasm cannot be solved by immunophenotyping. Under these circumstances, genotyping comes into play. The genotypic techniques are usually more sensitive than the phenotypic techniques. With the development of more modified or new techniques in molecular biology, the major disadvantage of genotyping for its time-consuming, cumbersome procedures has been overcome substantially. The following is a brief discussion of individual techniques.

IMMUNOPHENOTYPING

Immunophenotyping serves many different functions. When the features of cytology and histopathology are not diagnostic, immunophenotyping helps distinguish a benign lesion from a malignant one, thus achieving a definitive diagnosis. Even when diagnosis is not a major problem, immunophenotyping is still needed and plays an essential role in differential diagnosis, subclassification, and prediction of prognosis. These functions are well exemplified in the area of low-grade B-cell lymphomas, such as small lymphocytic lymphoma/chronic lymphocytic leukemia, hairy-cell leukemia, monocytoid B-cell lymphoma, splenic lymphoma with villous lymphocytes, and mantle-cell lymphoma, to name just a few. The continuing discovery of new monoclonal antibodies enables better refinement for the diagnosis and classification. For instance, the availability of CD23 antibody facilitates the distinction between small lymphocytic lymphoma and mantle-cell lymphoma. The prognosis for a certain lymphoma can be evaluated by quantifying the proliferation-associated antigens, such as Ki-67 and PCNA (proliferating cell nuclear antigen). A poor prognosis may also be expected when high percentages of activation antigens (e.g., CD25, CD38, CD71, HLA-DR) are present.[1] There are many other prognostic indicators, which will be discussed in subsequent chapters.

Among all the functions of immunophenotyping, the criteria for diagnosing hematologic neoplasms have drawn most attention. In the past decade, a great deal of experience has been accumulated in the subtle distinction of phenotypes between lymphoid hyperplasia and neoplasms (Table 3.1).[1,2]

1. *Immunoglobulin light-chain restriction:* The surface immunoglobulin/light-chain ratio is the most commonly used and reliable criterion for determining the clonality of a lymphoid population. When one light chain is dominant over the other (κ:λ ratio > 3:1 or λ:κ ratio > 2:1), it is referred to as light-chain restriction and is indicative of monoclonality. Monoclonality may also be expressed as one single-heavy-chain or double-heavy-chain (i.e., IgM/IgD) predominance; however, since a heavy chain can switch after rearrangement, this is not a routinely used criterion.

2. *Loss of surface immunoglobulin in a B-cell population:* In about 10–20% of lymphomas, B-cell antigens are demonstrated on tumor cells that show no surface immunoglobulin by immunohistochemical studies[2] or a low percentage of immunoglobulin-positive cells by flow cytometric analysis.[3] Since surface immunoglobulin is the antigen receptor on normal B-cells, the lack of it is demonstrated only on neoplastic cells.

3. *Coexistence of two different cell-lineage markers on the same cell population:* Double-cell lineage markers have become the hallmark of several lymphoid tumors. For instance, chronic lymphocytic leukemia carries a B-cell marker (either CD19 or CD20) and a T-cell

TABLE 3.1
Criteria for Diagnosis of Hematologic Neoplasms

1. Immunoglobulin light-chain restriction
2. Loss of surface immunoglobulin in a B-cell population
3. Coexistence of 2 cell-lineage markers on the same cell population (e.g., CD22 and CD11c in hairy-cell leukemia)
4. Expression of immature cell markers (e.g., TdT, CD10, and CD34) in a large number of cells
5. Selective loss of 1 or more cell-lineage antigens

Modified from Sun T: *Color Atlas/Text of Flow Cytometric Analysis of Hematologic Neoplasms,* New York, Igaku-Shoin, 1993, p 37.

marker (CD5), and hairy-cell leukemia bears a B-cell marker (CD22) and a monocyte marker (CD11c). On the other hand, the presence of a myeloid marker(s) in lymphoid leukemia or a lymphoid marker(s) in myeloid leukemia makes the tumor bilineal but does not indicate a special type of tumor.

4. *Expression of immature cell markers in a large number of cells:* The demonstration of terminal deoxynucleotidyl transferase (TdT) and CD10 (CALLA) on tumor cells of lymphoblastic lymphoma/acute lymphoblastic leukemia and CD34 on cells of acute myeloblastic leukemia are good examples. Therefore, double-staining with a lymphoid marker and TdT or CD10 may count the lymphoblastic tumor cells more accurately.

5. *Selective loss of one or more cell-lineage antigens:* This criterion is particularly useful for diagnosis of T-cell lymphomas because there are no clonal markers for T-cells analogous to light-chain restriction for B-cells. When three pan-T-cell markers (CD3, CD5, CD7) are included in a study panel, the early-appearing marker (CD7) is more frequently demonstrated in the tumor derived from early T-cell development stage, while the late-appearing marker (CD3) is more frequently seen in peripheral T-cell lymphoma.[4] The gradual decrease in CD7+ cells in contrast to the persistence of CD3+ cells in cases of mycosis fungoides is one of the most dramatic examples.[2]

Immunohistochemistry

Immunohistochemistry is still the most popular technique in a pathology laboratory for the following reasons: (a) the major advantage is that it allows the pathologist to correlate the marker results with morphology—in contrast, a flow cytometric analysis sometimes cannot determine whether a certain marker belongs to the tumor or the normal population because of the lack of morphologic correlation; (b) it is a relatively simple technique and can be performed in a routine pathology laboratory; and (c) although expansive immunohistochemical staining equipment is available, manual techniques can meet the demand in most laboratories—thus, it is cost-effective.

Immunohistochemical stains can be performed on either frozen or paraffin-embedded sections (Fig. 3.1). Paraffin-embedded sections usually show better morphology than do frozen sections, and retrospective studies can be performed on archival paraffin blocks. However, many monoclonal antibodies can apply only to frozen sections, and even the fixation and embedding-resistant antigens are partially damaged in paraffin sections; thus immunohistochemical techniques performed on paraffin sections are seldom as sensitive as those used in frozen sections.[5,6]

For frozen sections, the avidin–biotin complex (ABC) immunoperoxidase technique and the alkaline/antialkaline phosphatase (APAAP) technique are most commonly used.[7] ABC is also the preferred technique for paraffin sections. Recently, a double immunohistochemical technique, combining APAAP and immunofluorescence, has been used to demonstrate two different antigens, for instance, Epstein–Barr virus and a B-cell antigen, in the same cells.[8] Tissue fixed in B5 or formalin yield good results for immunohistochemical stains, but Zenker's fixation may cause high, nonspecific staining.

Occasionally, tissue imprints can be made for cytochemical staining, such as tartrate-resistant acid phosphatase in cases of hairy-cell leukemia, and terminal deoxynucleotidyl transferase in lymphoblastic lymphoma.[9]

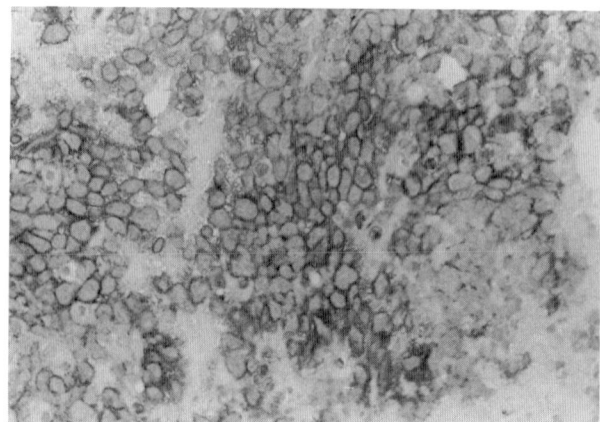

Fig. 3.1 A frozen section of lymph node biopsy showing a large-cell lymphoma stained positively for a B-cell antigen (CD20). Immunoperoxidase, ×500.

Flow Cytometry

About a decade ago, the surface antigens on lymphocytes were analyzed mainly by the manual immunofluoresence technique. However, this technique has gradually been replaced by an automated fluorescence detection device, generally referred to as the *flow cytometer*.[1] The demand for rapid, multimarker analysis in large numbers of cells makes this type of instrument an ideal tool for the study of lymphoid neoplasms and the distinction between malignant and benign conditions.

A flow cytometer is able to measure the physical properties (e.g., cell size and cytoplasmic granularity), surface and cytoplasmic antigens, and DNA/RNA contents of individual cells in a cell suspension. The physical properties of cells are determined through light scatter characteristics. The two major optical signals generated in flow cytometers are forward-angle (2–10°) light scatter, which is proportional to the cell size, and right-angle (90°) or side scatter, which is related to cytoplasmic granularity and nuclear configuration. The detection of surface and cytoplasmic antigens is by means of fluorochrome conjugated antibodies. A flow cytometer usually counts 3000–5000 cells for the study of each antigen in a few minutes, compared with 100–200 cells counted in manual techniques. Thus, flow cytometry produces more efficient, sensitive, accurate, and reproducible results than do any manual techniques used for immunophenotyping. The capability of measuring multiple parameters on the same cells is the most useful function of flow cytometry. With the availability of increasing numbers of fluorochromes with different emission spectra, the analytical capability of flow cytometer will, undoubtedly, expand rapidly.

In a flow cytometer, the specimen in the form of cell suspension travels through a fluid transport system (Fig. 3.2). In the flow chamber, the cells in the specimen form a single-cell file and meet the light source (mercury-arc lamp or laser) at the light interception point. The light signal thus generated is registered in an electronic system. The addition of a computer system further provides the instrument the capability of data storage and graphic display on a screen.

The most useful functions of a flow cytometer are the list-mode storage and the gating facility. All parameters measured can be stored on a floppy disk or a hard disk. All data can be combined and analyzed later and can be printed in graphic form as a permanent record. A "gate" in this context is an electronic window that can be set with a cursor on the screen to circumscribe a group of cells with similar characteristics (e.g., size and cytoplasmic granularity). Gating is used to isolate this special group of cells for analysis electronically, thus avoiding the difficult task of purifying the cell population by biologic or chemical means.

The graphs generated by the computer can be displayed in various forms. A *scattergram* is composed of

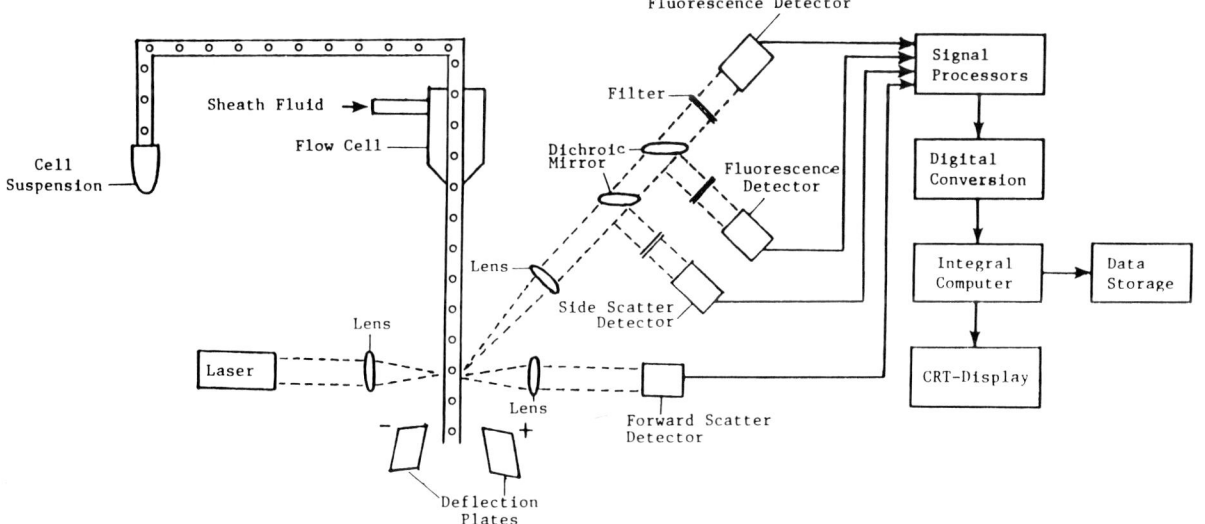

Fig. 3.2 The basic structure of a flow cytometer showing the fluid transport system, the optical system, and the electronic system. (From Sun T: *Color Atlas/Text of Flow Cytometric Analysis of Hematologic Neoplasms*, New York, Igaku-Shoin, 1993.)

multiple dots, each representing a single cell, and its position is determined by two related parameters along the x (abscissa; horizontal) and y (ordinate; vertical) axes (Fig. 3.3). When the scattergram is determined by the cell size and cytoplasmic granularity, for instance, the leukocytes can be separated in three clusters: the lymphocytes, monocytes and granulocytes. When cells are stained with fluorochrome-conjugated monoclonal antibodies, a *single histogram* provides the percentages of positive and negative populations (Fig. 3.4). The correlation of two monoclonal antibodies or DNA/RNA contents can be displayed in the form of a *contourgram* (Fig. 3.5). Instead of being represented by dots as in a scattergram, cells are represented by isocontour lines connecting elements of similar frequency of events. Finally an *isometric plot* is the display of three-dimensional isometric curves (Fig. 3.6). The isometric plot is most frequently used for simultaneous DNA/RNA analysis, but it can be used to display the correlation of any three parameters.

MOLECULAR GENETICS

Immunophenotyping may help distinguish malignant from benign conditions under most circumstances. However, some tumor cells may fail to express an im-

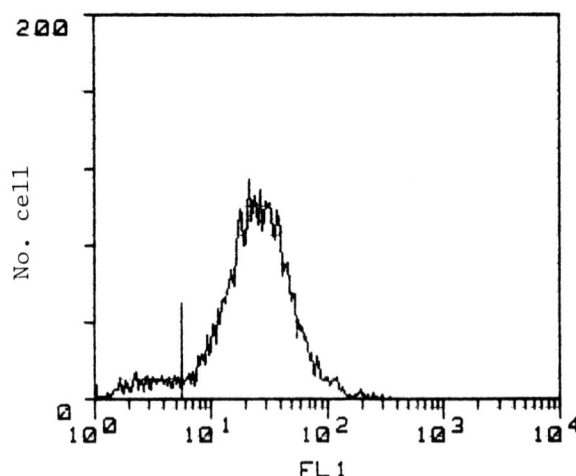

Fig. 3.4 Single histogram showing a prominent κ light-chain-positive population.

munophenotype either by their own nature or when tumor cells are in the minority of a lymphoid population and below the detectable level of a phenotyping technique. These are the conditions in which immunogenotyping comes into play. The major indication of immunogenotyping is for the diagnosis of T-cell neoplasms because there are no clonal markers

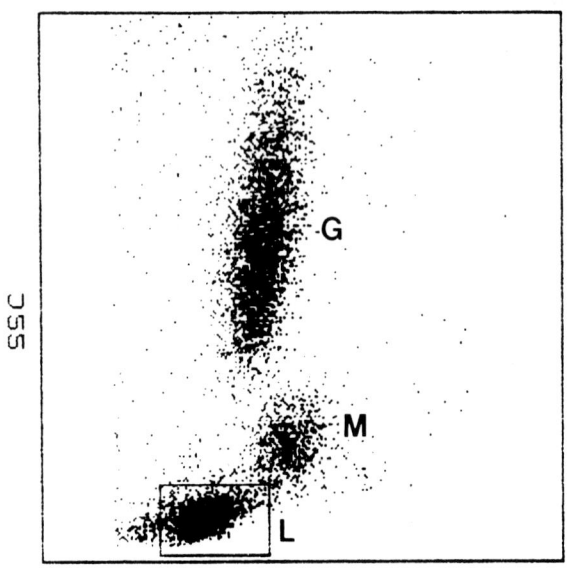

Fig. 3.3 Scattergram with side scatter (SSC) plotted against forward-angle light scatter (FSC), showing clusters of lymphocytes (L), monocytes (M), and granulocytes (G) in a peripheral blood specimen.

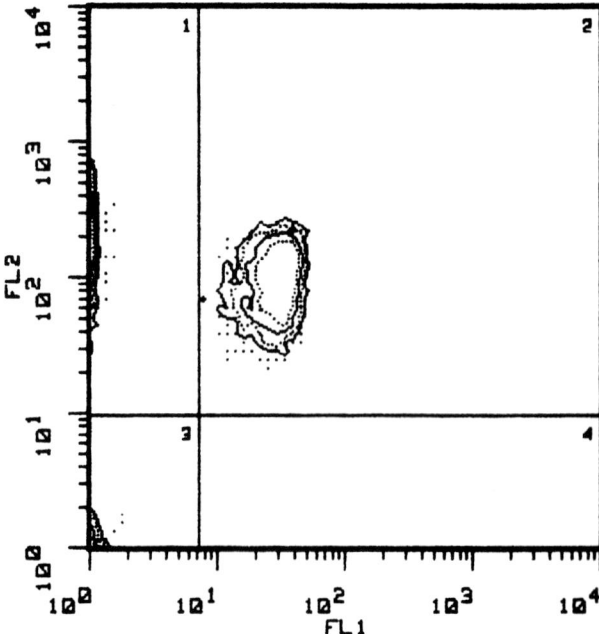

Fig. 3.5 Contourgram of a case of chronic lymphocytic leukemia showing the double-positive (CD19+ CD5+) leukemic population in quadrant 2.

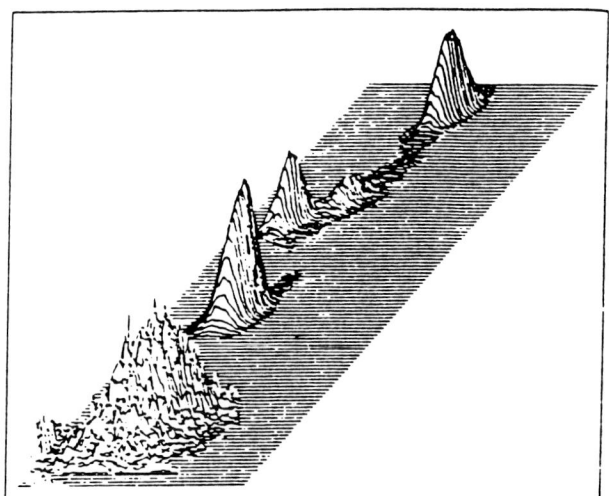

Fig. 3.6 A composite isometric plot combining individual two-parameter light-scatter histograms of platelets, red blood cells, lymphocytes, monocytes, and granulocytes. (From Martin GE: Diagnostic flow cytometry in hematology: The leukemias. *Pathol Immunopathol Res* 5:416–436, 1986.)

for T-cells analogous to surface immunoglobulin for B-cells. As immunogenotyping can also be performed with frozen blocks, it is possible to make retrospective studies when fresh specimen is no longer available for immunophenotyping. As will be discussed later, a DNA-rearranged band from a certain clone of lymphoid cells has a constant electrophoretic mobility when digested by the same restriction enzyme; therefore, immunogenotyping is an ideal tool for identifying the clonal origin of different tumors in cases of composite, biphenotypic, secondary, or recurrent lymphomas. In contrast, it is difficult for immunophenotyping to distinguish the clonal origin of different tumors, because most lymphomas have the same monoclonal IgM-κ phenotype, which can be distinguished only by the cumbersome production of antiidiotype monoclonal antibodies. The differences of immunophenotyping and immunogenotyping are summarized in Table 3.2.[10]

Immunoglobulin and T-Cell Receptor Gene Rearrangements

The definitive marker for B-cells is surface immunoglobulin, which serves as an antigen receptor for B-cells. Even in cases of surface-immunoglobulin-negative B-cell lymphoma, immunoglobulin gene rearrangement can be detected.[11] The definitive marker for T-cells is the T-cell receptor (TCR). These receptors are each encoded by two genes located at different chromosomes. Each gene contains 3–4 regions, which, in turn, consist of various numbers of segments (Table 3.3).[12,13] All antigen receptor genes contain the variable, joining, and constant regions, but a diversity region is present in the immunoglobulin heavy chain gene and in the TCR β- and δ-chain genes. The specific composition of these receptor proteins is the result of random selection of one segment from each region on the germline and recombination into an intact gene, a process referred to as *gene rearrangement*. The recombinant DNA will then be transcribed into RNA, and the messenger RNA, in turn, will be translated into protein (Fig. 3.7). Since these

TABLE 3.2
Comparison of Immunophenotyping and Immunogenotyping

	Immunophenotyping	Immunogenotyping
Result analysis	Quantifying % abnormal cells	DNA print of clonal population
Capability of monoclonal identification	95%	Nearly 100%
Identification of biclonality	Using antiidiotype monoclonal antibodies	Identifying more than 2 rearranged bands
Identification of secondary or recurrent tumor	Not reliable	Reliable
Reliable detectable level of clonal-cell population	20%	5%
Monitoring course of disease	Quantifying % clonal population	Visualizing rearranged bands
Specimen required	Fresh	Fresh/frozen
Minimal specimen size	0.5 mg of tissue	0.1 mg of tissue
Time required for testing	2 days	7 days

From Sun T: *Color Atlas/Text of Flow Cytometric Analysis of Hematologic Neoplasms*, New York, Igaku-Shoin, 1993, p 27.

TABLE 3.3
Characteristics of Receptor Genes

	Heavy chain	κ chain	λ chain	TCRα	TCRβ	TCRγ	TCRδ
Locus	14q32	2p12	22q11	14q11	7q34	7p15	14q11
Variable segments	100–200	40–80	40	50–100	75–100	8	4
Diversity segments	10	0	0	0	2	0	2
Joining segments	6	5	4	50–100	13	2	3
Constant segments	9	1	4	1	2	2	1

genes are composed of many segments and other mechanisms (insertion and deletion of nucleotides at the joining site and point mutations) also add to the diversity, the consequence of the recombination of immunoglobulin genes has the potential of producing more than 10^8 surface immunoglobulin receptors. Thus, a large number of varying antibodies can be synthesized by the mammalian host.

The immunoglobulin molecule is composed of a pair of heavy chains and a pair of light chains (either κ or λ). Therefore, each molecule is encoded by a heavy-chain gene and a light-chain gene. Immunoglobulin gene rearrangement takes place in every B-lymphocytes in an orderly fashion or developmental hierarchy: the immunoglobulin heavy-chain gene is rearranged early in B-cell development, which is followed by rearrangement of the κ light-chain gene. Only when the κ light-chain gene rearrangements are not productive will the λ light-chain alleles be rearranged. If the unproductive κ light-chain gene is not deleted, both κ- and λ-rearranged bands may be present in a lymphoma with a λ phenotype.

The structure of TCR is similar to that of immunoglobulin. It is a heterodimer composed of two dif-

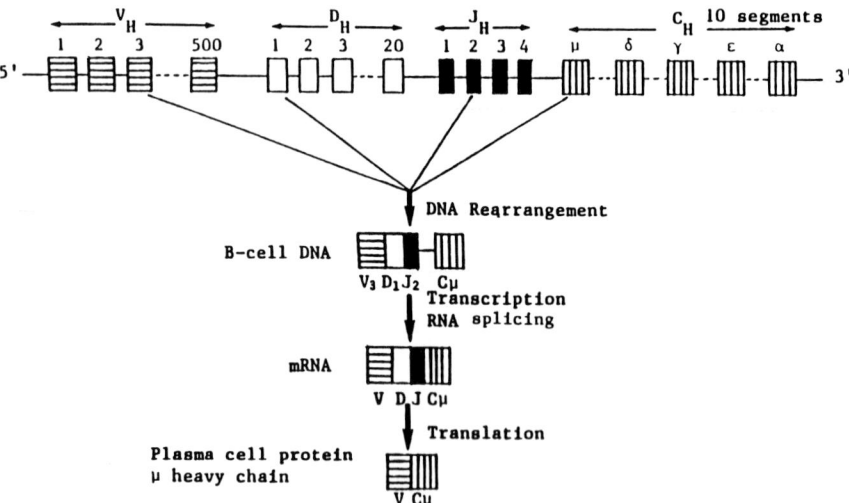

Fig. 3.7 Immunoglobulin heavy chain gene rearrangement. The germline heavy chain gene include four components: V (variable), D (diversity), J (joining) and C (constant). Each gene contains a certain number of segments. DNA rearrangement is the random selection of one segment from each gene. The selected gene segments are transcribed into messenger RNAs (mRNAs), which are, in turn, translated into proteins (immunoglobulins). (From Sun T: *Interpretation of Protein and Isoenzyme Patterns in Body Fluids*, New York, Igaku-Shoin, 1991.)

ferent polypeptide chains, each of which contains a variable region and a constant region. Approximately 95% of mature T-cells express TCR α/β that is composed of α and β polypeptides, encoded by the TCR α- and β-chain genes, respectively. The remaining 5% of mature T-cells express TCR γ/δ. The developmental hierarchy in TCR gene rearrangement is that TCRδ gene is rearranged first, followed by rearrangements of the TCRγ and TCRβ genes. The TCRα gene is the last to be rearranged.

Monoclonality as demonstrated by gene rearrangement analysis is usually seen in lymphoid neoplasms. However, in several conditions in which the patients have reduced immunoregulation, monoclonality may be present without coexisting lymphoid neoplasms. These conditions include angioimmunoblastic lymphadenopathy with dysproteinemia (AILD), congenital immunodeficiency syndrome, the plasma-cell variant of Castleman's disease, autoimmune diseases (e.g., Sjögren's syndrome, rheumatoid arthritis), iatrogenic immunosuppression (posttransplantation), and the acquired immunodeficiency syndrome (AIDS).[13] However, these diseases can be considered premalignant conditions, since patients with these diseases are at a high risk of developing lymphomas.

Another problem in gene rearrangement analysis is cross-lineage rearrangement. Rearrangement of heavy-chain gene was seen in 10% of patients with T-cell leukemia[14], whereas rearrangement of TCR was reported in 25% of patients with non-T-cell acute lymphoblastic leukemia.[15] TCR and immunoglobulin gene rearrangements were also seen in about 50% of cases of acute myelogenous leukemia with positive TdT, and in 10% of cases without TdT expression.[16] However, the rearranged bands in cross-lineage conditions are usually faint and represent partial (DJ joining) rearrangement.[17] Fortunately, immunoglobulin light-chain rearrangement is lineage-specific. Therefore, with coexistence of both TCR and light-chain gene rearrangement, B-cell lymphoproliferative disorder should be considered unless proven otherwise.

Although immunogenotyping is most useful in diagnosing T-cell neoplasms, TCR rearrangement is sometimes not demonstrated in T-cell tumors, and about 12% of T-cell tumors were negative for TCR gene rearrangement in one series.[18,19] Besides technical errors and low percentage of tumor cells, there are several factors that may cause false negative results. The most common one is that TCR probe is not compatible with the TCR gene rearranged (e.g., use TCRβ probe to test on cells with TCR γ/δ rearrangement).

Others include the rearranged band superimposed with the germline band, multiple rearrangements occur in a polyclonal fashion, and rearranged gene being deleted.[12,20] In a small number of T-cell tumors, the tumor cells may not go through the TCR rearrangement process.[18]

Southern Blotting

This is the classical technique for the identification of rearranged bands in a clonal population.[21] DNA is isolated from clinical specimens by phenol–chloroform extraction and ethanol precipitation. The DNA extract is then digested by restriction enzymes, most commonly BamHI, EcoRI, and HindIII. The resultant restriction fragments are size-fractionated by electrophoresis in 0.8% agarose gels. The DNA in the gel is treated with alkali to become single-stranded, transferred to a nitrocellulose or nylon membrane, and immobilized by heating. Bands containing DNA of the gene fragment of interest are detected by a DNA probe, usually labeled with a radioisotope and visualized by autoradiography. Normal lymphocytes show only germline bands, but clonal lymphoid cells reveal one or more bands not identical to the germlines, which are called *rearranged bands* (Fig. 3.8).

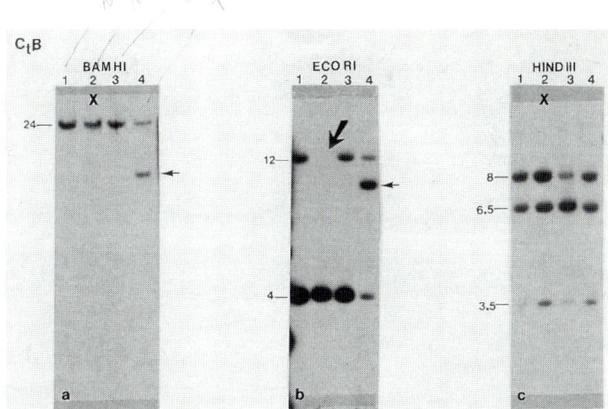

Fig. 3.8 Southern blot hybridization analysis of the T-cell receptor β-chain gene (CτB) in cases of thymoma (lane 2), B-cell lymphoma (lane 3), and T-cell lymphoma (lane 4). Lane 1 is a normal lymphocyte control. The EcoRI (*b*) digest shows a biallelic deletion of the 12kb fragments (large arrow) in the thymoma case and a rearranged band (small arrow) in the T-cell lymphoma case. BamHI (*a*) digest also reveals a rearranged band in the T-cell lymphoma case. (From Sun T, et al: *J Clin Lab Anal* 3:156–162, 1989.)

It is important to select the appropriate probes for this procedure.[13] The C (constant-region) probes were first cloned and used as the probes for heavy-chain gene, light-chain gene, and TCR genes. However, the J (joining region) segment is involved in most rearrangement and is limited in number; therefore, the use of J probes may have a higher positive yield, and these probes have gradually replaced the C probes for all gene rearrangement studies.

For TCR gene analysis, the TCRα-chain gene is composed of an enormous J region; therefore, it is impractical to test TCRα gene routinely by using either a J probe or C probe. On the other hand, TCRγ-chain gene is difficult to analyze because of its limited number of V (variable) segments. As a result, fewer than 10 different restriction fragments are generated after the digestion by restriction enzymes. Therefore, polyclonal T-cell population may produce a visibly rearranged band and sometimes obscure the neoplastic clone.

Polymerase Chain Reaction

Since the Southern blotting technique is tedious and time-consuming, the current trend is using a newer technique, polymerase chain reaction (PCR). PCR is an *in vitro* technique for enzymatic amplification of a DNA segment of interest that can provide sufficient material for the demonstration of the rearranged band(s).[22] The PCR products are assayed by gel electrophoresis. When the target DNA sequence is abundant in the specimen, a rearranged band can be visualized after the gel is stained by ethidium bromide.[12] If sufficient material is not available, the more sensitive Southern blotting technique should be used.

The PCR procedure is composed of repetitive cycling of three simple reactions: DNA denaturation, primer annealing, and primer extension (Fig. 3.9). All reactions take place in the same test tube at various temperatures. DNA denaturation is accomplished by a high temperature (90–95°C) which breaks the hydrogen bonds of the double-stranded DNA and produces single-stranded DNA. Two single-stranded oligonucleotides (primers), synthesized to be complementary to known sequences of the target DNA, are added with polymerases and excess deoxyribonucleoside triphosphates (nucleotides), as the building block for new DNA synthesis. At a lower temperature (45–55°C), the two primers anneal to opposite ends of two single-stranded DNA molecules derived from the first step. The polymerase then catalyzes the synthesis of a complementary second strand of the new DNA at 72°C, leading to the extension of each annealed primer. Two

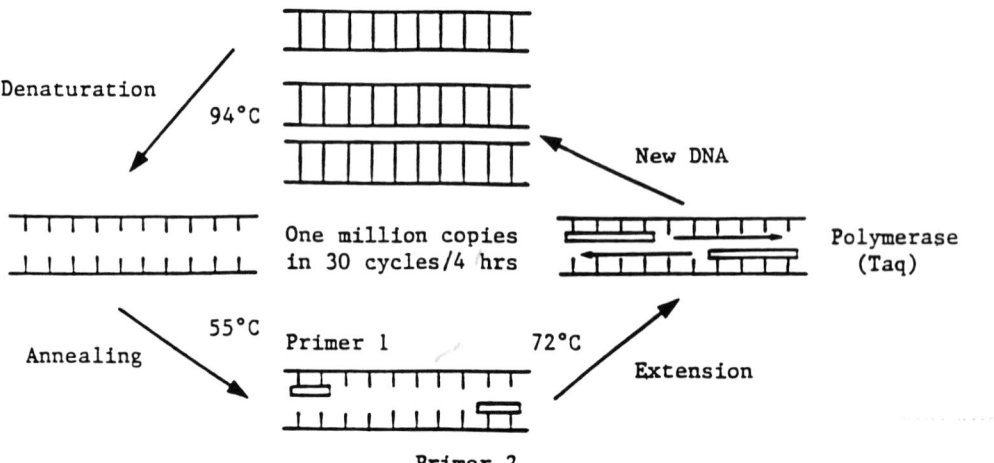

Fig. 3.9 Scheme of polymerase chain reaction showing the stages of denaturation, annealing, and extension with the reaction of primers and polymerase under different temperatures. (From Sun T: *Color Atlas/Text of Flow Cytometric Analysis of Hematologic Neoplasms*, New York, Igaku-Shoin, 1993.)

single-stranded DNA copies are produced in the first cycle, but DNA increases exponentially in subsequent cycles. After repeating the cycle 30 times, about 1 million copies of the target DNA segments are generated in 4 hr.

Assessment of clonality for antigen gene receptors can be accomplished by using a pair of oligonucleotides that are complementary to the consensus sequences common to V segments and J segments. A polyclonal population forms a smear in gel because there are numerous rearrangements that have different junctional sequences. On the other hand, a monoclonal population produces a distinct band due to the uniform junctional sequences in cells of the same clone. On the basis of the same principle, chromosomal translocation can be detected by the use of two primers complementary to two different chromosomes.

PCR is also a sensitive tool for the detection of minimal residual disease. However, sequence analysis and tumor-specific oligonucleotide synthesis are needed in this procedure; therefore this procedure is more time-consuming than the PCR procedure for other purposes.

The major disadvantage of PCR is contamination of the template DNA leading to false-positive results. PCR may also amplify nonspecific sequences creating spurious products.[12]

In situ Hybridization

The *in situ* hybridization technique provides a useful means for studying lymphoid neoplasms at the DNA/RNA levels.[13] This technique allows direct application of appropriate probes (DNA, RNA, or oligonucleotide) to cytology smears, frozen or paraffin sections. The probes are composed of single-stranded DNA or RNA that hybridizes with the denatured DNA or RNA in the smears or sections. The result can be detected by autoradiography when the probes are labeled with radioisotopes, or by regular immunohistologic or immunocytologic techniques when linked to biotin (Figs. 3.10, 3.11). Thus far, this technique is most frequently used to detect viral DNA or RNA. The correlation of EBV (Epstein–Barr virus) with lymphoproliferative disorders has been reported in many current studies.[23] Another major application of *in situ* hybridization is the detection of numeric and structural chromosomal abnormality by using fluorochrome-labeled, chromosome-specific probes.[24] This technique is called *fluorescent in situ hybridization* (FISH). It can de-

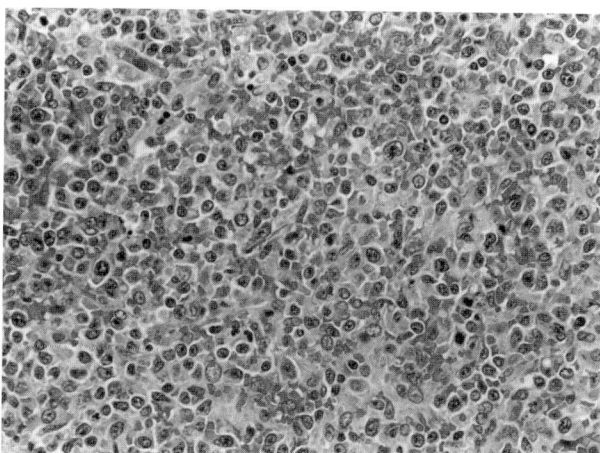

Fig. 3.10 Natural-killer-cell lymphoma in the spleen showing mixed small and large lymphoid cells. H&E, ×500.

tect chromosomes at interphase directly in intact cells on smears or sections. The same principle can be applied to RNA *in situ* hybridization (RISH).

CYTOGENETICS AND ONCOGENES

Although not directly proved in every individual neoplasm, it has been generally accepted that carcinogenic effects of both chemical and physical carcinogens are through the damage of DNA and that cytogenetic abnormality is the basis of carcinogenesis.[25] Those tumors that show no cytogenetic abnormalities are as-

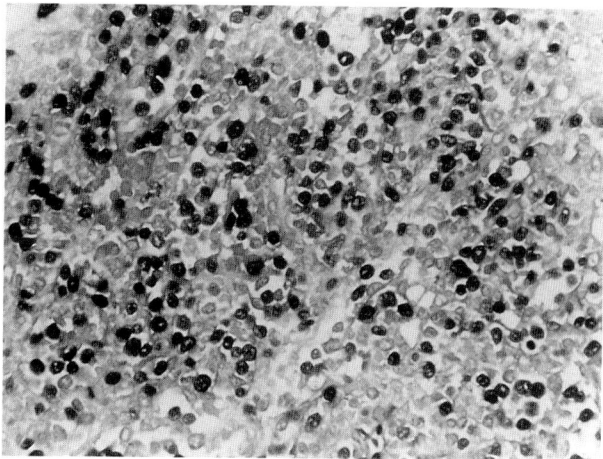

Fig. 3.11 The same specimen as in Fig. 3–10 demonstrating Epstein–Barr virus genome by RNA hybridization technique. ×500.

sumed to have subtle changes that are not detectable by current techniques. Therefore, the most important role for cytogenetic analysis is to determine the nature of a pathologic lesion when morphologic, immunophenotypic, and/or immunogenotypic studies are inconclusive.[26] However, nonrandom (recurring) cytogenetic abnormalities have been established only in a few lymphoid neoplasms, such as t(8;14) in Burkitt's lymphoma and t(14;18) in follicular lymphoma (Fig. 3.12); thus karyotyping can seldom be depended on for diagnosis.

It is now apparent that cytogenetics are a reliable predictor for prognosis. Generally speaking, neoplasms carrying a normal karyotype have a better prognosis than those with an abnormal one. One exception is childhood acute lymphoblastic leukemia, in which hyperdiploidy carries a better prognosis than diploidy.[27] The prediction of prognosis by karyotyping is sometimes associated with the histopathologic pattern. For instance, a favorable prognosis in lymphoma with t(14;18) is due to its association with follicular lymphoma, while the poor prognosis predicted by t(8;14) is due to its association with Burkitt's lymphoma.[28] Some numerical chromosomal abnormalities, such as +5, +6, or +18, are related to shorter survival in patients with non-Hodgkin's lymphoma.[29]

Cytogenetic studies are also useful in monitoring of clinical course. When the patient has a relapse, karyotyping is able to determine whether it is a recurrent or a secondary tumor.[3] Structural chromosomal abnormalities usually initiate malignant transformation, whereas numerical chromosomal abnormalities represent chromosomal evolution leading to the progression of disease.[30] The appearance of new abnormalities in the karyotype, no matter whether it is structural or numeric, signals transformation of tumor to higher-grade malignancy.[26]

Cytogenetic analysis is also able to detect residual minimal disease. As mentioned in a previous section, the detection of residual tumor cells is frequently based on the use of two primers to probe two translocated chromosomes.

Among all the genomic alterations, chromosomal translocation draws most attention. Translocation is frequently a nonrandom change and thus is diagnostic. It also frequently involves oncogenes and antigen receptors in translocation, thus helping to elucidate the mechanism of tumorigenesis, which varies in different tumors (Table 3.4). The mechanism of oncogene activation can be divided as follows:

1. *Fusion transcript:* The classical example is chronic myelogenous leukemia but the same pattern is encountered in cases of acute lymphoblastic leukemia. In these cases, the cytogenetic abnormality is t(9;22) (q34;q11), or the so-called Philadelphia chromosome. The translocation results in the fusion of *c-abl*, a protooncogene, on chromosome 9q34, and a restriction region on chromosome 22q11, called the breakpoint cluster region (*bcr*), leading to transcription to an aberrant hybrid *c-abl-bcr* RNA. The *bcr* domain activates the tyrosine kinase activity of the *c-abl* protein.[25] The abnormal activity of the tyrosine kinase may disturb the normal process of transduction in the cell and cause malignant transformation.

2. *Transcriptional deregulation:* The well-known example is Burkitt's lymphoma, in which the *c-myc* protooncogene is translocated from chromosome 8 to chromosome 14 and juxtaposed with the heavy-chain gene. As a result of the translocation, *c-myc* submits to the control of the transcriptional enhancer of the immunoglobulin gene and is thus activated or deregulated. Constitutive *myc* expression may prevent cells from entering the resting state (G_0 phase) and differentiating, leading to continuing proliferation of undifferentiated cells.[31]

3. *bcl-2 overexpression:* Follicular lymphoma is characterized by the genomic alteration of t(14;18), in which the protooncogene *bcl-2* (18q21) moves into the proximity of the immunoglobulin heavy-chain enhancer region (14q32). As a result, the protooncogene is activated (deregulated) and the functional *bcl-2*-Ig fusion protein is overexpressed. The *bcl-2* gene en-

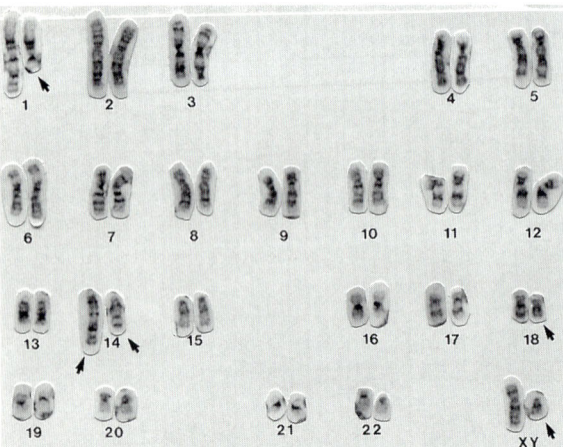

Fig. 3.12 A karotype of lymph node cells showing chromosomal 14; 18 translocation (arrows) and additional abnormalities: inv(Y) (q21;q32), t(1;14) (q23;q32). (Courtesy of Dr. Prasad Koduru.)

TABLE 3.4
Chromosomal Translocation in Lymphoid Neoplasms

Neoplasm	Protooncogene/chromosome	Antigen receptor gene/chromosome
B-ALL	c-abl/9q34	bcr/22q11
Burkitt's lymphoma/ALL	c-myc/8q24	IgH/14q32
Burkitt's lymphoma/ALL	c-myc/8q24	IgK/2p12
Burkitt's lymphoma/ALL	c-myc/8q24	IgL/22q11
T-ALL	c-myc/8q24	TCRα/14q11
T-ALL	tcl-2/11p13	TCRδ/14q11
T-ALL	tcl-3/10q24	TCRδ/14q11
T-ALL	tcl-4/9q32	TCRβ/7q34-36
T-ALL	tcl-5/1p32	TCRδ/14q11
T-ALL	lyl-1/19p13	TCRβ/7q34
T-ALL	tal-1/11p15	TCRδ/14q11
B-CLL	bcl-1/11q13	IgH/14q32
B-CLL	bcl-3/19q13	IgH/14q32
T-CLL	c-myc/8q24	TCRα/14q11
Mantle-cell lymphoma	bcl-1/11q13	IgH/14q32
Follicular lymphoma	bcl-2/18q21	IgH/14q32
Immunoblastic lymphoma	c-myc/8q24	IgK/2p12
Multiple myeloma	bcl-1/11q13	IgH/14q32

Abbreviations: ALL = acute lymphoblastic leukemia; CLL = chronic lymphocytic leukemia; IgH = immunoglobulin heavy-chain gene; IgK = immunoglobulin κ light-chain gene; IgL = immunoglobulin λ light-chain gene; TCR = T-cell receptor gene

codes for an inner mitochondrial membrane protein that plays a role in blocking programmed cell death (apoptosis).[32] Therefore, cells with abnormal expression of this protein remain in the G_0 stage and become immotalized.

4. *PRAD1 overexpression:* In mantle-cell lymphoma, the protooncogene bcl-1 (11q13) is juxtaposed to an Ig enhancer sequence located on chromosome 14. This translocation results in deregulation of a gene PRAD1 linked to the bcl-1 locus.[33] PRAD1 encodes for cyclin D1, a cell cycle protein. As a result of PRAD1 activation, the G_1–S transition of the cell cycle is disturbed and the t(11;14)-carrying cells cannot exit from the cell cycle, leading to an expanded B-cell department.[34]

5. *Activation by point mutation or gene amplification:* Mutation of the ras genes has been found in some hematologic neoplasia including acute myelogenous leukemia, chronic myelogenous leukemia, acute lymphoblastic leukemia, and multiple myeloma.[25] Amplification of the N-*myc* gene has been demonstrated in neuroblastoma, and *neu* gene in breast and ovarian carcinoma[25], but this mechanism of activation has not been detected in lymphoid neoplasms.

Finally, tumor suppressor gene, such as p53, has been reported to be involved in the tumorigenesis of Burkitt's lymphoma and Richter's transformation.[35] In view of the recent advances, molecular genetic techniques are expected to unveil more and more cytogenetic abnormalities in lymphoid tumors in the near future.

REFERENCES

1. Sun T: *Color Atlas/Text of Flow Cytometric Analysis of Hematologic Neoplasms*, New York, Igaku-Shoin, 1993, pp 3–17, 36–39.
2. Picker LJ, Weiss LM, Medeiros LJ, et al: Immunophenotypic criteria for the diagnosis of non-Hodgkin's lymphoma. *Am J Pathol* 128:181–201, 1987.
3. Sun T, Susin M: A practical approach to immunophenotyping of lymphomas: Comparison of immunohistologic and immunocytologic techniques. *Ann Clin Lab Sci* 17:14–16, 1987.
4. Sun T, Ngu M, Henshall J, et al: Marker discrepancy as a diagnostic criterion for lymphoid neoplasms. *Diagn Clin Immunol* 5:393–399, 1988.
5. Stetler-Stevenson M, Medeiros LJ, Jaffe ES: Immunophenotypic methods and findings in the diagnosis of lymphoproliferative diseases. In Jaffe ES (ed): *Surgical Pathology of the Lymph Nodes and Related Organs*, 2nd ed, Philadelphia, Saunders, 1995, pp 22–57.
6. Knowles DM, Chadburn A, Inghirami G: Immunophenotypic markers useful in the diagnosis and classification of

hematopoietic neoplasms. In Knowles DM (ed): *Neoplastic Hematopathology*, Baltimore, Williams & Wilkins, 1992, pp 73–167.
7. Sheibani K, Tubbs RR: Enzyme immunohistochemistry: Technical aspects. *Semin Diagn Pathol* 1:235–250, 1984.
8. Tao Q, Srivastava G, Loke SL, et al: Improved double immunohistochemical staining method for cryostat and paraffin wax sections, combining alkaline phosphatase antialkaline phosphatase and indirect immunofluorescence. *J Clin Pathol* 47:597–600, 1994.
9. Sun T, Li Y, Yam LT: *Atlas of Cytochemistry and Immunochemistry of Hematologic Neoplasms*, Chicago, American Society of Clinical Pathologists Press, 1985.
10. Sun T, Eisenberg A, Benn P, et al: Comparison of phenotyping and genotyping of lymphoid neoplasms. *J Clin Lab Anal* 3:156–162, 1989.
11. Brabndter LB, Smith CIE, Hammarstrom L, et al: Clonal immunoglobulin gene rearrangements in primary mediastinal clear cell lymphomas. *Leukemia* 3:122–129, 1989.
12. Sklar J: Antigen receptor genes: Structure, function, and techniques for analysis of their rearrangements. In Knowles DM (ed): *Neoplastic Hematopathology*, Baltimore, Williams & Wilkins, 1992, pp 215–244.
13. Medeiros LJ, Bagg A, Cossman J: Molecular genetics in the diagnosis and classification of lymphoid neoplasms. In Jaffe ES (ed): *Surgical Pathology of the Lymph Node and Related Organs*, 2nd ed, Philadelphia, Saunders, 1995, pp 58–97.
14. Kuchingham GR, Rovigatti U, Mauer AM, et al: Rearrangements of immunoglobulin heavy chain genes in T-cell acute lymphoblastic leukemia. *Blood* 65:725–729, 1985.
15. Tawa A, Hozumi N, Minden M, et al: Rearrangement of the T-cell receptor β-chain gene in non-T-cell non-B-cell acute lymphoblastic leukemia of childhood. *N Engl J Med* 313:1033–1037, 1985.
16. Seremetis SV, Pelicci PG, Tabilio A, et al: High frequency of clonal immunoglobulin on T-cell receptor gene rearrangements in acute myelogenous leukemia expressing terminal deoxynucleotidyl transferase. *J Exp Med* 165:1703–1712, 1987.
17. Griesser H, Takchuk D, Reis MD, et al: Gene rearrangements and translocations in lymphoproliferative diseases. *Blood* 73:1402–1415, 1989.
18. Weiss LM, Picker LJ, Grogan TM, et al: Absence of clonal beta and gamma T-cell receptor gene rearrangements in a subset of peripheral T-cell lymphomas. *Am J Pathol* 130:436–442, 1988.
19. O'Connor NTJ, Wainscoat JS, Weatherall DJ, et al: Rearrangement of the T-cell receptor δ-chain in the diagnosis of lymphoproliferative disorders. *Lancet* 1:1295–1297, 1985.
20. Willman CL, Griffith BB, Whittaker M: Molecular genetic approaches for the diagnosis of clonality in lymphoid neoplasms. *Clin Lab Med* 10:119–149, 1990.
21. Southern EM: Detection of specific sequences among DNA fragments separated by gel electrophoresis. *J Mol Biol* 98:503–517, 1975.
22. Eisenstein BI: The polymerase chain reaction: A new method of using molecular genetics for medical diagnosis. *N Engl J Med* 322:178–183, 1990.
23. Hamilton-Dutoit SJ, Pallesen G: Detection of Epstein–Barr virus small RNAs in routine paraffin sections using non-isotopic RNA/RNA in situ hybridization. *Histopathology* 25:101–111, 1994.
24. Anastasi J: Interphase cytogenetic analysis in the diagnosis and study of neoplastic disorders. *Am J Clin Pathol* 95:(suppl 1):S22–S28, 1991.
25. Gaidano G, Dalla-Favera R: Protooncogenes and tumor suppressor genes. In Knowled DM (ed): *Neoplastic Hematopathology*, Baltimore, Williams & Wilkins, 1992, pp 245–261.
26. Le Beau MM: The role of cytogenetics in the diagnosis and classification of hematopoietic neoplasms. In Knowled DM (ed): *Neoplastic Hematopathology*, Baltimore, Williams & Wilkins, 1992, pp 299–321.
27. Pui CH, Christ WM, Look AT: Biology and clinical significance of cytogenetic abnormalities in childhood acute lymphoblastic leukemia. *Blood* 76:1449–1463, 1990.
28. Kristoffersson U, Heim S, Mandahl N, et al: Prognostic implications of cytogenetic findings in 106 patients with non-Hodgkin's lymphoma. *Cancer Genet Cytogenet* 25:55–64, 1987.
29. Schouten HC, Sanger WG, Weisenburger DD, et al: Chromosomal abnormalities in untreated patients with non-Hodgkin's lymphoma. *Int J Cancer* 32:683–692, 1983.
30. Dewald GW, Noel P, Dahl RJ, et al: Chromosome abnormalities in malignant hematologic disorders. *Mayo Clin Proc* 60:675–689, 1985.
31. McKeithan TW: Molecular biology of non-Hodgkin's lymphoma. *Semin Oncol* 17:30–42, 1990.
32. Hockenberry D, Nunez G, Milliman C, et al: Bcl-2 is an inner-mitochrondrial membrane protein that blocks programmed cell death. *Nature* 348:334–336, 1990.
33. Rosenberg CL, Wong E, Petty E, et al: PRAD1, a candidate BCL-1 oncogene: Mapping and expression in centrocytic lymphoma. *Proc Natl Acad Sci (USA)* 88:9638–9642, 1991.
34. Rimokh R, Berger R, Delso G, et al: Detection of the chromosomal translocation t(11;14) by polymerase chain reaction in mantle cell lymphomas. *Blood* 83:1871–1875, 1994.
35. Gaidano G, Ballerini P, Gong JZ, et al: p53 mutations in human lymphoid malignancies: Association with Burkitt's lymphoma and chronic lymphocytic leukemia. *Proc Natl Acad Sci (USA)* 88:5413–5417, 1991.

4
Reactive Lymphoid Hyperplasias

Reactive lymphoid hyperplasias or reactive lymphadenopathies cover a broad spectrum of diseases. Although the etiology is unknown in most cases, the cause of reactive lymphadenopathy may be due to a large array of factors, including biologic, chemical, immunologic, and neoplastic components. Among the various clinical entities, most are associated with biologic agents or immunologic status of the patients, either immunodeficiency or hyperimmune reaction. Under most circumstances, the histologic pattern is characteristic although not specific. Therefore, correlation of clinical manifestation and laboratory findings is often required to achieve a definitive diagnosis. As an etiologic classification is impractical because of the lack of causes in most cases, a histologic classification is most popular and immunologic components, such as the cell lineage, are expected to be included in the future.[1-4] Traditionally, reactive lymphoid hyperplasias have been divided into four categories: follicular pattern (I), sinus pattern (II), diffuse pattern (III), and mixed pattern (IV) (Table 4.1).

FOLLICULAR PATTERN

Nonspecific reactive follicular hyperplasia is the most common form of reactive hyperplasia. Follicular hyperplasia and its distinction from follicular lymphoma will be discussed in Chapter 9. Another topic under follicular hyperplasia, Castleman's disease, will be discussed in Chapter 8.

Acquired Immunodeficiency Syndrome

In patients with HIV infection, persistent generalized lymphadenopathy (PGL) is a frequent manifestation. Most cases with PGL progress into AIDS. There are three histologic patterns of PGL, representing three progressive stages (Table 4.2).[4-6]

The early stage of PGL usually shows florid follicular hyperplasia (see Fig. 4.1). In this stage, the follicles are increased in both number and size. The enlarged follicles may coalesce and show a wide variation in shape. These follicles are characterized by the presence of patchy hemorrhages, necrosis, and small lymphocytic infiltration in the germinal centers, a phenomenon that is called *follicular fragmentation* or *follicular lysis*. In addition, there are numerous mitoses and tingible-body macrophages that confer a starry-sky appearance. The mantle zone is usually attenuated or absent. The parafollicular sinuses are filled with monocytoid B-lymphocytes and some neutrophils. The interfollicular and paracortical areas are infiltrated by small lymphocytes, plasma cells, immunoblasts, eosinophils, histiocytes, and monocytoid B-lymphocytes. Proliferation of arborizing high epithelial venules (HEVs) is also present in these areas. Multi-nucleated giant cells (polykaryocytes of the Warthin–Finkeldy type) may be present occasionally in the germinal centers or interfollicular areas.

Follicular hyperplasia may progress into follicular involution. In contrast to the early stage, the follicles in this stage become small with a hyaline vascular center resembling those seen in Castleman's disease. The follicle center lymphocytes are largely replaced by follicular dendritic cells and epithelioid histiocytes. The mantle zone is markedly reduced or absent. Sinus histiocytosis and capsular fibrosis may be present. The interfollicular and paracortical areas are infiltrated by plasma cells, histiocytes, and immunoblasts. Lymphocytes become sparse in these areas. Without a crowded cellular background, proliferation of HEVs stands out prominently (Figs. 4.2–4.4).

The final stage is lymphocyte depletion, which is usually seen in autopsy cases. In this stage, follicles are markedly decreased, or only a few sclerotic remnants are present. Mantle zones are absent. Sinus histiocytosis is present, sometimes with erythrophagocytosis. The interfollicular and paracortical areas are infiltrated mainly by plasma cells and histiocytes, as lymphocytes are markedly depleted. Excessive vascularization is present in these areas. The lymph node may have diffuse fibrosis with obliteration of the normal architecture.

In immunohistochemical studies of the lymphoid follicles, CD4 cells are progressively decreased, while CD8 cells are gradually increased and are often clustered around blood vessels. The distribution of the follicular dendritic reticulum cells, as demonstrated by DRC-1 (CD21) staining, is fragmented consistent with the pattern of follicle fragmentation. However, in the hyperplastic stage, 90% of the follicle center cells are CD19-positive B-cells that also show strong posi-

TABLE 4.1
Reactive Lymphoid Hyperplasias

I. Follicular pattern:
   Nonspecific reactive follicular hyperplasia
   Acquired immunodeficiency syndrome (AIDS)
   Rheumatoid arthritis (Felty's syndrome and Still's disease)
   Sjögren's syndrome
   Syphilis
   Progressive transformation of germinal centers
   Castleman's disease
   Kimura's disease
II. Sinus pattern:
   Sinus histiocytosis
   Sinus histiocytosis with massive lymphadenopathy (Rosai–Dorfman disease)
   Langerhans'-cell histiocytosis
   Hemophagocytic syndrome
   Monocytoid B-cell hyperplasia
   Whipple's disease
   Lymphangiographic effect
   Vascular transformation of sinuses
   Kaposi sarcoma
III. Diffuse pattern:
   Infectious mononucleosis
   Cytomegalovirus lymphadenitis
   Herpes zoster/herpes simplex lymphadenitis
   Postvaccinial lymphadenitis
   Measles lymphadenitis
   Posttransplantation lymphoproliferative disorders
   Drug-induced lymphadenopathy
   Angioimmunoblastic lymphadenopathy
   Bacillary angiomatosis
IV. Mixed pattern:
   Toxoplasmic lymphadenitis
   Dermatopathic lymphadenopathy
   Systemic lupus lymphadenopathy
   Granulomatous lymphadenitis
      Nonnecrotizing: sarcoidosis
      Necrotizing: cat-scratch disease, tuberculosis, atypical mycobacteriosis, brucellosis, tularemia, fungal infections, *Yersinia* infection, lymphogranuloma venereum
   Kikuchi–Fujimoto disease (histiocytic necrotizing lymphadenitis)
   Kawasaki disease (mucocutaneous lymph node syndrome)

tivity of Ki67 representing proliferating cells in G_1–G_2 phases. The major core HIV protein, p24, has been demonstrated in the follicles with distribution identical to that of the DRC-1-positive cells.[7] The HIV genome has been detected with the *in situ* hybridization technique in rare and isolated cells located in germinal centers and paracortical areas in a few cases of PGL.[8]

Rheumatoid Arthritis

Rheumatoid arthritis and its related disorders (Still disease and Felty syndrome) are frequently associated with generalized lymphadenopathy.[1,3,4] The incidence varies from 29% to 75% in different studies.[4] Since patients with rheumatoid arthritis are at high risk of developing lymphoma[4] and lymphadenopathy may precede arthritis,[3] it is important to have the enlarged lymph node examined histologically to rule out lymphoma in these patients.

The diagnostic triad in rheumatoid lymphadenopathy is follicular hyperplasia, interfollicular plasmacytosis, and intrasinus neutrophils (Figs. 4.5–4.7).[1] Hyperplastic follicles may be seen in both the cortex and medulla. The histologic features of the follicles are consistent with the general pattern of nonspecific hyperplasia, namely, the follicles are varying in size and shape, mitoses are prominent, and tingible-body macrophages are numerous. In addition, PAS (periodic-acid-Schiff)-positive, hyaline-like material may be present in the germinal centers. The mantle zone is reduced in size. The most striking feature is the presence of sheets of plasma cells, which may contain Russell bodies.

The histologic features in rheumatoid arthritis are characteristic but not specific, as the same features can be demonstrated in other autoimmune disorders, such as Sjögren's syndrome, Hashimoto thyroiditis, dermatomyositis, polyarteritis nodosa, and scleroderma.[3] The major exception is systemic lupus erythematosus (SLE), which will be discussed later. Immunologic studies of lymphocytes and plasma cells in these disorders usually demonstrate polyclonality. In Sjögren's syndrome, however, monoclonality has been identified in small lymphocytes and plasma cells by immunophenotyping and genotyping. Whether this phenomenon represents a premalignant condition or overt lymphoma is controversial.[1,9]

Syphilis

Luetic lymphadenitis is similar to rheumatoid lymphadenopathy in that marked follicular hyperplasia, interfollicular plasmacytosis, and intrasinus neutrophils are present in the lymph nodes (Fig. 4.8).[3,4] The differential features are (a) the presence of epithelioid-cell

TABLE 4.2
Histologic Patterns in AIDS-Related Lymphadenopathy

	Follicular hyperplasia	Follicular involution	Lymphocyte depletion
Number and size of follicles	Increased	Decreased	Markedly decreased
Shape of follicles	Variable with irregular margins	Atrophic with hyaline vascular center	Sclerotic
Follicular pattern	Patchy hemorrhages, necrosis, and lymphocytic infiltrate	Follicle center cells replaced by dendritic and epithelioid cells	Sclerotic remnants
Starry-sky appearance	Prominent	Inconspicuous	Inconspicuous
Mitosis	Prominent	Seldom seen	None
Mantle zone	Reduced or absent	Reduced or absent	Absent
Parafollicular sinuses	Monocytoid B-cell and neutrophils	Histiocytosis	Histiocytosis
Interfollicular and paracortical areas	Lymphocyte, plasma cell, immunoblast, histiocyte, and eosinophil infiltrate	Plasma cell, histiocyte immunoblast infiltrate	Plasma cell and histiocyte infiltrate
Vascular proliferation	Present	Prominent	Prominent
Fibrosis	Absent	Mild	Prominent

granulomas with or without multinucleated giant cells in the interfollicular or paracortical areas, (b) the consistent finding of arteritis and endarteritis with prominent perivascular plasma cell infiltrate, and (c) the demonstration of spirochetes by silver impregnation in tissues or by immunofluorescent techniques applied on lymph node imprints. In tertiary syphilis, gummas may be found in the lymph nodes. Spirochetes are seen mainly in the epithelioid-cell granulomas, blood vessel walls, and follicle centers. In chronic luetic lymphadenitis, fibrosis is prominent. The fibrous tissue involves the capsule and penetrates into the lymph node cortex.

Progressive Transformation of Germinal Centers (PTGC)

This is a histologic diagnosis made by identifying hyperplastic follicles with the germinal centers replaced by small lymphocytes (Figs. 4.9, 4.10).[1,2,4] The importance of PTGC lies on its association with nodular lymphocyte predominance Hodgkin's dis-

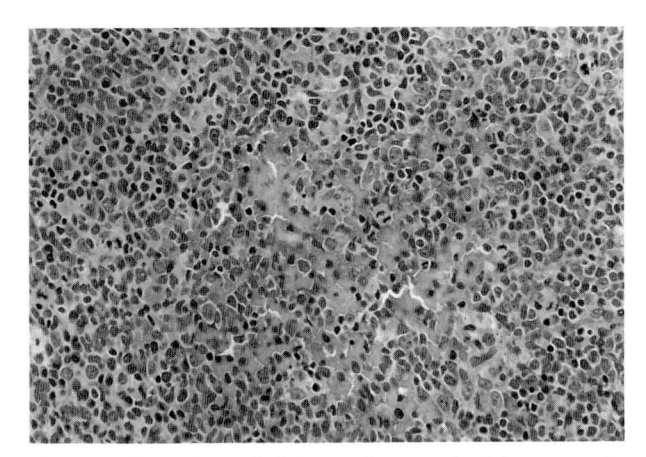

Fig. 4.1. Lymph node biopsy in acquired immunodeficiency syndrome showing follicular hyperplasia with patchy hemorrhages, necrosis, and small lymphocytic infiltration in the germinal centers. H&E, ×500.

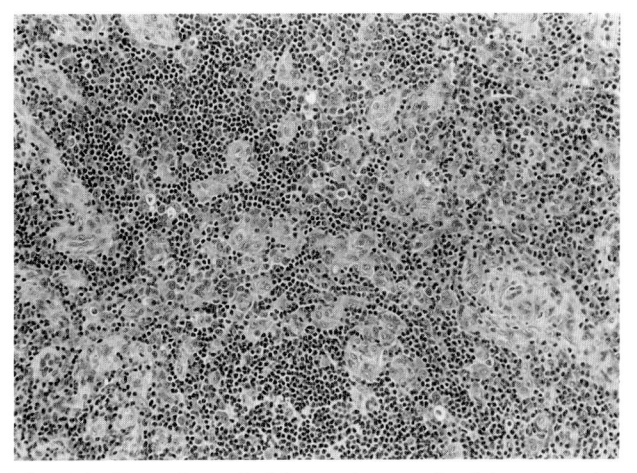

Fig. 4.2. Lymph node biopsy in acquired immunodeficiency syndrome showing depletion of lymphocytes and sinus histiocytosis. Proliferation of high endothelial venules stands out because of the hypocellular background. H&E, ×250.

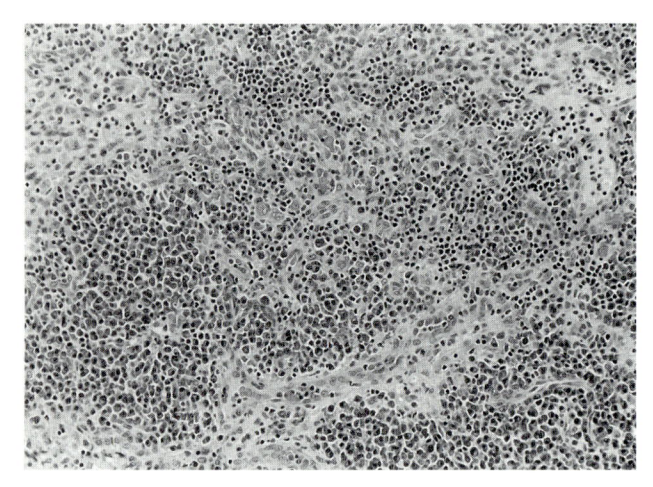

Fig. 4.3. Lymph node biopsy from the same case as Fig. 4.2 showing marked increase in plasma cells in addition to features described in Fig. 4.2. H&E, ×250.

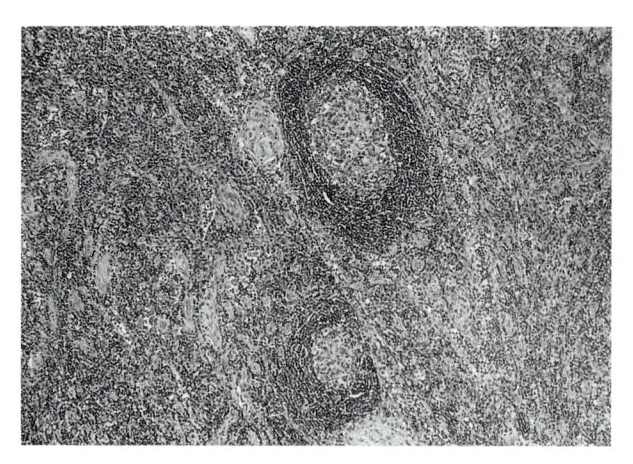

Fig. 4.5. Lymph node biopsy in rheumatoid arthritis showing hyperplastic germinal centers and increased vascularity. H&E, ×125.

ease (NLPHD). PTGC may be present before, after, or concomitantly with NLPHD. However, most cases of PTGC are seen in reactive lymphadenopathies unrelated to NLPHD. The follicles involved by PTGC are at least 2 or 3 times larger than the adjacent follicles, which are often hyperplastic. The small lymphocytes, which are the IgM+, IgD+ mantle-zone lymphocytes, gradually replace the germinal center cells and at the same time, expand the mantle zone. The demarcation between the germinal center and the mantle zone is therefore no longer discernible. In addition to the B-lymphocytes of the mantle zone, PTGCs also contain large numbers of CD4+, CD57+ T-lymphocytes and a network of follicular dendritic reticulum cells.

PTGC can be distinguished from NLPHD by the absence of L&H or "popcorn" cells, Reed–Sternberg cells, and epithelioid histiocytes. NLPHD frequently involves a large area with architectural effacement and interfollicular involvement.[1] In follicular lymphoma, the tumor cells in the germinal centers are small cleaved cells intermingled with various numbers of large lymphocyte; all of which are monotypic. The neoplastic follicles rarely reach the size of the transformed germinal centers, and there are no reactive follicles present between them.[4]

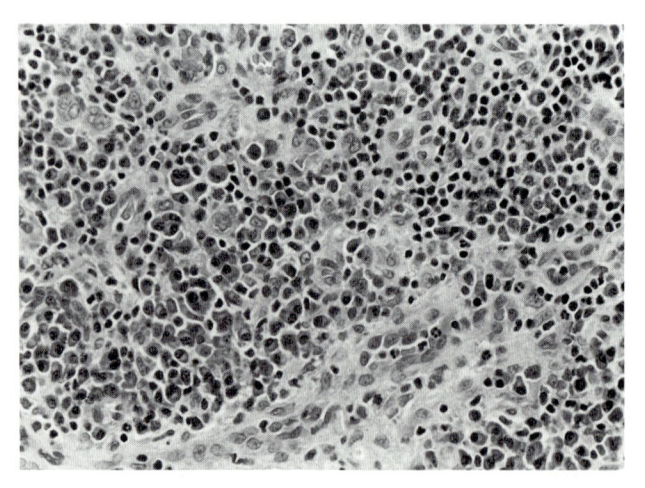

Fig. 4.4. A higher-power view of Fig. 4.3 showing lymphocyte depletion and increase in plasma cells and epithelioid histiocytes. H&E, ×500.

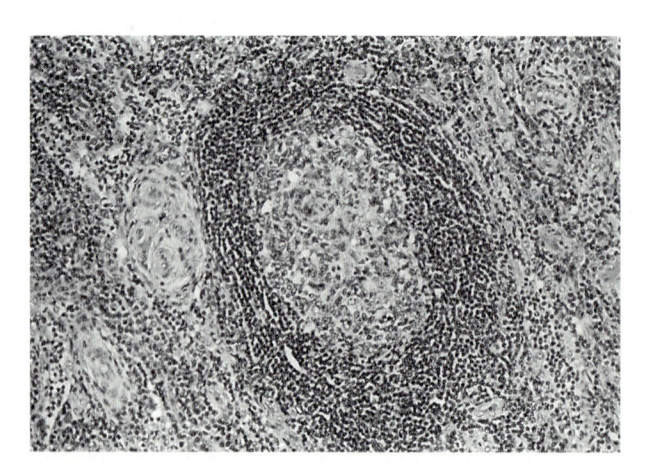

Fig. 4.6. A higher-power view of Fig. 4.5 showing hyperplastic germinal center with proliferation of vasculature. H&E, ×250.

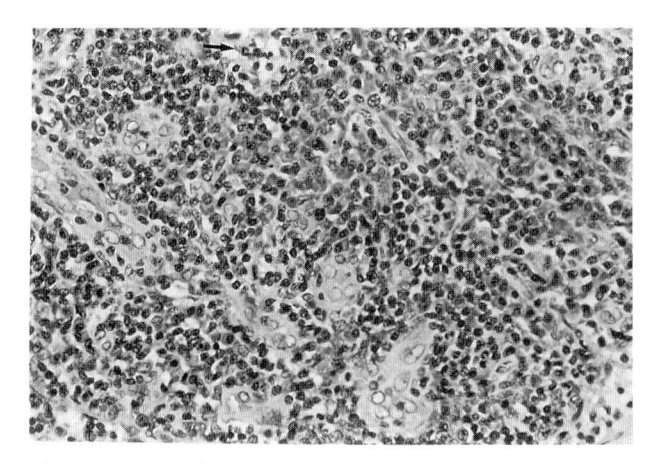

Fig. 4.7. A higher-power view of Fig. 4.5 showing increased plasma cells and scattered intrasinus neutrophils (arrow). H&E, ×500.

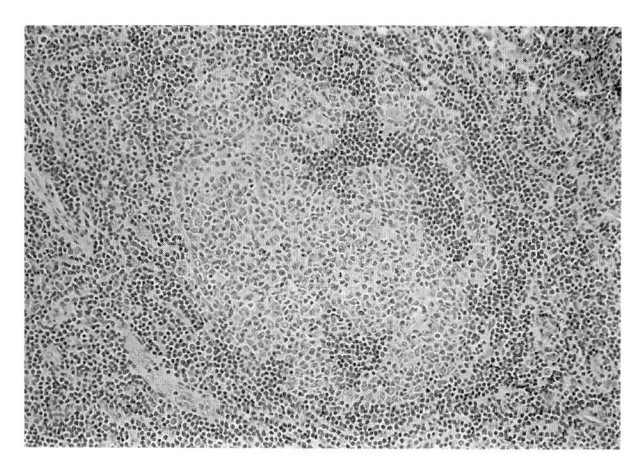

Fig. 4.9. Lymph node biopsy of progressive transformation of germinal centers (PTGC) showing small lymphocytes replacing part of the germinal center and expanding the mantle zone. H&E, ×250.

Kimura's Disease

Kimura's disease is a disorder of subcutaneous lymphogranuloma with esoinophilia and elevation of serum IgE.[10-13] Since this disease frequently (67-100%) involves the regional lymph nodes, it is included in the differential diagnosis of reactive lymphadenopathies.[10] The subcutaneous lesions are usually located in the head and neck regions. The underlying salivary glands are also frequently involved. There have been occasional reports of skeletal muscle and prostate lesions as well as nephrotic syndrome.[10,12]

The major histologic features in Kimura's disease include florid germinal centers with vascularization, increased postcapillary venules in the paracortex, esoinophilic infiltration in the interfollicular areas and sinusoids (Figs. 4.11-4.13), and the presence of polykaryocytes of the Warthin-Finkeldey type in germinal centers and the paracortex. Eosinophilic abscesses may be present in paracortex. When the germinal centers are infiltrated by eosinophils, Kimura's disease may progress into eosinophilic folliculolysis. In addition to eosinophils, plasma cells and mast cells are often increased in the paracortex and medullary cords. Charcot-Leyden crystals are sometimes present. Homoge-

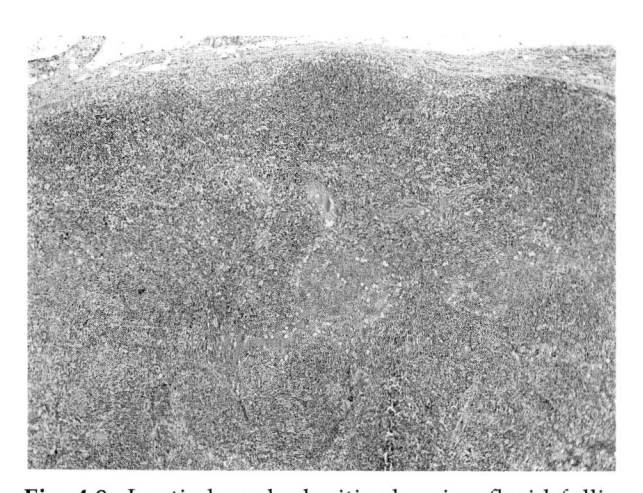

Fig. 4.8. Luetic lymphadenitis showing florid follicular hyperplasia with many tingible-body macrophages. There are interfollicular plasmacytosis and intrasinus neutrophilic infiltration not visible at this magnification. H&E, ×125. (AFIP 67-7354.)

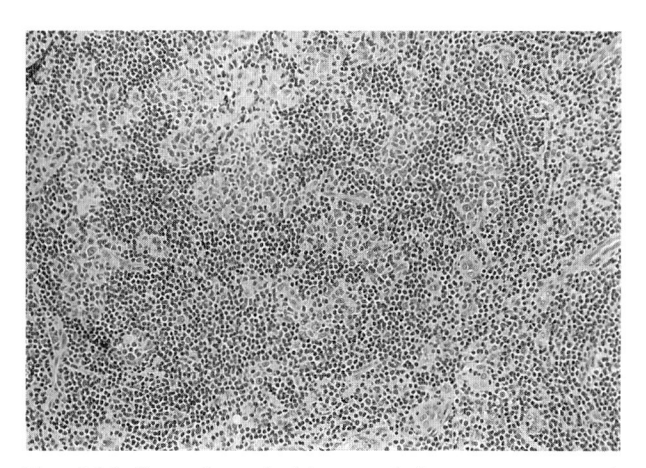

Fig. 4.10. Lymph node biopsy of the same case as in Fig. 4.9 showing a germinal center being largely replaced by small lymphocytes. H&E, ×250.

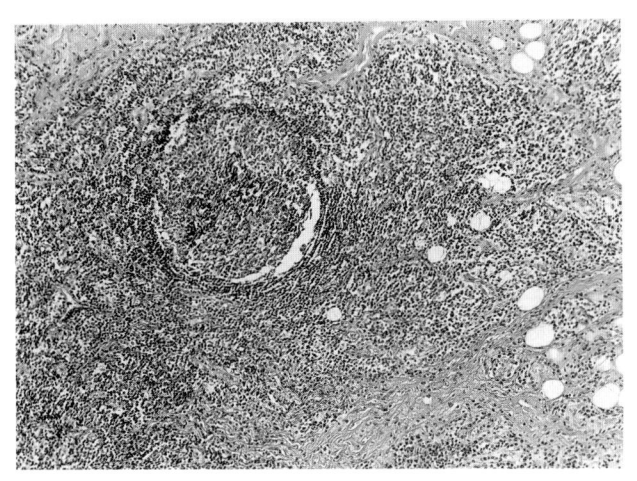

30 DIFFERENTIAL DIAGNOSIS OF LYMPHOID DISORDERS

Fig. 4.11. Subcutaneous lesion in Kimura's disease showing a hyperplastic lymphoid follicle with increased vascularity. The infiltrating cellular elements are not recognizable at this magnification. H&E, ×125. (Case contributed by Dr. T. T. Kuo.)

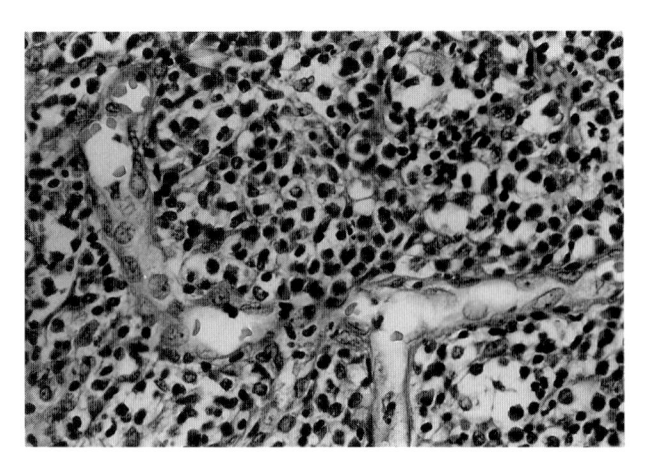

Fig. 4.13. Higher magnification shows plasma cells and eosinophils. The endothelial cells of the postcapillary venules appear normal. H&E, ×500.

neous proteinaceous material is sometimes demonstrated between the germinal center cells.[11] Sclerosis of variable degrees is also a frequent feature. The histologic features in the subcutaneous tissue are similar to those seen in lymph nodes: florid germinal centers, vascular proliferation, and eosinophilic infiltration.

Immunohistochemical stain may demonstrate an IgE reticular network in germinal centers as well as IgE-coated nondegranulated mast cells.[11] Variable amounts of IgG, IgM, and fibrinogen can also be demonstrated in the germinal center, but IgA, CIq, and C3 were not detected in one study.[10] The deposits of IgE in the germinal centers and the elevation of serum IgE and eosinophilia suggest that Kimura's disease is atopic in nature.[10,11]

Kimura's disease was first described in China by Kim and Szeto in 1937 as eosinophilic hyperplastic lymphogranuloma.[13] However, it was not until 1948 when Kimura et al. reported several similar cases in Japan that this entity became widely recognized in Asia. Since this disease is rare in the Western world, it had been confused with angiolymphoid hyperplasia with eosinophilia (ALHE) until Rosai et al. pointed out the differences between these two diseases and included ALHE in their unifying concept of histiocytoid hemangiomas.[14]

The major difference between Kimura's disease and ALHE is that the former is mainly a lymphoproliferative lesion and the latter, a vascular lesion (Table 4.3). Characteristically, ALHE shows thick-walled blood vessels with the so-called "histiocytoid" or "epithelioid" endothelial cells, which are hypertrophied and vacuolated endothelial cells protruding into or occluding the vascular lumen (Figs. 4.14–4.17). The proliferative vessels in Kimura's disease are thin-walled and never contain the histiocytoid endothelial cells. On the other hand, lymphoid hyperplasia and eosinophilic infiltrate are not prominent, and no lymphadenopathy is present in ALHE as in Kimura's disease. Peripheral eosinophilia and elevated serum IgE are also not constant features in ALHE as in Kimura's disease. Polykaryocytes of Warthin–Finkeldey type are rarely seen in ALHE. Patients with Kimura's disease are usually younger, and the skin lesions are larger and deeper (subcutaneous tis-

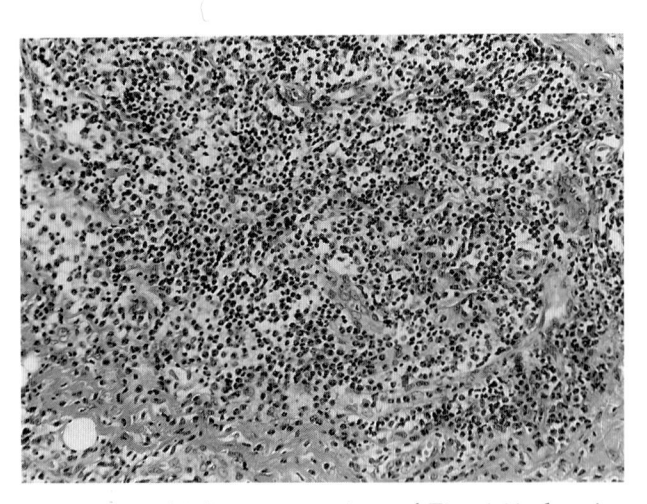

Fig. 4.12. A higher-power view of Fig. 4.11 showing extensive infiltration by plasma cells and eosinophils and increased vascularity. H&E, ×250.

TABLE 4.3
Comparison of Kimura Disease and Angiolymphoid Hyperplasia

	Kimura disease	*Angiolymphoid hyperplasia*
Geographic distribution	Mainly Asia	Worldwide
Sex	Male predominance	Male predominance
Age	7–53 yr	13–67 yr
Duration of disease	2 mo–24 yr	3 wk–12 yr
Lesion size	Large masses (2–10 cm)	Small papules or nodules (0.5–3.0 cm)
Lesion location	Subcutaneous	Dermal
Regional lymphadenopathy	Frequently present	Absent
Recurrence	25%	33%
Peripheral eosinophilia	Constant finding	Frequent finding
Serum IgE level	Elevated	Usually normal
Major histologic features	Follicular hyperplasia, eosinophilic infiltration, and increased blood vessels	Proliferation of thick-walled blood vessels with "histiocytoid" endothelial cells

sue) than those of ALHE. The duration of Kimura's disease is often longer than that of ALHE.

Other differential diagnosis includes Hodgkin's disease, because of the patchy sclerosis and eosinophilic infiltration, but the absence of Reed–Sternberg cells, the preserved nodal architecture, and the characteristic IgE staining pattern in Kimura's disease are the distinguishing features.[11] Eosinophilic infiltration in lymph nodes is also a common feature in drug reaction or allergy and parasitic infection such as filariasis. However, in drug reaction or allergy, vasculitis may be prominent, but there is no true vasculitis in Kimura's disease. In parasitic infection, segments of a parasite should be present, and eosinophilic granuloma is a common feature. Finally, vascularization of germinal centers and proliferation of venules are shared by Castleman's disease and Kimura's disease, but eosinophilia and florid germinal centers are not seen in Castleman's disease.

SINUS PATTERN

Sinus histiocytosis is a very common finding in lymph node biopsies (Figs. 4.18, 4.19). It may or may not be coexistent with follicular hyperplasia. Sinus histiocytosis may be the result of draining either inflammatory lesions or carcinoma, but in most instances, the cause is unknown. There are several special patterns of histiocytosis, such as sinus histiocytosis with massive

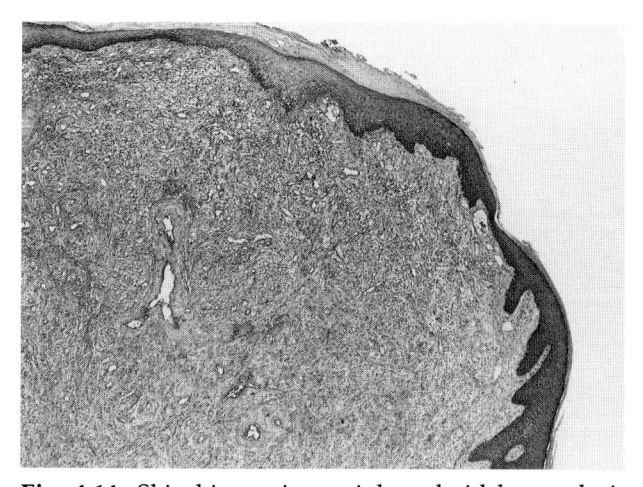

Fig. 4.14. Skin biopsy in angiolymphoid hyperplasia with eosinophilia showing marked vascular proliferation in the dermis. Lymphoid hyperplasia is not present. H&E, ×50. (Case contributed by Dr. T. T. Kuo.)

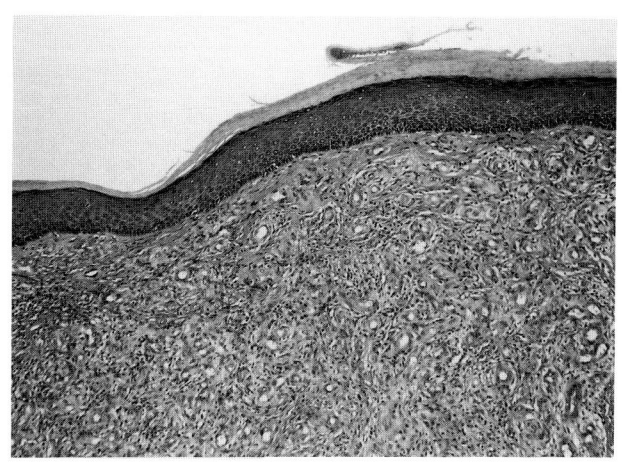

Fig. 4.15. A higher-power view of Fig. 4.14 showing vascular proliferation with scanty cellular infiltration. H&E, ×125.

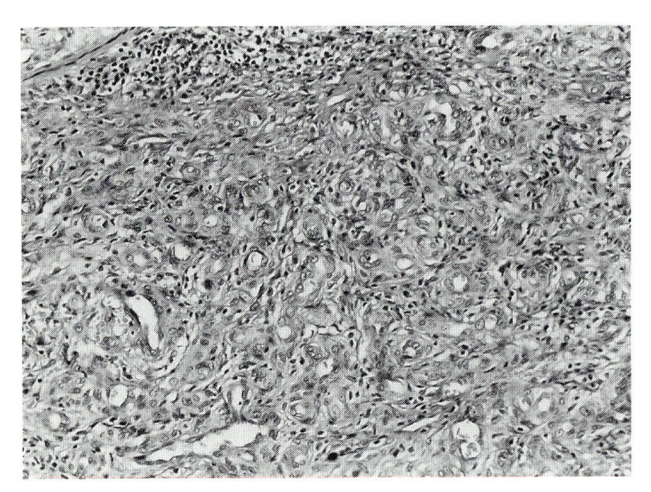

Fig. 4.16. A higher-power view of Fig. 4.15 showing thick-walled blood vessels. H&E, ×250.

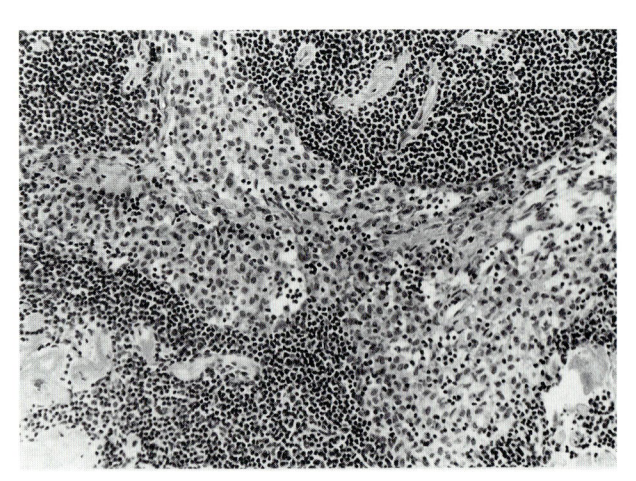

Fig. 4.18. Lymph node biopsy showing sinus histiocytosis. H&E, ×250.

lymphadenopathy (Rosai–Dorfman disease), Langerhans'-cell histiocytosis, and hemophagocytic syndrome, which are to be discussed in Chapter 17. Monocytoid B-cell hyperplasia is a reactive histologic pattern showing monocytoid B-cells in the sinuses of lymph nodes, which will be discussed in Chapter 12.

Whipple's Disease

The histologic features of the lymph nodes in Whipple's disease are similar to those seen after lymphangiography.[4] The sinuses are dilated, containing large vacuoles and vacuolated histiocytes (Fig. 4.20). These vacuoles represent lipid substances dissolved during tissue processing. Although these characteristic features are usually demonstrated in intraabdominal lymph nodes draining the small intestine, they may also be seen in enlarged peripheral lymph nodes. A definitive diagnosis is established by demonstrating the PAS-positive, diastase-resistant sickle-form particles in the cytoplasm of histiocytes. These particles represent the causative bacillary organisms that can be identified by electron microscopy.

Lymphangiographic Effect

After lymphangiography, the radiopaque lipid material used in this procedure may be present in the distended sinuses as large vacuoles.[4] It may also evoke sinus his-

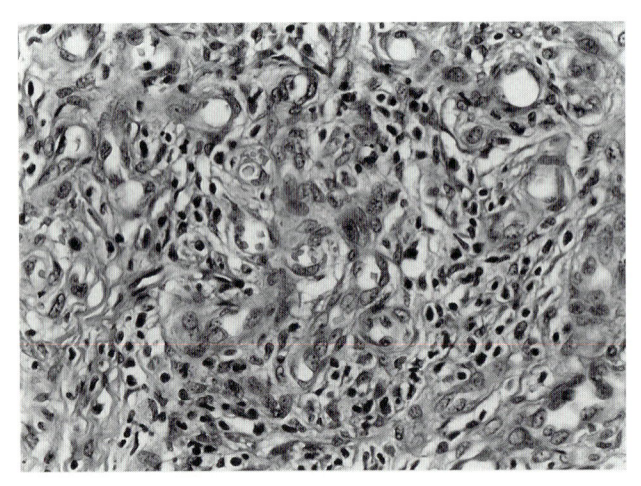

Fig. 4.17. A high magnification showing the histiocytoid endothelial cells. The infiltrating cells are mainly lymphocytes with a few eosinophils. H&E, ×500.

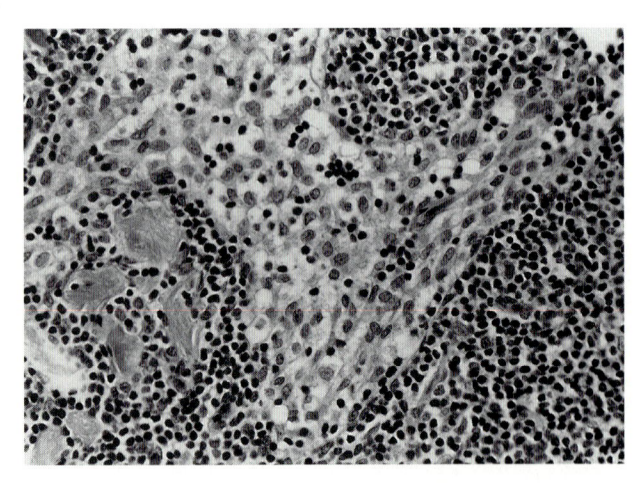

Fig. 4.19. A higher-power view of Fig. 4.18 showing histiocytes in the sinus. H&E, ×500.

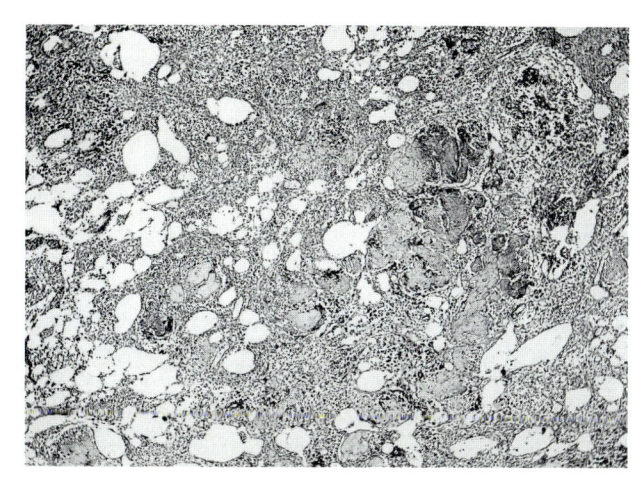

Fig. 4.20. Lymph node in Whipple's disease showing multiple vacuoles and clusters of foamy histiocytes. H&E, ×125. (AFIP 58-4674.)

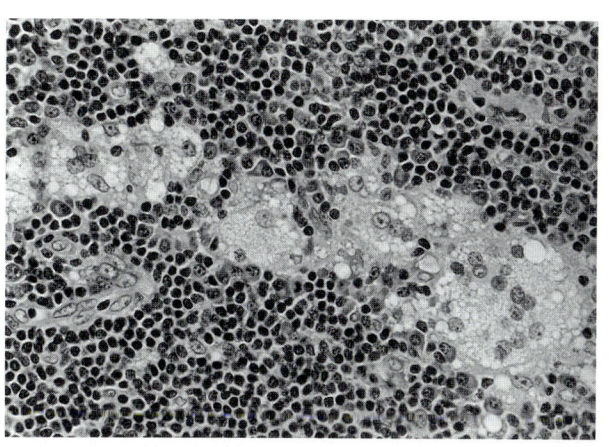

Fig. 4.22. A higher-power view of Fig. 4.21 showing large vacuoles and vacuolated histiocytes in the sinus. H&E, ×500.

tiocytosis, and the histiocytes may also contain vacuoles (Figs. 4.21, 4.22). In addition, multinucleated foreign-body giant cells are usually present with intracytoplasmic vacuoles and around large vacuoles. The presence of the foreign-body giant cells and the absence of PAS-positive sickle-form particles in the histiocytes distinguish this entity from Whipple's disease. However, similar features may be demonstrated in lymph nodes in the region of the porta hepatis and celiac axis following intestinal absorption of lipid substances.

Vascular Transformation of Sinuses

Vascular transformation of sinuses (VTS) is a rare condition. It is selectively located in the lymph node si-

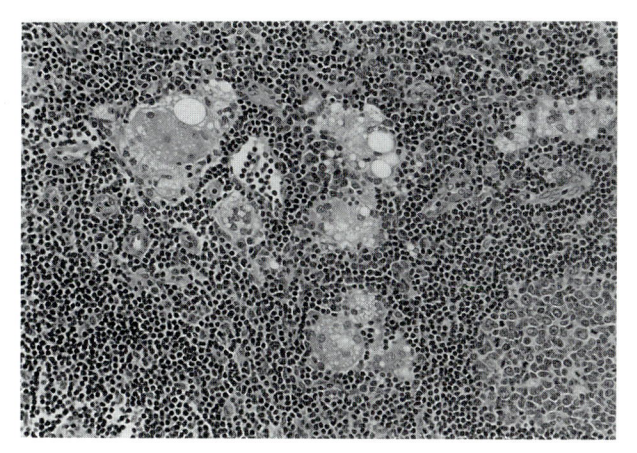

Fig. 4.21. Lymph node biopsy showing lipogranuloma after lymphangiography. H&E, ×250.

nuses without involving the parenchyma, capsule, or perinodal fibroadipose tissues. This condition was thought to be due to thrombosis of perinodal blood vessels, but a recent study showed that 71% of cases had lymphatic or venous obstruction at more distal sites caused by tumors, congestive heart failure, thrombosis of major vessels, surgical procedures, and radiotherapy.[15] Similar conditions can be seen in toxoplasmosis,[16] HIV infections,[17] and bacillary angiomatosis.[18] Ioachim has hypothesized that angiogenesis factors that are released by activated lymphoid cells under unknown conditions may be the mechanisms of VTS.[3]

The lesion is frequently located in the subcapsular sinuses, but intermediate and medullary sinuses can also be involved. Although the lymphoid follicles and paracortex are not replaced by the vascular network, the expansion of the sinuses may finally compress the parenchyma and alter the lymph node architecture. Four different histologic patterns are recognized: cleft-like spaces lined by flat endothelial cells (Fig. 4.23), rounded vascular spaces engorged with blood and lined by plumped endothelial cells, solid structure composed of spindle and plump cells, and plexiform structures formed by intercommunicating channels.[15] All patterns are associated with varying degrees of extravasation of erythrocytes, deposits of hemosiderin, and fibrosis.

The major differential diagnosis is Kaposi sarcoma, which is composed of spindle cells separated by slit-like spaces filled with red cells. Kaposi sarcoma also invades the capsule of lymph node that is not seen in VTS. Hemangioma and hemangioen-

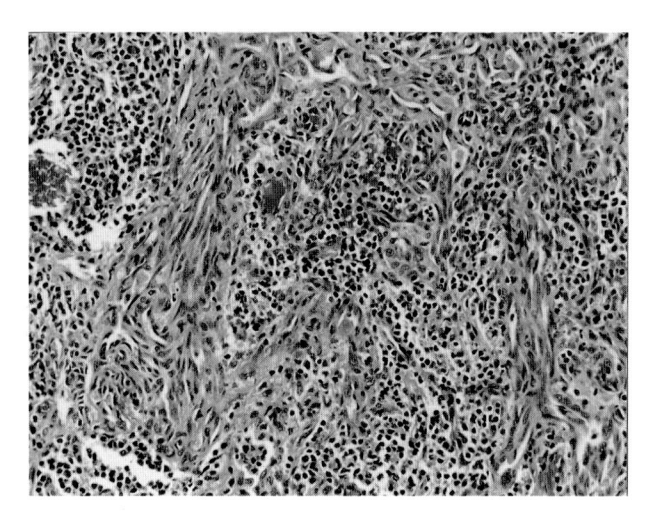

Fig. 4.23. Vascular transformation of sinuses in a lymph node showing anastomosing vascular clefts and stromal sclerosis. H&E. (Courtesy of Dr. John K. C. Chan; Pathology Institute of Hong Kong.)

dothelioma show well-circumscribed nodules composed of various types of blood vessels that replace the nodal parenchyma. The parenchyma is intact in VTS.

Kaposi Sarcoma

Kaposi sarcoma (KS) is divided into four clinical varieties.[19] The first one is classic KS, which is seen in North America and Europe among elderly men of Mediterranean or eastern European Jewish ancestry. The second variety is the African or endemic KS occurring in the sub-Saharan region of Africa among young black adult males and children. The third variety is iatrogenically immunosuppressed KS, seen mainly in renal transplant patients and patients receiving immunosuppressants. The last form is epidemic or HIV-associated KS, typically found in homosexual or bisexual young men with HIV infection.

Clinically, KS can be divided into four stages: stage I, locally indolent cutaneous KS; stage II, locally aggressive cutaneous KS with or without regional lymph nodes; stage III, generalized mucocutaneous and/or lymph node involvement; and stage IV, visceral KS.[19] The stages are subtyped by the absence (A) or presence (B) of weight loss, persistent fever, or night sweats.[20] As seen from this staging, lymph node involvement can be seen in stages II and III. In terms of clinical types, lymphadenopathy is rarely seen in classic and African types, is occasionally seen in iatrogenically immunosuppressed type, but is very common in the epidemic type. In the African type, however, there is a lymphadenopathic subtype found exclusively in children who present with ocular and salivary gland lesions and widespread dissemination to lymph nodes and viscera. In the epidemic type, KS occurs mainly in homosexual men but is much less common in intravenous drug users. A survey conducted in 1982 by the CDC (Centers For Disease Control and Prevention) showed that the incidence of KS in homosexual men was 36%, as compared with an incidence of 4.3% in intravenous drug users.[21] This phenomenon suggests that there must be cofactors in the pathogenesis of the epidemic KS. The cofactors under consideration are infectious agents, such as cytomegalovirus[22] and human papilloma virus. The p53 gene mutation may play an important role in the progression to malignancy.[23] The decline in KS incidence in homosexual and bisexual men from the peak of 61% in 1982 to 14% in 1990 also supports the coexistence of cofactors.[19]

For cutaneous KS lesions, the histopathologic pattern can be divided into the patch, plaque, and nodular stages. For lesions in lymph nodes, such division is not applicable. The lymph node lesions are usually in the form of tumor nodules with a whorled structure replacing normal lymphoid parenchyma.[3] Early involvement is usually limited to the capsule and subcapsular sinuses.[4] Later lesion may extend to the medulla.[3] The histologic criteria for the diagnosis of

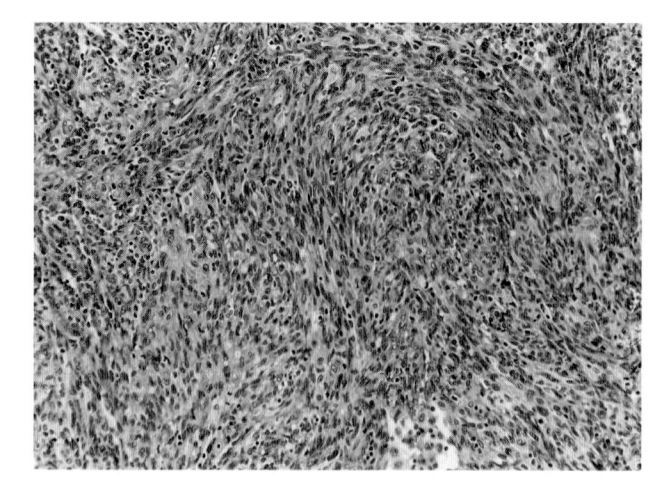

Fig. 4.24. Lymph node in Kaposi sarcoma showing replacement of normal architecture by spindle-shaped cells arranged in fascicles. H&E, ×250.

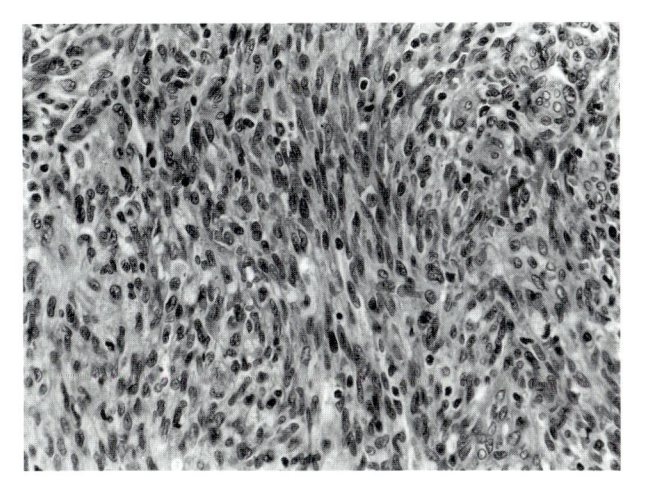

Fig. 4.25. A higher-power view of Fig. 4.24 showing spindle-shaped tumor cells, some of them forming vascular slits. H&E, ×500.

KS in Johns Hopkins Hospital includes two major criteria and three minor criteria (Figs. 4.24–4.26).[19] The major criteria are (a) proliferation of relatively uniform spindle-shaped cells between collagen bundles with at least some arrangement in fascicles and (b) vascular slits. The minor criteria include (a) hemosiderin deposition, (b) plasma cell in the inflammatory infiltrate, and (c) hyaline bodies.

Although the spindle-cell bundles are a constant feature in KS, the proliferating vasculature in between the bundles can be well-formed capillaries, ectatic vessels, or cleft-like structures. Most of these structures contain erythrocytes, or the red cells can be extravasated. Hemosiderin deposition and hemosiderin-laden macrophages are frequently present. Mitoses are usually present. There are also plasma-cell and lymphocyte infiltrates between the spindle cells or around the blood vessels. A relative special feature is the presence of hyaline or eosinophilic bodies (inclusions) within the macrophages and spindle cells; this may represent the altered erythrocytes. The uninvolved portion of the lymph node may show marked follicular hyperplasia and plasma-cell infiltration in the medullary cords.[3] Alternatively, depletion of lymphocytes and Castleman disease-like changes may be demonstrated.[4]

The major differential diagnosis is HIV lymphadenopathy, which may exhibit marked vascular proliferation. However, the blood vessels are well formed, and bundles or whorls of spindle cells are not present in HIV lymphadenopathy. The differences between KS and VTS have been discussed in the VTS section. The distinction between KS and other spindle-cell neoplasms can be substantiated by using factor VIII-RA and *Ulex europaeus* lectin to stain the KS cells and distinguish them from cells of nonendothelial origin.[3] A new monoclonal antibody against human placenta endothelial cells (QBEnd/10) may also serve the same purpose.[24] Demonstration of the eosinophilic hyaline bodies with Okajima stain is considered to be helpful in the diagnosis of KS, especially in AIDS-related cutaneous lesions, in which the inclusions are less apparent.[19]

DIFFUSE PATTERN

A diffuse pattern is frequently seen in viral infections. It also occurs in posttransplantation conditions, drug-induced hypersensitivity, and bacillary angiomatosis. One cause of the diffuse pattern, angioimmunoblastic lymphadenopathy, will be discussed in Chapter 16.

Infectious Mononucleosis

Infectious mononucleosis (IM) was originally classified by Dorfman and Warnke[25] under the mixed pattern, but it is currently classified under the diffuse pattern by Schnitzer.[4] In the early stage of IM, there is only follicular hyperplasia. In the later stage, because of the expansion of the paracortical region, the follicles are separated and are gradually replaced by the infiltrating cell population (Fig. 4.27a & b). Finally the fol-

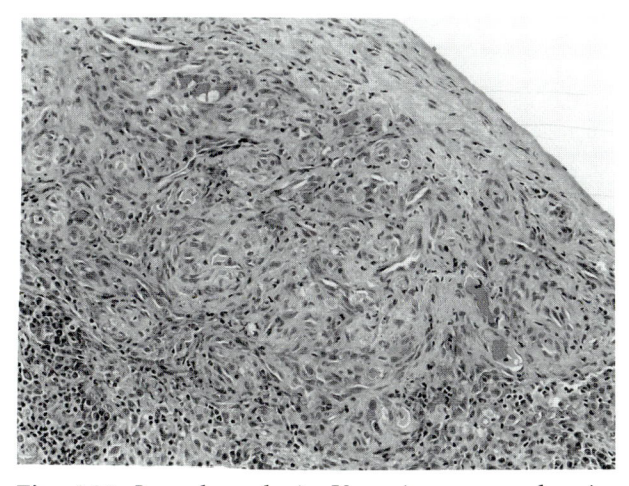

Fig. 4.26. Lymph node in Kaposi sarcoma showing vascular slits beneath the capsule. H&E, ×250.

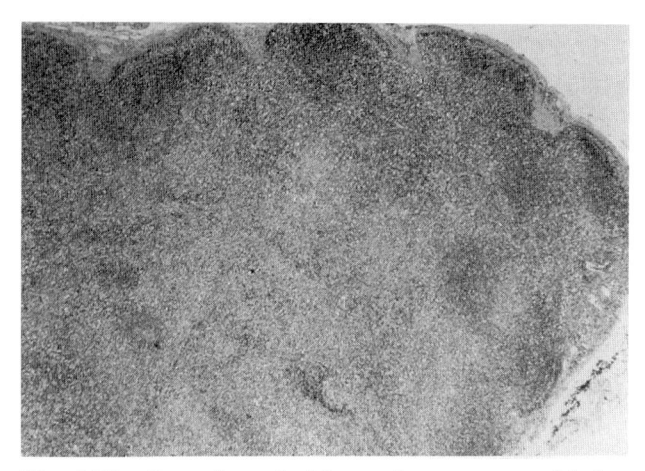

Fig. 4.27a. Lymph node biopsy from a case of infectious mononucleosis, showing follicular hyperplasia, expansion of paracortex and mottled appearance. H&E, ×125. (Courtesy of Dr. Glauco Frizzera of New York University Medical Center)

licles may become completely obliterated. Therefore, the histopathology of IM may, in fact, present as either mixed or diffuse pattern depending on the stages.

A characteristic pattern of IM is the coexistence of follicular hyperplasia, expansion of the paracortex, and dilatation of the sinuses.[3] In the enlarged germinal centers, multiple tingible-body macrophages are frequently present, giving a starry-sky appearance. The expanded paracortical region consists of sheets of immunoblasts, admixed with lymphocytes, histiocytes, and plasma cells, forming the mottled pattern. Mitotic figures are frequently seen among the immunoblasts. The immunoblasts are pleomorphic and sometimes, binucleated with prominent nucleoli resembling Reed-Sternberg cells. The cellular infiltration often extends into the capsule and perinodal fat. These features often make IM difficult to distinguish from non-Hodgkin's lymphoma and Hodgkin's disease. The dilated sinuses are filled with immunoblasts, plasma cells, lymphocytes, histiocytes, and monocytoid B-cells.[3,4] Focal areas of necrosis often occur.

IM is mainly the result of infection by Epstein–Barr virus (EBV), although a minority of cases may be caused by cytomegalovirus infection. By *in situ* hybridization techniques, EBV sequences were demonstrated in 1–10% of lymphocytes and 60–90% of immunoblasts in the interfollicular areas.[26] The immunoblasts are of different cell lineages reacting to B-cell (CD20, CD74, CDw75) and T-cell (CD43, CD45RO) antibodies. While the B-cells (with EBV receptor) are the infected cells, the T-cells are the predominant reactive population. The Reed–Sternberg-like cells are negative for CD15. As the histopathologic features of IM are so similar to those of malignant lymphoma, lymph node biopsy is not recommended, to avoid confusion.[4] In case of doubt, a clinical history, peripheral blood examination, and serologic tests are needed for a definitive diagnosis. The leukocyte count is usually about 10×10^9/L with atypical lymphocytes (Downey cells), which represent the reactive T-cells. The serologic tests include the heterophil antibody (Paul–Bunnell) test, monospot test (more sensitive test), and EBV-specific antibody tests. The EBV antibodies are specific for the viral capsid antigen (VCA), early antigen (EA), and Epstein–Barr nuclear antigen (EBNA), which appear at different stages of IM.

For the distinction from Hodgkin's disease, a negative anti-CD15 reaction to the Reed–Sternberg-like cells is helpful. The Reed–Sternberg-like cells in IM usually have basophilic nucleoli, which are adjacent to the nuclear membrane, and a paranuclear hof (the *hof* is the hollow area of cell cytoplasm in which the nucleus is embedded) representing the Golgi zone.[25] In addition, the mottled pattern in the paracortical region, the presence of monocytoid B-cells and transformed lymphocytes in the sinuses, and the presence of hyperplastic follicles, as seen in IM, are usually absent in Hodgkin's disease.

The large, pleomorphic immunoblasts, especially when present in the sinuses of a lymph node, in the case of IM may mimic large-cell anaplastic lymphoma

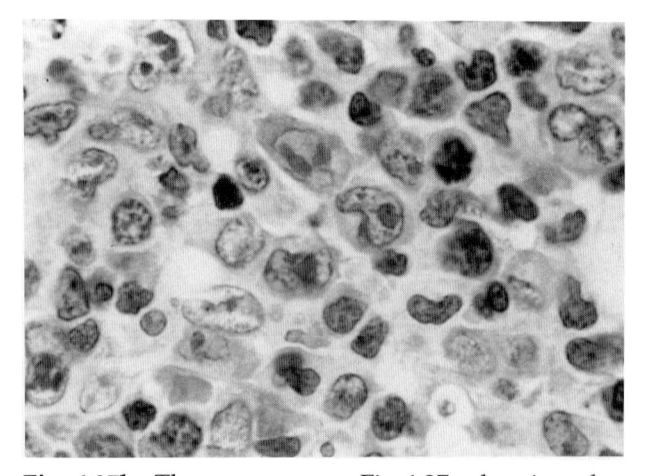

Fig. 4.27b. The same case as Fig 4.27a showing pleomorphic immunoblasts and histiocytes. H&E, ×1,250.

(Ki-1-positive lymphoma).[27] Although Ki-1 antigen (CD30) can be present in the immunoblasts of IM cases, only a few cells are reactive, and these cells are not present in the sinuses.[27] In lymphomas, the tumor cells show a monoclonal surface immunoglobulin pattern and the normal architecture of the lymph node is effaced. In IM, the immunoblasts bear a polyclonal immunoglobulin pattern and the lymph node architecture is generally preserved as demonstrated by a reticulin stain.[3]

Cytomegalovirus Lymphadenitis

Cytomegalovirus (CMV) infection may cause lymphadenopathy and atypical lymphocytosis in the peripheral blood similar to those seen in IM. Although the clinical features may not distinguish these two entities, serologic tests are helpful. In CMV lymphadenopathy with mononucleosis, the heterophil antibody tests are negative but the CMV antibody test is positive.[3]

The histopathologic pattern in the lymph node of CMV cases is also similar to that seen in IM: follicular hyperplasia and expansion of paracortex due to a mixed cellular infiltration consisting of immunoblasts, lymphocytes, plasma cells, and macrophage/histiocytes.[3,4] As in other viral infections, the mottled appearance of the lymph node, due to the presence of large immunoblasts among small lymphocytes, is characteristic. Reed–Sternberg-like cells are occasionally seen. A distinctive feature in CMV infection is the presence of a single prominent viral inclusion in the nucleus (Fig. 4.28) and multiple inclusions in the cytoplasm of infected cells, including endothelial cells and T-cells.[4] The inclusions are positive for Feulgen and PAS stains. More specifically, these inclusions are positive with immunohistochemical stain for CMV antigen and with *in situ* hybridization technique for CMV sequences (Fig. 4.29).[28] These special techniques may demonstrate CMV infection in apparently normal-looking lymphocytes. The CMV-positive cells are located mostly in the medulla or corticomedullar junction.[3]

As in IM, CMV lymphadenopathy should be distinguished from Hodgkin's disease and non-Hodgkin's lymphoma. The Reed–Sternberg-like cells in CMV infection may react to anti-CD15 antibody, a condition that may lead to the erroneous diagnosis of Hodgkin's disease, but these cells are CD30-negative. The infiltrating cell components, follicular hyperplasia, and the intranuclear and cytoplasmic inclusions in CMV may help distinguish it from Hodgkin's disease. Non-Hodgkin's lymphoma, especially anaplastic large-cell lymphoma, can be differentiated from CMV infection by its monoclonal surface immunoglobulin pattern and the rather monomorphic cell population in contrast to the polymorphous background in the lymph node of CMV-infected cases. In herpes simplex virus and herpes zoster virus lymphadenitis, the histologic pattern and the intranuclear inclusions may be indistinguishable from those due to CMV infection. Immunohistochemical stain with monoclonal antibodies specific for CMV and herpes simplex/herpes zoster virus may help differentiate these entities.

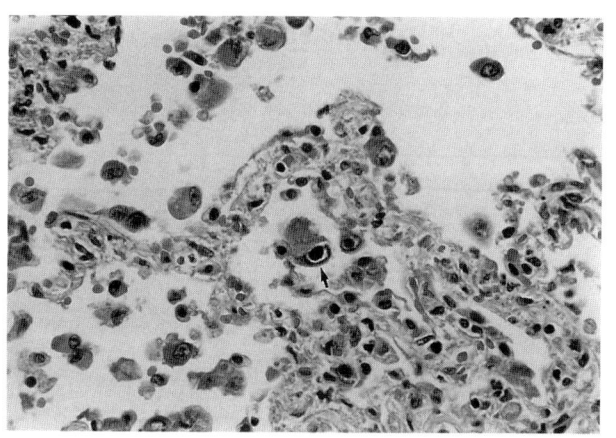

Fig. 4.28. A few intranuclear inclusions (arrow) of cytomegalovirus are demonstrated in a lung section. H&E, ×500.

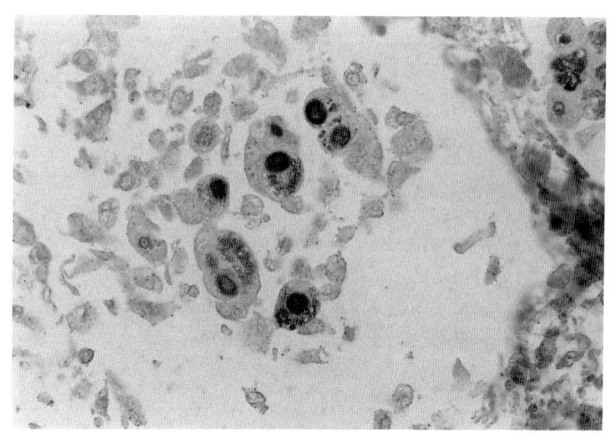

Fig. 4.29. In situ hybridization technique demonstrates DNA sequences of CMV in the nucleus and cytoplasm of infected cells. H&E, ×500.

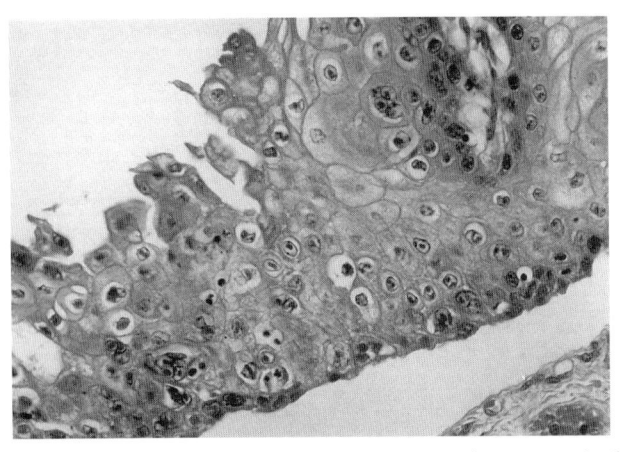

Fig. 4.30. Herpes simplex esophagitis showing viral inclusions in mononucleated and multinucleated epithelial cells. H&E, x 500. (Courtesy of Dr. H. Dincsoy.)

Herpes Zoster/Herpes Simplex (HZV/HSV) Lymphadenitis

The histopathologic patterns in both HZV and HSV lymphadenitis are similar to those in other viral infections in the presence of mottled appearance in the paracortex due to the presence of immunoblasts among small lymphocytes.[3] Follicular hyperplasia is seldom present in either condition, except in the recovery phase of HZV infection.[3,30] Both disorders may show intranuclear inclusions (Figs. 4.30 & 4.31) which are demonstrated in immunoblasts in HZV infection and in T-lymphocytes or stromal cells in HSV infection.[3] Multinucleated cells with ground-glass nuclei may be present in HSV infection. Foci of cellular necrosis is also seen in HSV lymphadenitis. The differentiation between various viral infections with intranuclear inclusions depends on the use of specific monoclonal antibody or *in situ* hybridization when available. The distinction between these two entities and Hodgkin's disease or non-Hodgkin's lymphoma is the same as that described for IM and CMV lymphadenitis.

Postvaccinial Lymphadenitis

Postvaccinial lymphadenitis (PL) is caused by inoculation of vaccinia virus for the prevention of smallpox. Since smallpox has been eliminated globally, PL no longer exists. The histologic pattern can be follicular hyperplasia and diffuse or combined follicular and diffuse pattern.[3,4] The diffuse pattern may appear early, and the follicular pattern occurs more than 15 days after vaccination. The characteristic feature is similar to those of other viral infections in that the lymph node shows a mottled appearance because of the presence of many immunoblasts among small lymphocytes and plasma cells. Cellular infiltration includes also eosinophils and mast cells which are seldom seen in other viral infections. Proliferation of blood vessels and dilated sinuses filled with immunoblasts, plasma cells, and proteinaceous fluid are also commonly seen in this entity. Reed–Sternberg-like cells may be present and, if so, must be distinguished from those seen in Hodgkin's disease.

Measles Lymphadenitis

Measles lymphadenitis is also similar to other viral infections with a mottled appearance usually demonstrable in the lymph node, due to diffuse immunoblastic infiltration among small lymphocytes. The characteristic polykaryocytes originally described by Warthin and Finkeldey (Fig. 4.32) can be found in tonsils, adenoids, lymph nodes, spleen, appendix, and thymus. However, this polykaryocyte is not specific for measles and can be seen in other benign lymphadenopathies as well as in malignant lymphomas.[3] The polykaryocytes of Warthin and Finkeldey react with CD3, CD4, and CD43 and are considered to be helper T-cell in origin.[31] Cellular inclusions are infrequently found in the cytoplasm of polykaryocytes and endothelial cells. When the histologic pattern is indistinguishable from those of other viral infections, clini-

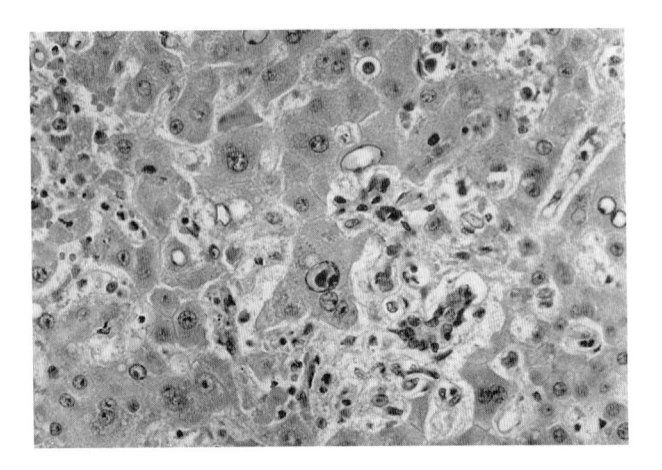

Fig. 4.31. Herpes simplex inclusion in a hepatocyte. H&E, x 500. (Courtesy of Dr. H. Dincsoy.)

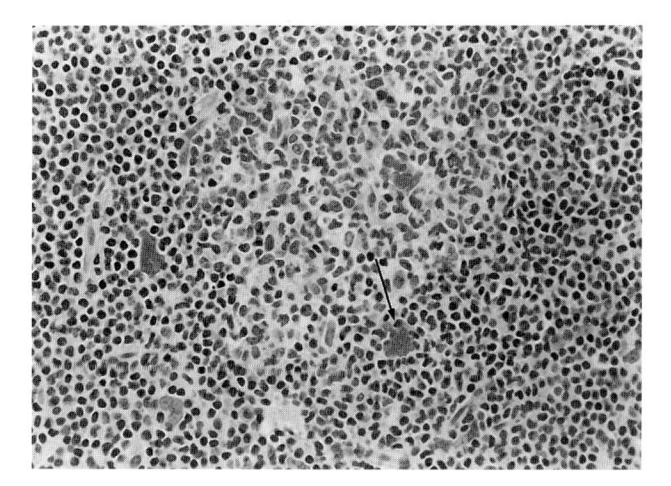

Fig. 4.32. A few polykaryocytes of Warthin and Finkeldey (arrow) are present in a lymph node. H&E, ×500.

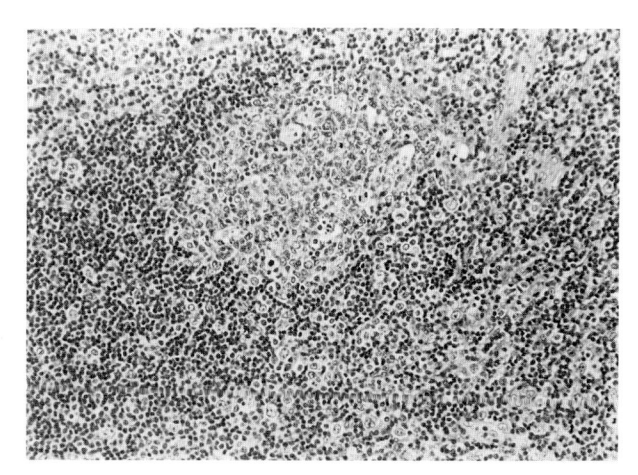

Fig. 4.33. Posttransplantation lymphoproliferative disorder (PTLD) in lymph node showing follicular hyperplasia and a mottled paracortex due to immunoblastic infiltration on a small lymphocyte background. H&E, ×250.

cal manifestation and serology may be helpful in establishing the diagnosis of measles lymphadenopathy.

Posttransplantation Lymphoproliferative Disorders

The incidence of lymphoma in allograft recipients was estimated to be 350 times greater than in their normal counterpart.[3] Current statistics of posttransplantation lymphoproliferative disorders (PTLD) represents approximately 2% of all organ allograft recipients.[32] The acronym PTLD is used because a wide spectrum of lymphoid proliferations from benign reactive lymphoid hyperplasia to high-grade non-Hodgkin's lymphoma has been encountered in allograft recipients, and the demarcation between benign and malignant lesions is sometimes difficult to define. The frequency of PTLD is 1.8–20% in patients after cardiac transplantation, 1–5% after renal graft, and 0.6% after bone marrow transplantation.[32]

PTLD shares many common features with other immunodeficient disorders. Besides the great variation in morphology, these lesions have a predilection for extranodal sites, are frequently associated with EBV infection, often lack immunophenotypic or genotypic evidence of monoclonality, and respond poorly to chemotherapy or radiation therapy.[32] Unlike other immunodeficiency-related lymphoproliferative disorders, PTLD resolves or regresses following the cessation of immunosuppression. The latency period for the development of PTLD is directly related to the immunosuppressive regimen used; it occurs 4–5 years with aza-

thioprine but only 5–7 months with cyclosporin A or CD3 antibody.[3] The former regimen is frequently associated with extranodal lesions, mainly the gastrointestinal (GI) tract and the brain; the latter regimen is associated with more lymph node involvement.[3]

The histopathologic pattern may range from one with a mottled paracortex with mixed immunoblasts and lymphocytes resembling infectious mononucleosis to one that shows a monomorphic immunoblastic population similar to that of large-cell lymphoma (Figs. 4.33–36). Reed–Sternberg-like cells, a high mitotic rate, and focal necrosis can be demonstrated in

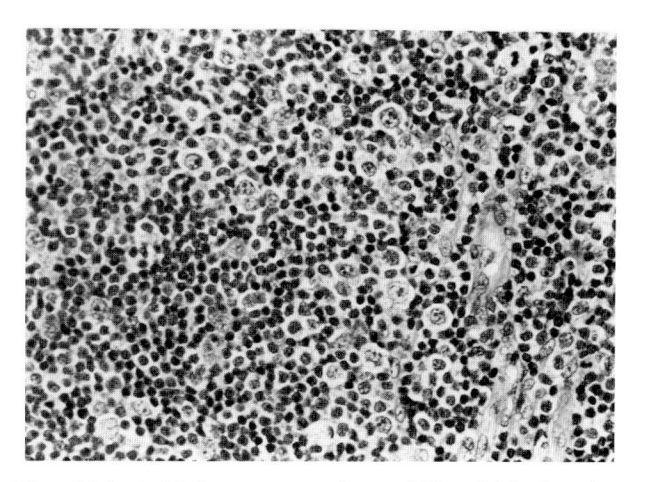

Fig. 4.34. A higher-power view of Fig. 4.33 showing the mottled appearance of the paracortex. H&E, ×500.

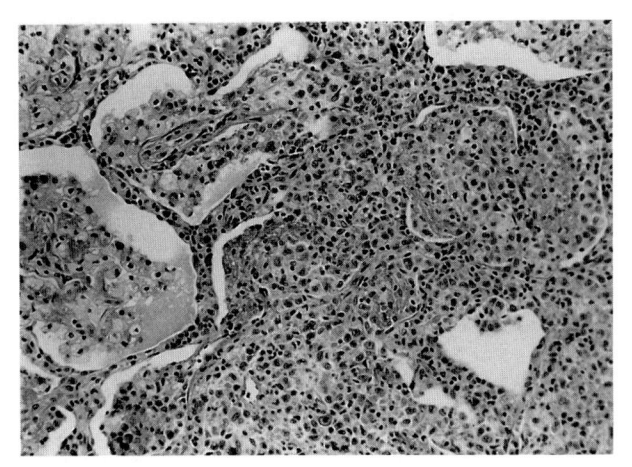

Fig. 4.35. PTLD in the lung showing diffuse atypical lymphoid infiltration in the alveolar space. H&E, ×250. (Case contributed by Dr. Kevin Basham.)

the lymphoma-like lesions. Although cellular atypia, necrosis, and focal invasion were used as criteria for malignancy in these lesions, they are not as reliable diagnostically as in lesions seen in immunocompetent patients, since many "malignant" lesions may be reversible on reduction of immunosuppression.

Frizzera et al. divided PTLD into four categories: nonspecific reactive lymphoid hyperplasia, polymorphic diffuse B-cell hyperplasia, polymorphic diffuse B-cell lymphoma, and immunoblastic sarcoma of B-cells.[33] Although this classification is still popular, it does not correlate well with immunophenotyping and genotyping, nor does it reliably predict the outcome of the patient after reduced immunosuppression. Therefore, Craig et al. suggested simplifying the classification into polymorphic PTLD and monomorphic PTLD and considered the only reliable predictor of a good outcome a favorable response to reduced immunosuppression.[32]

The majority of PTLD are of B-cell type, and a minority are of T-cell type. In one study, the ratio of B-cell to T-cell PTLD was 86:14%.[34] Immunogenotyping in cardiac-transplant recipients showed polyclonal, oligonclonal, and monoclonal patterns.[35] Locker and Nalesnik found that nonresponsiveness to reduced immunosuppression can be predicted only when a strong monoclonal band was identified by the Southern blot techniques.[35] The clonality of PTLD can also be demonstrated by molecular genetic analysis of the episomal EBV DNA.[35] The association of *c-myc* oncogene rearrangement in PTLD has also been reported.[35]

The pathogenesis of PTLD is hypothesized to undergo three steps.[32] The first step is the activation and immortalization of B-lymphocytes by EBV. This step may depend on the expression of bcl-2 and a BHRF1 gene in EBV genome as a result of EBV infection. Cyclosporin A may act synergistically with EBV to block apoptosis. The second step is proliferation of EBV-infected cells due to immunosuppression. The third step involves a genetic event that may cause irreversible transformation of the lymphocytes into malignant cells. The translocation of *c-myc* oncogene has been found in PTLD and may be associated with this process.

Drug-Induced Lymphadenopathy

Although lymphadenopathy has been reported in association with many drugs such as paraaminosalicylic acid, iron dextran, phenylbutazone, methyldopa, and meprobamate, the most important drugs are diphenylhydantoin (dilantin) and carbamazepine.[3] It is important to recognize anticonvulsant-therapy-associated lymphadenopathy because the histopathologic features in this lesion may mimic non-Hodgkin's lymphoma or Hodgkin's disease.[3,4] Sometimes the only way to distinguish this entity from malignancy is the regression of lymphadenopathy after withdrawal of the drug. Therefore, a history of using anticonvulsant drug is important in cases of lymphoid malignancy, especially in young patients. However, long-term anticonvulsant therapy may also be associated with lymphoid neoplasms.[36] Fortunately, only 1.6% of patients with lymphoid tumors have a history of prolonged phenyltoin therapy.[3]

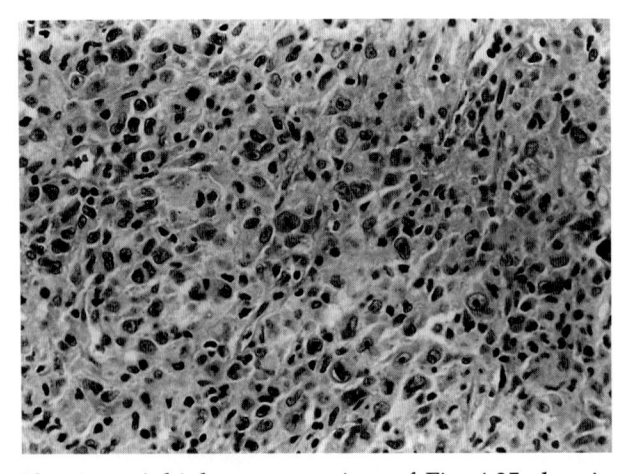

Fig. 4.36. A higher-power view of Fig. 4.35 showing polymorphic infiltration by mixed small and large lymphoid cells containing large nuclei and prominent nucleoli. H&E, ×250.

The histopathologic feature in this entity is mainly that of a mottled paracortex with polymorphous infiltrate composed of immunoblasts, eosinophils, plasma cells, lymphocytes, and neutrophils.[3,4,36] Reactive follicular hyperplasia may also be seen. As a result, there are varying degrees of architectural effacement. In addition, the large immunoblasts may show nuclear atypia as well as frequent mitosis, and scattered small foci of necrosis are also present. These features may lead to the misdiagnosis of non-Hodgkin's lymphoma. The presence of Reed–Sternberg-like cells in some cases may be confused with Hodgkin's disease. It may be indistinguishable from angioimmunoblastic lymphadenopathy (AILD), especially because AILD may also be drug-induced. However, when vascular proliferation and proteinaceous substance precipitation are prominent, the diagnosis of AILD should be considered. Immunohistochemical studies usually show polyclonal lymphoid population in drug-related lymphadenopathy. A few cases with monoclonal B-cell pattern have been reported and may represent lymphomatous transformation.[37]

Bacillary Angiomatosis

Bacillary angiomatosis (BA) is a relatively new entity, first described in the early 1980s in patients with AIDS.[38] It involves skin primarily in the form of multiple papules and nodules, resembling verruga peruana, but lymph node, spleen, liver, bone, and soft tissue may also be involved. The etiologic agent was identified only recently as *Rochalimaea henselae* by polymerase chain-reaction analysis of the RNA gene sequences.[39]

The lymph node lesion is characterized by the formation of vascular nodules that replace the lymphoid parenchyma (Fig. 4.37).[18] The blood vessels are of varying sizes and shapes. Some vessels are round and dilated, while others are small with barely visible lumens. Erythrocytes are seen in some vessels or are extravasated. Solid sheets of endothelial cells may be present without vascular formation. The endothelial cells lining the vessels are hyperplastic. Some are vacuolated or have an epithelioid appearance.[2] The diagnostic feature is identification of clumps of bacilli in the granular amphophilic material between the vascular structure by Warthin–Starry stain. These bacilli are negative with the Gram, PAS, Ziehl–Nielsen, and silver methenamine stains.[18] The bacilli are frequently mixed with inflammatory cells, mainly neutrophils. Similar histopathologic features are demonstrated in skin and visceral organs. Immunohistochemical study

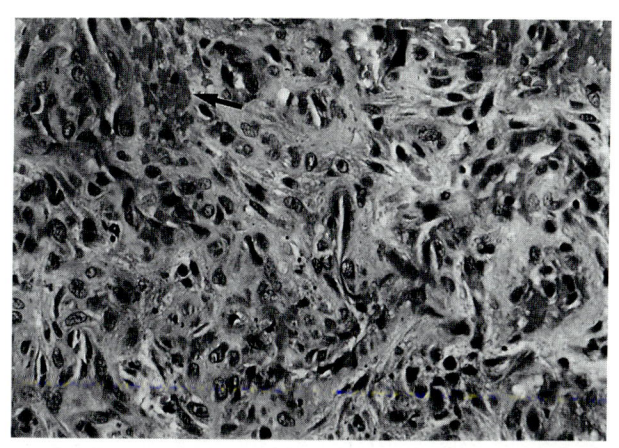

Fig. 4.37. A case of bacillary angiomatosis showing capillary proliferation and amorphous interstitial material (arrow), which represents clusters of bacilli. H&E, ×500. (Case provided by Dr. Harry Ioachim.)

may show factor VIII-related antigen, *Ulex europaeus* antigen, and α-1-antichymotrypsin in the endothelial cells.

The major differential diagnosis for BA is KS, which is also composed of blood vessels of various sizes and shapes. However, the vessels in KS are characteristically cleft-like, and the endothelial cells are spindle-shaped. In addition, the endothelial cells in KS are negative for factor VIII-related antigen in contrast to the positive reaction seen in BA.[38] Bacilli with positive Warthin–Starry stain are not present in KS. The differential diagnoses of various vascular tumors of lymph nodes other than KS are summarized in a recent article.[40]

MIXED PATTERN

"Mixed pattern" includes lesions showing both follicular and sinus patterns. Granulomatous lymphadenitis, for instance, belongs to this pattern, but this group is composed of multiple entities and will be discussed in Chapter 5.

Toxoplasmic Lymphadenitis

Toxoplasmosis is a protozoal infection prevalent in warm and humid regions. A common disease in developed countries, the disease is contracted by ingestion of raw or undercooked meat or by contact with the feces of infected cats. In immunocompetent pa-

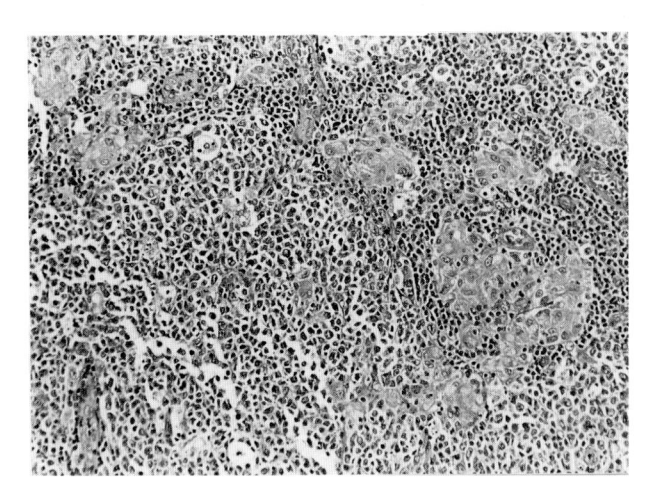

42 DIFFERENTIAL DIAGNOSIS OF LYMPHOID DISORDERS

Fig. 4.38. Toxoplasmic lymphadenopathy showing clusters of epithelioid histiocytes encroaching and penetrating the germinal center. H&E, ×250.

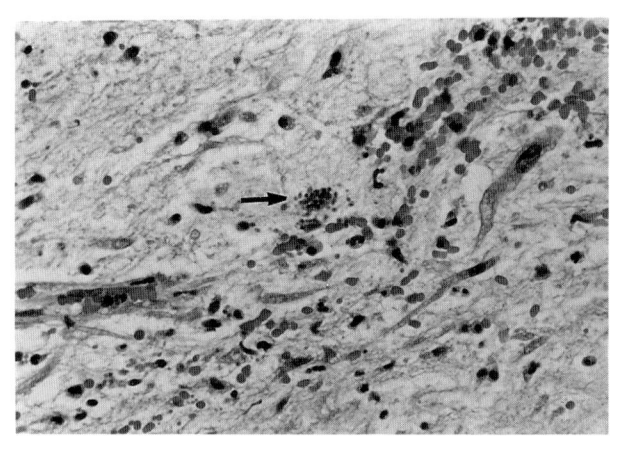

Fig. 4.40. A pseudocyst of *Toxoplasma* (arrow) is present in the brain. H&E, ×500.

tients, the most common clinical presentation is cervical lymphadenitis. In immunocompromised patients, especially in patients with AIDS, encephalitis is the most frequent symptom.[41]

The characteristic features in the lymph node are reactive follicular hyperplasia, aggregates of epithelioid histiocytes in the interfollicular areas, and filling of monocytoid B-cells in the subcapsular and trabecular sinuses (Figs. 4.38, 4.39).[42] The follicular centers are enlarged, containing immunocytes, tingible-body macrophages, and multiple mitotic figures. The epithelioid histiocytes usually form small clusters (< 20 cells), do not form well-defined granulomas, and there are no multinucleated giant cells in the aggre-

gates. Typically, the histiocytic clusters encroach on and penetrate the germinal centers, leading to a blurred contour of the latter structures. In the dilated sinuses, many monocytoid B-cells are present. These cells have abundant pale cytoplasm, well-demarcated cell borders, and usually centrally located nuclei.

These features are characteristic of toxoplasmic lymphadenitis, but a definitive diagnosis requires serologic confirmation because the organism is seldom found in the lymph node lesions. In other organs, especially the brain (Fig. 4.40) and the lungs (Fig. 4.41), free tachyzoites, pseudocysts, and/or cysts may be detected and a diagnosis is more readily established. The most frequently used serologic test is the indirect immunofluorescent test, which may be

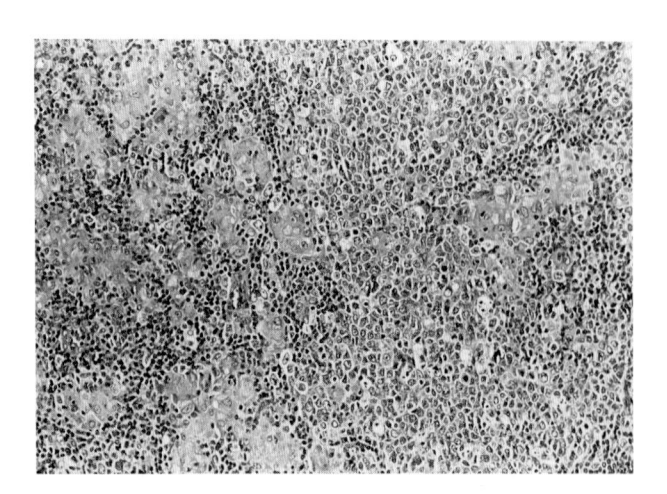

Fig. 4.39. Toxoplasmic lymphadenopathy showing blurred contour of the germinal center due to epithelioid histiocyte penetration. H&E, ×250.

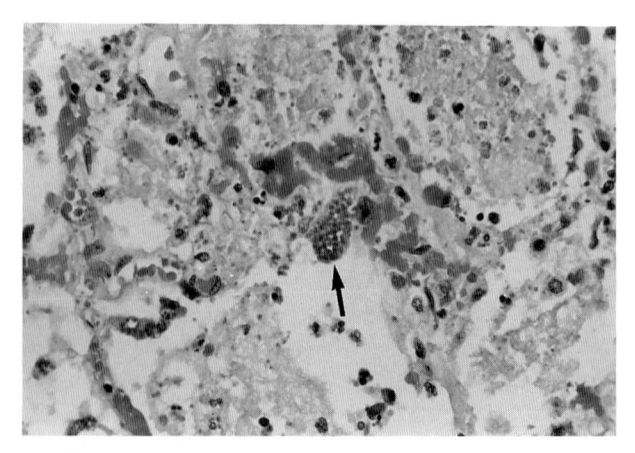

Fig. 4.41. A pseudocyst of *Toxoplasma* (arrow) is demonstrated in the alveolar wall of the lung. Many free tachyzoites are also seen in the alveolar space. H&E, ×500.

used for the detection of either the IgM or IgG antibodies. The former is more specific but not sensitive. The latter is very sensitive but cannot distinguish a past infection from current infection, unless rising titers are demonstrated.

There are several disorders that show aggregates of epithelioid histiocytes, including sarcoidosis, mycobacterial infections, syphilis, and Lennert's lymphoma, which may mimic toxoplasmic lymphadenitis.[4] However, the histiocytic encroaching to the germinal center, the absence of multinucleated giant cells and the presence of monocytoid B-cells in the dilated sinuses in toxoplasmosis may help distinguish it from the above-mentioned disorders. Monocytoid B-cells can be seen in other reactive lymphadenopathy especially in HIV infections, but the characteristic histiocytic aggregate and serologic tests may distinguish them. A more difficult differential diagnosis is leishmania lymphadenitis, which may show epithelioid cells extending into the follicular centers. A thorough search for Leishman–Donovan bodies (Fig. 4.42) is required to distinguish it from toxoplasmosis. The presence of multinucleated giant cells can be seen in leishmania but not in toxoplasmic lymphadenitis.[4] Immunoperoxidase stain for toxoplasma is helpful for the diagnosis of toxoplasmosis in other organs, but is seldom helpful in lymph nodes.

Dermatopathic Lymphadenopathy

Dermatopathic lymphadenopathy (DL) is associated with skin diseases, especially exfoliative and eczematoid lesions, such as pemphigus, psoriasis, neurodermatitis, eczema, and atropia senilis.[3] It may also be seen in cutaneous T-cell malignancies, namely, mycosis fungoides and Sézary syndrome. The characteristic feature in DL is proliferation of histiocytes that contain melanin, lipid, and/or hemosiderin in the paracortex of lymph node (see Figs. 19.7–19.10).[3,4] These histiocytes have abundant pale-staining cytoplasm, and their aggregation conveys an appearance of "alopecia-like" patches. There are three types of histiocytes present: the phagocytic histiocyte, Langerhans' cell, and interdigitating reticulum cell; the latter two represent antigen presenting cells. Varying numbers of immunoblasts, plasma cells, and eosinophils may be scattered among the histiocyte–lymphocyte background. In severe cases, the great expansion of the paracortex may compress the follicles. In less severe cases, follicular hyperplasia and sinus histiocytosis may be present.

DL in Sézary syndrome/mycosis fungoides may show only a small number of tumor cells with convoluted or cerebriform nuclei in the paracortex. In later stages, however, the nodal architecture may be partially or entirely replaced by the neoplastic cells.

Melanin pigment, hemosiderin, and lipid in the histiocytes can be demonstrated by Fortana, Prussian blue, and Sudan black B stains, respectively. The interdigitating reticulum cells and Langerhans' cells are positive for surface HLA-DR and CD1a antigens.[43] Both cells are also positive for intranuclear and intracytoplasmic S-100 protein, which demonstrates spider-like processes in both cell types. Birbeck granules can be detected by electron microscopy in Langerhans' cells but are absent in interdigitating reticulum cells.

Systemic Lupus Lymphadenopathy

In 30–60% of cases of systemic lupus erythematosus (SLE), enlarged lymph nodes are detected, either locally or generalized. Although the diagnosis of SLE depends on clinical and serologic evidence, lymph node biopsy is needed from time to time because patients with SLE are prone to develop non-Hodgkin's lymphoma.[4]

It is not difficult to distinguish lymphoma from SLE lesions. The latter show massive or segmental necrosis and lymphoid hyperplasia. The major hyperplastic change is in the follicles, but the interfollicular areas are also infiltrated by plasma cells and immunoblasts. Varying degrees of necrosis, sometimes accompanied by hemorrhage and edema, are characteristic in SLE

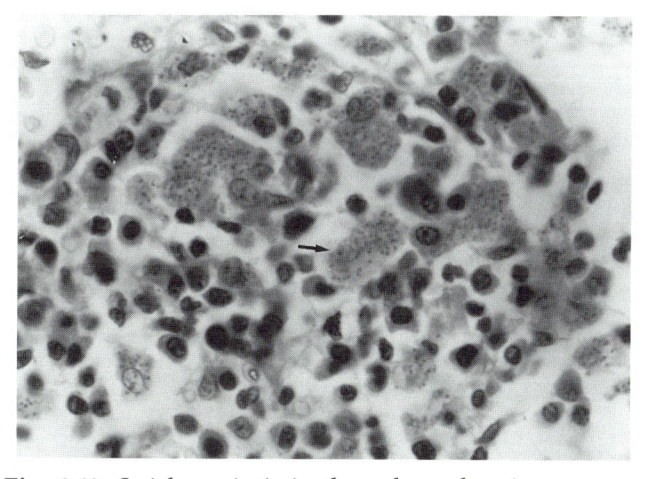

Fig. 4.42. Leishmaniasis in the spleen showing many amastigote forms (Leishman–Donovan bodies) (arrow) in the macrophages. The presence of kinetoplast and nucleus is barely visible in some organisms. H&E, ×1250.

lymphadenopathy.[3,4] The nodal architecture may be effaced. The necrosis is usually of the coagulative type, containing amorphous eosinophilic material and nuclear debris. Neutrophils are typically absent.[4] However, the pathognomonic feature in SLE is the presence of hematoxylin bodies. These are amorphous particles, 5–12 μm in diameter, stained strongly with hematoxylin, PAS, and Feulgen stains. The hematoxylin bodies are composed of DNA, polysaccharides, and immunoglobulins. They are present extracellularly, in necrotic areas and sinuses. The blood vessels in the lymph node may show fibrinoid necrosis and "onion-skin" appearance due to perivascular deposition of collagen fibers and immunoglobulins.[3]

Immunohistochemical studies revealed two predominant cell populations within and surrounding the paracortical zones of necrosis: CD15-positive histiocytes and CD8-positive T-suppressor cells. In the nonnecrotic interfollicular areas, the CD4-positive T-helper cells are predominant.

While the immunohistologic pattern and the histopathology of multiple necrotic foci in LE lymphadenopathy are indistinguishable from those of Kikuchi–Fujimoto disease (histiocytic necrotizing lymphadenopathy), the presence of hematoxylin bodies and vascular fibrinoid necrosis in SL lymphadenopathy may help exclude the diagnosis of the latter. Other lymphadenopathies with necrotic lesions, including cat-scratch disease, histoplasmosis, tuberculosis, leprosy, and luetic lymphadenitis may also be excluded by the presence of the two features mentioned above, while the identification of the corresponding pathogens by silver stain or acid-fast stain in these lesions may confirm their diagnoses.

Kikuchi–Fujimoto Disease

Kikuchi–Fujimoto disease (KFD) is also called *histiocytic necrotizing lymphadenitis* because histiocytosis and necrosis are the major features in the full-blown stage. However, it is now realized that KFD covers a broad morphologic spectrum and necrosis is not always present in the early stages.[44–46] On the other hand, several cytologic variants may make it more difficult to reach a correct diagnosis. Diagnosing KFD is important because it is a benign, self-limited disease and yet is easily misdiagnosed as malignant lymphoma.

This disease was first reported in Japan in 1972, but it has since been reported in the Western world, although most cases are of Asian extraction. Most patients are young female under age 40 years. Cervical lymph nodes are most frequently affected. The patients may have fever, chills, skin rash, myalgia, sore throat, leukopenia, and atypical lymphocytes in their peripheral blood. Most patients recover spontaneously in a few months. There is only one reported case of a patient who died of necrotizing myocarditis.[44] The etiology of KFD is still unknown, but the presence of tuboreticular structures in histiocytes, lymphocytes, and endothelial cells in the affected areas, and the elevation of 2'5'-oligoadenylate synthetase, in conjunction with the clinical and histologic patterns, are consistent with viral infection.[47]

Nathwani has suggested three histologic stages in KFD.[45] The first stage is a proliferative phase characterized by the presence of plasmacytoid monocytes (previously called *plasmacytoid T-cells*), immunoblasts, and histiocytes, with little or no overt necrosis. The second stage is characterized by large areas of necrosis with extensive karyorrhexis and karyolysis. The third stage is characterized by resorption and a return to normal histology. Tsang et al. postulated that the fibrogranulation areas observed in some of their cases represented the organizing phase of KFD.[44]

Although in the early phase, the major feature is cellular aggregate, small foci of karyorrhexis is invariably present and may extend into perinodal tissue in the later phase. The necrosis is characterized by eosinophilic fibrinoid deposits, admixed with nuclear debris (Fig. 4.43) and surrounded by histiocytes, plasmacytoid monocytes, and immunoblasts (Figs. 4.44, 4.45). Neutrophils, plasma cells, and eosinophils are typically absent or scarce.[45] The lesions are present mainly in the paracortex. The follicles may be partly replaced, lymphocyte-depleted, or infiltrated by histiocytes or plasmacytoid monocytes in rare cases.[44]

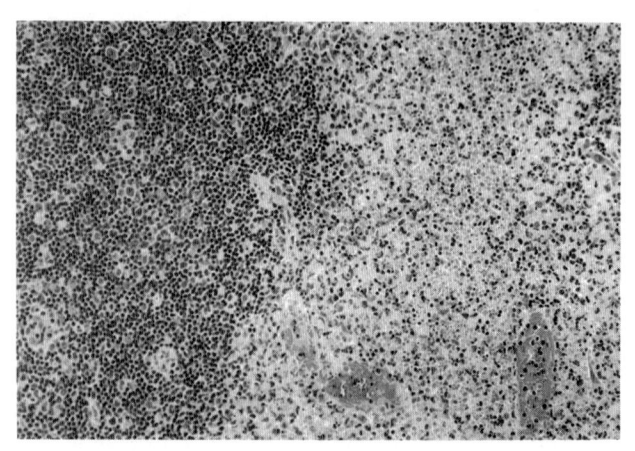

Fig. 4.43. Kikuchi–Fujimoto disease in lymph node showing necrotic foci with extensive karyorrhexis. No granulocytes are present. H&E, ×250.

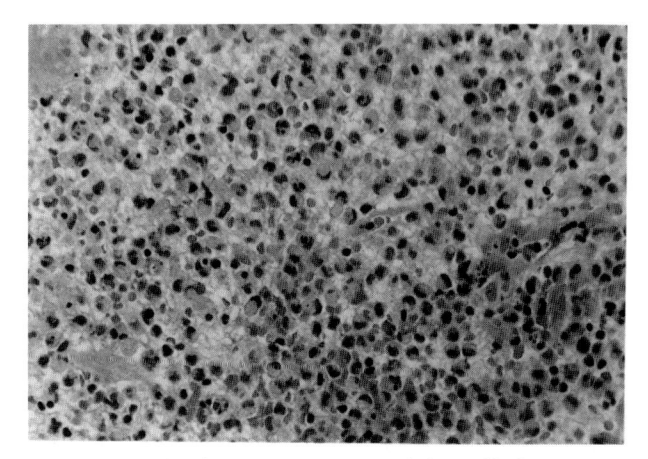

Fig. 4.44. A higher-power view of the cellular components in Kikuchi–Fujimoto disease showing crescentic histiocytes (arrow), immunoblasts and plasmacytoid monocytes. H&E, ×500.

Recognition of the special cytologic features of various cell components is very important for the diagnosis of KFD. The special type of histiocytes in KFD have peripherally placed c-shaped nuclei and abundant cytoplasm, containing karyorrhectic debris. This type of histiocyte is designated by Tsang et al. as crescentic histiocyte.[44] There are also nonphagocytic histiocytes with twisted or reniform nuclei that are frequently mistaken as lymphoma cells. The second important cell type is plasmacytoid monocyte. These cells have eccentrically placed round nuclei with dispersed chromatin, mimicking plasma cells, but they have proved to be monocytes by cytochemical studies. Although plasmacytoid monocytes can be present in a variety of reactive lymphoid proliferations, their presence substantiates the diagnosis of KFD. The third prominent cell type is immunoblast, which is exclusively of T-cell origin.

Kikuchi has suggested dividing the histologic pattern into four types: lymphohistiocytic, phagocytic, necrotic, and foamy cell.[46] Lymphohistiocytic type is composed mainly of cellular aggregates, frequently mimicking a malignant lymphoma (Fig. 4.46). The other three types also have the lymphohistiocytic background but with additional features such as numerous phagocytes, overt necrosis, and aggregates of foamy histiocytes, respectively. Another rare cell type reported by Tsang et al. is the signet-ring-cell type.[44]

Immunohistochemical studies have identified three major cell types in the affected area: the lysozyme-positive histiocytes; CD3+, CD8+, CD11b- cytotoxic T-cells; and CD4+, Ki-M1p+ plasmacytoid monocytes.[47] Ki-M1P is a new monoclonal antibody for plasmacytoid monocytes, but it also reacts with histiocyte. When double-staining with CD4 and Ki-M1p, most histiocytes can be excluded. This staining pattern also clarifies the difference between plasmacytoid monocytes and plasmacytoid lymphocytes, which are CD4/Ki-M1P negative.

The major differential diagnosis is non-Hodgkin's lymphoma, because the pleomorphic histiocyte, plasmacytoid monocytes, and immunoblasts may be misinterpreted under different conditions as lymphoma cells.[45] The presence of frequent mitoses, pericapsular infiltration, extensive necrosis, and obliteration of lymphoid sinuses may also add to the confusion. However, the presence of reactive follicles and patent sinuses in the uninvolved areas, the mottled pattern in interfollicular areas, and the identification of differ-

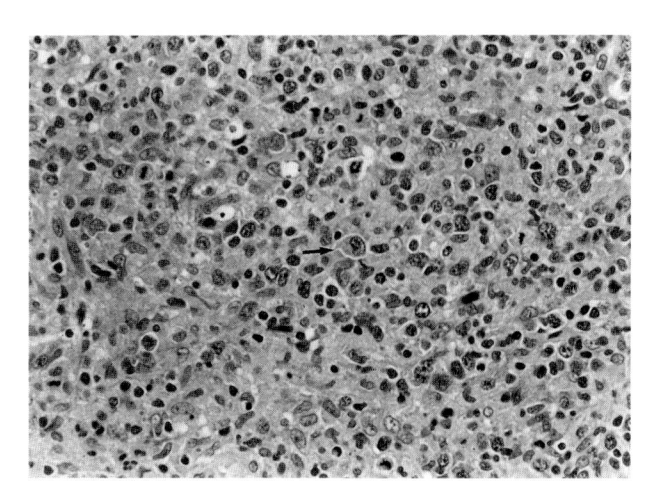

Fig. 4.45. Another field of the same case of Fig. 4.43 showing plasmacytoid monocytes (arrow) immunoblasts and histiocytes. H&E, ×500.

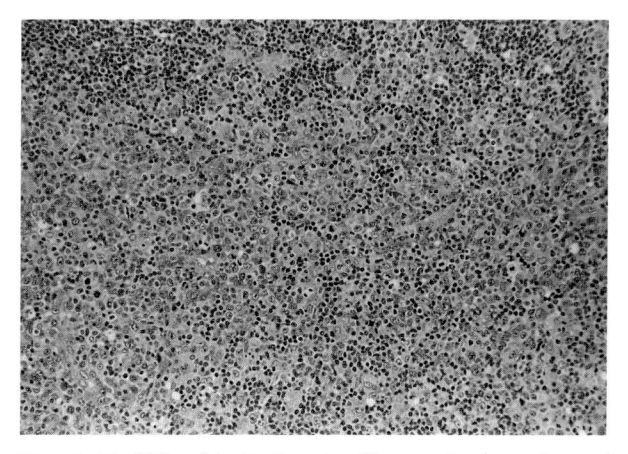

Fig. 4.46. Kikuchi–Fujimoto disease in lymph node showing immunoblastic proliferation mimicking lymphoma. H&E, ×250.

ent cell types by immunohistochemical techniques may help establish the diagnosis of KFD.[45] A monoclonal surface immunoglobulin pattern, on the other hand, is in favor of malignant lymphoma.

SLE may mimic KFD because it is usually seen in young female patients, and the involved lymph node also shows extensive necrosis. However, the special type of histiocytes and plasmacytoid monocytes are not present in SLE, which is characterized by the hematoxylin bodies and vascular fibrinoid necrosis.

Kawasaki Disease (Mucocutaneous Lymph Node Syndrome)

Kawasaki disease (KD) was described in 1967 by Kawasaki as acute febrile mucocutaneous syndrome with lymphoid involvement, but it is generally called *mucocutaneous lymph node syndrome* in the current literature. As the term indicates, the patients have fever, cervical lymphadenopathy and mucocutaneous lesions, namely, bilateral conjunctival congestion, erythematous or fissured lips, strawberry tongue, congested oropharynx, erythema or edema of hands and feet, periungual desquamation during convalescent phase, and polymorphous skin rash involving primarily the trunk.[48,49] The original group of patients were from Japan, but KD has now been reported in many other countries. The average age of KD patients in the United States is about 3 years, while KD patients in Japan are mostly 9–12-months old. Most of the patients recovered in 3–4 weeks, but 1–2% of the affected children die of complications of coronary arteritis such as thrombosis or rupture of coronary aneurysm. Empirically, intravenous gammaglobulin may reduce systemic inflammation and prevent cardiac complications. The etiology of KD is still unknown.

In spite of the name, mucocutaneous lymph node syndrome, lymph node biopsy is seldom performed in patients with KD. Most early reports stressed nonspecific changes in lymph nodes from KD patients.[49,50] A few reports described the presence of focal necrosis and thrombosis,[50,51] which, according to Giesker et al.,[50] is the most specific feature in KD.

The necrosis is multifocal, accompanied by different degrees of neutrophilic infiltration. Fibrin microthrombi are invariably demonstrated in small vessels adjacent to the necrotic foci. Concentric perivascular infiltrates of lymphocytes and histiocytes (onion-skin appearance) may also be seen. The histologic findings in the biopsies of skin, kidney, and muscle, as part of the workup of vasculitis, are usually noncontributory to the diagnosis of KD. Since the incidence of KD has increased in the Western world and there is no specific test or clinical symptoms to help the diagnosis, cervical lymph node biopsy should be attempted.[50] A recent study of antineutrophil cytoplasmic and anti-endothelial-cell antibodies in patients with KD or other febrile disease revealed no statistically significant difference between these two groups of patients.[52]

Histologically, KD should be distinguished from SLE, cat-scratch disease, and other necrotizing lymphadenitis. However, the presence of thrombotic vasculitis and the absence of granulomas and microorganisms, demonstrated by either silver stain or acid-fast stain, should be helpful in the differential diagnosis. The absence of cluster of peculiar histiocytes and plasmacytoid monocytes can help exclude KFD. However, since KD is seen in only very young children, many of the abovementioned diseases can be easily eliminated.

REFERENCES

1. Swerdlow SH, Sukapanichant S, Glick AD, et al: Reactive states in lymph nodes resembling lymphomas or progressing to lymphomas: A selective review. *Mod Pathol* 6:378–391, 1993.
2. Krishman J, Danon AD, Frizzera G: Reactive lymphadenopathies and atypical lymphoproliferative disorders. *Am J Clin Pathol* 99:385–396, 1993.
3. Ioachim HL: *Lymph Node Pathology*, 2nd ed, Philadelphia, Lippincott, 1994.
4. Schnitzer B: Reactive lymphoid hyperplasias. In Jaffe ES (ed): *Surgical Pathology of the Lymph Nodes and Related Organs*, 2nd ed, Philadelphia, Saunders, 1995, pp 98–132.
5. Knowles DM, Chadburn A: Lymphadenopathy and the lymphoid neoplasms associated with the acquired immune deficiency syndrome (AIDS). In Knowles DM (ed): *Neoplastic Hematopathology*, Baltimore, Williams & Wilkins, 1992, pp 773–835.
6. Baroni CD, Uccini S: The lymphadenopathy of HIV infection. *Am J Clin Pathol* 99:397–408, 1993.
7. Uccini S, Monardo F, Vitolo D, et al: HIV and Epstein–Barr virus (EBV) antigens and genome in lymph nodes of HIV positive patients affected by persistent generalized lymphadenopathy (PGL). *Am J Clin Pathol* 92:729–735, 1989.
8. Baroni CD, Pezzella F, Pezzella M, et al: Expression of HIV in lymph node cells of LAS patients: Immunohistology, in situ hybridization and identification of target cells. *Am J Pathol* 133:498–506, 1988.
9. Fishleder A, Tubbs R, Hesse B, et al: Uniform detection of immunoglobulin gene rearrangement in benign lymphoepithelial lesions. *N Engl J Med* 316:1118–1121, 1987.

10. Kuo TT, Shih LY, Chan HL: Kimura's disease: Involvement of regional lymph nodes and distinction from angiolymphoid hyperplasia with eosinophilia. *Am J Surg Pathol* 12:843–854, 1988.
11. Hui PK, Chan JKC, Ng CS, et al: Lymphadenopathy of Kimura's disease. *Am J Surg Pathol* 13:177–186, 1989.
12. Allen PW, Ramakrishna B, MacCormac LB: The histiocytoid hemangiomas and other controversies. *Pathol Annu* 27(pt 2):51–87.
13. Kung ITM, Gibson JB, Bannatype PM: Kimura's disease: A clinicopathological study of 21 cases and its distinction from angiolymphoid hyperplasia with eosinophilia. *Pathology* 16:39–44, 1984.
14. Rosai J, Gold J, Landy R: The histiocytoid hemangiomas. A unifying concept embracing several previous described entities of skin, soft tissue, large vessels, bone and heart. *Hum Pathol* 10:707–730, 1979.
15. Chan JKC, Warnke RA, Dorfman RF: Vascular transformation of sinuses in lymph nodes. A study of its morphological spectrum and distinction from Kaposi's sarcoma. *Am J Surg Pathol* 15:732–743, 1991.
16. Rousselet MC, Saint-Andre JP, Beaufils JM, et al: Benign vascular proliferation in a lymph node following acute toxoplasmosis. A differential diagnosis from Kaposi's sarcoma. *Arch Pathol Lab Med* 112:1264–1266, 1988.
17. Ioachim HL, Cronin W, Roy M, et al: Persistent lymphadenitis in individuals at high risk for HIV infection: Clinicopathologic correlations and long-term follow-up in 29 cases. *Am J Clin Pathol* 93:208–218, 1990.
18. Chan JKC, Lewin KJ, Lombard CM, et al: Histopathology of bacillary angiomatosis of lymph nodes. *Am J Surg Pathol* 15:430–437, 1991.
19. Martin RW, Hood AF, Farmer ER: Kaposi sarcoma. *Medicine* 72:245–261, 1993.
20. Krigel RL, Laubenstein LJ, Muggia FM: Kaposi's sarcoma: A new staging classification. *Cancer Treat Rep* 67:531–534, 1983.
21. Centers for Disease Control: Epidemiologic aspects of the current outbreak of Kaposi's sarcoma and opportunistic infections. *N Engl J Med* 306:248–252, 1982.
22. Siegal B, Levinton-Kriss S, Schiffer A, et al: Kaposi's sarcoma in immunosuppression. Possibly the result of a dual viral infection. *Cancer* 65:492–498, 1990.
23. Scinicariello F, Dolan MJ, Nedelcu I, et al: Occurrence of human papillomavirus and p53 gene mutations in Kaposi's sarcoma. *Virology* 203:153–157, 1994.
24. Sankey EA, More L, Dhillon AP: QB End/10: A new immunostain for the routine diagnosis of Kaposi's sarcoma. *J Pathol* 161:267–271, 1990.
25. Dorfman RF, Warnke R: Lymphadenopathy simulating the malignant lymphomas. *Hum Pathol* 5:519–550, 1974.
26. Strickler JG, Fedeli F, Horwitz CA: Infectious mononucleosis in lymphoid tissue-histopathology, in situ hybridization differential diagnosis. *Arch Pathol Lab Med* 117:269–278, 1993.
27. Abbondanzo SL, Sato N, Strauss SE, et al: Acute infectious mononucleosis: CD30 (Ki-1) antigen expression and histologic correlations. *Am J Clin Pathol* 93:698–702, 1990.
28. Strickler JG, Manivel JC, Copenhauer CM, et al: Comparison of in situ hybridization and immunohistochemistry for detection of cytomegalovirus and herpes simplex virus. *Hum Pathol* 21:443–448, 1990.
29. Rushin JM, Riordan GP, Heaton RB, et al: Cytomegalovirus-infected cells express Leu M1 antigen. A potential source of diagnostic error. *Am J Pathol* 136:989–995, 1990.
30. Tamaru JI, Mikata A, Horie H, et al: Herpes simplex lymphadenitis. Report of two cases with review of the literature. *Am J Surg Pathol* 14:571–577, 1990.
31. Kamel OW, LeBrun DP, Berry GJ, et al: Warthin–Finkeldey polykaryocytes demonstrate a T-cell immunophenotype. *Am J Clin Pathol* 97:179–183, 1992.
32. Craig FE, Gulley ML, Banks PM: Post-transplantation lymphoproliferative disorders. *Am J Clin Pathol* 99:265–276, 1993.
33. Frizzera G, Hanto DW, Gajl-Peczalska KJ, et al: Polymorphic diffuse B-cell hyperplasias and lymphomas in renal transplant recipients. *Cancer Res* 41:4262–4279, 1981.
34. Penn I: The changing pattern of posttransplant malignancies. *Transplant Proc* 23:1101–1103, 1991.
35. Locker J, Nalesnik M: Molecular genetic analysis of lymphoid tumors arising after organ transplantation. *Am J Pathol* 135:977–987, 1989.
36. Abbondanzo SL, Irey NS, Frizzera G: Dilantin (DN)-associated lymphadenopathy. Spectrum of histopathologic patterns. *Mod Pathol* 5:73A, 1992.
37. Katzin WE, Julius CJ, Tubbs RR, et al: Lymphoproliferative disorders associated with carbamazepine. *Arch Pathol Lab Med* 114:1244–1248, 1990.
38. LeBoit PE, Berger TG, Egbert BM, et al: Bacillary angiomatosis. The histopathology and differential diagnosis of a pseudoneoplastic infection in patients with human immunodeficiency virus disease. *Am J Surg Pathol* 21:567–569, 1989.
39. Relman DA, Loutit JS, Schmidt TM, et al: The agent of bacillary angiomatosis: An approach to the identification of uncultured pathogens. *N Engl J Med* 323:1573–1580, 1990.
40. Chan JKC, Frizzera G, Fletcher CDM, et al: Primary vascular tumors of lymph nodes other than Kaposi's sarcoma: Analysis of 39 cases and delineation of two new entities. *Am J Surg Pathol* 16:335–350, 1992.
41. Sun T: Current topics in protozoal diseases. *Am J Clin Pathol* 102:16–29, 1994.
42. McCabe RE, Brooks RG, Dorfman RF, et al: Clinical spectrum in 107 cases of toxoplasmic lymphadenopathy. *Rev Infect Dis* 9:754–774, 1987.
43. Gould E, Porto R, Albores-Saavedra J, et al: Dermatopathic lymphadenitis: The spectrum and significance of its morphologic features. *Arch Pathol Lab Med* 112:1145–1150, 1988.

44. Tsang WYW, Chan JKC, Ng CS: Kikuchi's lymphadenitis: A morphologic analysis of 75 cases with special reference to unusual features. *Am J Surg Pathol* 18:219–231, 1994.
45. Nathwani BN: Kikuchi–Fujimoto disease. *Am J Surg Pathol* 196–197, 1991.
46. Kikuchi M: Histiocytic necrotizing lymphadenitis (Kikuchi–Fujimoto disease) in Japan. *Am J Surg Pathol* 15:197–198, 1991.
47. Sumiyoshi Y, Kikuchi M, Takeshita M, et al: Immunohistologic studies of Kikuchi's disease. *Hum Pathol* 24:1114–1119, 1993.
48. Sundel RP, Newburger JW: Kawasaki disease and its cardiac sequelae. *Hosp Pract* 28:51–66, 1993.
49. Yanagihara R, Todd JK: Acute febrile mucocutaneous lymph node syndrome. *Am J Dis Child* 134:603–614, 1980.
50. Giesker DW, Pastuszak WT, Forouhar FA, et al: Lymph node biopsy for early diagnosis in Kawasaki disease. *Am J Surg Pathol* 6:493–501, 1982.
51. Marsh WL Jr, Bishop JW, Koenig HM: Bone marrow and lymph node findings in a fatal case of Kawasaki's disease. *Arch Pathol Lab Med* 104:563–567, 1980.
52. Guzman J, Fung M, Petty RE: Diagnostic value of antineutrophil cytoplasmic and anti-endothelial cell antibodies in early Kawasaki disease. *J Pediatr* 124:917–920, 1994.

5
Differential Diagnosis of Granulomatous Lymphadenitis

A granulomatous lesion is a common finding in lymph nodes. Many entities may cause such a lesion in lymph nodes, and there may be subtle differences between these lesions. However, these interlesion differences are seldom specific, and special stains, particularly acid-fast and silver stains, should be routinely performed to rule out infectious agents. Granulomatous lymphadenitis can be divided into nonnecrotizing and necrotizing categories. Sarcoidosis is representative of nonnecrotizing granulomatous lymphadenitis. However, foreign-body reaction, reactions to lymphomas and carcinomas, and even fungal infections may manifest as nonnecrotizing lesions.

Sarcoidosis

Sarcoidosis is a multisystem granulomatous disease with unknown etiology.[1] The female:male frequency ratio is ~2:1, but it is mostly seen in blacks, about 10 times more frequent than in whites. The most common site of involvement is the pulmonary hilar lymph nodes and lungs, but peripheral lymph nodes, liver, eye, skin, and any other organs can also be involved. Sarcoidosis may begin with alveolitis; however, the pulmonary lesions are frequently masked by thoracic lymphadenopathy. On the other hand, the presence of peribronchial lymphadenopathy without obvious pulmonary lesion and enlarged lymph nodes in other sites is a strong indication of sarcoidosis. Patients with acute symptoms such as fever, weight loss, and erythema nodosum have better prognoses than do those with chronic symptoms involving the lungs and myocardium.

The histopathologic features are essentially those of noncaseating, noncalcified granulomas (Figs. 5.1, 5.2). The nodular granulomas are usually evenly spaced and closely packed, but the margin of the granulomas are sharp and are seldom coalescent. The granuloma is formed by multiple epithelioid histiocytes and a few multinucleated giant cells of the Langhans type. Inside the epithelioid histiocytes and multinucleated giant cells, three types of inclusion bodies can sometimes be found: asteroid bodies, Schaumann bodies, and Hamuzaki–Wesenberg bodies, with frequency ranges of 2–9%, 48–88%, and 11–68%, respectively.[1]

The asteroid bodies are 10–25-μm spider-like inclusions and are stained red in hematoxylin–eosin (H&E) preparations (Fig. 5.3). The Schaumann bodies are concentric, basophilic, oval structures, consisting of calcium phosphate, carbonate, or iron in a protein matrix. The Hamazaki–Wesenberg bodies are giant lysosomes extruded extracellularly at or near the peripheral sinus and outside the granulomas. The presence of these inclusion bodies is characteristic but not diagnostic of sarcoidosis. In between the granuloma are lymphocytes, plasma cells, and fibroblasts. The lymphoid follicles may be partially or completely replaced by granulomas. In a late stage, fibrosis may occur.

Immunohistochemical studies have demonstrated large numbers of CD4+ (helper) cells in the lesion during the active stage.[2,3] In the later stage, CD8+ (suppressor) cells become predominant. There are also numerous B-cells and frequent plasma cells identified in the intergranulomatous regions, which are probably responsible for the production of polyclonal immunoglobulins and immune complexes.[4] The epithelioid histiocytes and multinucleated giant cells in the granulomas may be positive for lysozyme and angiotensin-converting enzyme, but are negative for CD15 and HAM-56. The Hamazaki–Wesenberg bodies are positive for PAS and acid-fast stains.

Besides histologic studies, the elevation of angiotensin-converting enzyme and lysozyme in serum, hypercalcemia, hypergammaglobulinemia, and a favorable response to corticosteroid therapy are helpful in substantiating the diagnosis of sarcoidosis.

However, before a final diagnosis is made for sarcoidosis, infections should be excluded by special stains or culture. Acid-fast stain should be performed to exclude tuberculosis and nontuberculous mycobacterial infection. Gomori methenamine silver (GMS) and PAS stains should be routinely used to rule out fungal infections. A granulomatous reaction to lymphoma and carcinoma should also be considered. Finally, berylliosis is very similar to sarcoidosis histologically, as Schaumann bodies can also be demonstrated in this entity. The demonstration of birefringent crystals of beryllium under polarized microscopy is helpful for the diagnosis of berylliosis.

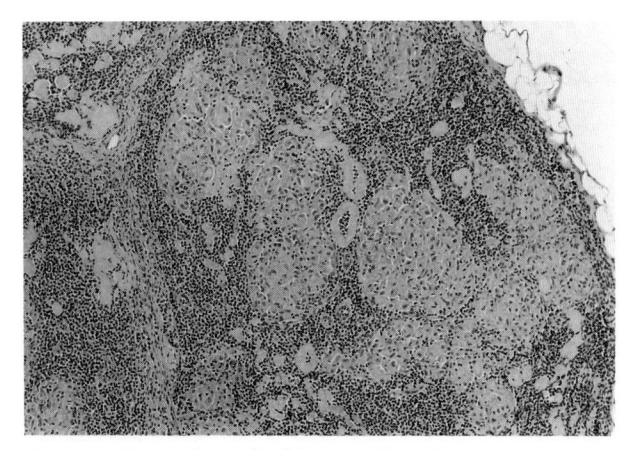

Fig. 5.1. Lymph node biopsy showing noncaseating, noncalcified granulomas with sharp margins consistent with sarcoidosis. H&E, ×125.

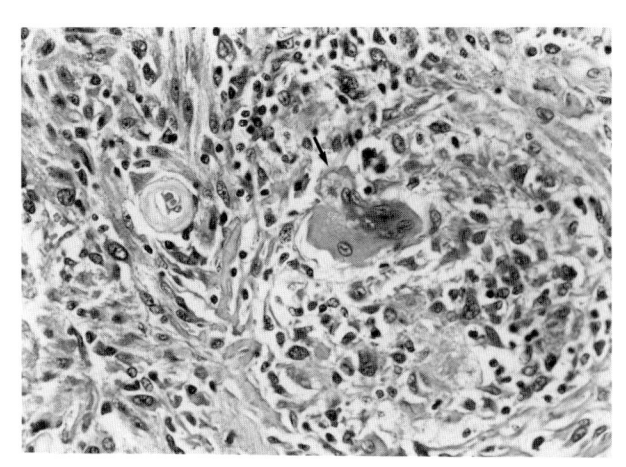

Fig. 5.3. An asteroid body showing the spider-like structure (arrow) present in a multinucleated giant cell. H&E, ×500.

Cat-Scratch Disease

Cat-scratch disease (CSD) is caused by *Afipia felis*[5] and *Rochalimaea henselae*.[6,7] About 90% of patients have a history of cat scratch or cat bite.[6] It usually presents as a local skin lesion in the extremities with regional lymphadenopathy, most frequently involving axillary, cervical, epitrochlear, and inguinal lymph nodes. In patients with AIDS, CSD can be presented as a severe systemic disease.[8]

The histopathologic feature in the lymph node during the early stage is follicular hyperplasia without distortion of the normal architecture.[1] The germinal centers may contain tingible-body macrophages and amorphous, pink, intercellular proteinaceous material. The sinuses may be packed with monocytoid B-cells. Microabscesses and focal necrosis first occur in the subcapsular sinus, and later spread to the cortex and medulla. Finally, there are well-formed granulomas composed of a central abscess surrounded by palisaded epithelioid histiocytes, and a few Langhans giant cells (stellate necrotizing granulomas) (Figs. 5.4, 5.5). In this stage, the nodal architecture is distorted to varying degrees and the abscesses may rupture through the capsule.

These features, although characteristic for CSD, are

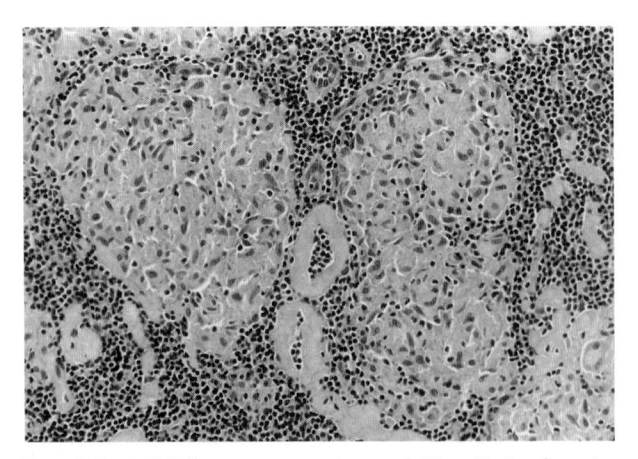

Fig. 5.2. A higher-power view of Fig. 5–1 showing epithelioid histiocytes in the granulomas. H&E, ×250.

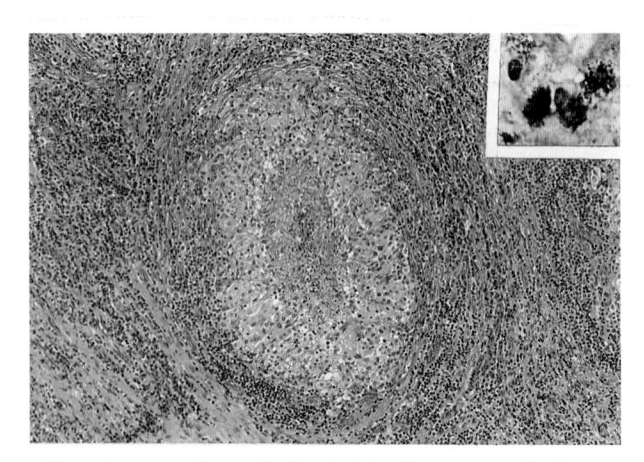

Fig. 5.4. Lymph node biopsy of cat-scratch disease showing a well-formed granuloma composed of a central abscess surrounded by palisaded epithelioid histiocytes. H&E, ×125. Inset: clusters of CSD bacilli are demonstrated by Warthin–Starry silver stain. x 1250.

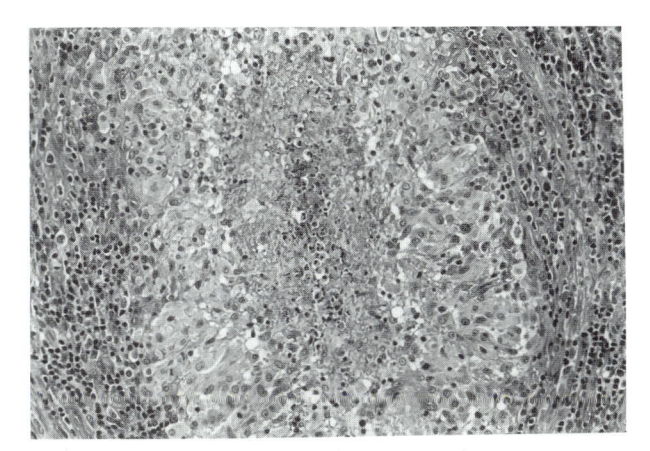

DIFFERENTIAL DIAGNOSIS OF LYMPHOID DISORDERS 51

Fig. 5.5. A higher-power view of Fig. 5.4 showing a few Langhans giant cells among the epithelioid histiocytes. H&E, ×250.

not specific, as the same features can be demonstrated in other necrotizing granulomatous lymphadenopathy. A definitive diagnosis depends, therefore, on the identification of the CSD bacilli. This organism is gram-negative, stained faintly by the Brown–Hopps Gram stain, but not by the Brown–Brenn Gram stain. The organisms are best demonstrated by the Warthin Starry silver impregnation, but it does not react to the Dieterle silver stain.[9] Successful immunoperoxidase stain with CSD bacilli antibody and isolation of the organisms from lymph nodes have been reported.[10] The CSD bacilli are coccobacilli with the presence of L-shaped forms, and are located usually in the necrotic foci, the blood vessel walls, and the vicinity of collagen fibers. *Rochalimaea henselae* can now be identified by indirect immunofluorescence[6] and immunohistochemical techniques.[1]

Without special stains to identify the specific organisms, it is very difficult, if not impossible, to distinguish CSD from lymphogranuloma venereum, tularemia, and brucellosis. It is also important to exclude tuberculosis and fungal infection in equivocal cases.

Lymphogranuloma Venereum

Lymphogranuloma venereum (LGV) is a sexually transmitted disease caused by *Chlamydia trachomatis*. This organism can also cause trachoma, urethritis, and conjunctivitis. Only *C. trachomatis* of the serotypes L-1, L-2, and L-3 are responsible for the development of LGV.[12] The primary site of infection is usually in the genital organs or the uterine cervix, where it presents as herpetiform vesicle, and its subsequent rupture leads to a superficial ulcer. The clinical symptoms are usually caused by regional lymphadenopathy, which occurs most frequently in the inguinal lymph nodes in male patients, but in the perianal or deep pelvic lymph nodes in the female patients. There may be chronic sinus tract formation, secondary to rupture of lymph nodes, and lymphangiectasis as a result of lymphatic obstruction. The sequelae are more severe in female patients, as chronic vulvar edema and rectal stricture may occur. However, LGV is seen in males 2–20 times more frequently than in females, partly because the genital lesions in women are often unnoticed by the patients.[1]

The histopathologic features in the lymph nodes are essentially those described in the CSD section: central necrosis with a large number of neutrophils, surrounded by palisaded epithelioid cells, macrophages, and Langhans giant cells (Fig. 5.6). Lymphocytes and plasma cells may also infiltrate the affected areas. The unaffected regions may show follicular hyperplasia. The lymph node capsule and the perinodal tissues are frequently involved by the supurative process and become fibrosed.

LGV is indistinguishable from CSD, tularemia, and brucellosis histologically. However, the diagnosis of LGV can be substantiated by serologic tests, cytology, immunofluorescent test, and tissue culture.[13,14] The most commonly used serologic test is the complement-fixation test, but the microimmunofluorescence

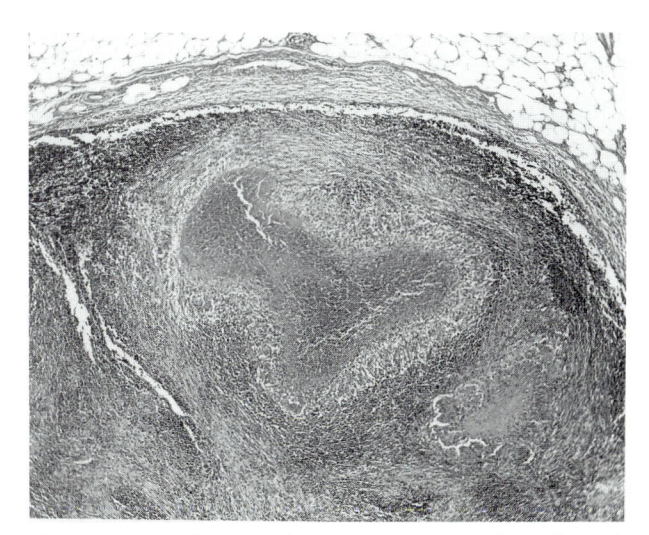

Fig. 5.6. Lymphogranuloma venereum in lymph node showing stellate abscesses surrounded by palisading epithelioid cells and a wide zone of lymphocytes and plasma cells. H&E, ×50. (AFIP 72-1434.)

test and counterimmunoelectrophoresis are more sensitive and specific, although seldom used in routine clinical laboratories. Cytology preparations with Papanicolaou and Giemsa stains may demonstrate the cytoplasmic inclusions of chlamydia, but a monoclonal antibody staining is more specific. In cases of doubt, tissue culture with McCoy or HeLa cells for chlamydia should be performed (Fig. 5.7). The availability of enzyme-linked immunosorbent assays using monoclonal antibodies should greatly facilitate the diagnosis of LGV.[14]

Tularemia

Tularemia is caused by *Francisella tularensis*, a gram-negative rod. Its transmission can be through insect vectors (ticks or deer flies), handling infected rabbits, animal bites, inhalation of infected aerosols, or ingestion of infected animal tissue.[15] The most common clinical presentation is the combination of focal skin ulcer, enlargement of regional lymph nodes, and constitutional symptoms, which are collectively referred to as *ulceroglandular-form tularemia*.[9] When cutaneous lesions are not visible, the tularemia is called *glandular form*. The oculoglandular form involves the eyes and regional lymph nodes. An enteric or typhoidal form shows typhoid-like symptoms and is probably contracted through the oral route. The pulmonary form can be obtained by inhaling infected aerosols or is secondary to bacteremia. Regardless of the clinical forms, lymph nodes are invariably involved.

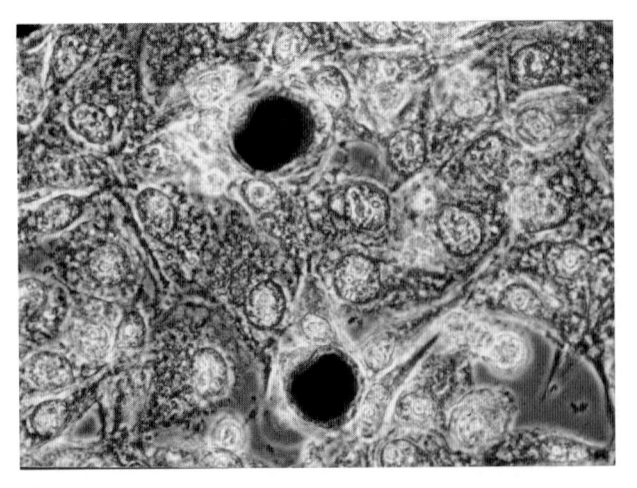

Fig. 5.7. Tissue culture with McCoy cells showing two large cytoplasmic inclusions of chlamydia. Iodine stain, phase-contrast microscopy, ×500.

The histopathologic feature in lymph node is indistinguishable from those of CSD, LGV, and brucellosis, as they all show necrotizing granulomas. The organism is gram-negative but is more easily demonstrated with a modified Dieterle stain.[9] A positive culture of the blood or tissue (lymph nodes) will confirm the diagnosis. An agglutination test is helpful to establish the diagnosis of tularemia, but there is cross-reaction between tularemia and brucellosis.

Brucellosis

Brucellosis is also called *Malta fever, Mediterranean fever,* and *undulant fever*. It is a zoonosis caused mainly by *Brucella melitensis, B. abortus,* and *B. suis* and is transmitted by goats, cows, and pigs, respectively. Ingesting unpasteurized milk from goats or unfermented cheese is the usual source of human infection. The high-risk group includes farmers, veterinarians, meat handlers (butchers, etc.), hunters, and microbiology laboratory workers, who have frequent contact with infected animals or cultures.[16] The bacteria invade through the gastrointestinal (GI) tract, lungs, conjunctiva, and skin and spread through the bloodstream to organs of the reticuloendothelial system including the spleen, liver, lymph nodes, and bone marrow.[17] The organism multiplies inside monocytes and histiocytes. Therefore, histiocytic hyperplasia with noncaseating granulomas is the major finding in the early stage. In later stages, central necrosis develops in the epithelioid granulomas (Fig. 5.8), a feature indistinguishable from those of CSD, LGV, and tularemia. In the liver, there is lymphocytic and mononuclear infiltration in the portal tracts.

Clinically, the patient may manifest as acute malignant type, recurrent undulant fever type, or intermittent (chronic) type. The best means for diagnosis is culture of the blood or tissue. More frequently, however, a diagnosis is based on a rising serologic titer. The tradition serologic test is the agglutination test, but the ELISA (enzyme-linked immunosorbent assay) technique is now available.[9] The organism is a gram-negative bacillus and can be demonstrated occasionally inside histiocytes by MacCallum–Goodpasture stain in tissue sections. As there is reemergence of brucellosis in different parts of the world, this entity should be included in the differential diagnosis when necrotizing granulomatous lymphadenitis is encountered.

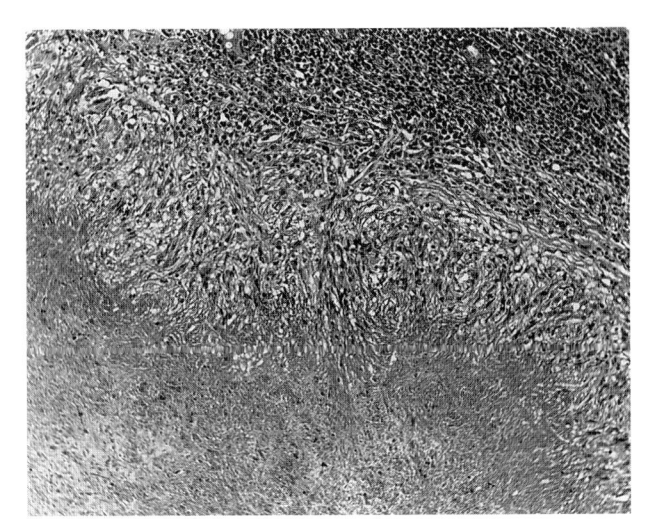

Fig. 5.8. Brucellosis in kidney showing palisading epithelioid cells at the margin of a caseous granuloma. H&E, ×135. (AFIP 74-5782.)

Mycobacterial Lymphadenitis

Pulmonary tuberculosis was previously the major problem for mycobacteria infection, caused by *Mycobacterium tuberculosis* and occasionally, *M. bovis*. Its incidence had steadily decreased in the past 30 years, but a resurgence trend has gradually become apparent since 1985.[1] The reasons for this trend is multiple, including the epidemics of AIDS, drug abuse, influx of infected immigrants, increased immunosuppressive therapy, and other social conditions related to poverty.[18] In the past 15 years, the incidence of nontuberculous (atypical) mycobacterial infections has increased faster than that of tuberculosis.[19] Lymphadenitis is a common feature in these infections. *Mycobacterium tuberculosis* is still the most common species isolated from lymph nodes of both HIV-seropositive and HIV-seronegative patients. However, in United States-born patients with HIV infection, nontuberculous mycobacterial infection is predominant.[18]

Among the nontuberculous mycobacteria, the *M. avium/M. intracellulare* complex (MAC) is the most common human pathogen. Although MAC infection can be seen in non-AIDS patients, it is often demonstrated in AIDS patients because MAC has little virulence in the normal host.[20] Whereas *M. scrofulaceum* is commonly seen in children with cervical lymphadenitis, it seldom causes disease in adults. Other species (*M. fortuitum/M. chelonae* complex, *M. kansasii*, and *M. haemophilum*) have been implicated occasionally in cases of lymphadenitis.

The characteristic histopathologic feature in tuberculous or mycobacterial lymphadenitis is the presence of multiple granulomas composed of epithelioid histiocytes, Langhans giant cells, and lymphocytes with central necrosis (Fig. 5.9). These granulomas may coalesce and form irregular-shaped areas of necrosis, surrounded by epithelioid cells, multinucleated giant cells, lymphocytes, plasma cells, and fibroblasts. The necrosis is typically caseous, i.e., exhibiting complete coagulative necrosis without a trace of cellular configuration and nuclear debris. In the healing stage, the granulomas or tubercles become fibrosed, hyalinized, or calcified.

In nontuberculous infections, granuloma formation may not be present. When MAC infection occurs in AIDS patients, the nodal architecture is replaced in varying degrees by sheets or clusters of pale-stained histiocytes with abundant foamy cytoplasm and eccentrically placed nuclei. These histiocytes are loaded with acid-fast bacilli (AFB) (Fig. 5.10). In lesions caused by *M. tuberculosis*, on the other hand, only a few bacilli can be detected except in patients with HIV infection in whom AFB are easily demonstrated.[18] AFB are usually seen at the periphery of necrotic areas or in the granulomas.

AFB can be demonstrated by Ziehl–Neelsen, Kinyoun, or rhodamine–auramine fluorescent stains. In cases with MAC infection, the organisms are also positive for PAS and GMS stains (Figs. 5.11, 5.12).[1,20] However, since staining techniques may not show the

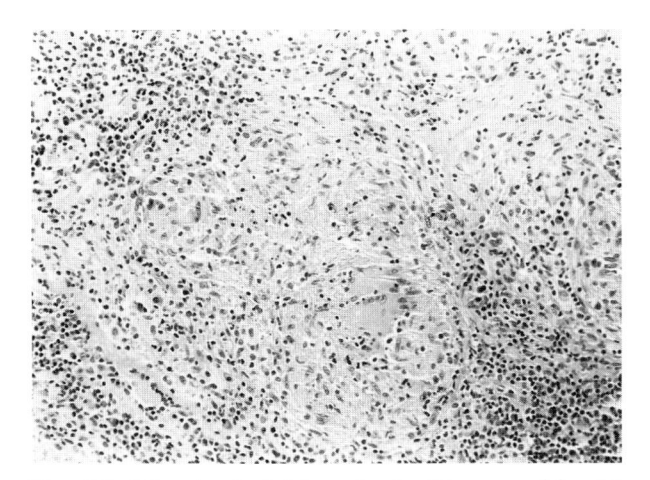

Fig. 5.9. Mycobacterial lymphadenitis caused by *Mycobacterium tuberculosis* showing granulomas and caseating necrosis. H&E, ×125.

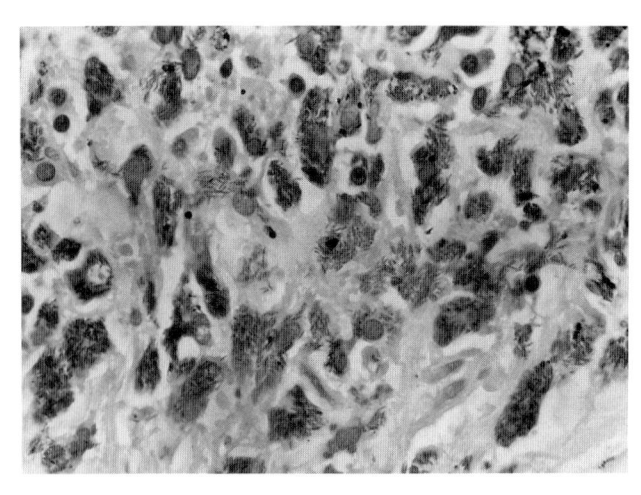

Fig. 5.10. *Mycobacterium avium-intracellularae* infection in the spleen showing many macrophages containing numerous acid-fast bacilli. Acid-fast, ×500.

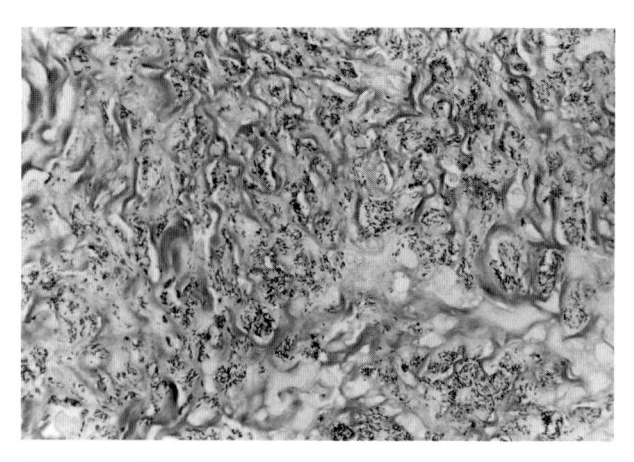

Fig. 5.12. The same specimen as in Fig. 5.10 showing silver-stain-positive bacilli inside the macrophages. Gomori's methenamine silver, ×500.

organism until it is over 10,000 per milligram (> 10,000 mg) of tissue, the sensitivity of the staining technique is only about 22%, while the culture technique has a sensitivity of about 69%.[1] Therefore, the absence of AFB in smears or tissue sections cannot rule out mycobacterial lesions. When caseation is present, other means, such as chest x-ray and skin test, should be used to confirm the diagnosis. DNA probes and polymerase chain reaction (PCR) may help identify the mycobacterial species after culture.[19] Recently, PCR is applied directly to formalin-fixed, paraffin-embedded tissues, thus making a rapid, specific diagnosis possible.[21]

Mycobacterial lymphadenitis should be distinguished from all the necrotizing granulomatous lymphadenitis mentioned in this chapter. Caseation is a hallmark of tuberculosis, but it may be seen in some fungal infections, such as histoplasmosis. In nontuberculous lymphadenitis or in immunocompromised patients, granuloma may be poorly formed or absent.[22] Therefore, every effort has to be made to search for AFB, and whenever there is doubt, a mycobacterial culture should be done. The availability of the PCR technique in the near future for a rapid diagnosis may make the pathologist's job much easier.

Mycobacterium leprae Lymphadenitis

Leprosy, caused by *Mycobacterium leprae*, is primarily a skin disease associated with nerve involvement. As *M. leprae* grows preferentially in low temperature, the lesions of leprosy are often distributed in cooler parts of the body, namely, the skin (Fig. 5.13), mucous membranes of the upper respiratory tract, the anterior part of the eye, testes, superficial nerves, and lymph nodes that drain skin lesions.[1] Leprosy is very different from other nontuberculous mycobacterial infections clinically and pathologically and is thus discussed separately.

Leprosy is divided into two major categories: the lepromatous type, which is seen in patients with minimal cellular immunity; and the tuberculoid type, which is seen in patients with high cellular immunity. The lepromatous type is highly contagious, as the lesion contains numerous leprosy bacilli, clinically pro-

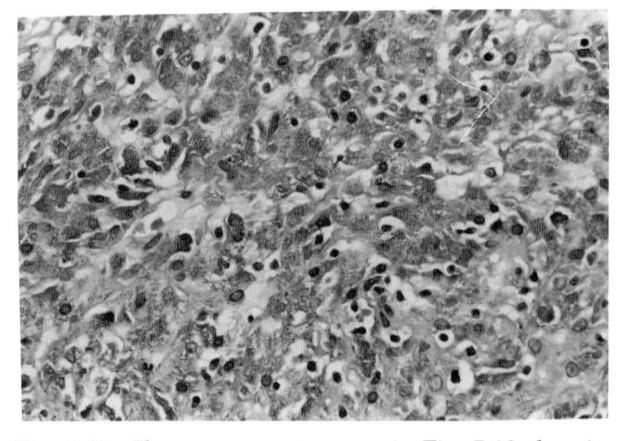

Fig. 5.11. The same specimen as in Fig. 5.10 showing PAS-stain-positive bacilli inside the macrophages. PAS, ×500.

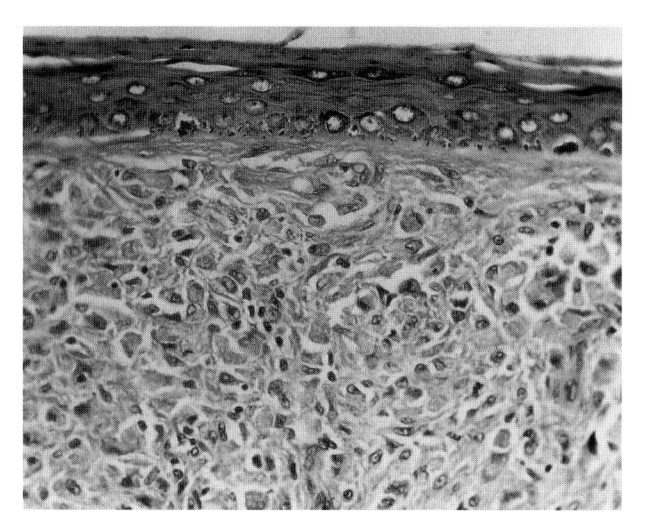

Fig. 5.13. A lepromatous nodule of the skin showing extensive infiltrate of the upper dermis by vacuolated histiocytes containing leprosy bacilli (not shown). H&E, ×350. (AFIP 74-2725.)

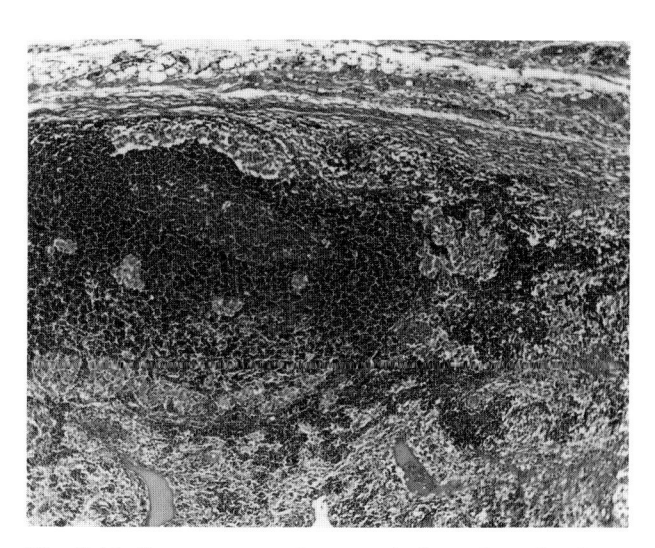

Fig. 5.14. Lepromatous leprosy in lymph node showing numerous foamy macrophages in the subcapsular sinuses and parafollicular and medullary areas. H&E, ×90. (AFIP 72-12505.)

gressive, and the lepromin skin test is usually negative in this type. On the other hand, the tuberculoid lesion has few bacilli, limited clinical manifestation, and the skin test is often positive. In between these two extremes are borderline leprosy and indeterminate leprosy.

In the lymph nodes, the histopathologic features also consist of a spectrum of changes between lepromatous and tuberculoid types. In the lepromatous type, there is marked lymphocyte depletion in the paracortex where sheets of foamy histiocytes or lepra cells are present (Fig. 5.14). In the early stage, the leprosy bacilli are frequently arranged in parallel bundles. In a later stage, the bacilli form dense masses in the cytoplasm of the lepra cells, and these clusters of organisms are called *globi*. When the globi are released from the degenerated lepra cells and engulfed by giant cells, they coalesce and form giant globi. The bacilli may also be seen in endothelial cells and blood vessel walls.

In the tuberculoid type, lepra cells are not seen and leprosy bacilli are rarely found. The major feature is nonnecrotizing granulomas composed of epithelioid cells and multinucleated Langhans giant cells and surrounded by thick cuffs of lymphocytes. A rare histologic feature has been described as histoid leprosy, in which the spindle-shaped histiocytes replace the epithelioid histiocytes. The clinical significance of this type is not known.

The lymphocytes in the tuberculoid type are mainly CD4+ T-cells, while those in the lepromatous type are CD4+ and CD8+ T-cells in similar proportions.[23] The cytokines released by the T-lymphocytes play an important role in stimulating the transformation of epithelioid cells, multinucleated giant cells, and granulomas. The interferon γ (IFNγ) is responsible for activating bactericidal mechanisms within the phagocytized macrophages.[23]

Mycobacterium leprae is best demonstrated by the Fite–Faraco stain on lymph node smears, touch preparations, and tissue sections. The organism can also grow in the footpad of the mouse, and the armadillo is also susceptible to *M. leprae* infection. Thus far, there is no *in vitro* technique for cultivation of the leprosy bacilli. However, the organism has been demonstrated by the PCR technique in tissue sections successfully.[24,25]

Mycobacterium leprae lymphadenitis should be distinguished from other forms of granulomatous lymphadenitis. Particularly, MAC infection is very similar to lepromatous leprosy, while tuberculoid leprosy mimics sarcoidosis.

Cryptococcus Lymphadenitis

Cryptococcosis is caused by *Cryptococcus neoformans*, which has two variants: var. *neoformans* and var. *gattii*. The absolute majority of human infections are induced by *C. neoformans* var. *neoformans*,[26] and *C. neoformans* var. *gattii* is seen mainly in African countries. Cryptococcosis was a rare disease until immunosuppressive therapy and chemotherapy became popular in the 1970s. From early 1980s, AIDS has become the leading predisposing factor in cryptococcosis, accounting for 50% of clinical cases in the United States. Cryptococcosis is now one of the leading causes of death in AIDS patients. The most important natural source of *C. neoformans* is avian (mainly pigeons) droppings in the soil or old buildings. Patients may inhale the dust or airborne particles that are created by wind current or mechanical disturbance. Therefore, pulmonary infection is supposed to be the primary infection. However, the most common and severe clinical manifestation is cryptococcal meningitis, which is frequently the cause of death in patients with cryptococcosis. Cryptococcal pneumonia is the second common infection. Other tissues and organs, including skin, bone, eyes, kidneys, heart valves, prostate, adrenals, liver, and draining lymph nodes, may also be involved occasionally.[1,26]

The lesion in lymph nodes is most frequently a nonnecrotizing granuloma composed of epithelioid cells, lymphocytes, and multinucleated giant cells. The diagnostic feature is the presence of budding yeast cells with great variation in size. Most of the organisms are between 4 and 7 μm, but yeasts from 2 to 15 μm may be encountered occasionally. Cryptococcus differs from other yeasts by a thick capsule, resembling a large halo (Fig. 5.15) and separating the cryptococcal cells from each other and from the cytoplasm of the macrophage, when ingested. A multinucleated giant cell may contain a cluster of several cryptococcal cells. The presence of budding yeast cells, the great variation in size, and the recognition of suspected capsule on the yeast cells outside and inside the macrophages may lead to a preliminary diagnosis of cryptococcosis. However, a definitive diagnosis depends on special stains and culture.

The most simple special stain is the Indian ink preparation, which works well for cerebrospinal fluids, bronchoalveolar lavage specimens, and tissue imprints. The special stains for fungi in tissue sections are GMS and PAS. These two stains may identify the organism as fungus, but Mayer's mucicarmine stain for the capsule distinguishes cryptococcus from other yeasts. With the mucicarmine stain, delicate, radiating spines can be demonstrated projecting from the yeast cell wall (Fig. 5.16). This so-called sunburst effect is due to the shrinkage of the mucinous capsules caused by fixation, but this feature is diagnostic for cryptococcosis. For capsule-deficient cryptococcus, a new stain, Masson–Fontana melanin stain, should be used for differential diagnosis.[27] Culture from tissue specimen should always be attempted when possible. The restriction fragment-length polymorphism (RFLP) analysis may help identify different strains of *Cryptococcus*,[28] a technique that is potentially useful for diagnostic purposes when the organism is

Fig. 5.15. Cryptococcus lymphadenitis showing many yeast cells surrounded by halos. Thick capsule is seen in a few cells (arrow). H&E, ×500.

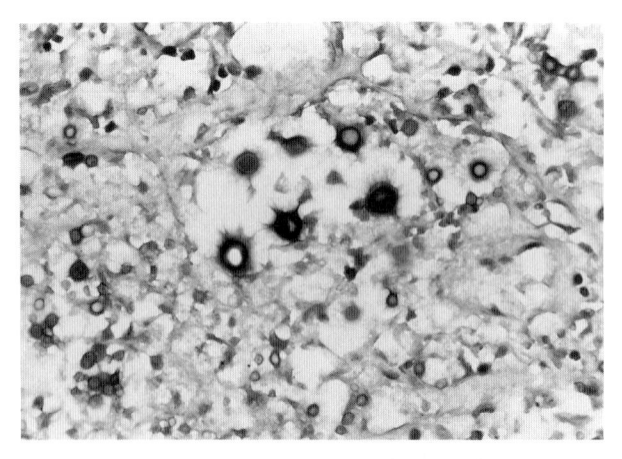

Fig. 5.16. Cryptococcus lymphadenitis showing many organisms stained with mucicarmine. Note multiple delicate, radiating spines projecting from the yeast cell wall (sunburst effect). Mayer's mucicarmine, ×1250.

too sparse to be identified by histologic or even cultural techniques. Detection of cryptococcal antigen in CSF and serum by serologic techniques is helpful in diagnosing cryptococcal meningitis or systemic dissemination of cryptococcosis.

The major differential diagnoses are histoplasmosis and blastomycosis. *Histoplasma capsulatum* is smaller (2–4 μm in diameter), mucicarmine-stain-negative and predominantly intracellular. Necrotizing granuloma is much more commonly seen in histoplasmosis than in cryptococcosis. *Blastomyces dermatitidis* is larger (8–15 μm in diameter), with thicker cell wall (double contour) and multiple nuclei (Fig. 5.17). A broad base is present between mother and daughter cells. This fungus can be weakly carminophilic in a small percentage of cells. *Rhinosporidium* is the only other fungus that is strongly carminophilic, but its huge size (100–350 μm), endospores, and absence of budding distinguish it from cryptococcus. Rhinosporidiosis is usually present in the nose. In the lung tissue, *Pneumocystis carinii* should be distinguished from *Cryptococcus*, not only because they are similar in size but also because both react to GMS and PAS. However, *P. carinii* is not identifiable in H&E-stained sections, is negative for mucicarmine stain, and contains sporozoites, which can be demonstrated by Giemsa stain. In *Pneumocystis* lymphadenitis, the characteristic lesion is a well-confined area of necrosis similar to the eosinophilic foamy exudate in the alveoli of patients with *Pneumocystis carinii* pneumonia (Figs. 5.18, 5.19).

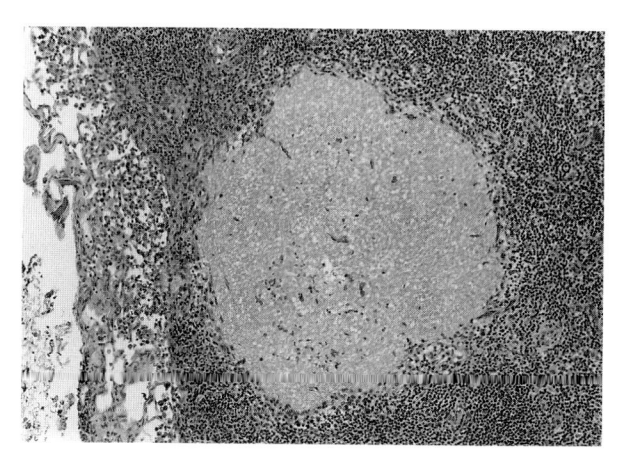

Fig. 5.18. A case of *Pneumocystis* lymphadenitis showing focal necrosis mimicking the eosinophilic foamy exudate seen in alveoli of *Pneumocystis carinii* pneumonitis. H&E, ×125.

Histoplasma Lymphadenitis

Histoplasmosis is caused by *Histoplasma capsulatum*, which has two variants: *H. capsulatum* var. *capsulatum* and *H. capsulatum* var. *duboisii*. The latter variant is seen exclusively in Africa. The natural source of *H. capsulatum* is mainly from the soil, and patients contract the infection by inhalation of airborne conidia of the fungus.[26] Therefore, the major clinical manifestation is pulmonary infection, acute or chronic. Hematogenous dissemination can be seen in immunocompromised patients, such as patients with AIDS, with hematologic neoplasms, or with

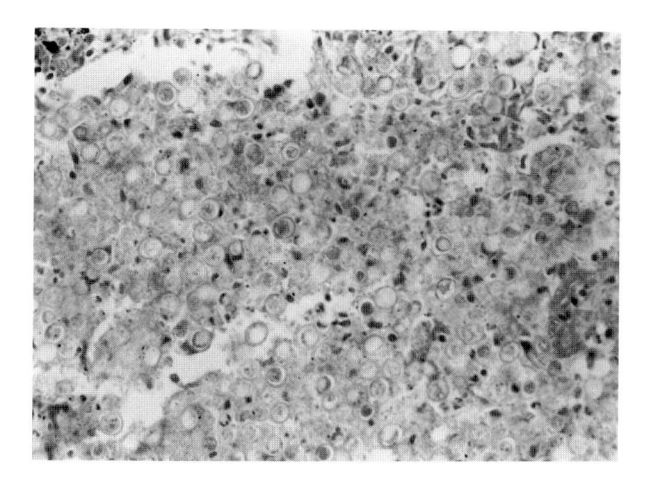

Fig. 5.17. Pulmonary blastomycosis showing an area loaded with *Blastomyces dermatitidis* cells. Some yeast cells show broad-base connection and double-contour cell wall. H&E, ×500.

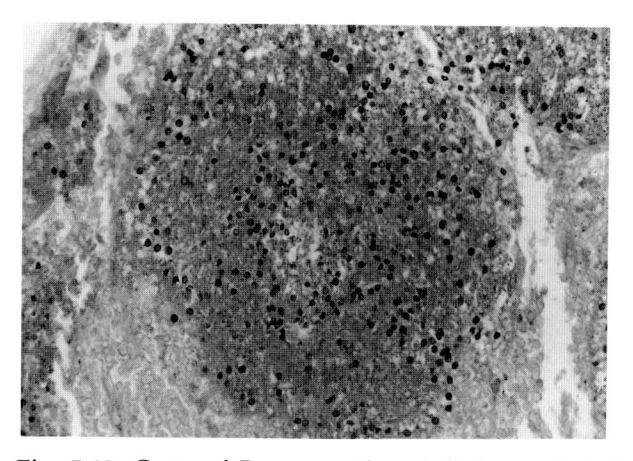

Fig. 5.19. Cysts of *Pneumocystis carinii* demonstrated by silver stain. Gomori methenamine silver (GMS), ×500.

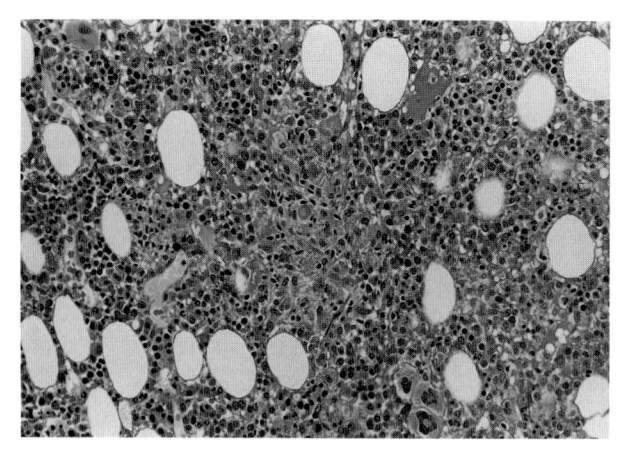

Fig. 5.20. Bone marrow biopsy showing a granuloma caused by *Histoplasma capsulatum* in the center of the field. H&E, ×250.

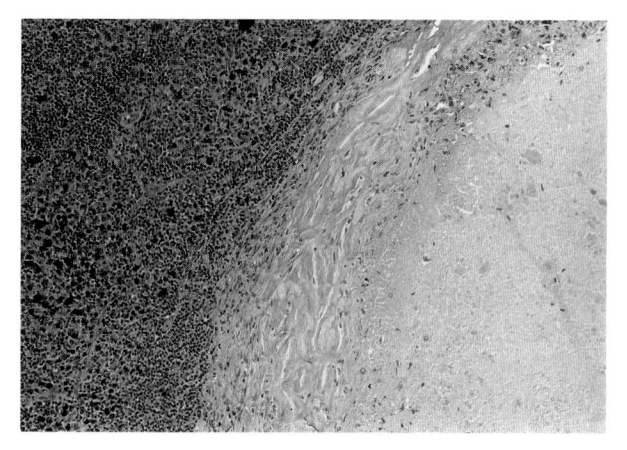

Fig. 5.21. Pulmonary histoplasmosis showing caseous necrosis, dense fibrous capsule and calcification, and intensive lymphocytic infiltration. H&E, ×125.

immunosuppressive therapy. In these patients, hepatosplenomegaly and lymphadenopathy may occur. The organism may be detected in the blood and bone marrow. These clinical features are due to the special affinity of *H. capsulatum* to the reticuloendothelial system. In cases of pulmonary histoplasmosis, the hilar of mediastinal lymph nodes may also be involved.

The histopathologic features in histoplasmosis differ between immunocompetent host and immunocompromised host. The reaction in normal hosts is well-formed epithelioid granulomas (Fig. 5.20). In patients with immunodeficiency, the main feature is large numbers of macrophages and other phagocytic cells that contain numerous histoplasma cells.[29] Necrotizing granulomas develop in later stages and gradually replace the nodal architecture.[26] Finally, large areas of caseous necrosis, dense bands of collagen fibers, and calcification may be the only discernible features (Fig. 5.21) in the lymph node that are very similar to tuberculosis. Under this condition, only acid-fast stain and fungal stains can help distinguish between these two entities morphologically.

Histoplasma organisms measure 2–4 μm in diameter. Although the size of cryptococcus may overlap with that of histoplasma, the former shows great variation in size while the latter is more homogeneous (Table 5.1). In addition, the protoplasm of histoplasma usually retracts from the cell wall and leave a space that appears like a capsule; thus the erroneous name *H. capsulatum*.[29] Histoplasma is positive for GMS (Fig. 5.22) and PAS stains but negative for mucicarmine. These fungal stains help differentiate histoplasma from two intracellular protozoa—leishmania and toxoplasma, which are negative for GMS and PAS.

TABLE 5.1
Comparison of Histoplasma with Similar Organisms

	Histoplasma	Cryptococcus	Toxoplasma	Leishmania
Major tissue form	Intracellular	Extracellular	Extracellular	Intracellular
Size (diameter, μm)	2–4	2–15	4–7	2–3
Characteristic	Eccentric protoplasm	Thick capsule	Nucleus	Kinetoplast
Budding form	Present	Present	Absent	Absent
Tissue reaction	Granuloma	Granuloma	Acute inflammation[a]	Histiocytosis
Common site	Lung	Brain	Brain	Liver/spleen
GMS/PAS	Positive	Positive	Negative	Negative
Mucicarmine	Negative	Positive	Negative	Negative

[a]Acute inflammation is seen in tissues other than lymph nodes, which seldom show toxoplasma organisms.

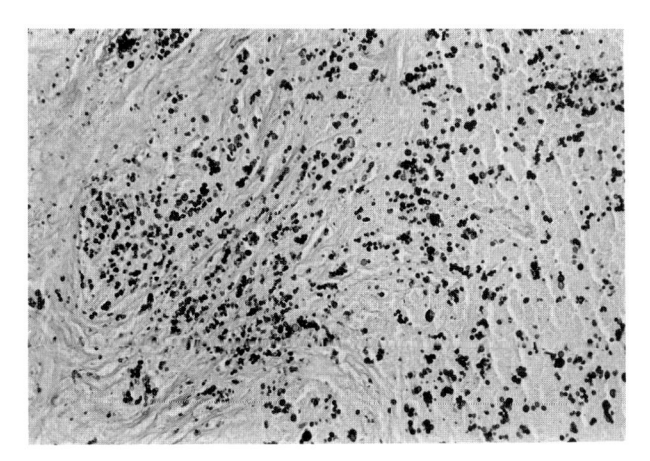

Fig. 5.22. Pulmonary histoplasmosis showing numerous GMS-positive organisms in the necrotic area as shown in Fig. 5.21. Note most organisms form clusters representing intracellular location and a few budding yeast cells are present. GMS, ×500.

The amastigote form (Leishman–Donovan body) of leishmania shows a kinetoplast in addition to its nucleus. The intracellular toxoplasma usually forms a pseudocyst, and its nucleus is well demonstrated in a Giemsa stain preparation.

In cases of doubt, a culture should be obtained. Blood and bone marrow are the most frequent positive sources.[30] The isolate can be identified with a chemiluminescent DNA probe.[31] A radioimmunoassay for histoplasma polysaccharide antigen in serum and urine is a useful technique for a rapid diagnosis of disseminated disease.[30] It is now possible to type *Histoplasma capsulatum* with the RFLP technique.[32]

Coccidioides Lymphadenitis

Coccidioidomycosis is caused by *Coccidioides immitis*. Its natural habitat is in the soil. In a dry climate, a large number of arthrospores, the infective stage, are formed. When the airborne arthrospores are inhaled, patients become infected. Therefore, the primary lesion is usually in the lungs.[26] Hilar lymphadenopathy is found in 20% of cases with pulmonary coccidioidomycosis, and its persistence after resolution of the lung lesion may be confused with lymphoma.[33] Lymphadenitis is a common finding in all forms of coccidioidomycosis, including disseminated disease.

Once in the host, the arthrospores transform into sporangia (spherules), which are about 20–60 μm in diameter and have thick cell walls. Within each spherule, multiple endospores, 2–4 μm in diameter, develop. A mature spherule may rupture and release the endospores, which finally grow into spherules. This developmental process may stimulate both pyogenic and granulomatous reactions.[26] Eosinophilic infiltration may also be present. the granulomas are composed of epithelioid histiocytes, Langhans giant cells, lymphocytes, and plasma cells. the granulomas may develop central caseous necrosis. In AIDS patients, granulomas are poorly formed. Mature, ruptured spherules often attract a neutrophilic exudate, and small abscesses can be present. In a later stage, there may be only extensive necrosis surrounded by a broad fibrotic band. However, the spherules may still be identifiable even though the normal architecture of the host tissue is no longer preserved.

A thick-walled sporangium containing multiple endospores is diagnostic of coccidioidomycosis (Figs. 5.23–5.25). However, the lymph node or other tissue may show only endospores of various sizes that may mimic *Histoplasma*, *Cryptococcus*, *Blastomyces dermatitidis*, or *Paracoccidioides brasiliensis*. Therefore, painstaking search for an intact or ruptured sporangium is important to reach a correct diagnosis. A negative mucicarmine stain may help rule out cryptococcosis. The finding of multiple budding or daughter cells indicates the diagnosis of paracoccidiodomycosis (Fig. 5.26). *Rhinosporidium seeberi* is most similar to *Coccidioides* with the pres-

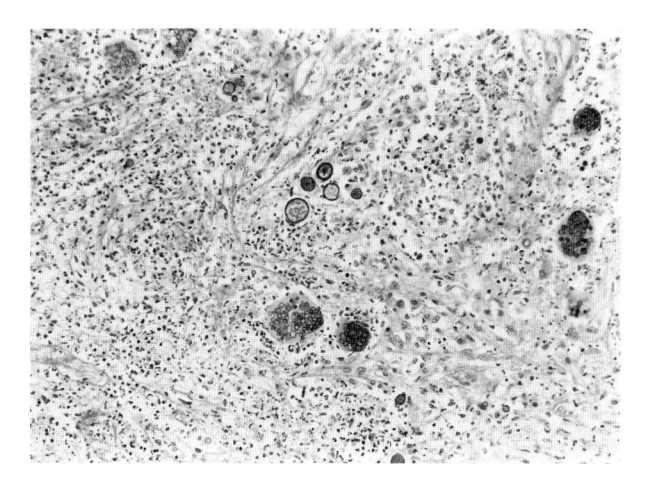

Fig. 5.23. Coccidioidomycosis in pulmonary hilar lymph node showing multiple spherules (sporangia) of varying sizes. PAS, ×250. (Courtesy of Dr. Michael DeMartino.)

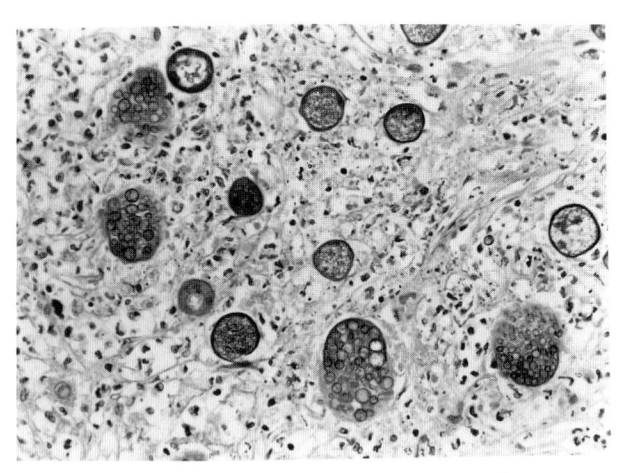

Fig. 5.24. A higher-power view of Fig. 5.23 showing the details of the spherules that contain multiple endospores. Many free endospores are also present. PAS, ×500.

ence of sporangia and endospores. However, its sporangia are larger and have thicker walls, and endospores are larger and more numerous in *Rhinosporidium* than in *Coccidioides*.[26] Furthermore, *Rhinosporidium* is seen exclusively in the nose and nasopharynx and cannot be cultured. A successful culture result is most definitive for a final diagnosis of different fungal infections. The culture can be confirmed within 48 hr by a positive DNA probe assay for the ribosomal RNA of *Coccidioides*.[34] Serologic tests, such as complement-fixation test and immunodiffusion test, may help but cannot distinguish previous from current infections.

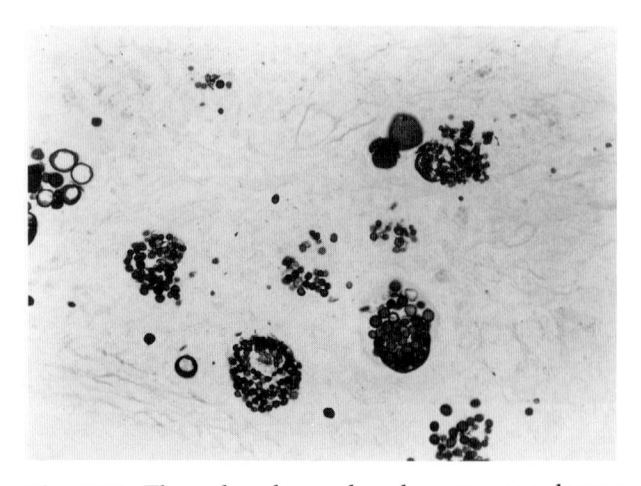

Fig. 5.25. The spherules and endospores are demonstrated by GMS stain. ×500.

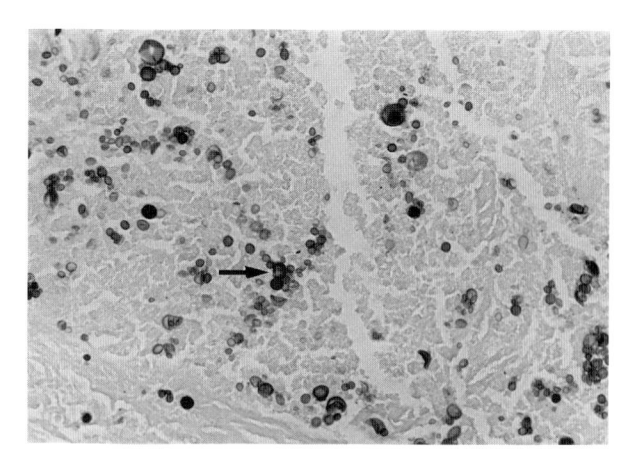

Fig. 5.26. Pulmonary paracoccidioidomycosis showing multiple-budding yeast cells (arrow). GMS, ×500.

REFERENCES

1. Ioachim HL: Lymph Node Pathology, 2nd ed, Philadelphia, Lippincott, 1994.
2. Semenzata G, Zezzutto A, Pizzolo G, et al: Immunohistological study in sarcoidosis: Evaluation at different sites of disease activity. *Clin Immunol Immunopathol* 30:29–40, 1984.
3. Chilosi M, Menestrina F, Capelli P, et al: Immunohistochemical analysis of sarcoid granulomas. Evaluation of Ki67+ and interleukin-1+ cells. *Am J Pathol* 131:191–198, 1988.
4. Fazel SB, Howie SE, Krajewski AS, Lamb D: B lymphocyte accumulations in human pulmonary sarcoidosis. *Thorax* 47:964–967, 1992.
5. Brenner DJ, Hollis DG, Moss CW, et al: Proposal of Afipia gen. nov., with *Afipia felis* sp. nov. (formerly the cat scratch disease bacillus) *Afipia clevelandensis* sp. nov. (formerly the Cleveland Clinic Foundations strain), *Afipia broomeae* sp. nov., and three unnamed genospecies. *J Clin Microbiol* 29:2450–2460, 1991.
6. Adal KA, Cockerell CJ, Petri WA Jr: Cat scratch disease, bacillary angiomatosis, and other infections due to Rochalimaea. *N Engl J Med* 330:1509–1515, 1994.
7. Schwartzman WA: Infections due to Rochalimaea: The expanding clinical spectrum. *Clin Infect Dis* 15:893–902, 1992.
8. Koehler JE, LeBoit PE, Egbert BM, et al: Cutaneous vascular lesions and disseminated cat-scratch disease in patients with the acquired immunodeficiency syndrome (AIDS) and AIDS-related complex. *Ann Intern Med* 109:449–455, 1988.
9. von Lichtenberg F: *Pathology of Infectious Diseases*, New York, Raven Press, 1991, pp 146–147, 149–150.
10. English CK, Wear DJ, Margileth AM, et al: Cat-scratch disease: Isolation and culture of the bacterial agent. *JAMA* 259:1347–1352, 1988.

11. Min KW, Reed JA, Welch DF, et al: Morphologically variable bacilli of cat scratch disease are identified by immunocytochemical labeling with antibodies to *Rochalimaea henselae*. *Am J Clin Pathol* 101:607–610, 1994.
12. Tenenbaum MJ, Greenspan J: Sexually transmitted disease caused by *Chlamydia trachomatis*. In Sun T (ed): *Sexually Related Infectious Diseases: Clinical and Laboratory Aspects*, New York, Field-Rich, 1986, pp 153–159.
13. Hipp S: Laboratory techniques for identification of *Chlamydia trachomatis*. In Sun T (ed): *Sexually Related Infectious Diseases: Clinical and Laboratory Aspects*, New York, Field-Rich, 1986, pp 161–171.
14. Joseph AK, Rosen T: Laboratory techniques used in the diagnosis of chancroid, granuloma inguinale, and lymphogranuloma venereum. *Dermatol Clin* 12:1–8, 1994.
15. Capellan J, Fong IW: Tularemia from a cat bite: Case report and review of feline-associated tularemia. *Clin Infect Dis* 16:472–475, 1993.
16. Gilbert GL: Brucellosis: Continuing risk. *Med J Aust* 159:147–148, 1993.
17. Belter LF: Brucellosis. In Binford CH, Connor DH (eds): *Pathology of Tropical and Extraordinary Diseases*, Washington DC, Armed Forces Institute of Pathology, 1976, pp 174–177.
18. Shriner KA, Mathisen GE, Goetz MB: Comparison of mycobacterial lymphadenitis among persons infected with human immunodeficiency virus and seronegative controls. *Clin Infect Dis* 15:601–605, 1992.
19. Wolinsky E: Mycobacterial diseases other than tuberculosis. *Clin Infect Dis* 15:1–12, 1992.
20. Horsburgh CR Jr: *Mycobacterium avium* complex infection in the acquired immunodeficiency syndrome. *N Engl J Med* 324:1332–1338, 1991.
21. Cook SM, Bartos RE, Pierson CL, et al: Detection and characterization of atypical mycobacteria by the polymerase chain reaction. *Diagn Mol Pathol* 3:53–58, 1994.
22. Pinder SE, Colville A: Mycobacterial cervical lymphadenitis in children: Can histological assessment help differentiate infections caused by non-tuberculous mycobacteria from *Mycobacterium tuberculosis*? *Histopathology* 22:59–64, 1993.
23. Britton WJ: Leprosy 1962–1992: 3. Immunology of leprosy. *Trans Roy Soc Trop Med Hyg* 87:508–514, 1993.
24. Colston MJ: Leprosy 1962–1992: 2. The microbiology of *Microbacterium leprae*; progress in the last 30 years. *Trans Roy Soc Trop Med Hyg* 87:504–507, 1993.
25. Sung KJ, Kim SB, Choi JH, et al: Detection of mycobacterium leprae DNA in formalin-fixed, paraffin-embedded samples from multibacillary and paucibacillary leprosy patient by polymerase chain reaction. *Int J Dermatol* 32:710–713, 1993.
26. Kwon-Chung K, Bennett JE: *Medical Mycology*, Philadelphia, Lea & Febiger, 1992.
27. Ro JY, Lee SS, Ayala AG: Advantage of Fontana-Masson stain in capsule deficient cryptococcal infection. *Arch Pathol Lab Med* 111:53–57, 1987.
28. Currie BP, Freundlich LF, Casadevall A: Restriction fragment length polymorphism analysis of *Cryptococcus neoformans* isolated from environmental (pigeon excreta) and clinical sources in New York City. *J Clin Microbiol* 32:1188–1192, 1994.
29. Binford CH, Dooley JR: Deep Mycoses. In Binford CH, Connor DH (eds): *Pathology of Tropical and Extraordinary Diseases*, Washington DC, Armed Forces Institute of Pathology, 1976, pp 551–599.
30. Case records of the Massachusetts General Hospital, Case 5-1994. *N Engl J Med* 330:273–280, 1994.
31. Hall GS, Pratt-Rippin K, Washington JA: Evaluation of a chemiluminescent probe assay for identification of *Histoplasma capsulatum* isolated. *J Clin Microbiol* 30:3003–3004, 1992.
32. Keath EJ, Kobayashi GS, Medoff G: Typing of *Histoplasma capsulatum* by restriction fragment length polymorphisms in a nuclear gene. *J Clin Microbiol* 30:2104–2107, 1992.
33. Case Records of the Massachusetts General Hospital. Case 21-1994. *N Engl J Med* 330:1516–1522, 1994.
34. Beard JS, Benson PM, Skillman L: Rapid diagnosis of coccidioidomycosis with a DNA probe to ribosomal RNA. *Arch Dermatol* 129:1589–1593, 1933.

6
Differential Diagnosis of Storage Histiocyte Disorders

Storage histiocyte disorders are a group of diseases with inborn errors of metabolism resulting in accumulation of the intermediate product within the histiocytes (monocytes, macrophages). The organs of the mononuclear phagocyte or the reticuloendothelial system (the lymph nodes, spleen, liver, and bone marrow) are frequently involved.[1] The metabolic error is usually due to an inherited deficiency of a hydrolytic enzyme that is normally present in lysosomes. This chapter will discuss three major disease groups: Gaucher disease, Niemann–Pick disease, and the mucopolysaccharidoses (Table 6.1).

CLINICAL MANIFESTATION

Gaucher Disease

Gaucher disease (GD) is an autosomal recessive disorder.[1-4] The metabolic error is due to a deficiency of glucocerebrosidase leading to accumulation of glucocerebroside (glucosylceramide) in the lysosomes of histiocytes (macrophages/monocytes). In rare occasions, it may be due to the deficiency of a cofactor of glucocerebroside called *saposin*. The gene for glucocerebrosidase is located on chromosome 1 in the region of q21. In GD patients, the common mutations are found at nucleotides 84, 1226, and 1448.[3,5] The genotype 1226G/1226G is usually associated with a mild clinical course. The genotypes 1226G/84GG and 1226G/1448C are associated with more severe clinical manifestations. However, there are great variations within the same genotype. On the basis of clinical manifestations, GD is divided into three types: type I (nonneuronopathic adult GD), which has a benign clinical course without neurologic involvement and is seen in about 99% of patients; type II (acute neuropathic), which defines a fulminating clinical course with severe neurologic manifestations (patients with GD type II usually die in the first 18 months of life); and type III (subacute neuropathic), which is the juvenile form of the disorder. Type III is characterized by a later onset of neurologic symptoms than in type II disease and by a longer clinical course.

The glycolipid-laden macrophages are responsible for all the nonneurologic clinical manifestations in GD. Therefore, hepatosplenomegaly is the most frequent physical finding in these patients. Splenomegaly and the associated thrombocytopenia may contribute to the most common presenting symptoms: the bleeding tendency.[3] Bone marrow is also commonly involved. A specific sign of bone involvement in GD is the "Erlenmyer flask" deformity of the distal femur. Pulmonary symptoms are frequently demonstrated in chronic stage.

Patients with type I disease may be asymptomatic or have mild clinical symptoms. In type II disease, patients may show neurologic symptoms in the middle of the first year of life. In patients with type III disease, neurologic symptoms occur in the first few years of life or even later.

GD can now be treated effectively with enzyme replacement, but the cost is prohibitive for most patients. Bone marrow transplantation is curative, but the high risk of this procedure deters its use in patients with mild disease (type I). Gene transfer is a promising therapeutic procedure, although it can provide only a short-term benefit at this stage.[2,3,5]

Niemann–Pick Disease

Niemann–Pick disease (NPD) is an autosomal recessive metabolic disorder. Patients with NPD type I disease have a deficiency of sphingomyelinase, resulting in accumulation of sphinomyelin in visceral organs, such as spleen, liver, bone marrow, lungs, and brain.[6] Type I disease was divided into subtypes IA and IB, which are now respectively redesignated as type A and type B. The type II disease (now designated type C) differs from types A and B in pathogenesis and the stored substance.[7-9] It is characterized by delayed and impaired homeostatic responses to exogenous low-density lipoprotein (LDL) cholesterol loading with lysosomal accumulation of unesterified cholesterol (LDL receptor defect).

Patients with type A disease, the most common form, usually show clinical symptoms, such as hepatosplenomegaly as well as physical and mental retardation, by 6 months of age. Diffuse pulmonary infiltration may also be present in early life. Death occurs in early childhood due to central nervous system (CNS) involvement. In type B disease, the patient may have visceral involvement by lipid-laden macrophages, but the CNS is spared. Therefore, the clinical course is more benign in type B than in type A. Type C disease may be manifested as severe neonatal jaundice, hepatosplenomegaly, dementia, and dystonic posturing

TABLE 6.1
Comparison of Storage Histiocyte Disorders

	Gaucher disease	Niemann–Pick disease	Mucopolysaccharidosis
Enzyme defect	Glucocerebrosidase	Sphingomyelinase[a]	Mucopolysaccharidosis
Accumulated substance	Glucocerebroside	Sphingomyelin	Mucopolysaccharide
Hereditary pattern	Autosomal recessive	Autosomal recessive	Autosomal recessive[b]
Age group	Children	Children	Children
Mild clinical type[c]	Type I	Type B	Variable
Neurologic involvement	Types II, III	Types A, C	Types I–III, VII
Hepatosplenomegaly	Present	Present	Present
Lymph node involvement	Present	Present	Present
Bone marrow involvement	Present	Present	Present
Cytoplasmic characteristic	Striation	Well-defined vacuoles	Minute vacuoles
Positive cytochemical stains	PAS, TRAP,[d] nonspecific esterase	PAS, fat, and phospholipid stains	PAS, toluidine blue O

[a]In Niemann–Pick type C, the defect is LDL receptor on cell surface with accumulation of unesterified cholesterol.
[b]The only exception is Hunter's syndrome, which is X-linked.
[c]Mild type can be seen in young adults.
[d]TRAP = tartrate-resistant acid phosphatase.

in childhood.[7] However, the onset of neurologic symptoms is extremely variable, and patients may not have neurologic changes until the 5th decade.

Mucopolysaccharidoses

Mucopolysaccharidoses are a group of metabolic disorders caused by a deficiency of the lysosomal enzymes involved in the degradation of mucopolysaccharides (MPS).[1,10] This group includes Hurler's syndrome, Scheie's syndrome, Hunter's syndrome, Sanfilippo's syndrome, Morquio's syndrome, Maroteaux–Lamy syndrome, and Sly's syndrome. Besides Hunter's syndrome, which is X-linked, all other syndromes are autosomal recessive disorders. Mental retardation is seen in patients with Hurler's, Hunter's, Sanfilippo's and Sly's syndromes. Patients in various syndromes may also have hydrocephalus, ocular disease, hearing impairment, joint stiffness, obstructive-airway disease, and cardiovascular disease.[10]

PATHOLOGY

Gaucher Disease

The major histopathologic feature is the infiltration of the mononuclear phagocyte system (spleen, liver, bone marrow, and intrathoracic and intraabdominal lymph nodes) by the glucocerebroside-laden macrophages (Gaucher cells) (Figs. 6.1–6.2). The Gaucher cells are round or polyhedral histiocytes, 20–100 μm in diameter, with an eccentrically or centrally located nucleus and abundant pale cytoplasm. The cytoplasm has a striated or fibrillary pattern, like wrinkled tissue paper or "crumpled silk."[4,11] The Gaucher cells may form small focal lesions to nearly total replacement of the bone marrow. Marked reticulin fibrosis may be present in areas of Gaucher cell proliferation. In children with the acute neuronopathic type, Gaucher cells are seen in the Virchow–Robin spaces. Neurons and glial cells may show progressive degeneration but no evidence

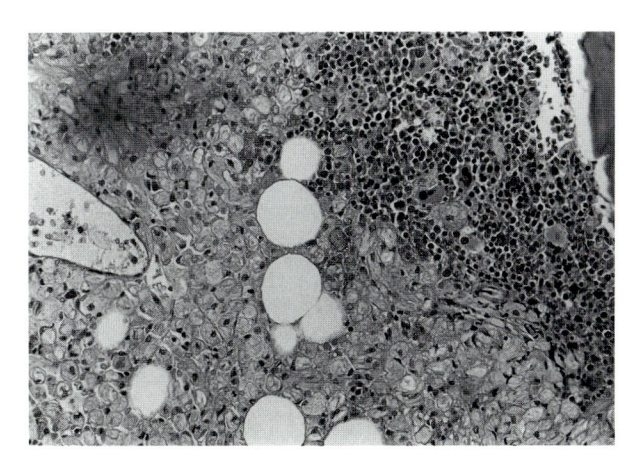

Fig. 6.1. A bone marrow biopsy showing the normal elements are partially replaced by a sheet of Gaucher cells which have eccentrically located nucleus and abundant cytoplasm. H&E, ×250.

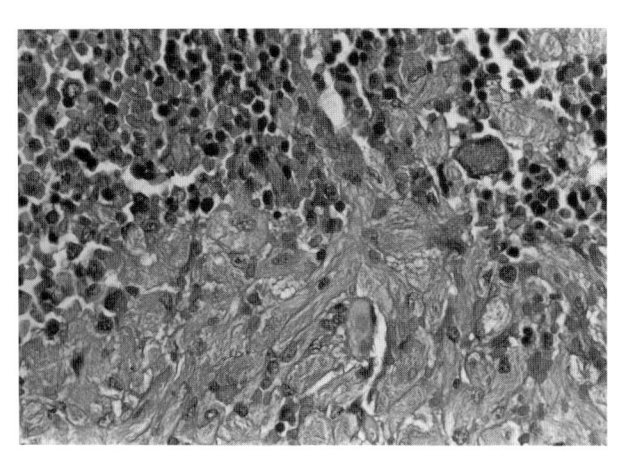

Fig. 6.2. A higher-power view of Fig. 6.1 showing the striated or fibrillary cytoplasmic pattern of the Gaucher cells. H&E, ×500.

of lipid storage. Other internal organs such as lungs, kidney, thymus, tonsils, thyroid, and adrenals may also be infiltrated by Gaucher cells. The incidence of lymphoproliferative disorders (e.g., myeloma and chronic lymphocytic leukemia) is significantly increased in patients with GD and should be ruled out by examination of bone marrow or lymph nodes when suspected.[2]

Under electron microscopy, the intracytoplasmic fibrils appear to be membrane-bound hollow tubules, measuring 250–725 angstroms (Å) in diameter (Fig. 6.3). Cytochemically, the Gaucher cells are positive for periodic-acid Schiff (PAS) reaction (Fig. 6.4), tartrate-resistant acid phosphatase (TRAP), and nonspecific esterase, but are weakly positive or negative for fat stains.[1,4]

Niemann–Pick Disease

As mentioned before, patients with NPD types A and B may have accumulation of sphingomyelin and patients with NPD type C, cholesterol. The lipid-laden phagocytic cells, varying from 20 to 50 μm in diameter, contain numerous sharply defined small vacuoles and sometimes nuclear debris in the cytoplasm, imparting a foamy appearance (Figs. 6.5, 6.6). Sea-blue histiocytes may also be present (Fig. 6.7). These foamy cells are found in the spleen, liver, lymph nodes, bone marrow, tonsils, GI tract, and lungs.[1,6,9]

Unlike GD neurons, the neurons in NPD patients are involved, showing vacuolation and ballooning. The accumulation of lipid substance in neurons finally leads to cell death and loss of brain substance. Because of extensive infiltration by the foamy cells, the spleen is usually markedly enlarged and the liver is moderately enlarged. The size changes in lymph nodes may vary from moderate to marked. In some cases, patients develop hepatocellular damage, cirrhosis, and portal hypertension.

Ultrastructurally, the cytoplasmic vacuoles appear to be engorged secondary lysosomes that contain membranous cytoplasmic bodies resembling concentric lamellated bodies. The vacuoles are positive for fat stains, such as Sudan black (Fig. 6.8) and oil red O, PAS, and Pearce's phospholipid staining.[12]

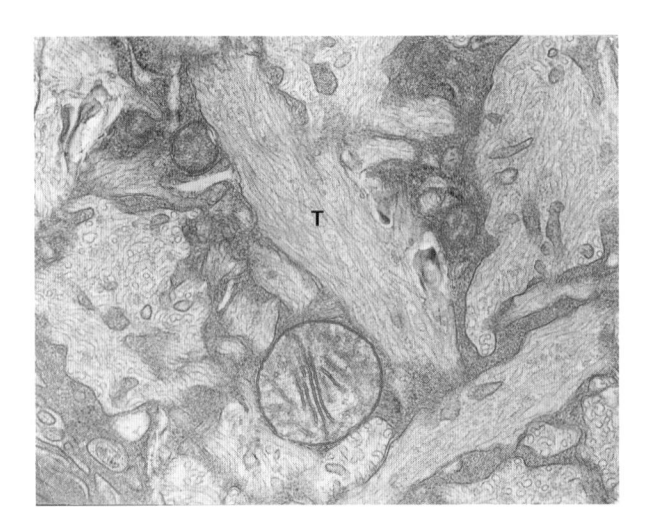

Fig. 6.3. Electron micrograph of a Gaucher cell showing intracytoplasmic membrane-bound hollow tubules (T). ×40,500. (Courtesy of Dr. S. Teichberg and Beth Roberts.)

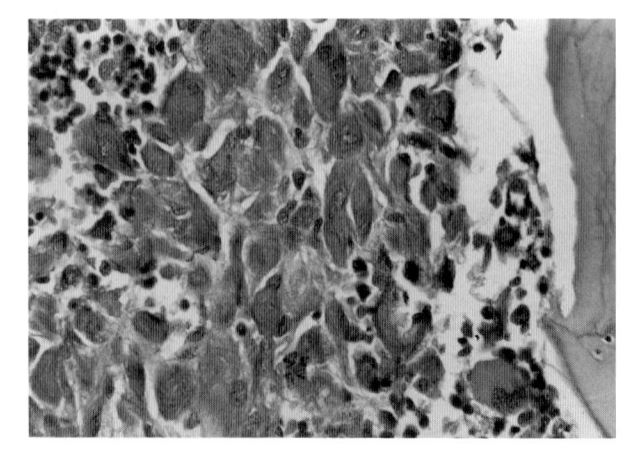

Fig. 6.4. Gaucher cells in the bone marrow showing positive PAS staining. ×500.

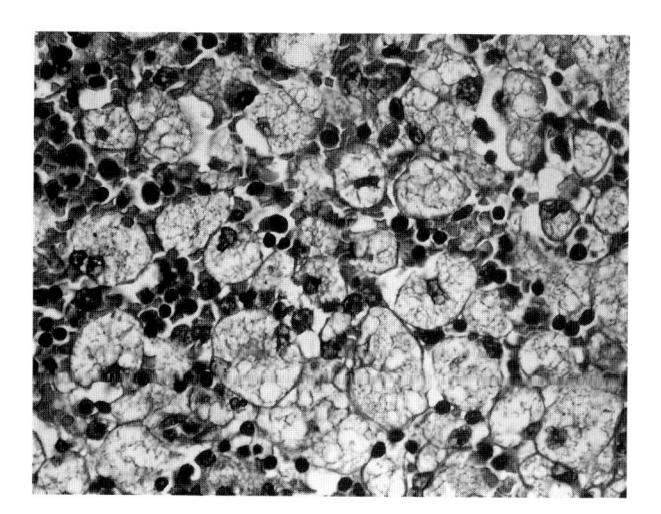

Fig. 6.5. A case of Niemann–Pick disease showing foamy cells in the spleen. H&E, ×280. (Courtesy of Dr. Takeo Narita, from Mod Pathol 7:416, 1994.)

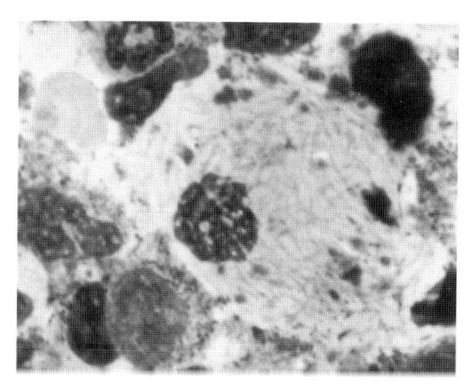

Fig. 6.7. A sea-blue histiocyte in a bone marrow aspirate. Wright-Giemsa, ×1,250.

Mucopolysaccharidosis

As in the other two disorders, the major histopathologic feature is systemic infiltration of multiple organs by the MPS-laden macrophages.[1,10,11] In addition, the endothelial cells, intimal smooth-muscle cells, and fibroblasts may also contain MPS. The organs commonly involved include the liver (Figs. 6.9, 6.10), spleen (Fig. 6.11), bone marrow, lymph nodes (Fig. 6.12), blood vessels, and heart. When the CNS is involved, the neuron may also contain MPS (Fig. 6.13).

The MPS-laden cells show large amounts of clear cytoplasm and are called the "balloon cells." The vacuoles in the cytoplasm are minute and delicate, in contrast to the large vacuoles seen in the foamy histiocytes in NPD. Ultrastructurally, the small vacuoles are swollen lysosomes filled with finely granular, PAS-positive material. The neurons in patients with Hunter's or Hurler's syndrome may also contain a membrane-bound cytosome enclosing many parallel transverse lamellae designated "zebra bodies" (Fig. 6.14).[13] The formation of zebra bodies is the result of ganglioside accumulation.

The bone marrow may contain various numbers of histiocytes packed with basophilic inclusions of varying size, but massive proliferation of histiocytes is rarely seen. These granules stain metachromatically with toluidine blue O, which causes these histiocytes

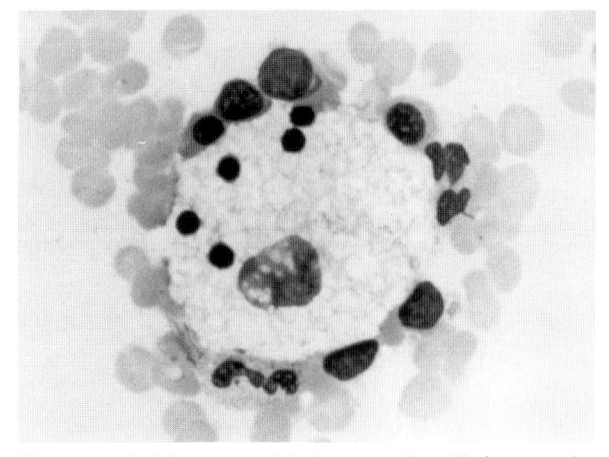

Fig. 6.6. A Niemann–Pick type C cell from a bone marrow. May-Grunwald-Giemsa stain, ×1040. (Courtesy of B.D. Lake, Professor of Histopathology, Great Ormond Street Hospital, London, U.K.)

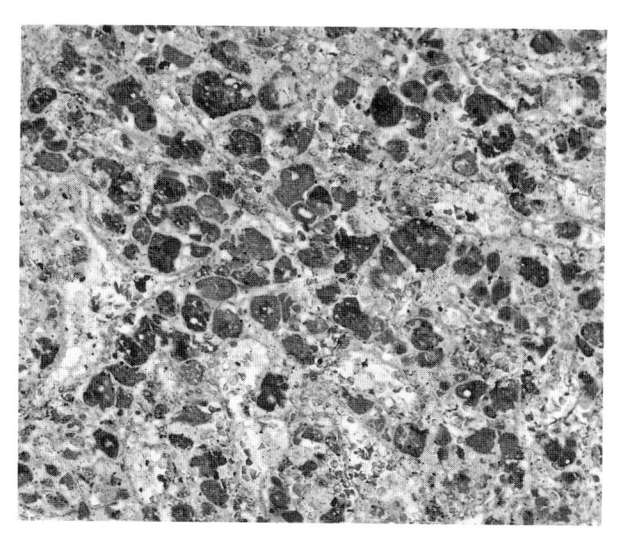

Fig. 6.8. Niemann–Pick cells from spleen showing positive stain for Sudan black B. ×100. (From the same source as Fig. 6.5).

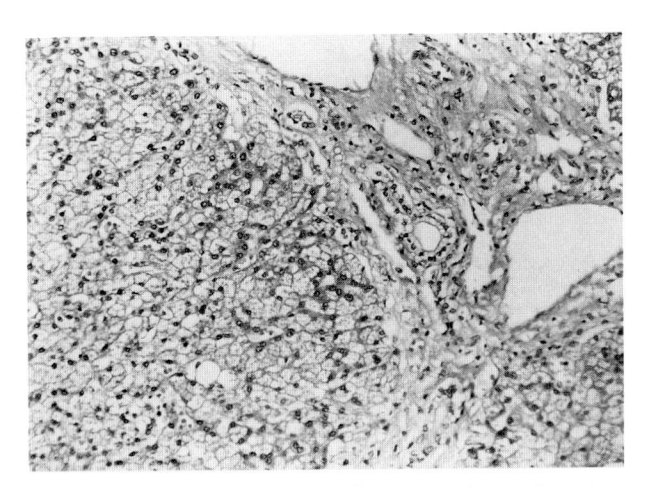

Fig. 6.9. Liver in a case of mucopolysaccharidosis (Hunter syndrome) showing all liver cells and the epithelial cells of the bile duct with clear cytoplasm (balloon cells). H&E, ×250. (Case contributed by Barbara McHeffey-Atkinson, M.D.)

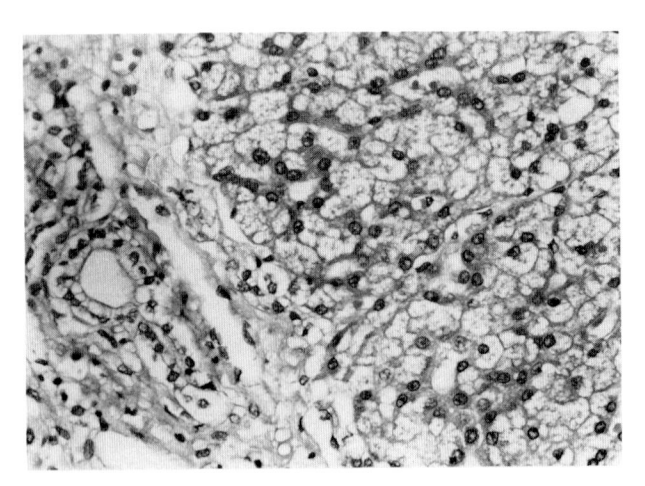

Fig. 6.10. A higher-power view of Fig. 6.9 showing the balloon cells. H&E, ×500.

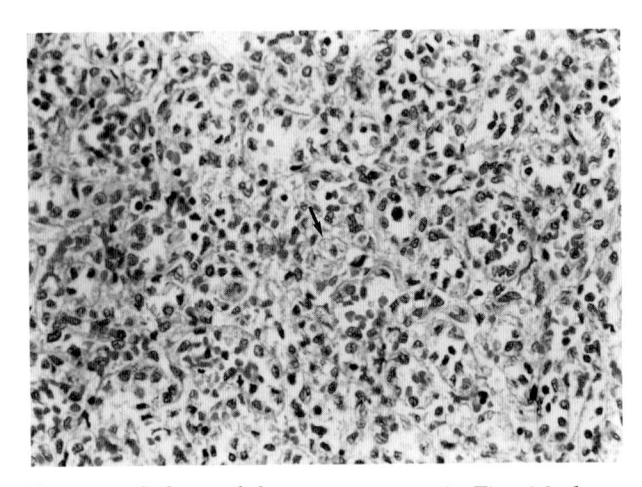

Fig. 6.11. Spleen of the same case as in Fig. 6.9 showing macrophages with clear cytoplasm (balloon cells) (arrow). H&E, ×500.

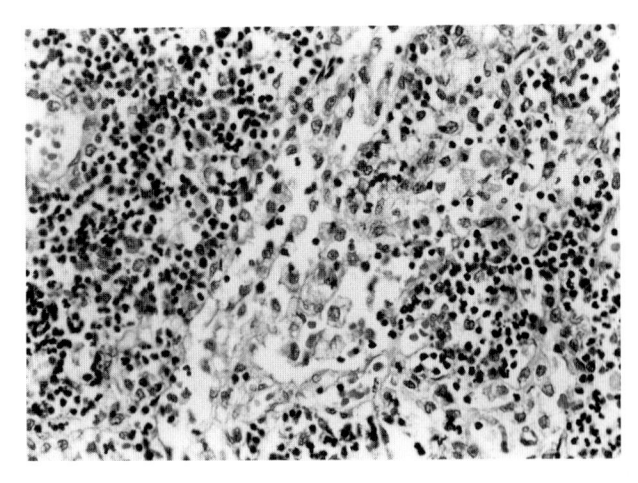

Fig. 6.12. Lymph node of the same case as in Fig. 6.9 showing dilated sinuses containing macrophages with clear cytoplasm (balloon cells). H&E, ×500.

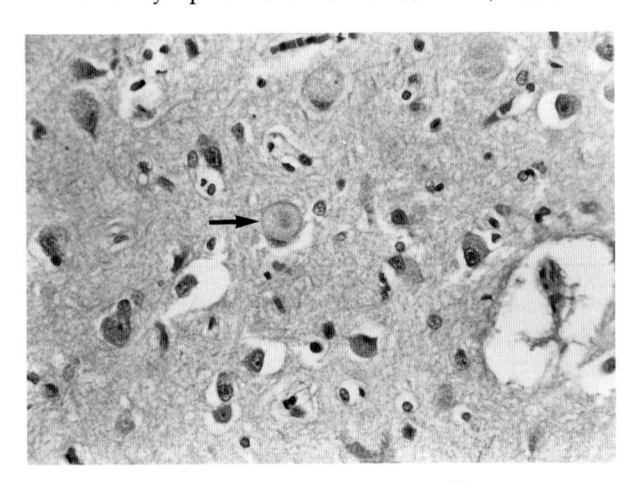

Fig. 6.13. Brain of the same case as in Fig. 6.9 showing ballooning and granularity of the neurons (arrow). H&E, ×500.

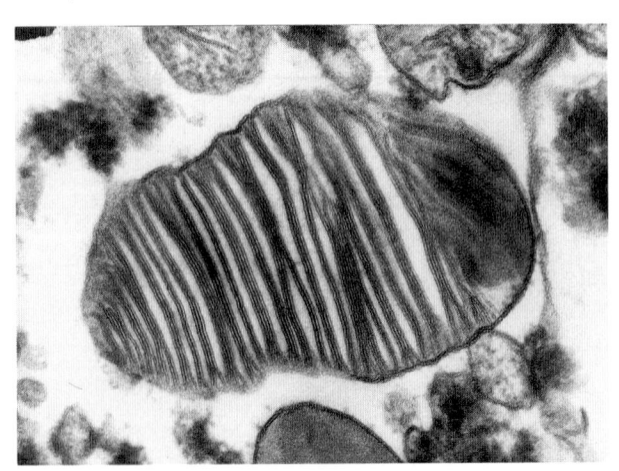

Fig. 6.14. Electron micrograph of a "zebra body" membrane-delimited inclusion inside a neuron from a patient with Hunter syndrome. The banding pattern is formed by the adherence of parallel membranes. ×77,000. (Courtesy of Dr. S. Teichberg and Beth Roberts.)

to resemble mast cells. In some cases, plasma cells may also contain the same granules. In the blood smears, the lymphocytes may contain dark basophilic granules that stain metachromatically with the toluidine blue O stain. The granulocytes may contain Alder–Reilly granules in some cases.

LABORATORY FINDINGS

Gaucher Disease

GD is usually diagnosed by the finding of Gaucher cells in the bone marrow, liver, or spleen. However, the bone marrow is most frequently examined because it is a relatively simple approach. Nevertheless, pseudo-Gaucher cells may be found in the bone marrow of various hematologic disorders, including chronic myelogenous leukemia, acute leukemia, and congenital dyserythropoietic anemia.[1] The simple and reliable way to make the diagnosis of GD is to determine the blood leukocyte β-glucosidase activity, which is decreased.[2] The increased serum acid phosphatase and angiotensin-converting enzyme are not specific for GD but may help substantiate the diagnosis. The most precise tool is the detection of specific mutations at nucleotides 84, 1226, and 1448 by the polymerase chain reaction.

Niemann–Pick Disease

A diagnosis of NPD can be made by identifying the characteristic foamy histiocytes in the liver, bone marrow, or spleen. In the liver, Kupffer cells are typically involved with sphingomyelin or cholesterol storage. Lipid storage may also be demonstrated in the ganglion cells of the rectum.[7] However, foamy histiocytes can also be seen in hyperlipidemia and other conditions; therefore, their demonstration is not entirely specific. A definitive diagnosis should be established by showing a decreased sphingomyelinase activity in liver or bone marrow biopsies, leukocyte extracts, or cultured skin fibroblasts.[1] The sphingomyelinase gene can be detected by DNA probe analysis.[1]

Mucopolysaccharidoses

In mucopolysaccharidoses, basophilic cytoplasmic inclusions can be demonstrated in the lymphocytes in the peripheral blood and in bone marrow histiocytes. These inclusions are metachromatic when stained with toluidine blue O. Histiocytes in viscera assume the balloon appearance showing numerous minute vacuoles. The granulocytes may contain Alder–Reilly granules.

An accurate diagnosis can be achieved by performing a specific enzyme assay characteristic of a particular syndrome, using fibroblasts, leukocytes, or serum (Table 6.2).[14] Glycosaminoglycanuria is the basis for most of the screening test.[10] A recent study showed that quantitative test for glycosaminoglycan may miss some cases and should be complemented by qualitative analysis with cellulose acetate electrophoresis and oligosaccharide screening.[15] Prenatal diagnosis is possible for most mucopolysaccharidoses by measuring enzyme activity in cultured amniotic cells obtained by amniocentesis.[10]

TABLE 6.2
Enzyme Deficiency in Various Types of Mucopolysaccharidoses

Classification	Syndrome	Enzyme Deficiency
MPS I H/S	Hurler–Scheie	α-L-Iduronidase
MPS II	Hunter	Iduronate sulfatase
MPS IIIA	Sanfilippo A	Heparon N-sulfatase
MPS IIIB	Sanfilippo B	α-N-Acetylglucosaminidase
MPS IIIC	Sanfilippo C	Acetyl-CoA: 2-glucosaminide acetyltransferase
MPS IIID	Sanfilippo D	N-Acetylglucosamine 6-sulfatase
MPS IVA	Morquio A	Galactose 6-sulfatase
MPS IVB	Morquio B	β-Galactosidase
MPS VI	Maroteaux–Lamy	N-Acetylgalactosamine 4-sulfatase (arylsulfatase B)
MPS VII	Sly	β-Glucuronidase

REFERENCES

1. Brunning RD, McKenna RW: *Atlas of Tumor Pathology: Tumors of the Bone Marrow*, Washington DC, Armed Forces Institute of Pathology 1994, pp 439–443.
2. Beutler E: Gaucher's disease. *N Engl J Med* 325:1354–1360, 1991.
3. Zimran A, Kay A, Gelbart T, et al: Gaucher disease: Clinical, laboratory, radiologic, and genetic features of 53 patients. *Medicine* 71:337–353, 1992.
4. Kolodny EH: Gaucher disease. In Wyngaarden JB, Smith LH, Bennett JC (eds): *Cecil Textbook of Medicine*, 19th ed, Philadelphia, Saunders, 1992, pp 1091–1093.
5. Beutler E: Gaucher's disease: New molecular approaches to diagnosis and treatment. *Science* 256:794–799, 1992.
6. Putterman C, Zelingher J, Shouval D: Liver failure and the sea-blue histiocyte/adult Niemann–Pick disease: Case report and review of the literature. *J Clin Gastroenterol* 15:146–149, 1992.
7. Kelly DA, Partmann B, Mowat AP, et al: Niemann–Pick disease type C: Diagnosis and outcome in children, with particular reference to liver disease. *J Pediatr* 123:242–247, 1993.
8. Higgins JJ, Patterson MC, Dambrosia JM, et al: A clinical staging classification for type C Niemann–Pick disease. *Neurology* 42:2286–2290, 1992.
9. Elleder M: Niemann–Pick disease. *Pathol Res Pract* 185:293–328, 1989.
10. Muenzer J: Mucopolysaccharidoses. *Adv Pediatr* 32:269–302, 1986.
11. Cotran RS, Kumar V, Robbins SL: *Pathologic Basis of Disease*, 5th ed, Philadelphia, Saunders, 1994, pp 142–145.
12. Narita T, Nakazawa H, Hizawa Y, et al: Glycogen storage disease associated with Niemann–Pick disease: Histochemical, enzymatic and lipid analysis. *Mod Pathol* 7:416–421, 1994.
13. Aleu FP, Terry RD, Zellweger H: Electron microscopy of two cerebral biopsies in gargoylism. *J Neuropathol Exp Neurol* 24:304–317, 1965.
14. Neufield EF, Muenzer J: The mucopolysaccharidoses. In Scriver CR, Beaudet AL, Sly WS, et al (eds): *The Metabolic Basis of Inherited Diseases*, 6th ed, New York, McGraw-Hill, 1989; pp 1565–1588.
15. Piraud M, Boyer S, Mathieu M, et al: Diagnosis of mucopolysaccharidoses in a clinically selected population by urinary glycosaminoglycan analysis: A study of 2,000 urine samples. *Clin Chim Acta* 221:171–181, 1993.

7
Hodgkin's Disease vs. Lymphomas with Reed–Sternberg-Like Cells

Hodgkin's disease (HD) was originally considered to represent a granulomatous inflammation, but its malignant nature has now been well established. However, as the malignant component—the Reed—Sternberg cell—is not the predominant cell population, its isolation and identification have been problematic. Therefore, the cell lineage of Reed–Sternberg cell is still unresolved.

Historically, there have been three important schemes for the classification of HD. The earliest one is that of Jackson and Parker, who divided HD into three types: paragranuloma, granuloma, and sarcoma.[1] Lukes and Butler further divided HD into lymphocytic and/or histiocytic (subtype nodular and diffuse), nodular sclerosis, mixed cellularity, diffuse fibrosis, and reticular.[2] Finally, a simplified classification was adopted at an international meeting in Rye, New York, dividing HD into lymphocyte predominance (LP), nodular sclerosis (NS), mixed cellularity (MC), and lymphocyte depletion (LD).[3] The relationship between these three schemes of classification is summarized in Table 7.1.[4] Although the Rye classification has become most popular, the Lukes–Butler scheme is still used and is incorporated into the Rye classification as subtypes; thus there are nodular and diffuse subtypes in the lymphocytic predominance type as well as diffuse fibrosis and reticular subtypes in the lymphocytic depletion type. The definition of HD as "the identification of diagnostic Reed–Sternberg cells in the appropriate cellular environment," given by Lukes and Butler, is still the most appropriate definition.

CLINICAL FEATURES

Patients with HD have a bimodal age distribution with the first peak in the age group of 15–35 years and the second peak at 50 years and older.[4] However, the age range in various types of HD differs. In general, most patients are male except for the nodular sclerosis type, in which there is a female predominance.

On the basis of the extent of nodal and/or extranodal disease, HD is divided into four stages by the Ann Arbor classification (Table 7.2).[5] Essentially, a single lymph node region or extranodal site involvement is classified as stage I; two or more lymph node regions on the same side of diaphragm, stage II; lymph node regions on both sides of the diaphragm, stage III, and disseminated disease, stage IV. In addition, on the basis of absence or presence of constitutional symptoms, such as fever, sweats, and/or weight loss of 10% of body weight, the disease is further divided into substages A and B, respectively.

Lymphocyte Predominance

LP is seen in approximately 5% of cases of Hodgkin's disease.[4,6,7] It is characteristically seen in young (<35 years of age) males (Table 7.3). Most patients are asymptomatic. About 80% of patients are stage I or II at presentation. The most frequently involved lymph nodes are in the cervical and axillary region, followed by inguinal. The prognosis of LP is very favorable, but it may transform into MC or LD type with subsequent widespread extranodal disease. It is generally believed that the diffuse subtype of LP seldom relapses, while the nodular subtype has a high incidence of relapse. However, more recent studies suggested that these two subtypes may have a similar natural history.[8,9]

Nodular Sclerosis

NS is the most common type of HD, accounting for 60% of the total cases.[4,6,7] This is the only type of HD with female predominance. Patients are usually under 50 years of age, and 60% are stage I or II at presentation. The clinical manifestation is often cervical or supraclavicular lymphadenopathy or a mediastinal mass. NS has a greater histologic stability than do other types of HD. The prognosis is usually good except for the lymphocyte-depletion subtype, which is more frequently seen in men with symptoms and advanced stage of disease.

Mixed Cellularity

MC is the second common type of HD, accounting for approximately 30% of the total cases.[4,6,7] This is considered to be an intermediate form between LP and LD. Therefore, the age range of patients, the clinical

TABLE 7.1
Relation Between Various Histologic Classifications of Hodgkin's Disease

Rye	Lukes & Butler	Jackson & Parker
Lymphocyte predominance	Lymphocytic and/or histiocyte (L&H) Nodular Diffuse	Paragranuloma Granuloma
Nodular sclerosis	Nodular sclerosis	Granuloma
Mixed cellularity	Mixed cellularity	Granuloma
Lymphocyte depletion	Diffuse fibrosis Reticular	Granuloma Sarcoma

course, and the prognosis are all in between LP and LD. The stage at presentation is usually II or III. MC frequently transforms into the LD type of HD.

Lymphocyte Depletion

LD is a rare type of HD, seen in only 5% of total cases.[4,6,7] It is usually encountered in elderly patients with a median age of 50–57 in different reports. Male patients are predominant in this type. Most patients have constitutional symptoms, namely, night sweats in 30% of patients, fever in 60%, and weight loss in 67%.[6] Patients may also have peripheral lymphadenopathy, hepatosplenomegaly, lymphopenia, and subdiaphragmatic disease.[7] Vascular invasion and extranodal spread are common autopsy findings. About 80% of the patients are found to have stage IIIb or IVb at presentation. The prognosis is very poor, especially for patients with the reticular subtype.

PATHOLOGY

The most important criterion for the diagnosis of HD is the identification of the Reed–Sternberg cell and its variants in histologic sections. The diagnostic or classic Reed–Sternberg cell is characterized by its large size, bilobed or polylobated nuclei or multinucleation with prominent acidophilic inclusion-like nucleoli, and abundant amphophilic cytoplasm (Fig. 7.1). There are several variants of Reed–Sternberg cells. The presence of the variants alone is not diagnostic, but it should be an indication for further search of the diagnostic cells. The mononuclear variant is a large cell with a single nucleus that contains a prominent nucleolus. This cell, also called *Hodgkin's cell*, is not diagnostic in an unknown case, but its presence is sufficient for the diagnosis of extranodal HD in patients with known nodal HD. The degenerated form is a dark smudged cell, which is also called a "mummified cell."

The other two variants are also not diagnostic of HD but are characteristic of certain types of HD. The L&H variant or popcorn cells are large cells with folded, convoluted, or lobated nuclei, thin nuclear membrane, vesicular chromatin pattern, and inconspicuous nucleoli (Fig. 7.2). The cytoplasm of these cells is usually abundant and pale-staining. The L&H cells are characteristically seen in the LP type. The lacunar variant is a large cell located in a lacuna-like space (Fig. 7.3). This phenomenon is considered to be an artifact due to formalin fixation, as the lacuna-like space is not seen in other forms of fixation. The lacunar cells have polylobated nuclei, delicate nuclear chromatin, small nucleoli, and abundant water-clear or pale eosinophilic cytoplasm. These cells are typically found in the NS type of HD.

Lymphocyte Predominance

LP is divided into diffuse and nodular subtypes, with the former seen in 2/3 of cases. In the diffuse subtype, the nodal architecture is completely replaced by a diffuse lymphocyte/histiocyte infiltration with a predominance of histiocytes.[4] The histiocytes may form clusters mimicking epithelioid granulomas. The characteristic cell type is the L&H cells (Fig. 7.2), which is

TABLE 7.2
Ann Arbor Staging System of Hodgkin's Disease

Stage	Degree of Involvement
I	Involvement of a single lymph node region (I) or a single extralymphatic site (IE)
II	Involvement of two or more lymph node regions on the same side of the diaphragm (II) or localized involvement of an extralymphatic site (IIE)
III	Involvement of lymph node regions on both sides of the diaphragm (III) or localized involvement of an extralymphatic site (IIIE) or spleen (IIIS) or both (IIISE) when both sides of the diaphragm are involved
IV	Disseminated involvement of one or more extralymphatic sites with or without lymph node involvement

Key: substage A = asymptomatic patients; substage B = patients with fever, sweats, and/or weight loss of >10% of body weight; E = Extranodal disease; S = Splenic involvement.

DIFFERENTIAL DIAGNOSIS OF LYMPHOID DISORDERS 71

TABLE 7.3
Comparison of Four Types of Hodgkin's Disease

	Lymphocyte predominance	Nodular sclerosis	Mixed cellularity	Lmphocyte depletion
Incidence	5%	60%	30%	5%
Peak age group	35 years median	<50 years	35–55 years	55 years median
Predominant sex	Male	Male	Female	Male
Stage at presentation	I or IIa	I or II	II or III	IIIb or IVb
Prognosis	Good	Depends on grades	Intermediate	Poor
Histologic pattern	Diffuse (67%); nodular (33%)	Nodules surrounded by collagen bands	Diffuse infiltrate	Diffuse fibrosis and reticular
Nodal effacement	Complete	Partial	Complete or focal	Complete
Necrosis	Absent	Present	Present	Present
Predominant cells	Diffuse—histiocytes; nodular—lymphocytes	Lymphocyte or mixed	Mixed	Diffuse fribrosis—spindle cells; reticular—pleomorphic RS
Characteristic cell	L&H cell	Lacunar cell	Classic RS[a]	Sarcomatous RS
Reed–Sternberg cell	Rare	Rare to moderate	Moderate	Diffuse fibrosis—rare; reticular—abundant

[a]RS = Reed–Sternberg cell.

frequently admixed with the background infiltrate. In addition, there are mononuclear Hodgkin's cells, mummified cells, abnormal ring-shaped mitosis, and occasional polykaryocytes of the Warthin–Finkeldey type.[7] The classic Reed–Sternberg cells are scarce in LP type, and sometimes a painstaking search for these cells is needed for a definitive diagnosis. Residual germinal centers, if present, are usually found in the subcapsular region.

The nodular subtype differs from the diffuse subtype in the presence of a vague nodular pattern, and the predominant lymphocytic background (Fig. 7.4). Reticulin stain may accentuate the nodular configuration. As in the diffuse subtype, abundant L&H cells, mononuclear Hodgkin's cells, mummified cells, and abnormal mitosis may be present. Classic Reed–Sternberg cells are hard to find. If Reed–Sternberg cells are easily identified, the classification is more

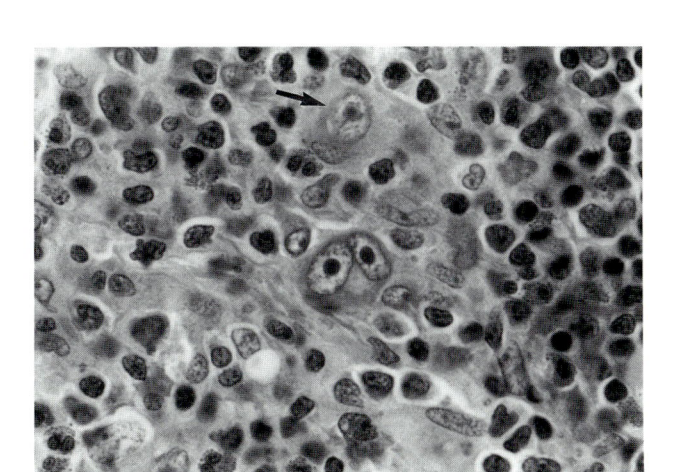

Fig. 7.1. Lymph node biopsy showing a classic Reed–Sternberg cell with a bilobed nucleus, prominent inclusion-like nucleoli, and abundant cytoplasm and a mononuclear Hodgkin's cell (arrow). H&E, ×1250.

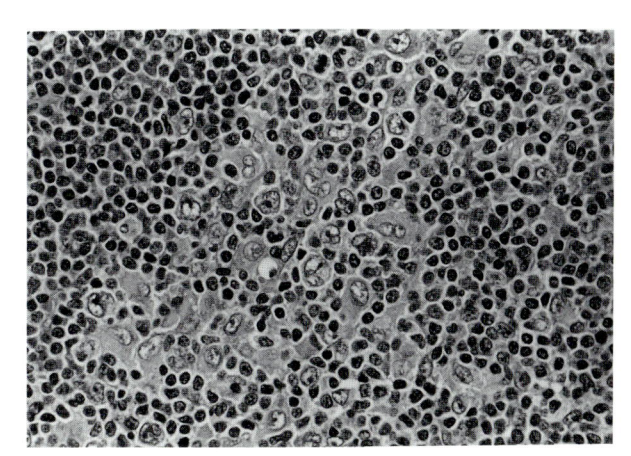

Fig. 7.2. A cluster of L&H variant or popcorn cells in a case of lymphocyte predominance type showing folded, convoluted, or lobated nuclei; vesicular chromatin pattern; inconspicuous nucleoli; and abundant cytoplasm. H&E, ×500.

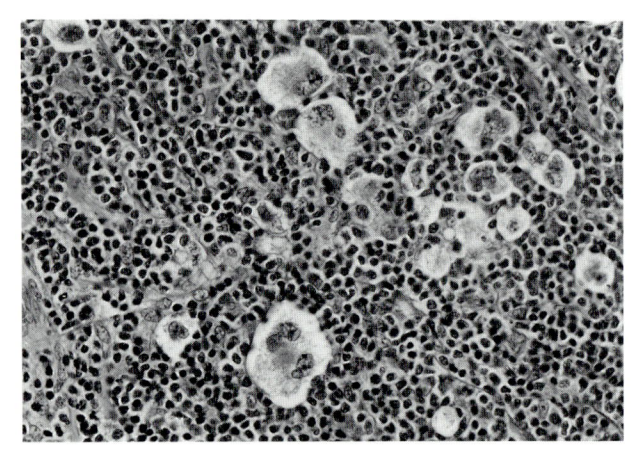

72 DIFFERENTIAL DIAGNOSIS OF LYMPHOID DISORDERS

Fig. 7.3. Multiple lacunar cells are seen in a case of nodular sclerosis type showing polylobated nuclei, delicate nuclear chromatin, small nucleoli, and water-clear cytoplasm. Each cell is located in a lacuna-like space. H&E, ×500.

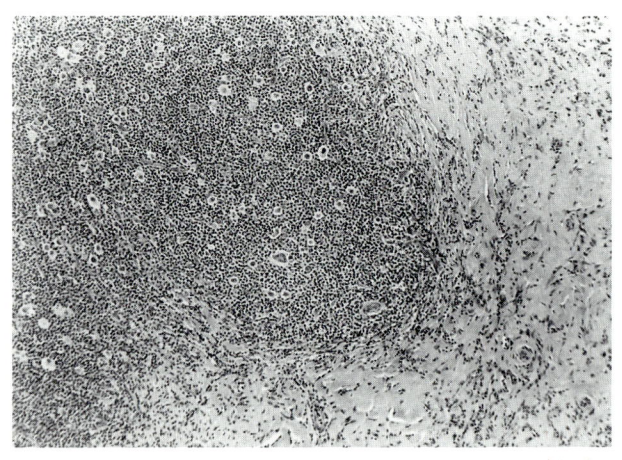

Fig. 7.5. A nodular sclerosis type showing cellular lymphoid nodules surrounded by dense collagenous bands. Many lacunar cells are visible in the lymphoid nodule. H&E, ×125.

likely to be MC rather than LP.[4] Eosinophils, plasma cells, and necrosis are rare in LP.

The LP type, especially its nodular subtype, draws considerable recent interest because its immunophenotype differs from that of other types of HD[10,11] and also because its relationship with progressive transformation of germinal centers (PTGC).[12,13] PTGC is a condition in which the germinal center enlarges to 2–40 times the size of the surrounding normal germinal centers, due to the replacement of the germinal center cells by small lymphocytes with a polyclonal T- or B-cell phenotype. This nodular pattern mimics the nodular pattern of LP. In addition, PTGC may exist before, simultaneously with, or after the presence of nodular LP, leading to the assumption that PTGC is a premalignant state related to this type of HD. However, 80% of PTGC cases do not correlate with HD.

Nodular Sclerosis

The characteristic histologic pattern of NS (see Figs. 7.5, 7.6) is the presence of interconnecting bands of collagen fibers separating lymphoid tissue into cellular

Fig. 7.4. A nodular subtype of lymphocyte predominance type showing complete replacement of nodal architecture by a diffuse lymphocyte/histiocyte infiltration. Note a vague nodular pattern and multiple clusters of pale-stained L&H cells. H&E, ×125.

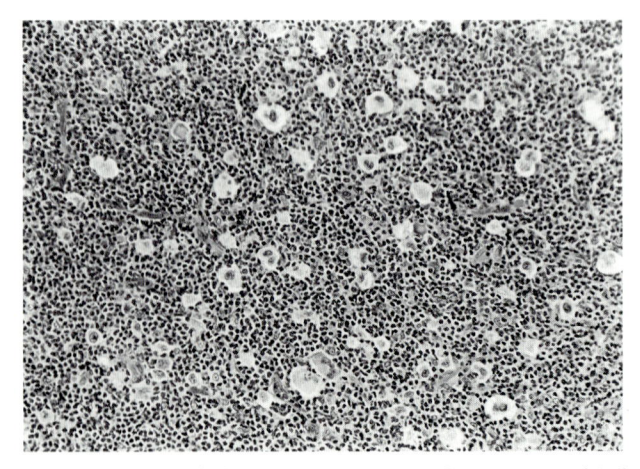

Fig. 7.6. A nodular sclerosis type showing multiple lacunar cells. H&E, ×250.

nodules. The collagen bands can be identified by their birefringent character when examined under polarized light. The characteristic cells of NS are the lacunar variants of Reed–Sternberg cells, which have subtle differences in number and in morphology among various subtypes. The number of classic Reed–Sternberg cells also varies in different subtype of NS. The background cellular components may be predominantly lymphocytes or mixed populations of lymphocytes, granulocytes, and eosinophils. Eosinophilic abscess and areas of central necrosis may be encountered in some cases. When necrosis occurs, Reed–Sternberg cells are more abundant and form cohesive clusters. They are also frequently found in the form of mummified cells. NS is a stable histologic type; therefore, it is proposed that the diagnosis of NS takes precedence over other histologic types when more than one type of histology is present in the same lymph node.[4,7]

On the basis of the cellular background of the nodules, NS can be divided into subtypes of lymphocyte predominance, mixed cellularity, and lymphocyte depletion with predominantly Reed–Sternberg cells.

In the lymphocyte-predominance subtype, the lacunar cells form cohesive clusters mixed with predominantly mature lymphocytes. The nuclei of the lacunar cells are rarely lobulated, and the nucleoli are inconspicuous. Classic Reed–Sternberg cells are scarce.

In the mixed-cellularity subtype, lacunar cells are abundant, are pleomorphic, and have conspicuous nucleoli. Classic Reed–Sternberg cells are easy to find. Focal necrosis is common. The cellular background includes neutrophils, eosinophils, and plasma cells.

In the lymphocyte-depletion subtype, the classic Reed–Sternberg cells are predominant and pleomorphic. The lacunar cells, on the other hand, are rare. Stellate necrosis is frequently present.

In addition, there are several variants of NS. The cellular variant is called the "cellular phase of NS Hodgkin's disease" by Lukes and associates. In this variant, sheets of lacunar cells and occasional Reed–Sternberg cells are present, but no collagen bands are identified. This variant usually shows clinical features and a survival rate closer to MC type than NS type.[14] Therefore, it is more reasonable to be classified as MC. The definition of NS, as some suggested, should include the presence of at least one single band of collagen extending from a thick capsule.[14] The syncytial variant exhibits sheets of lacunar cells and other variants of Reed–Sternberg cells (Figs. 7.7, 7.8). This variant is frequently present in the mediastinum and may be mistaken for thymoma, large-cell lymphoma, and metastatic carcinoma. Under these circumstances, immunophenotyping is often needed for the differential diagnosis. Another variant is obliterative sclerosis or fibrosis (Figs. 7.9, 7.10), in which the lymph node is replaced by extensive fibrosis. The connective tissue between the nodules remain collagenous, but the fibrous tissue inside the nodules is not birefringent. When fibroblasts are predominant, it is called *fibroblastic variant*.

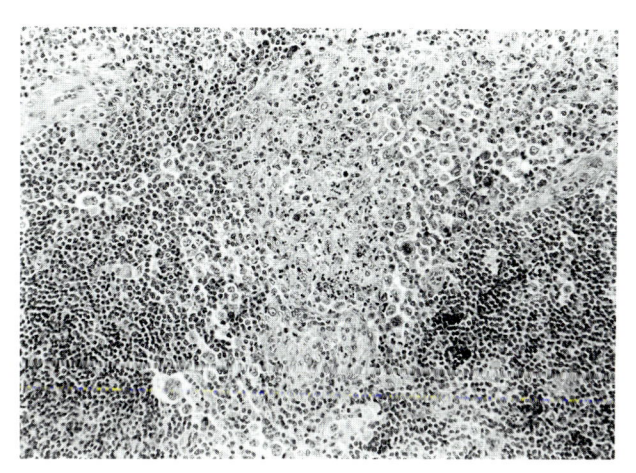

Fig. 7.7. The syncytial variant of nodular sclerosis type showing sheets of lacunar cell surrounding a necrotic area. H&E, ×250.

Mixed Cellularity

MC was originally described by Lukes and Butler[2] as an intermediate form between LP and LD types of HD. While this still holds true, several more unclassi-

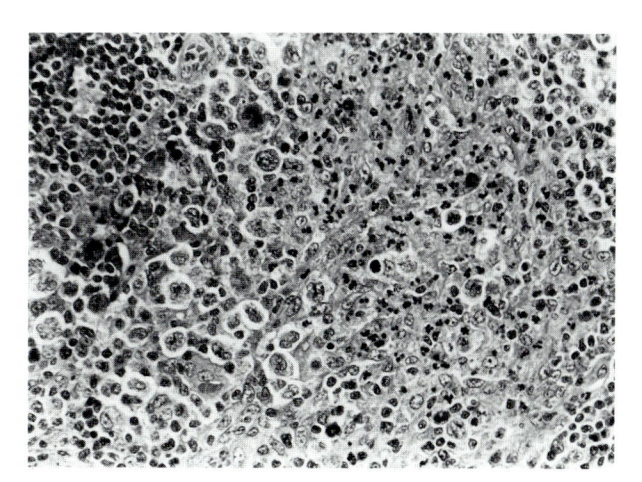

Fig. 7.8. A high-power view of Fig. 7.7 showing lacunar cells adjacent to a necrotic area. H&E, ×500.

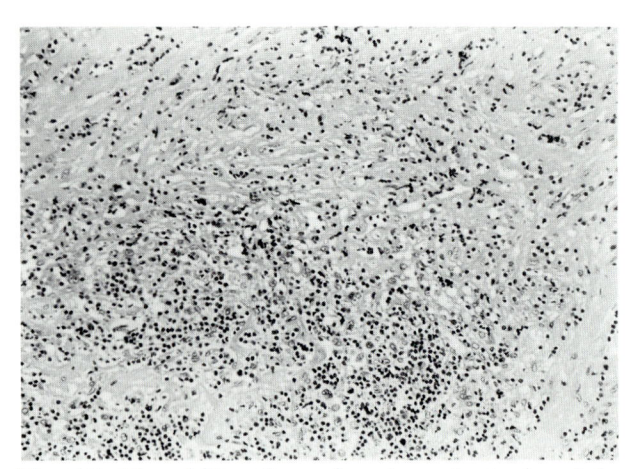

74 DIFFERENTIAL DIAGNOSIS OF LYMPHOID DISORDERS

Fig. 7.9. The obliterative sclerosis variant of nodular sclerosis type showing areas of dense sclerosis. H&E, ×250.

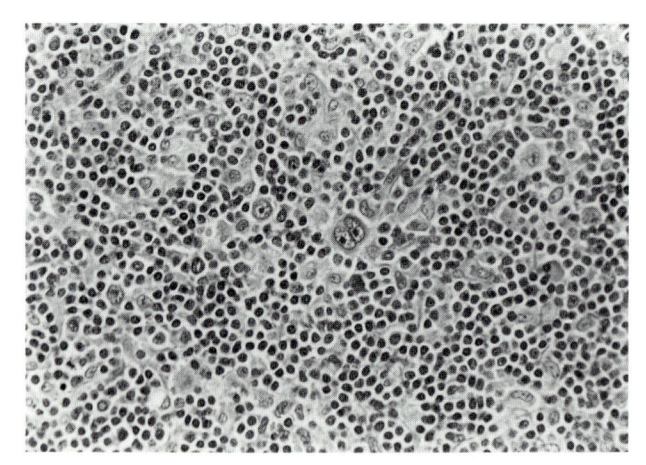

Fig. 7.11. Mixed-cellularity type showing a classic Reed–Sternberg cell in the center with a few mononuclear Hodgkin's cells on a lymphocyte/histiocyte background. H&E, ×500.

fied forms of HD are now included in the MC category. These include focal nodal and extranodal HD (except for NS type), HD with abundant lacunar cells but no collagen fibers, HD with excessive histiocytes, and interfollicular HD. However, the major diagnostic criteria remain in that the numbers of classic Reed–Sternberg cells as well as mature lymphocytes in MC is intermediate between LP and LD types and that there is a mixed cellular background (Figs. 7.11–7.13).[7] As a result of losing mature lymphocytes, the stroma, including noncollagenous fibrous tissue and venules, becomes more distinct in MC. Necrosis may be present in MC type, but this is seldom conspicuous.

A quantitative definition of MC type in terms of numbers of classic Reed–Sternberg cells and mononuclear Hodgkin's cells has been suggested and proved useful.[15,16] The MC type should have 5–15 classic Reed–Sternberg cells and mononuclear Hodgkin's cells per high-power field; while LP should have less than 5, LD should have more than 15 per high-power field. The cellular background in MC usually includes plasma cells, eosinophils, histiocytes, and mature lymphocytes. The number of classic Reed–Sternberg cells are inversely proportional to that of plasma cells and eosinophils. In cases when the mixed cellular background is absent or inconspicuous, the numbers

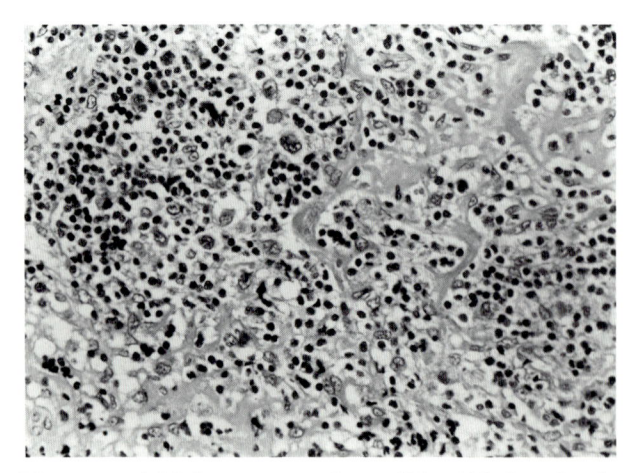

Fig. 7.10. A higher-power view of Fig. 7.9 showing lacunar cells and mononuclear Hodgkin's cells in sclerotic area. H&E, ×500.

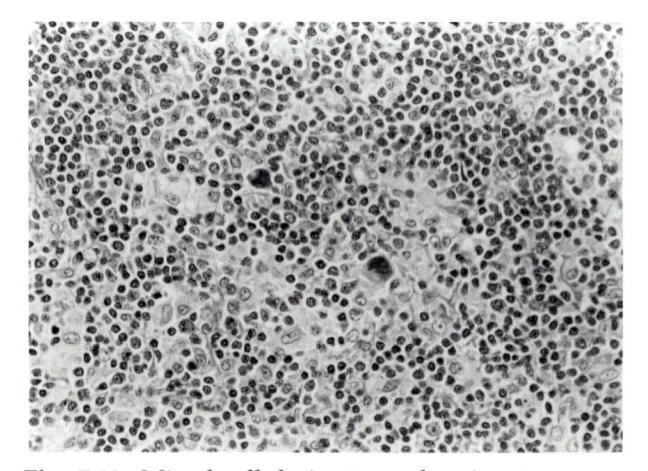

Fig. 7.12. Mixed-cellularity type showing two mummified cells in the center on a mixed cellular background, including lymphocytes, histiocytes, plasma cells, and eosinophils. H&E, ×500.

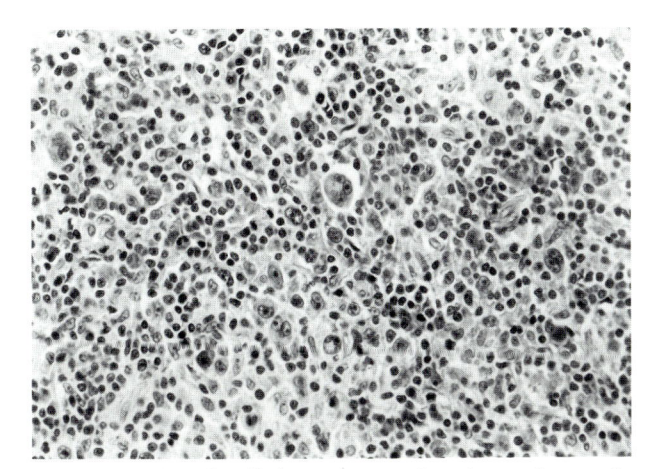

Fig. 7.13. Mixed-cellularity type showing a few polyloblated Reed–Sternberg cells, and mononuclear Hodgkin cells on a mixed cellular background. H&E, ×500.

of classic Reed–Sternberg cells and mono-nuclear Hodgkin's cells become the major criterion.[7]

There are no subtypes in MC, but two variants have been described. The nodal architecture in MC is usually completely effaced, but in the interfollicular variant (Figs. 7.14–7.16), the background is a florid reactive hyperplasia, features of HD are demonstrated only in interfollicular and paracortical areas. The histiocyte-abundant variant is characterized by the existence of a large number of epithelioid histiocytes, which form cohesive clusters, sometimes around areas of necrosis. Occasionally, frank granulomas with Langhans giant

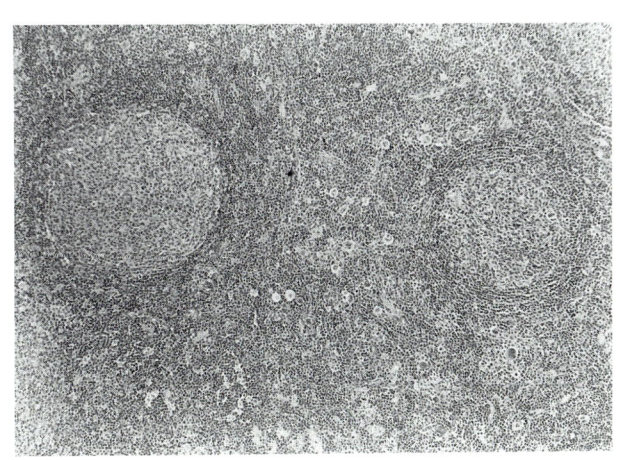

Fig. 7.14. An interfollicular variant of mixed-cellularity type showing two hyperplastic follicles and numerous lacunar cells in the interfollicular areas. H&E, ×125.

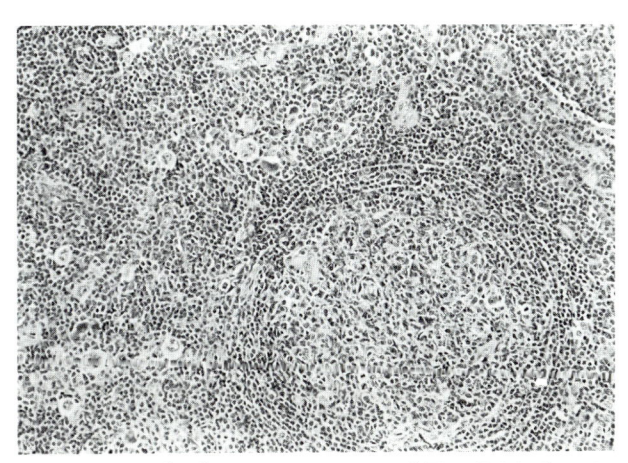

Fig. 7.15. A higher-power view of Fig. 7.14 showing many lacunar cells adjacent to a hyperplastic follicle. H&E, ×250.

cells may be encountered. In the histiocyte-abundant variant, classic Reed–Sternberg cells and mononuclear Hodgkin's cells are easily detected, but L&H cells are seldom found. This phenomenon distinguishes MC from the diffuse subtype of LP. This variant also differs from Lennert's lymphoma by the presence of small, mature lymphocyte instead of the atypical lymphoid cells present in Lennert's lymphoma.

Lymphocyte Depletion

LD is considered to be the last histologic phase of HD, in which tumor cells predominate and reactive lymphocytes diminish.[7] Thus, the classic Reed–Sternberg

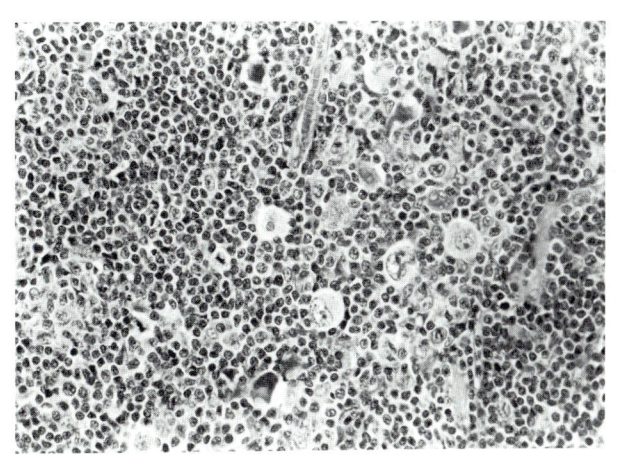

Fig. 7.16. A higher-power view of Fig. 7.14 showing two mummified cells and many lacunar cells. H&E, ×500.

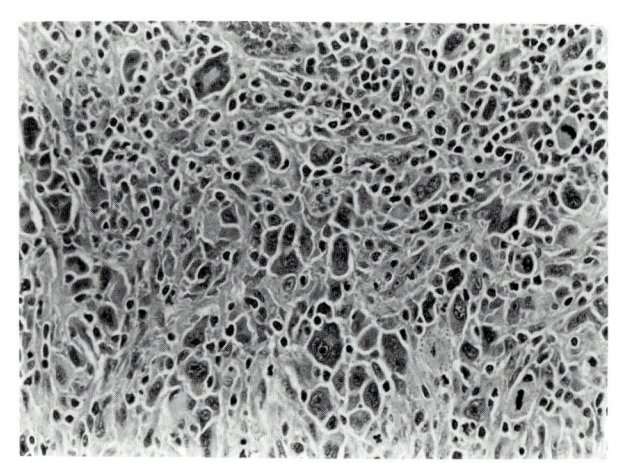

Fig. 7.17. Lymphocyte depletion type showing a large number of Reed–Sternberg cells. H&E, ×500.

cells become abundant and lymphocytes are depleted along with fibrosis (Figs. 7.17, 7.18). On the basis of variations in Reed–Sternberg cells and in the fibrotic pattern, LD type is subdivided into the reticular and diffuse fibrosis subtypes.

The reticular subtype is characterized by the presence of abundant classic Reed–Sternberg cells or of bizarre, multinucleated Reed–Sternberg cells, referred to as *sarcomatous* Reed–Sternberg cells. The latter pattern is called the *sarcomatous variant*. In this variant, there are occasional mononuclear Hodgkin's cells, mummified cells, and scattered aberrant mitoses. In the background, lymphocytes are scarce and plasma cells, eosinophils, histiocytes, and neutrophils are also rare or absent. The fibrosis is diffuse, patchy, irregular, and fibrillar in nature. The fibrous tissue is not birefringent and thus not collagenous. Focal necrosis is common in this subtype. When the sarcomatous variant shows cellular fibroblastic proliferation with a whorled, storiform pattern, it is classified as HD with a fibrosarcoma pattern. The nonsarcomatous variant of the reticular subtype also shows abundant Reed–Sternberg cells, but only a few of them exhibit the bizzare morphology. The fibrosis is rather acellular and inconspicuous.

In the subtype of diffuse fibrosis, lymphocytes are depleted, fibrosis is diffuse and disorderly, the number of Reed–Sternberg cells is variable and focal necrosis is frequently present. A distinctive variant in this subtype is characterized by an acellular fibrosis along the reticular network of the lymph node forming a sinusoidal pattern. In this subtype, classic Reed–Sternberg cells may be rare. The extensive fibrosis should be distinguished from the nonneoplastic fibrous scars following treatment of HD.

Extranodal Hodgkin's Disease

Primary extranodal HD was extremely rare before the AIDS epidemic. It is more frequently seen in the spleen, liver, and lungs than other organs. When the spleen is involved, it is usually secondary to nodal HD. The requirement for the diagnosis of extranodal HD is the same as nodal HD. The mere presence of granuloma in extranodal sites does not indicate involvement of these organs by HD.[4] On the other hand, extranodal organs, such as liver or bone marrow, may show only atypical changes. However, if the patient is known to have HD, the presence of mononuclear Hodgkin's cells should be sufficient to establish the diagnosis.[4,7]

In the spleen, the white pulp is exclusively involved, whereas the red pulp is characteristically spared. The detection of more than 4 nodules in the spleen usually indicates poor prognosis.[4,7] On the other hand, in patients with normal-sized or small-sized spleens, multiple sectioning is required to determine whether the spleen is involved with HD. In mild cases, the liver may show only lymphocytic infiltration of the portal areas with slight architectural alteration, and a bone marrow biopsy may reveal only foci of fibrosis. Under these circumstances, serial sections should be examined to achieve accurate staging.

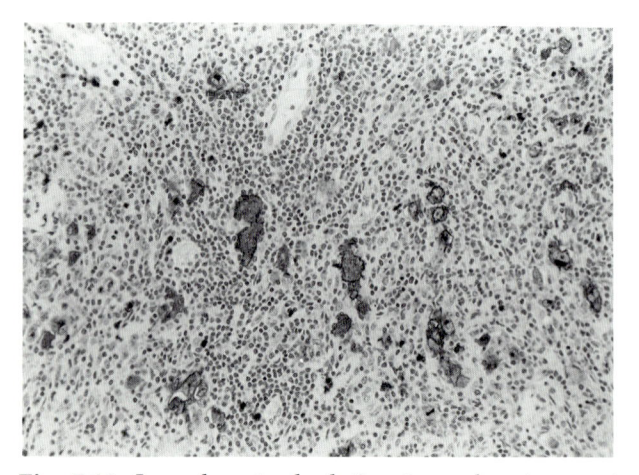

Fig. 7.18. Lymphocyte depletion type showing positive CD15 (LeuM1) staining of Reed–Sternberg cells and mononuclear Hodgkin's cells. Immunoperoxidase, ×250.

LABORATORY FINDINGS

Immunophenotyping

The origin of Reed–Sternberg cells has been speculated to be macrophages, histiocytes, interdigitating reticulum cells, dendritic reticulum cells, myelocytes, and lymphocytes. Although still not entirely conclusive, current immunophenotypic studies strongly suggest a lymphoid origin of the Reed–Sternberg cells, which is supported by immunogenotyping and karyotyping.[17,18] Although almost all myelomonocytic markers tested are negative for Reed–Sternberg cells, CD15 (LeuM1), a granulocytic marker, is consistently positive for Reed–Sternberg cells in the NS, MC, and LP types and serves to distinguish these types from the nodular subtype of LD (Table 7.4). CD15 has been demonstrated in non-Hodgkin's lymphoma of T-cell lineage; thus its reaction to Reed–Sternberg cells does not necessarily contradict the lymphoid origin of the latter. Another consistent marker for Reed–Sternberg cells is CD30 (Ki-1, Ber-H2). Although CD30 can be positive in some cases of non-Hodgkin's lymphomas and is consistently positive for a special type of anaplastic large-cell lymphoma, it is one of the most reliable markers for Reed–Sternberg cells both *in vitro* and *in vivo*.[19] Again, CD30 is positive for Reed–Sternberg cells only in NS, MC, and LD types but negative in LP type.

It turns out that CD30 is an activation antigen for lymphocytes. Subsequently, several other activation antigens have also been found positive for Reed–Sternberg cells, such as CD25 (IL-2 receptor), CD71 (transferin receptor), and HLA-DR (Ia). Proliferative markers, including Ki-67 and proliferating cell nuclear antigen (PCNA), are also frequently found in the nuclei of Reed–Sternberg cells.[17]

In terms of lymphoid markers, the nodular subtype of LP differs distinctly from NS, MC, and LD types. The nodular subtype of LP is positive for CD45 (LCA), CD20 (L26), J-chain, and polyclonal surface immunoglobulin but negative for CDw75 (LN1), the reactions to these antigens are exactly the opposite to those in NS, MC, and LD types.[11,17,18] Besides the activation antigens, the only lymphoid marker these four types share is CD74 (LN2). The phenotypic results of nodular LP subtype are mainly demonstrated in the L&H cells and occasionally classic Reed–Sternberg cells. Recently, monoclonal light chain in RNA has been successfully demonstrated by *in situ* hybridization techniques in nodular LP subtype of HD[20] despite the fact that these same techniques failed to demonstrate immunoglobulin light chain in RNA in 10 similar cases.[10]

Because of the specific phenotype of the Reed–Sternberg cells in the nodular LP subtype, the question has been raised as to whether they are real Reed–Sternberg cells.[7,11] In addition, the nodular LP subtype has several distinctive clinical features, such

TABLE 7.4
Phenotypes of Four Types of Hodgkin's Disease

	Lymphocyte predominance[a]	Nodular sclerosis	Mixed cellularity	Lmphocyte depletion
CD45 (LCA)	+	−	−	−
CD15 (LeuM1)	−	+	+	+
CD20 (L26)	+	−	−	−
CD25 (IL-2R)	+	+	+	+
CD30 (BerH2)	±	+	+	+
CD43 (MT1)	−	−	−	−
CD45RO (UCHL-1)	−	−	−	−
CD71 (OKT9)	+	+	+	+
CD74 (LN2)	+	+	+	+
CDw75 (LN1)	−	+	+	+
Surface Ig[b]	+	−	−	−
J chain	+	−	−	−
HLA-DR (Ia)	+	+	+	+
EMA	+	−	−	−

[a] The phenotype of lymphocytic predominance is based on its nodular subtype. The phenotype of its diffuse subtype is intermediate between the nodular subtype and the other three types.
[b] Ig = immunoglobulin.

as indolent clinical course, long-term survival, unimodal age distribution, a predilection to involve single lymph nodes, and a low incidence of thymic involvement.[11] The nodular LP subtype also tends to transform to diffuse, large-B-cell lymphoma as evidenced by the presence of epithelial membrane antigen (EMA) in both nodular LP and the secondary neoplasm.[11] EMA is seldom present in lymphomas. Therefore, nodular subtype is now considered to be a clinicopathologic entity distinct from other types of Hodgkin's disease.

With immunohistochemical techniques, T-cell antigens, such as CD43 (MT1) and CD45RO (UCHL-1), are usually negative for all types of HD. However, certain reports demonstrated CD2, CD3, and CD4 in NS and MC types or CD1, CD2, CD3, and CD4 in NS, MC, and LD types.[17]

Immunogenotyping

Rearrangements of immunoglobulin genes and T-cell receptor genes have been demonstrated in some cases of HD. However, the results varied widely; the range is 10–50% in studies of immunoglobulin genes, for instance.[17] In addition, these results differ from those seen in non-Hodgkin's lymphomas in several aspects.[17,18] First, the intensity of the rearranged bands does not correlate with the population size of Reed–Sternberg cells. Many studies showed only oligoclonal bands. Second, there is frequent discrepancy between phenotyping and genotyping results (e.g., B-cell phenotype but T-cell genotype), as well as between heavy-chain and light-chain genes (e.g., germline heavy-chain gene but rearranged light-chain gene). These studies may support the contention that Reed–Sternberg cells are of lymphoid origin, but it is not yet certain whether they are stem cells, B-cells, or T-cells and whether they are of clonal population.

Cytogenetics

Clonal chromosomal abnormalities in CD15+, CD30+ cells (i.e., Reed–Sternberg cells) have been demonstrated in a few studies.[21,22] Most clonal chromosomal abnormalities are numeric alterations, involving many different chromosomes. Structural abnormalities are rare, and no predominant pattern has been identified. The demonstration of t(14;18) translocation is particularly interesting as it further supports the lymphoid nature of the Reed–Sternberg cells. A recent study revealed that 2 out of 32 cases of HD had t(14;18) and expression of *bcl-2* oncogene; both cases had a prior history of follicular lymphoma, suggesting that a small proportion of HD cases may evolve from follicular lymphoma.[23]

Oncogene Alterations

The most commonly expressed oncogene in HD is *bcl-2*, with a frequency varying from 9% to 53%.[17,24,25] Other oncogenes found occasionally in HD include *c-ets*, *c-myb*, *c-myc*, *c-jun*, *c-raf*, and *N-ras*.[17,18] The tumor suppressor gene p53 is expressed on Reed–Sternberg cells with high frequency, but its expression does not correlate with clinical staging, B-symptoms, probability of relapse, or disease-free survival.[26] High-level p53 expression in most cases of Ki-1-positive anaplastic large-cell lymphoma was not accompanied by mutation in p53 exons 5 through 9.[27] It is probably also true for HD that over-expression of p53 does not necessarily indicate p53 mutation.

Relationship between Epstein–Barr Virus (EBV) and Hogkin's Disease

A larger-than-expected proportion of patients with HD showed elevated antibody titers against EBV capside antigen (VCA).[17,18] In tissue involved by HD, EBV antigens, EBV DNA, and EBV-encoded RNA can be demonstrated by various techniques, including immunoperoxidase stain, Southern blotting, *in situ* hybridization, and polymerase chain reaction. The demonstration of monoclonal EBV in the nuclei of Reed–Sternberg cells proves the monoclonality of these cells.[28,29] A high prevalence of EBV in the Reed–Sternberg cells has been shown in HIV-associated Hodgkin's disease.[30] On the other hand, EBV genome is seldom detected in the nodular LP subtype of HD. EBV-induced *bcl-2* activation with subsequent suppression of apoptosis is a possible mechanism of HD development.[17]

DIFFERENTIAL DIAGNOSIS

HD may mimic many different diseases, but only diseases with Reed–Sternberg-like cells are discussed in this chapter. Differential diagnosis with other diseases are discussed in Chapters 8, 14, and 15.

Lennert's Lymphoma

Lennert's lymphoma (LL) was originally considered a type of HD. It may occasionally show large pleomorphic lymphoma cells mimicking Reed–Sternberg cells.[7] The diffuse histiocytic infiltrate in LL is similar to that of diffuse subtype of LP. When the background is composed of plasma cells, eosinophils, and histiocytes, the MC type of HD should be distinguished. However, the atypical, angular lymphoid cells in LL with its CD45-positive, T-cell antigen phenotype can help establish the diagnosis of LL. A few cases of LL can be of B-cell phenotype, in which a monoclonal B-cell pattern should be helpful in differential diagnosis.

Other Peripheral T-Cell Lymphomas

Other peripheral T-cell lymphomas (see Chapters 16, 17, and 21), including angioimmunoblastic lymphadenopathy-like lymphoma and angiocentric T-cell lymphoma, often have Reed–Sternberg-like cells. However, the atypical small lymphocytes in the background in T-cell lymphomas help distinguish them from HD. Furthermore, T-cell lymphomas usually show loss of one or more pan-T-cell markers and presence of CD43 and CD45RO.[18]

Ki-1 Positive Anaplastic Large Cell Lymphoma (ALCL)

ALCL (see Chapter 14), as its name indicates, is a large-cell lymphoma with an anaplastic appearance. Some tumor cells may show inclusion-like nucleoli resembling Reed–Sternberg cells. The tumor often has a sinus infiltration pattern and may mimic the syncytial variant of the NS type. As most cases of ALCL are of T-cell lineage, the tumor cells are usually in the paracortical areas with sparing of B-cell regions. The presence of collagen fibers in ALCL makes it difficult to distinguish from the NS type of HD[7]. However, lacunar cells are not present in ALCL. The immunophenotype of ALCL is also similar to that of HD, as it is always CD30 positive and sometimes CD15-positive. However, the positive reactions to CD45 (LCA), CD43 (MT-1), and EMA help distinguish ALCL from HD.[4,7,18] In genotyping, ALCL may show clearcut rearranged bands for T-cell receptor genes, while HD may not.

Large-Cell Immunoblastic Lymphoma

Large-cell immunoblastic lymphoma (LCIL), especially the polymorphous subtype, may show Reed–Sternberg-like cells and it is sometimes difficult to distinguish from the LD type of HD. Grogan emphasized the morphology of the mononuclear Hodgkin's cells as the key factor in differentiation of these two entities.[7] In LCIL, the ratio of mononuclear to multinuclear cells is higher and the nuclei of the mononuclear cells are more regular than those seen in HD. On the other hand, the background lymphocytes are more irregular in LCIC than in HD. The immunophenotypes of positive CD45, CD20 (in B-cell cases), or CD43/CD45RO/CD3 (in T-cell cases) readily distinguish LCIC from HD. The demonstration of gene rearrangement in either immunoglobulin or T-cell receptor genes favors LCIC.

T-Cell Rich B-Cell Lymphoma

T-cell-rich B-cell lymphoma (TRBL) (see Chapter 11) is probably an early stage of a large-B-cell lymphoma. The large tumor cells may mimic Reed–Sternberg cells. The background lymphocytes, however, are usually more irregular than those seen in HD. The Reed–Sternberg-like cells are B-cells that stain positive for CD45, CD20, and monotypic surface immunoglobulin. Although the nodular subtype of LP type may express a B-cell lineage, monotypic surface immunoglobulin is usually absent in the HD cases. Genotyping may help distinguish these two entities, but in TRBL cases with extremely low numbers of tumor cells, immunoglobulin gene rearrangement may not be demonstrated.

Richter's Syndrome

In Richter's syndrome (RS) (see Chapter 10), the large-cell lymphoma component may be morphologically similar to Reed–Sternberg cells and the component of chronic lymphocytic leukemia may resemble the background lymphocytes in the LP type of HD. Immunophenotype may demonstrate two monoclonal B-cell populations (large-cell and small-cell) and immunogenotyping may show immunoglobulin gene rearrangement in RS.

Mediastinal Large B-Cell Lymphoma with Sclerosis

This lymphoma, because of its location in the mediastinum, and because of the presence of large immunoblast-like cells surrounded by bands of collagen, should be distinguished from NS type of HD.[7] However, no lacunar cells are present in the mediastinal B-cell lymphoma. The demonstration of its B-cell lineage by both immunophenotyping or genotyping can also distinguish it from HD. Nevertheless, this tumor is frequently surface-immunoglobulin-negative, so that a monotypic surface immunoglobulin pattern may be absent.[31]

Benign Immunoblastic Proliferations

Benign immunoblastic proliferations (see Chapters 4 and 16), such as virus-induced lymphadenitis, AIDS-associated lymphadenopathy, and angioimmunoblastic lymphadenopathy, may show Reed–Sternberg-like cells and a mixed cellular background, mimicking MC-type HD. Viral lymphadenitis usually reveals a mottled pattern with the immunoblasts scattered in a lymphoid background. The reactive lymphocytes in the benign lesions are usually a mixture of T- and B-cells, while the Reed–Sternberg-like cells are often negative for CD30 and CD15 with probably the exception of CMV infection in which CD15 is frequently positive.

Small Lymphocytic Lymphoma

Small lymphocytic lymphoma is seldom a diagnostic problem in distinction from HD. However, Reed–Sternberg-like cells and L&H cells can be occasionally demonstrated in this entity[7], and thus it should be considered in the differential diagnosis. Immunophenotyping or immunogenotyping to demonstrate a monoclonal B-cell population is instrumental in establishing the diagnosis of small-cell lymphocytic lymphoma.

REFERENCES

1. Jackson H Jr, Parker F Jr: *Hodgkin's Disease and Allied Disorders*, New York, Oxford University Press, 1947.
2. Lukes RJ, Butler JJ: The pathology and nomenclature of Hodgkin's disease. *Cancer Res* 26:1063–1081, 1966.
3. Lukes RJ, Craver LF, Hall TC, et al: Report of the nomenclature committee. *Cancer Res* 26:1311, 1966.
4. Burke JS: Hodgkin's disease: Histopathology and differential diagnosis. In Knowles DM (ed): *Neoplastic Hematopathology*, Baltimore, Williams & Wilkins, 1992; pp 497–533.
5. Carbone PP, Kaplan HS, Musshoff K, et al: Report of the committee on Hodgkin's disease staging classification. *Cancer Res* 31:1860–1861, 1971.
6. Lukes RJ, Collins RD: *Atlas of Tumor Pathology: Tumor of the Hematopoietic System*, Washington DC, Armed Forces Institute of Pathology, 1992, pp 225–272;.
7. Grogan TM: Hodgkin's disease, in Jaffe ES (ed): *Surgical Pathology of the Lymph Nodes and Related Organs*, 2nd ed, Philadelphia, Saunders, 1995, pp 133–192.
8. Borg-Grech A, Radford JA, Crowther D, et al: A comparative study of the nodular and diffuse variants of lymphocyte-predominant Hodgkin's disease. *J Clin Oncol* 7:1303–1309, 1989.
9. Tefferi A, Zellers RA, Banks PM, et al: Clinical correlates of distinct immunophenotypic and histologic subcategories of lymphocyte-predominance Hodgkin's disease. *J Clin Oncol* 8:1959–1965, 1990.
10. Momose H, Chen YY, Ben-ezra J, et al: Nodular lymphocyte-predominant Hodgkin's disease: Study of immunoglobulin light chain protein and mRNA expression. *Hum Pathol* 23:1115–1119, 1992.
11. Mason DY, Banks PM, Chan J, et al: Nodular lymphocyte predominance Hodgkin's disease: A distinct clinicopathological entity. *Am J Surg Pathol* 18:526–530, 1994.
12. Dorfman RF: Progressive transformation of germinal centers: Clinical significance and lymphocytic predominant Hodgkin's disease—the Stanford experience. *Am J Surg Pathol* 11:150–151, 1987.
13. Hansmann ML, Fellbaum C, Hui PK, et al: Progressive transformation of germinal centers with and without association to Hodgkin's disease. *Am J Clin Pathol* 93:219–226, 1990.
14. Colby TV, Hoppe RT, Warnke RA: Hodgkin's disease: A clinicopathologic study of 659 cases. *Lancet* 49:1848–1858, 1982.
15. Mann RB, Jaffe ES, Berard CW: Malignant lymphomas: A conceptual understanding of morphologic diversity. *Am J Pathol* 94:105–192, 1979.
16. Correa P, O'Connor GT, Berard DW, et al: International comparability and reproducibility in histologic subclassification of Hodgkin's disease. *J Natl Cancer Inst* 50:1429–1435, 1973.
17. Haluska FG, Brufsky AM, Canellos GP: The cellular biology of the Reed–Sternberg cell. *Blood* 84:1005–1019, 1994.
18. Kadan ME: Hodgkin's disease: Immunobiology and pathogenesis. In Knowles DM (ed): *Neoplastic Hematopathology*, Baltimore, Williams & Wilkins, 1992, pp 535–554.
19. Falini B, Flenghi L, Fedeli L, et al: In vivo targeting of Hodgkin and Reed–Sternberg cells of Hodgkin's disease with monoclonal antibody Ber-H2 (CD30): Im-

munohistological evidence. *Br J Haematol* 82:38–45, 1992.
20. Hell K, Pringle JH, Hansmann ML, et al: Demonstration of light chain in RNA in Hodgkin's disease. *J Pathol* 171:137–143, 1993.
21. Teerenhovi L, Lindholm C, Pakkala A, et al: Unique display of a pathologic karyotype in Hodgkin's disease by Reed–Sternberg cells. *Cancer Genet Cytogenet* 34:305–311, 1988.
22. Schlegelberger B, Weber-Matthiessen K, Himmler A, et al: Cytogenetic findings and results of combined immunophenotyping and karyotyping in Hodgkin's disease. *Leukemia* 8:72–80, 1994.
23. LeBrun DP, Ngan BY, Weiss LM, et al: The bcl-2 oncogene in Hodgkin's disease arising in the setting of follicular non-Hodgkin's lymphoma. *Blood* 83:223–230, 1994.
24. Stetler-Stevenson M, Crush-Stanton S, Cossman J: Involvement of bcl-2 gene in Hodgkin's disease. *J Natl Cancer Inst* 82:855–858, 1990.
25. Gupta RK, Whelan JS, Lister TA, et al: Direct sequence analysis of the t(14;18) chromosomal translocation in Hodgkin's disease. *Blood* 79:2084–2088, 1992.
26. Xerri L, Bouabdallah R, Camerlo J, et al: Expression of the p53 gene in Hodgkin's disease: Dissociation between immunohistochemistry and clinicopathological data. *Hum Pathol* 25:449–454, 1994.
27. Cesarman E, Inghirami G, Chadburn A, et al: High levels of p53 protein expression do not correlate with p53 gene mutations in anaplastic large cell lymphoma. *Am J Pathol* 143:845–856, 1993.
28. Weiss L, Movahed L, Warnke R, et al: Detection of Epstein–Barr viral genomes in Reed–Sternberg cells of Hodgkin's disease. *N Engl J Med* 320:502–506, 1989.
29. Gulley ML, Eagan PA, Quintanilla-Martinez L, et al: Epstein–Barr virus DNA is abundant and monoclonal in the Reed–Sternberg cells of Hodgkin's disease: Association with mixed cellularity subtype and hispanic American ethnicity. *Blood* 83:1595–1602, 1994.
30. Herndier BG, Sanchez HC, Chang KL, et al: High prevalence of Epstein-Barr virus in the Reed-Sternberg cells of HIV-associated Hodgkin's disease. *Am J Pathol* 142:1073–1079, 1993.
31. Sun T: *Color Atlas/Text of Flow Cytometric Analysis of Hematologic Neoplasms*, New York, Igaku-Shoin, 1993, pp 55–58.

8
Differential Diagnosis of Castleman's Disease (Angiofollicular Hyperplasia)

Castleman's disease is also called *angiofollicular hyperplasia, giant lymph node hyperplasia, benign giant lymphoma, angiomatous lymphoid harmatoma,* and *follicular lymphoreticuloma*. This entity was first described by Castleman in 1959 as a localized mediastinal lymph node hyperplasia resembling thymoma.[1] As the term *angiofollicular hyperplasia* implies, the basic lesion is follicular hyperplasia and capillary proliferation with endothelial hyperplasia. This histologic pattern has been classified as hyaline–vascular type to distinguish it from the plasma-cell type described later by Flendrig and Schilling in 1969.[2] The plasma-cell type is characterized by hyperplastic follicles and a dense interfollicular plasmacytosis. Some authors recognized a third localized type, called variably the *intermediate* type, *transitional* type, or *mixed* type.[3] More recently, a systemic lymphoproliferative disorder with morphologic features of Castleman's disease has been reported and designated as the *multicentric* or *systemic* type.[4,5]

CLINICAL FEATURES

Hyaline–Vascular Type

This is the most common type of Castleman's disease, accounting for 90% of cases in one large series.[3] In this series, the ages of patients ranged from 12 to 69 years (median age 33 years) with no predilection for either sex.[6] Patients with this type of Castleman's disease are usually asymptomatic unless the lesion obstructs or compresses a neighboring structure, such as a bronchus. The lesion is usually a solitary, slow-growing mass, and 52% of the lesions are confined to the mediastinum.[6] The prognosis for this type is excellent. Once the lesion is removed, the patient may have complete recovery.

Plasma-Cell Type

This type represents about 10% of the cases of Castleman's disease.[3] The ages of patients ranged from 8 to 62 years (median age 22 years) with no sex predilection.[6] Patients in this group usually have constitutional symptoms such as fever, night sweats, weight loss, and fatigue.[3,6,7] Hepatomegaly, splenomegaly, nephromegaly, and systemic amyloidosis have been reported in this type,[6,8] but some of those cases probably belong to the multicentric type. A case of nephrotic syndrome secondary to renal amyloidosis recovered from the syndrome 10 months after the resection of a giant axillary lymph node with features of Castleman's disease.[9] In pediatric cases, the patients may have growth failure, sexual retardation, and short stature.[8] Cutaneous lesions, including pemphigus, lichenoid eruptions, nodular eruptions, miscellaneous maculopapular eruptions, cutaneous necrotizing vasculitis, and plane xanthomas, have also been associated with this type.[10,11] There are also many abnormal laboratory findings: anemia, polyclonal gammopathy, elevated erythrocyte sedimentation rate (ESR), leukocytosis, and thrombocytosis.[3,6,8] The clinical symptoms usually disappear, and abnormal test results return to the normal after excision of the mass. The lesion is usually located in the abdominal lymph nodes (mesenteric, mesocolon, and retroperitoneal) instead of the mediastinum, as seen in the hyaline–vascular type.[6] Extranodal involvement has not been found in the plasma-cell type.

Intermediate Type

This rare type is classified on histologic basis. Clinically, the intermediate type is similar to the hyaline–vascular type; patients are usually asymptomatic. In two recently reported cases, however, both patients showed constitutional symptoms, systemic amyloidosis, anemia, and elevation of acute phase reactants in the plasma.[12]

Multicentric Type

In a study of 67 cases of Castleman's disease, 21 were unicentric and 26 were multicentric.[13] However, there is no large series for the documentation of an accurate incidence of the multicentric type. The multicentric type shows morphologic features similar to those of the plasma-cell type, but multiple lymph nodes and multisystem are involved.[5,14,15] In a summary of 38 reported cases, the patients' ages ranged from 19 to 85 years with a median age of 64 years.[5] The male:female ratio is about 2:1.[5] In the Mayo Clinic study of 26 multicentric cases, 13 were with neuropathy and 13 were without.[13]

In contrast to the local types, the multicentric type always involves the peripheral lymph nodes, but about half of the patients also have abdominal or mediastinal lymph node lesions.[5,14] Constitutional symptoms, such as malaise, weakness, fever, night sweats, weight loss, anorexia or nausea, are seen in 95% of patients. Other common clinical manifestations include cough, neurologic symptoms, skin rashes, and GI symptoms. Physical examination of the patient may show lymphadenopathy, hepatosplenomegaly, edema or efusions, skin rash, and abnormal neurologic signs. The common abnormal laboratory findings are anemia, hypoalbuminemia, elevated ESR, proteinuria, hypergammaglobulinemia, abnormal liver function tests, thrombocytopenia, leukopenia, and a variety of nonspecific serologic manifestations of rheumatic diseases.[5,14]

Patients with the multicentric type have been associated with several syndromes, namely, the POEMS syndrome (polyneuropathy, organomegaly, endocrinopathy, monoclonal gammopathy, and skin lesions), nephrotic syndrome, peripheral neuropathy, myelofibrosis, vasculitis, and sicca syndrome.[5,13,14,16]

Most patients with this type have an aggressive, rapidly fatal course, but some patients may have a chronic course or one with recurrent exacerbations and remissions. In a summary of the reported cases, about 50% of the patients died, with a median survival time of 27 months. In the Mayo Clinic series, 10 of 26 patients died after an 8-year follow-up, and 7 of them had neuropathy.[13] Patients with neuropathy are usually resistant to steroids and chemotherapy.[13]

PATHOLOGY

Hyaline–Vascular Type

The histology of the hyaline–vascular type is characterized by the presence of abnormal follicles and increased vascularity.[1,3,6,7] The follicles contain germinal centers of varying sizes, shapes, and numbers. The mantle zones are prominently expanded consisting of concentrically arranged small lymphocytes (onion-skin) (Fig. 8.1). Frequently, the germinal centers enclose one or more small blood vessels

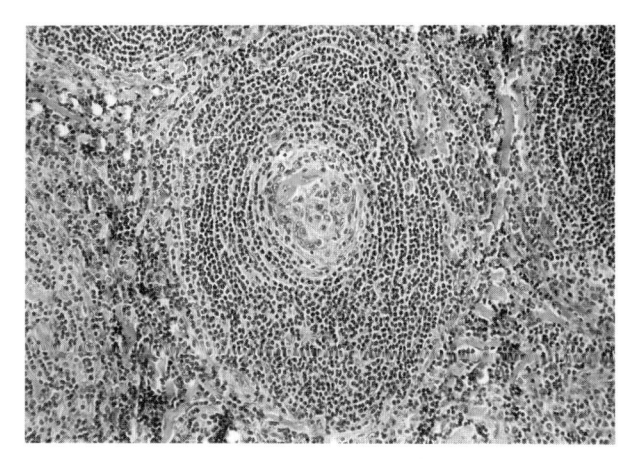

Fig. 8.1. A case of Castleman's disease showing a lymphoid follicle with expanded mantle zone consisting of concentrically arranged small lymphocytes (onion-skin). Many small blood vessels with hyalinized wall are present in the interfollicular area. H&E, ×250.

entering from the perifollicular tissue (Figs. 8.2, 8.3). Some of these blood vessels have thickened, hyalinized walls, which make the germinal centers superficially resemble Hassell's corpuscles (Fig. 8.4). These abnormal follicles are thus called "burned out" or "regressively transformed" or angiosclerotic follicles. In the interfollicular areas, there are varying but usually increasing numbers of small blood vessels. In between the vessel network are predomi-

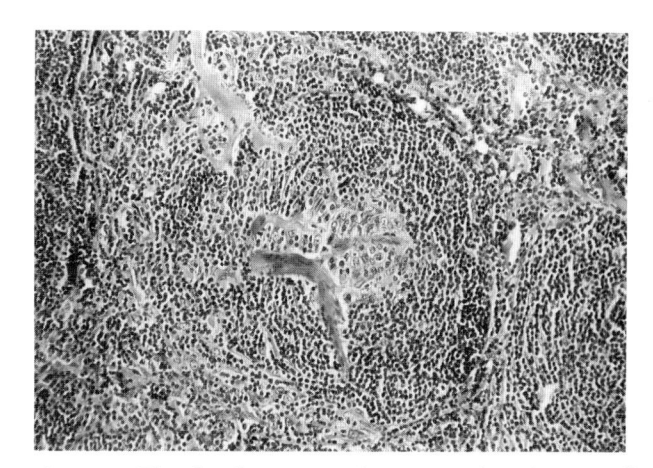

Fig. 8.2. The hyaline–vascular type showing small blood vessels with thickened, hyalinized wall entering from the perifollicular area to the germinal center. H&E, ×250.

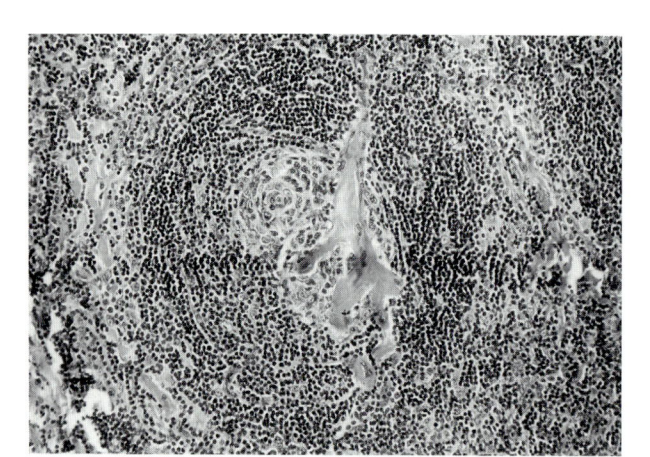

84 DIFFERENTIAL DIAGNOSIS OF LYMPHOID DISORDERS

Fig. 8.3. The hyaline–vascular type showing vascular penetration of the germinal center and onionskin pattern in the mantle zone. H&E, ×250

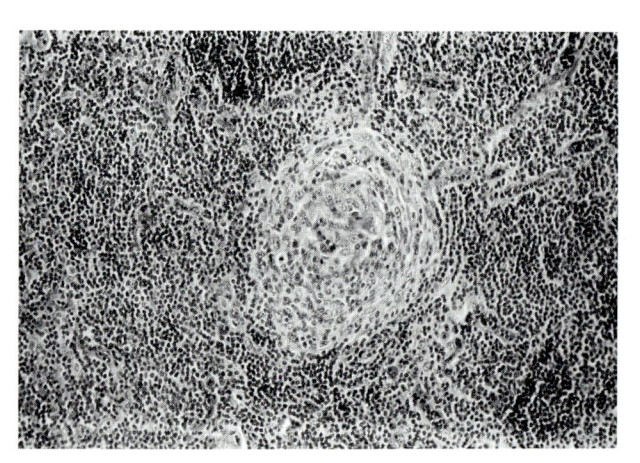

Fig. 8.5. The hyaline–vascular type showing a small follicle surrounded predominantly by lymphocytes. There is also increase in vascularity. H&E, ×500.

nantly small lymphocytes (Fig. 8.5), a few plasma cells, and rare immunoblasts.

A recent AFIP study has added the lack of sinuses and the presence of large numbers of KP1-positive plasmacytoid monocytes in the interfollicular areas as common diagnostic features for the hyaline–vascular type.[17] The same study has also noted the presence of actin-positive cells (fibroblastic reticulum cells or myoid cells) and KP1-positive dendritic cells in the interfollicular areas. According to the proportion of follicles to interfollicular tissue, the AFIP group divided the hyaline–vascular type into follicular, classic, and stroma-rich variants.[17] In the stroma-rich variant, there are decreased plasmacytoid monocytes and increased fibroblastic reticulum cells and dendritic cells.

Plasma-Cell Type

The histology of the plasma-cell type also shows follicular hyperplasia.[1,3,6,7] Unlike the hyaline–vascular type, there are no small vascular germinal centers. The germinal centers in the plasma-cell type are similar to those of nonspecific follicular hyperplasia, containing cleaved and noncleaved small and large lymphocytes, varying numbers of tingible-body macrophages, and considerable mitotic figures. The mantle zone is normal and not expanded. The most striking feature is the presence of sheets of mature plasma cells in the interfollicular area (Figs. 8.6, 8.7). A few immunoblasts may be present. Vascular proliferation is inconspicuous or absent.

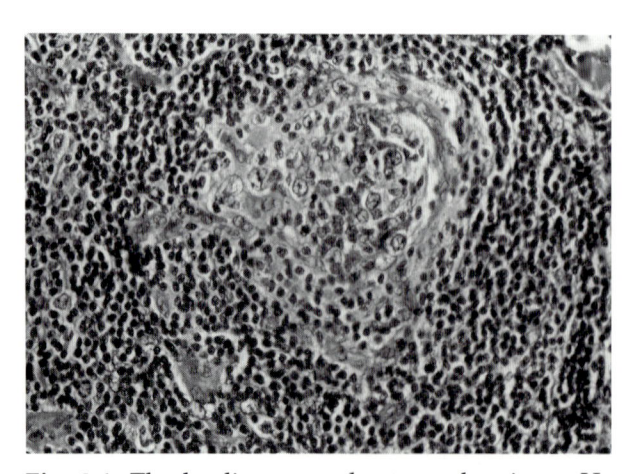

Fig. 8.4. The hyaline–vascular type showing a Hassell's corpuscle-like structure in a germinal center. H&E, ×500.

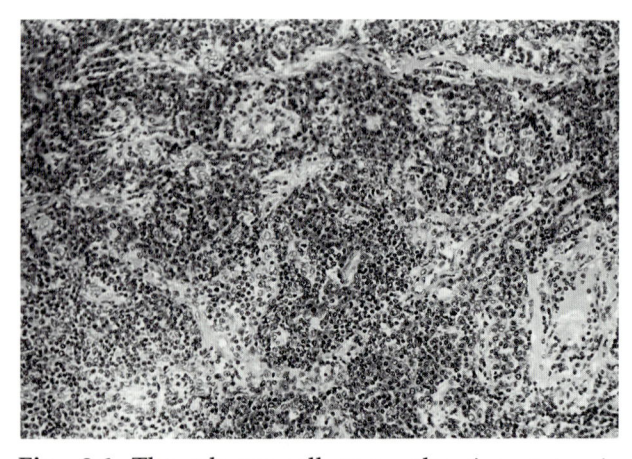

Fig. 8.6. The plasma-cell type showing extensive plasma-cell infiltration in the interfollicular area. H&E, ×250.

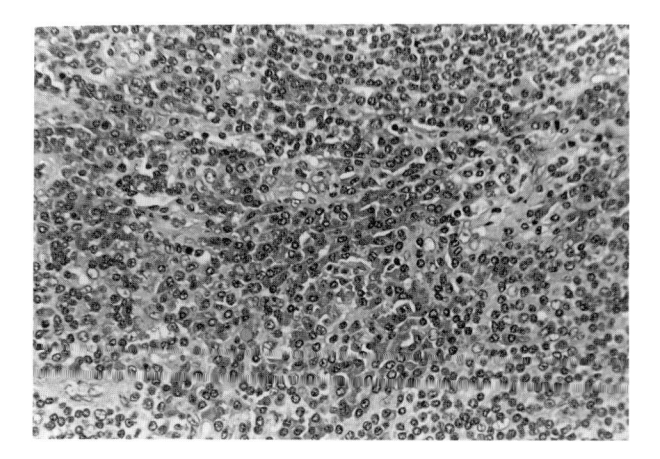

Fig. 8.7. A higher-power view of Fig. 8.6 showing plasma-cell infiltrate. H&E, ×500.

Intermediate Type

Most cases show predominant features of the hyaline–vascular type with foci of numerous plasma cells and some large, normal-appearing germinal centers (Fig. 8.8).[3] The less common feature is predominantly of the plasma-cell type with hyaline–vascular germinal centers (Fig. 8.9).

Multicentric Type

Although the histologic pattern in the multicentric type is usually referred to as the *plasma-cell type*, it shows frequently mixed features of the plasma-cell type and the hyaline—vascular type, namely, recognizable nodal architecture, germinal center abnormalities, and plasmacytosis.[5] Frizzera and associates have observed three patterns that are considered successive phases of the disease.[5,14] In the proliferative phase, there is a striking increase of activated high endothelial venules and immunoblasts, in addition to plasma cells, in the interfollicular areas. In the accumulative phase, mature plasma cells predominate and vascular proliferation is absent. In the burned-out phase, there are small vascular germinal centers, collapsed and often hyalinized blood vessels, and only a sparse plasma-cell component in the interfollicular areas (Figs. 8.10, 8.11). The last phase is frequently mistaken for the hyaline–vascular type.

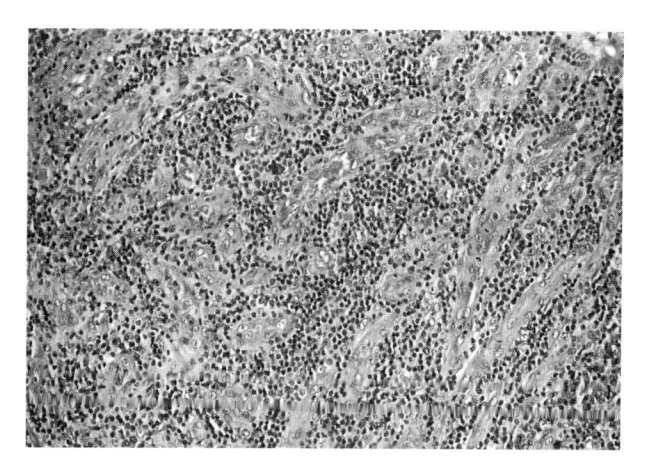

Fig. 8.9. The intermediate type showing marked proliferation of thick-walled blood vessels and lymphoplasmacytic infiltrate in the interfollicular area. H&E, ×250.

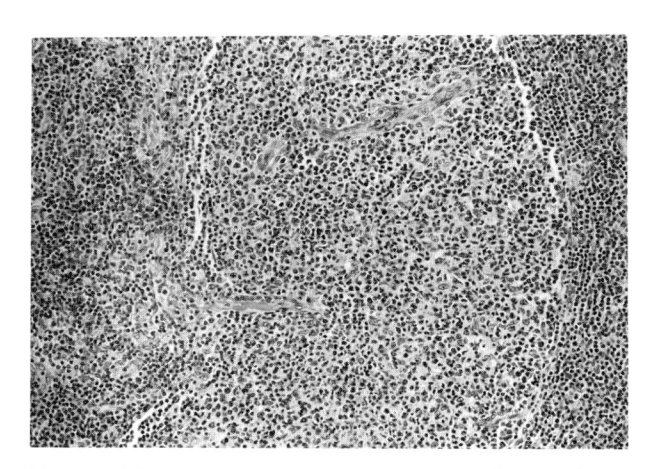

Fig. 8.8. The intermediate type showing hyperplastic, vascular follicular center and plasma-cell infiltrate in the interfollicular area. H&E, ×250.

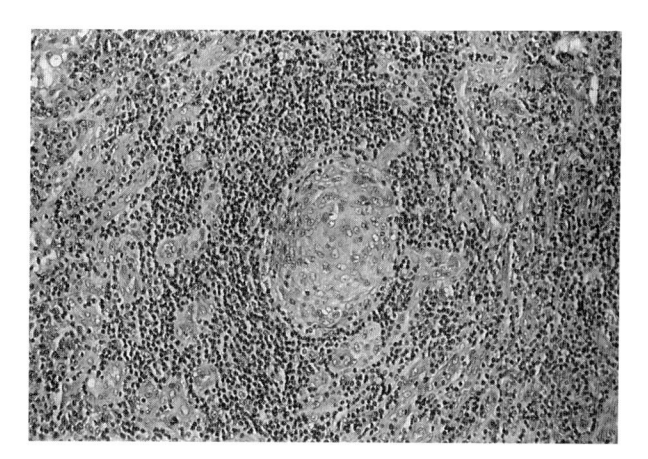

Fig. 8.10. The burned-out phase of the multicentric type showing a small germinal center surrounded by collapsed and hyalinized blood vessels and predominantly lymphocytic infiltration. H&E, ×250.

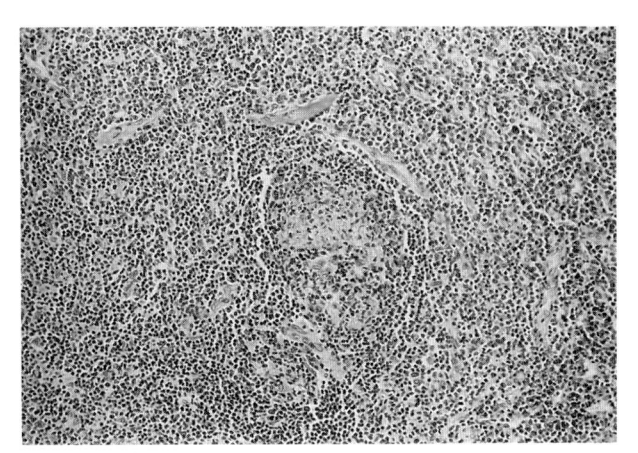

Fig. 8.11. The burned-out phase of the multicentric type showing an atrophic follicle, collapsed blood vessels, and lymphocytic infiltration. A few plasma cells are also present. H&E, ×250.

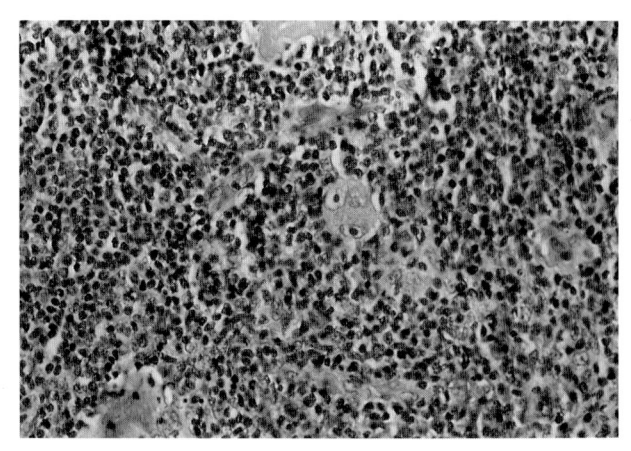

Fig. 8.13. Another area of the same case as in Fig. 8.12 showing a Reed–Sternberg cell in the center. H&E, ×500.

Neoplasms Associated with Castleman's Disease

Several neoplasms are associated with various types of Castleman's disease. Malignant lymphoma, vascular neoplasms, angiolipomatous hamartoma, and follicular dendritic cell tumor have been seen with the hyaline–vascular type; plasmacytoma, with the plasma-cell type; and Kaposi's sarcoma, glomeruloid hemangioma, malignant lymphoma, and plasmacytoma, with the multicentric type.[5,6,18,19] Approximately one-third of Castleman's disease cases are complicated by malignancies. Although these malignancies may be a coincidental finding in elderly patients with Castleman's disease, the incidence of Kaposi's sarcoma and non-Hodgkin's lymphoma is higher than expected in the general population.[5] These two malignancies are also a common cause of death in this group of patients. On the other hand, the coexistence of Hodgkin's disease and Castleman's disease are frequently present in the same lymph node,[5] and these cases are thus considered to be Hodgkin's disease with coexistent Castleman-like histologic features (Figs. 8.12–8.14).[20] In other words, the histologic pattern simply represents a tissue reaction to the malignancy.

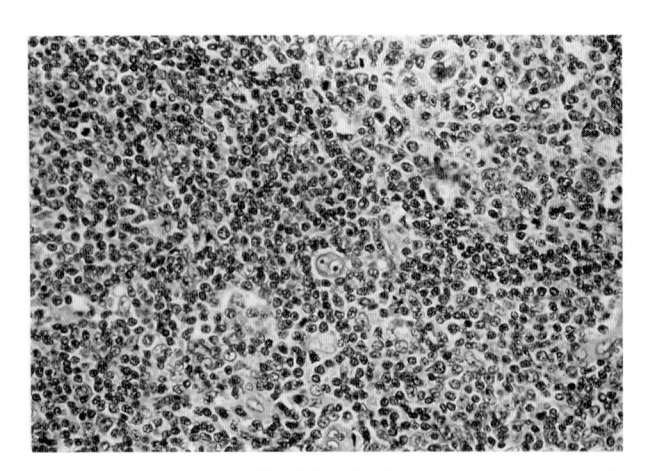

Fig. 8.12. A case of Hodgkin's disease coexistent with Castleman-like histologic features showing a Reed–Sternberg cell in the center. H&E, ×500.

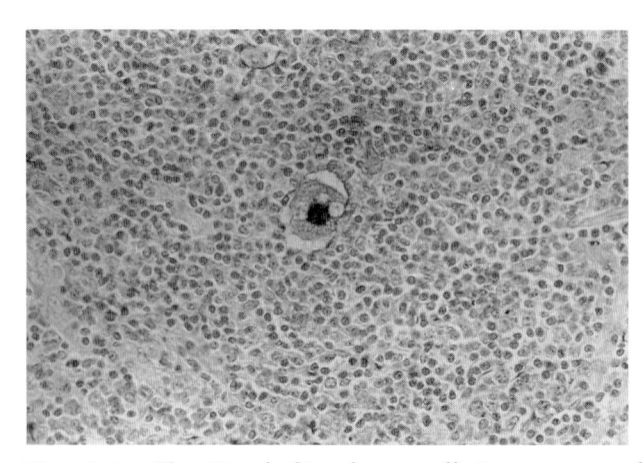

Fig. 8.14. The Reed–Sternberg cell in a case of Hodgkin's disease with coexistent Castleman-like histologic features showing intracytoplasmic (Golgi zone) staining by CD15 antibody. Immunoperoxidase, ×500.

Pathogenesis of Castleman's Disease

Castleman's disease is an idiopathic disorder; its etiology is still unknown. However, many hypothesis have developed over the years. The histopathologic features of the lymph nodes in multicentric Castleman's disease are indistinguishable from those seen in both acquired and congenital immunodeficiency.[5,6] Some of these patients also show decreased T-cells, inversion of the CD4:CD8 ratio, and T-cell unresponsiveness to mitogens. They also have high incidence of intercurrent infections and "opportunistic" neoplasms, such as Koposi's sarcoma. Therefore, there is sufficient evidence to indicate the existence of immunodeficiency in patients with Castleman's disease.

Other facts for the explanation of the pathogenesis include the presence of CD5-positive B-lymphocytes in the hyperplastic follicles[21] and the production of interleukin-6 (IL-6) by the germinal center cells.[22] The CD5-positive B-cell subset is associated with autoantibody production, while IL-6 stimulates B-cell differentiation into plasma cells and immunoglobulin production. In addition, IL-6 also regulates acute-phase reactants, serum albumin, and hematopoiesis. When anti-IL-6 antibody was used to treat a patient with Castleman's disease, the symptoms and signs of disease resolved, and most of the abnormal laboratory values (anemia, hypergammaglobulinemia, elevation of acute phase reactants, and hypoalbuminemia) markedly improved within a few days.[23] However, the therapeutic effects did not persist.

Peterson and Frizzera summarized the pathogenesis of Castleman's disease by linking all these factors together and stated that Castleman disease is "a lymphoproliferation of a specific autoantibody-producing B-cell subset, driven toward plasma-cell differentiation by abnormal IL-6 production and unregulated by a defective immune system."[5]

Another theory postulated by the AFIP group is that a developmental block in plasmacytoid monocytes is the mechanism for the development of Castleman's disease.[17] As plasmacytoid monocytes are the precursors of both follicular dendritic reticulum cells and sinus lining cells, this defect results in their accumulation with poor formation of germinal centers and sinuses.

LABORATORY FINDINGS

The immunophenotype of various histologic types are similar.[13,15,17,21,24–27] The lymphocytes in the mantle zone show polyclonal surface immunoglobulins (IgM+, IgD+) with positive CD45, CD19, CD20, CD22, HLA-DR, and CD5.[21] This phenotype represents an autoantibody-producing B-cell subset. Most follicles show a normal ratio of CD4- and CD8-positive T-cells.[14,21,26] However, the characteristic T-cell zoning and CD57-positive cells are absent in abnormal follicles.[21,26] The germinal centers contain mainly dendritic reticulum cells as detected by the DRC-1[27] or R4/23 antibody[21] and endothelial cells, detected by factor VIII-related antigen.[21] A large amount of IL-6 is also demonstrated in the germinal centers.[27]

The interfollicular areas are composed mainly of a CD4 helper-cell-predominant T-cell population,[21,26] admixed with plasma cells in the plasma-cell type. The plasma cells are frequently polyclonal. However, monoclonal plasma-cell population has also been demonstrated, especially in those with the POEMS syndrome.[13,24] Most plasma cells express λ light chains, and some cases may be associated with a serum paraprotein. The presence of monoclonal λ light chain was considered to be associated with poor prognosis as it was found almost exclusively in patients with neuropathy, probably due to its neurotoxicity.[13]

Molecular genetic analysis has been performed in 11 cases of multicentric Castleman's disease, and gene rearrangements have been identified in 8.[21,25,28–30] Five cases showed rearrangement of heavy-chain gene alone, one case had both heavy chain gene and T-cell receptor β-chain gene rearrangement, and one case revealed rearrangement of λ light-chain gene alone. Only one case demonstrated complete heavy chain and light-chain gene rearrangement.[28] Gene rearrangement was not detected in all 4 cases of localized type studied.[28] Although EBV genome was identified in 4 cases of multicentric Castleman's disease, the etiologic role of EBV in this disease has not been established.[28]

DIFFERENTIAL DIAGNOSIS

Acquired Immunodeficiency Syndrome (AIDS)-Related Lymphadenopathy

The lymphoid depletion type of lymph node from human immunodeficiency virus (HIV)-infected patients (see Chapter 4) may mimic the hyaline–vascular type of Castleman's disease.[7] When plasma cell infiltrate increases in the later stage of AIDS, the morphology may be similar to the plasma-cell type. In both conditions, the interfollicular vascular network, as seen in

Castleman's disease, is not present.[7] Serologic test for HIV and clinical symptoms may readily distinguish AIDS from Castleman's disease.

Mantle-Cell Lymphoma

Mantle cell lymphoma (see Chapter 9), especially the nodular type, is similar to Castleman's disease in terms of the prominent mantle zone. In mantle-cell lymphoma, however, the mantle-zone lymphocytes are neoplastic, showing irregular nuclear configuration and a monoclonal surface immunoglobulin pattern.

Autoimmune Disorders (Rheumatoid Arthritis, Systemic Lupus Erythematosus) or Syphillis

These diseases (see Chapter 4) may show follicular hyperplasia with plasma-cell infiltration in the interfollicular areas mimicking the plasma-cell type. Although the sinuses are more often obscured by the infiltrating plasma cells in Castleman disease than in these diseases,[7] there is no clearcut histologic distinction between these two groups of diseases. To make the matter more complicated, is serologic tests for autoimmune diseases are frequently positive in Castleman's disease. Therefore, the diagnosis of Castleman's disease is established only after exclusion of all conditions that may cause reactive hyperplasia in the lymph nodes.

Plasmacytoma or Lymphoplasmacytic Lymphoma

(See Chapter 22.) Plasmacytoma or metastatic multiple myeloma in the lymph node and lymphoplasmacytic lymphoma may masquerade as Castleman's disease, especially the multicentric type, in which the plasma cells can be monotypic. However, the effacement of nodal architecture and the lack of follicular hyperplasia distinguish this entity from Castleman's disease.

Angioimmunoblastic Lymphadenopathy (AIL)

(See Chapter 16.) The lymph node in Castleman's disease may sometimes show increase of immunoblasts in addition to increased vascularity. These features may be mistaken as AIL, but AIL does not have abnormal germinal centers and diffuse plasmacytosis.[14]

REFERENCES

1. Castleman B, Iverson L, Menendez VP: Localized mediastinal lymph node hyperplasia resembling thymoma. *Cancer* 9:822–830, 1959.
2. Flendrig JA, Schilling PHM: Benign giant lymphoma: The clinical sign and symptoms. *Folia Med Neerl* 12:119–120, 1969.
3. Keller AR, Hochholzer L, Castleman B: Hyaline–vascular and plasma-cell type of giant lymph node hyperplasia of mediastinum and other locations. *Cancer* 29:670–683, 1972.
4. Bartoli E, Massarelli G, Soggia G, et al: Multicentric giant lymph node hyperplasia. A hyperimmune syndrome with a rapidly progressive course. *Am J Clin Pathol* 73:423–426, 1980.
5. Peterson BA, Frizzera G: Multicentric Castleman's disease. *Semin Oncol* 20:636–647, 1993.
6. Frizzera G: Castleman's disease and related disorders. *Semin Diagn Pathol* 5:346–364, 1988.
7. Schnitzer B: Reactive lymphadenopathies. In Knowles DM (ed): *Neoplastic Hematopathology*, Baltimore, Williams & Wilkins, 1992; pp 427–457.
8. Hung IJ, Kuo TT, Lin JN: New observations in a child with angiofollicular lymph node hyperplasia (Castleman's disease) originated from the mesenteric root. *Am J Pediatr Hematol/Oncol* 14:255–260, 1992.
9. Perfetti V, Bellotti V, Maggi A, et al: Reversal of nephrotic syndrome due to reactive amyloidosis (AA-type) after excision of localized Castleman's disease. *Am J Hematol* 46:189–193, 1994.
10. Sherman D, Ramsay B, Thodorou NA, et al: Reversible plane xanthoma, vasculitis and peliosis hepatis in giant lymph node hyperplasia (Castleman's disease): A case report and review of the cutaneous manifestations of giant lymph node hyperplasia. *J Am Acad Dermatol* 26:105–109, 1992.
11. Kubota Y, Noto S, Takakuwa T, et al: Skin involvement in giant lymph node hyperplasia (Castleman's disease). *J Am Acad Dermatol* 29:778–780, 1993.
12. Ordi J, Grau JM, Junque A, et al: Secondary (AA) amyloidosis associated with Castleman's disease: Report of two cases and review of the literature. *Am J Clin Pathol* 100:394–397, 1993.
13. Menke DM, Camoriano JK, Banks PM: Angiofollicular lymph node hyperplasia: A comparison of unicentric, multicentric, hyaline–vascular and plasma cell type of disease by morphometric and clinical analysis. *Mod Pathol* 5:525–530, 1992.
14. Frizzera G: Atypical lymphoproliferation disorders. In Knowles DM (ed): *Neoplastic Hematopathology*, Baltimore, Williams & Wilkins, 1992, pp 459–495.

15. Weisenburger DP, Nathwani BN, Winberg CD, et al: Multicentric angiofollicular lymph node hyperplasia: A clinicopathologic study of 16 cases. *Hum Pathol* 16:162–172, 1985.
16. Adelman HM, Cacciatore ML, Pascual JF, et al: Case report: Castleman disease in association with POEMS. *Am J Med Sci* 307:112–114, 1994.
17. Danon AD, Krishman J, Frizzera G: Morpho-immunophenotypic diversity of Castleman's disease, hyaline–vascular type: With emphasis on a stroma-rich variant and a new pathogenetic hypothesis. *Virchows Archiv A Pathol Anat* 423:369–382, 1993.
18. Chan JKC, Tsang WYW, Ng CS: Follicular dendritic cell tumor and vascular neoplasm complicating hyaline–vascular Castleman's disease. *Am J Surg Pathol* 18:517–525, 1994.
19. Vasef M, Katzin WE, Mendelsohn G, et al: Report of a case of localized Castleman's disease with progression to malignant lymphoma. *Am J Clin Pathol* 98:633–636, 1992.
20. Zarate-Osorno A, Medeiros LJ, Danon AD, et al: Hodgkin's disease with coexistent Castleman-like histologic features: A report of three cases. *Arch Pathol Lab Med* 118:270–274, 1994.
21. Hall PA, Donaghy M, Cotter FE, et al: An immunohistological and genotypic study of the plasma cell form of Castleman's disease. *Histopathology* 14:333–346, 1989.
22. Hsu SM, Waldron JA, Xie SS, et al: Expression of interleukin-6 in Castleman's disease. *Hum Pathol* 24:833–839, 1993.
23. Beck JT, Hsu SM, Wijdenes J, et al: Brief report: Alleviation of systemic manifestations of Castleman's disease by monoclonal anti-interleukin-6 antibody. *N Engl J Med* 330:602–605, 1994.
24. Radaszkiewicz T, Hansman ML, Lennert K: Monoclonality and polyclonality of plasma cells in Castleman's disease of the plasma cell variant. *Histopathology* 14:11–24, 1989.
25. Ohyashiki JH, Ohyashiki K, Kawakubo K, et al: Molecular genetic, cytogenetic and immunophenotypic analysis in Castleman's disease of the plasma cell type. *Am J Clin Pathol* 101:290–295, 1994.
26. Martin JME, Bell B, Ruether BA: Giant lymph node hyperplasia (Castleman's disease) of hyaline vascular type. Clinical heterogeneity with immunohistologic uniformity. *Am J Clin Pathol* 84:439–446, 1985.
27. Yoshizaki K, Matsuda T, Nishimoto H, et al: Pathogenic significance of interleukin-6 (IL-6/BSF-2) in Castleman's disease. *Blood* 74:1360–1367, 1989.
28. Hanson CA, Frizzera G, Patton DF, et al: Clonal rearrangement for immunoglobulin and T-cell receptor genes in systemic Castleman's disease. Association with Epstein-Barr virus. *Am J Pathol* 131:84–91, 1988.
29. Nagai M, Irino S, Uda H, et al: Molecular genetic and immunohistochemical analysis of a case of multicentric Castleman's disease. *Jpn J Clin Oncol* 18:149–157, 1988.
30. Gould SJ, Diss T, Isaacson PG: Multicentric Castleman's disease in association with a solitary plamacytoma: A case report. *Histopathology* 17:135–140, 1990.

9
Follicular Lymphoma vs. Follicular Hyperplasia vs. Mantle-Cell Lymphoma

The distinction between follicular hyperplasia (FH) and follicular lymphoma (FL) is considered one of the classic diagnostic dilemmas in hematopathology.[1] The problem is related not only to their morphologic similarity but also to technical difficulties in immunophenotyping and time-consuming in immunogenotyping for their distinction. Mantle-cell lymphoma (MCL) or centrocytic lymphoma is another entity that could potentially be confused with FH and FL. The recent availability of new monoclonal antibodies and the improvement of molecular and cytogenetic techniques not only facilitate the differential diagnosis but also enable the elucidation of the cellular origin and the pathogenesis of these neoplasms.[2,3]

CLINICAL MANIFESTATION

Follicular Hyperplasia

FH represents a reactive state in lymph nodes as a response to various antigenic stimuli, including biologic, chemical, autoimmune, and neoplastic but in most cases, idiopathic (see Chapter 4). As its etiology varies, the clinical manifestation depends on the cause. If it is due to a biologic cause, for instance, the clinical manifestation will be that of acute or chronic infectious diseases. In general, the onset of diseases with FH is insidious, the symptoms are mild, the clinical course is indolent, and the prognosis is good. However, acute infectious diseases may have fulminating clinical features, and an autoimmune disease can be protracted and progressive, mimicking neoplasms. Therefore, the distinction between FH and FL depends on the histologic pattern and laboratory findings.

Follicular Lymphoma

FL is a lymphoma of older age groups. It is seldom seen in patients before age 20 and almost never encountered in young children.[4] It occurs with equal frequency in both sexes. The incidence of FL varies in different geographic locations. It is a common form of lymphoma in the United States, accounting for 20–30% of all non-Hodgkin's lymphoma and 40–50% of adult non-Hodgkin's lymphoma.[4,5] In European countries, the incidence ranges from 13% to 22%.[4,6] This tumor is uncommon in Japan.[4]

FL has an insidious onset; therefore, when a diagnosis is made, the disease is already in an advanced stage; about 67% of patients are in stage III or IV at the time of diagnosis.[6] Constitutional symptoms, such as fever, weight loss, and night sweats, are present in only 17% of patients. The major clinical presentation is peripheral lymphadenopathy, involving mostly the cervical and inguinal lymph nodes.[4,6] Extranodal involvement is rare but can be present in the spleen, Waldeyer's ring, or gastrointestinal (GI) tract. Skin and soft-tissue presentations are very rare; bone and CNS have not been reported as primary sites. In advanced stages, however, bone marrow and liver are most commonly invaded.[4] About 33% of patients show a leukemic blood picture,[6] but circulating lymphoma cells have been demonstrated with the polymerase chain reaction in 75% of patients who are in stages I and II.[7]

Although patients with FL have an indolent clinical course, FL is not a curable disease. Most patients may respond well to chemotherapy or radiation therapy at the beginning, but the disease gradually becomes refractory to treatment, leading to the death of the patient.[4] The cause of death in some cases may be due to transformation to high-grade lymphoma. Some patients may develop acute lymphoid or myeloid leukemia.[4]

Mantle-Cell Lymphoma

MCL is seen in elderly patients with a median age of about 60 years, and the male:female ratio has been reported to range from 2.7:1 to 5:1.[6,8,9] The incidence of MCL in the United States is 2.5–4.0% of all non-Hodgkin's lymphomas, but is 7–9% in Europe.[9]

Most (73%) patients present with generalized lymphadenopathy, and about 50% of patients have systemic symptoms. About 50% of patients have splenomegaly at presentation, and 80% of patients with the mantle-zone subtype of MCL may show prominent splenomegaly.[9] As in FL, most patients with MCL are in stage III or IV at diagnosis, and bone marrow and liver involvement are common findings. Hepatomegaly is seen in 20% of patients.[8] Primary extranodal presentation has been occasionally reported in the lungs, GI tract, and conjunctiva.[8] A peripheral lymphocytosis of >4 x 10^9/L occurs in 20–40% of cases, but seldom exceeds 20 x 10^9/μL.[9] Mild anemia and thrombocytopenia are seen in some cases. Hypogammaglobulinemia, monoclonal gammopathy, and positive Coombs test have been occasionally reported.

The median survival of all patients with MCL has ranged from 30 to 56 months.[9] Longer median survival (77–80 months) has been demonstrated in the mantle-zone subtype as compared to that of the diffuse intermediate lymphocytic lymphoma subtype (30–33 months).[9]

PATHOLOGY

Follicular Hyperplasia

FH is manifested as proliferation of lymphoid follicles with resultant increases in both number and size of the follicles. The expansion of the follicles is usually due to the enlargement of the germinal centers, which may vary in both size and shape. Mantle zones are usually intact, but frequently attenuated and occasionally increased in size.[10–12]

To distinguish FH from FL, the first feature to look for is whether the normal nodal architecture is preserved or effaced (Table 9.1). In FH, the nodal architecture is usually well preserved. However, the hyperplastic follicles are more irregular in size, shape, and distribution than the follicles of FL are (Figs. 9.1, 9.2). In addition, the benign follicles have lower density than the malignant ones. For instance, the median number of follicles per unit area for FH was 30 and that for FL, 47 in one study.[12] Under lower magnification, the demarcation between the germinal center and mantle zone should be recognizable in hyperplasia, but this demarcation becomes blurred in lymphoma, which may sometimes show a complete or partial loss of mantle zones. The capsule of the lymph node is usually not infiltrated by lymphocytes in FH.

The cytologic features may further distinguish FH from FL. In FH, the germinal centers contain mixed large and small cleaved and noncleaved lymphoid cells and phagocytic histiocytes. Polarization of the lymphoid cells is frequently demonstrated in the germinal centers in FH; small and large cleaved lymphoid cells are on one pole (light zone) and small and large noncleaved (transformed) lymphoid cells are on another pole (dark zone). In the dark zone, the mitotic rate is high and there are many tingible-body macrophages, forming a starry-sky pattern.

TABLE 9.1
Differentiation between Follicular Hyperplasia and Follicular Lymphoma

	Follicular hyperplasia	Follicular lymphoma
Lymph node architecture	Well preserved	Completely or partially effaced
Size and shape of germinal centers	Variable	Uniform
Distribution of follicles	Irregular, well separated	Even, back-to-back pattern
Density of follicles	Low	High
Margin of follicles	Sharp	Poorly defined
Mantle zone	Intact	Absent or incomplete
Infiltration of capsule	Absent or minimal	Present
Cells within germinal centers	Polymorphic	Monomorphic
Polarization in germinal centers	Present	Absent
Mitotic rate	High	Low
Tingible-body macrophages	Prominent	Rare
Cells in interfollicular area	Normal lymphocytes	Atypical lymphoid cells
Surface immunoglobulin pattern	Polyclonal	Monoclonal
CD45RA (MT2)	Negative	Positive
bcl-2 antibody	Negative	Positive
Cytogenetic finding	Normal karyotype	t (14;18) (q32;q21)
Molecular biology	No oncogene	bcl-2
Immunoglobulin gene	Germline	Rearrangement

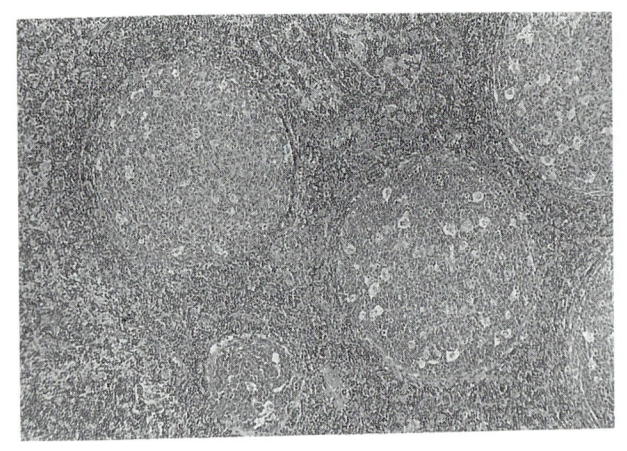

Fig. 9.1. Lymph node biopsy of follicular hyperplasia showing follicles of varying sizes with many tingible-body macrophages forming a starry-sky pattern. The demarcation between the germinal center and mantle zone is distinct. The follicles are separated by prominent areas of interfollicular lymphoid tissue containing small lymphocytes and pale-staining large lymphocytes. H&E, ×125.

In FH, the follicles are usually separated by prominent areas of interfollicular lymphoid tissue where predominantly small lymphocytes and scattered large lymphocytes are present. Inflammatory cells can be seen in either FH or FL.[11] When atypical cleaved lymphoid cells are found in the interfollicular area, the possibility of FL should be considered.

In spite of the existence of all these morphologic criteria for the distinction between FH and FL, none of them alone is infallible. When a definitive diagnosis cannot be made on morphologic basis, further ancillary studies should be performed. If such studies are not available or the results are inconclusive, the case under study should be regarded as atypical follicular hyperplasia (Fig. 9.3).[11]

Follicular Lymphoma

FL is classified as follicular, small cleaved, mixed, or large cell in the Working Formulation and as centroblastic/centrocytic follicular lymphoma in the Kiel classification. In 1994, the International Lymphoma Study Group proposed a new term, "follicle center lymphoma," to include follicular centroblastic lymphoma in this category.[13]

FL is sometimes difficult to distinguish from FH.[4,11,12] However, as mentioned in the section of FH, there are multiple morphologic criteria that can facilitate differential diagnosis. The lymph node architecture is usually effaced, completely or partially, in FL (Fig. 9.4). The neoplastic follicles are often uniform in both size and shape. These follicles are evenly distributed frequently with a back-to-back pattern so that the density of follicles is higher than that in FH and there is sparse intervening interfollicular tissue. The margin of the tumor follicles is usually poorly defined. The mantle zone is usually absent or incomplete. The capsule of the lymph node is frequently infiltrated by the lymphoma cells, which may spread into the perinodal soft tissue (Figs. 9.5, 9.6). The sub-

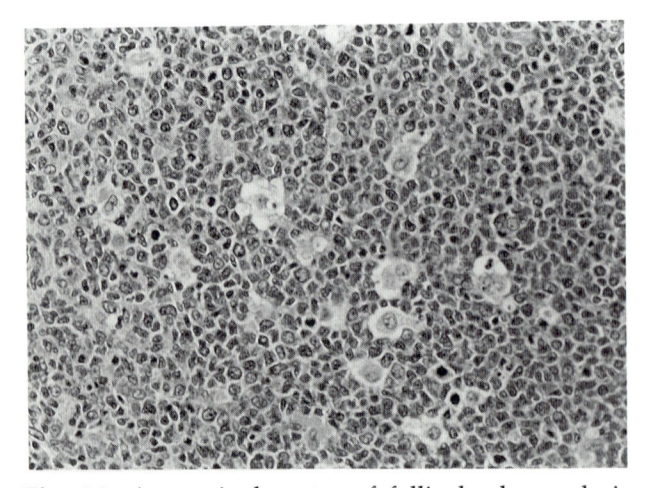

Fig. 9.2. A germinal center of follicular hyperplasia showing tingible-body macrophages and a high mitotic rate. H&E, ×500.

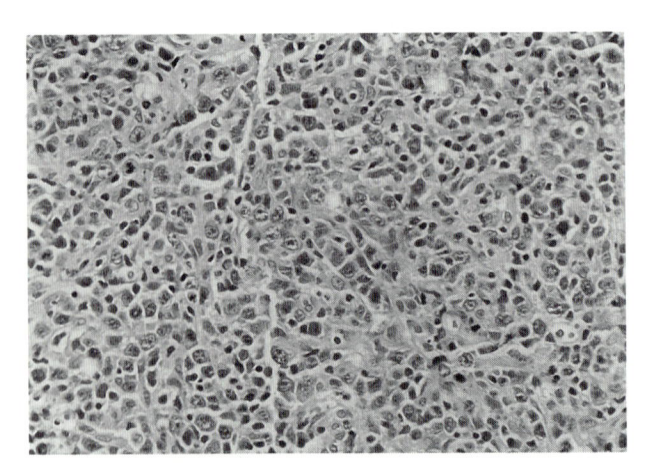

Fig. 9.3. A case of atypical hyperplasia showing effacement of normal architecture by lymphocytes, plasma cells, and immunoblasts. H&E, ×500.

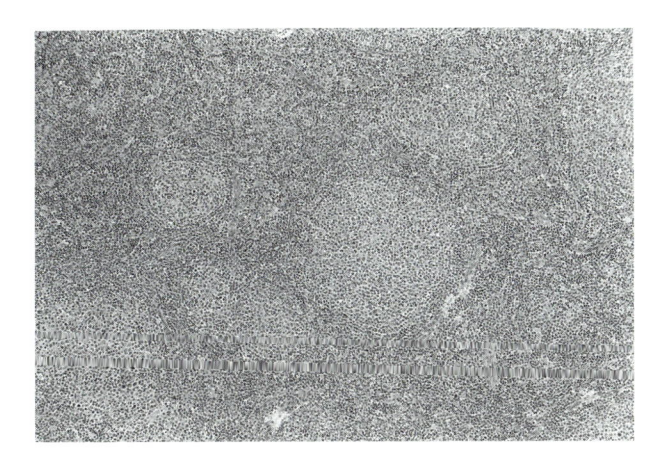

Fig. 9.4. Lymph node biopsy of follicular lymphoma showing effacement of normal architecture, ill-defined follicles, back-to-back pattern, absence or incomplete formation of mantle zone, and no tingible-body macrophages in the germinal centers. H&E, ×125.

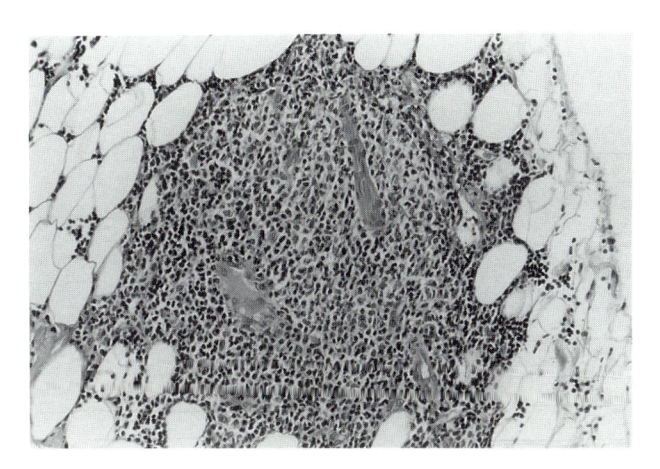

Fig. 9.6. A higher magnification showing the aggregate of small cleaved lymphoid cells in the perinodal adipose tissue from a case of follicular lymphoma. H&E, ×250.

capsular and medullary sinuses are often obliterated by the tumor infiltrate.

Cytologically, FL is composed of small cleaved lymphocytes and large transformed lymphoid cells in varying proportions, but it usually shows a monomorphic appearance without a polarization pattern of lymphoid cells. In most cases of FL, the mitotic rate is low and tingible-body macrophages are seldom seen except for the large-cell subtype. The presence of atypical lymphoid cells in the interfollicular region is helpful for the diagnosis of FL, although inflammatory cells may also be present.

In the Working Formulation, FL is divided into three subtypes: (a) predominantly small-cleaved-cell type; (2) mixed small-cleaved and large-cell type; and (3) predominantly large-cell type.[14]

The predominantly small-cleaved-cell type is the most common form, accounting for 40–50% of all FL cases. The characteristic nuclei may show prominent clefts, indentation, or linear infoldings (Fig. 9.7). The nuclear chromatin is condensed, and small nucleoli are present. The cytoplasm of the tumor cells is scant. Mitotic figures are rarely seen. A few large cells may be present, but they should constitute less than 20% of the tumor population and should not be more than 5 cells per high-power field.

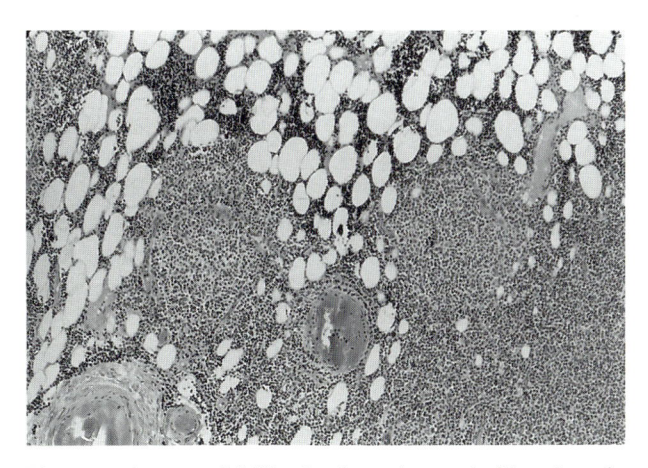

Fig. 9.5. A case of follicular lymphoma infiltrating the perinodal adipose tissue. H&E, ×125.

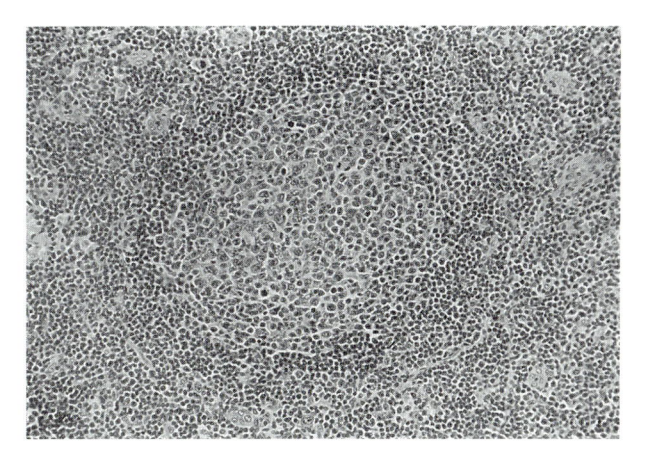

Fig. 9.7. Lymph node biopsy of follicular lymphoma of the small-cleaved-cell type. H&E, ×250.

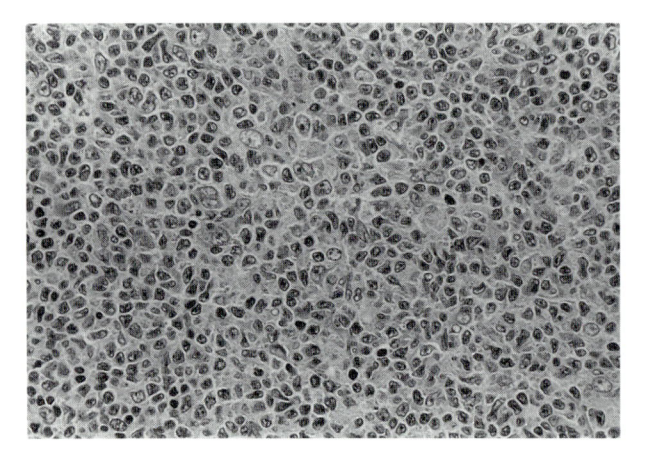

Fig. 9.8. Lymph node biopsy of follicular lymphoma of the mixed small-cleaved/large-cell type. H&E, ×500.

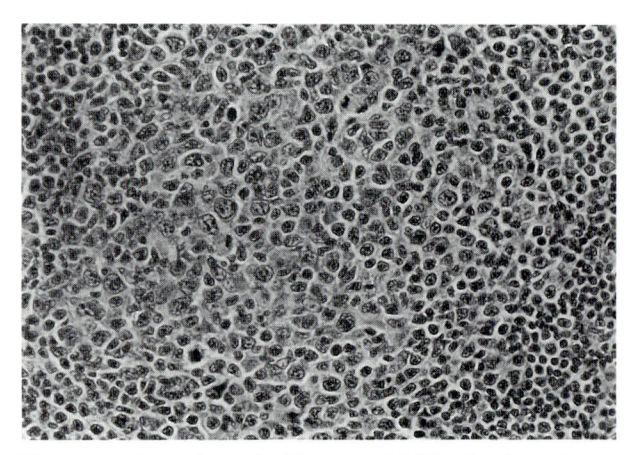

Fig. 9.10. Lymph node biopsy of follicular lymphoma of the large-cell type showing cleaved and noncleaved cells. H&E, ×500.

The mixed small-cleaved and large-cell type may have approximately equal numbers of small cleaved cells and large cells (Fig. 9.8). The large cells should account for 20–50% of the tumor cells or 5–15 cells per high-power field. The large tumor cells are 2–3 times as large as normal lymphocytes. They have a thin rim of cytoplasm, round or irregular, vesicular nuclei, and 1–3 nucleoli, which are typically opposed to the nuclear membrane.

The predominantly large-cell type is the least common among the three subtypes. The large cell in this type accounts for more than 50% of the neoplastic population or more than 15 cells per high-power field (Figs. 9.9, 9.10). In contrast to the other 2 types, the mitotic rate is high and tingible-body macrophages are frequently seen.

Generally speaking, the proportion of large cells is an important factor in prediction of the prognosis. Thus, the predominantly large-cell type has the worst prognosis and the predominantly small-cleaved-cell type predicts a much better prognosis. The International Lymphoma Study Group is of the opinion that these three subtypes are a continuous gradation in the number of large cells and are difficult to reproduce among groups of pathologists. Therefore, this group proposes these subtypes to be a grading system rather than subclassification.[13]

In some cases of FL, diffuse areas are present side-by-side with the follicular pattern. The proportions of follicular and diffuse areas are also associated with prognosis; a worse prognosis can be predicted in cases with larger diffuse areas.[13] Other cases of FL may show increased collagen fibers in the interfollicular region or diffuse areas, resulting in a characteristic nodular sclerotic pattern (Fig. 9.11). The association of sclerosis with prognosis is controversial.[11]

There are several rare variants of FL. The signet-ring-cell lymphoma is characterized by the presence of cytoplasmic vacuoles or Russell bodies in the tumor cells, which form a follicular pattern (Figs. 9.12, 9.13).[15] The cytoplasmic vacuoles usually contain monoclonal IgG or light chains, and the Russell bodies often show monoclonal IgM. Some cases of FL contain large numbers of plasma cells in the interfollicular region or diffuse area which may mimic FH, but the presence of atypical cleaved lymphocytes in the follicles may help exclude the possibility of FH.

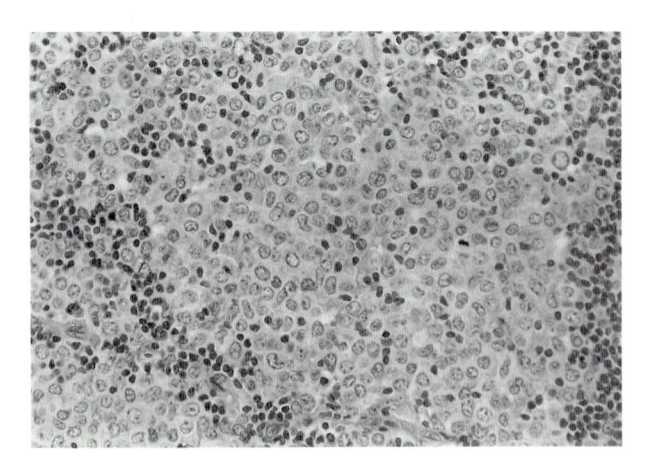

Fig. 9.9. Lymph node biopsy of follicular lymphoma of the large-noncleaved-cell type. H&E, ×500.

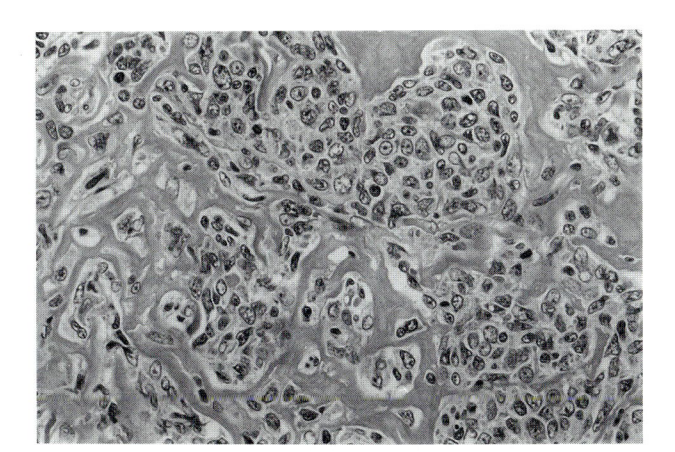

Fig. 9.11. A case of follicular lymphoma showing clusters of lymphoma cells separated by collagen fibers forming a nodular sclerosing pattern. H&E, ×500.

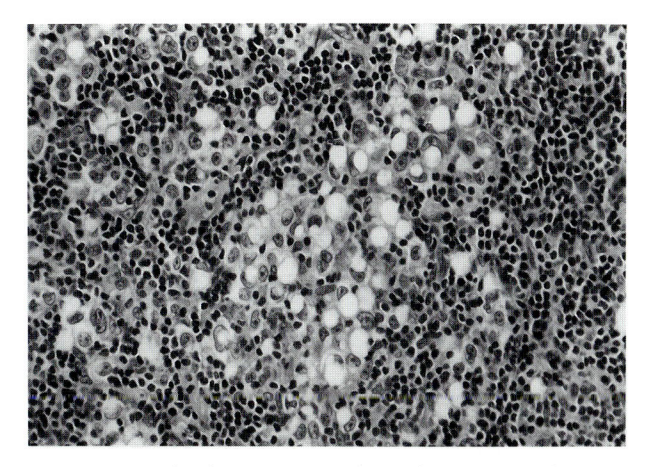

Fig. 9.13. A higher-power view of Fig. 9.12 showing signet-ring tumor cells. H&E, ×500.

These plasma cells may be monoclonal, and monoclonal gammopathy has been reported.[16] Other cases of FL may show amorphous extracellular precipitate (Fig. 9.14). This precipitation is usually seen in the follicles and is eosinophilic and often PAS-positive. By electron-microscopic and immunohistochemical studies, this material represents degradated membrane products of the tumor cells.[17] The so-called "reverse" variant has been reported in a few cases, in which the follicles have dark-staining center and pale-staining mantle zone owing to the presence of large lymphoid cells at the periphery of the follicles.[18] Finally, a floral variant of follicular lymphoma that is characterized by the neoplastic follicles being surrounded and penetrated by the small lymphocytes, imparting a floral appearance (Fig. 9.15) has recently been described.[19]

A primary diagnosis of FL cannot be made by examining specimens from an extranodal site as lymphoid aggregates or prominent follicle formation in the bone marrow, spleen, or liver can be seen in other types of lymphomas. However, certain characteristics are frequently demonstrated in FL occurring in these organs.

1. *Bone marrow:* The histologic pattern of bone marrow involvement by FL is characterized by the presence of well-defined lymphoid aggregates in the paratrabecular location (Fig. 9.16).[4,11] The cytologic features

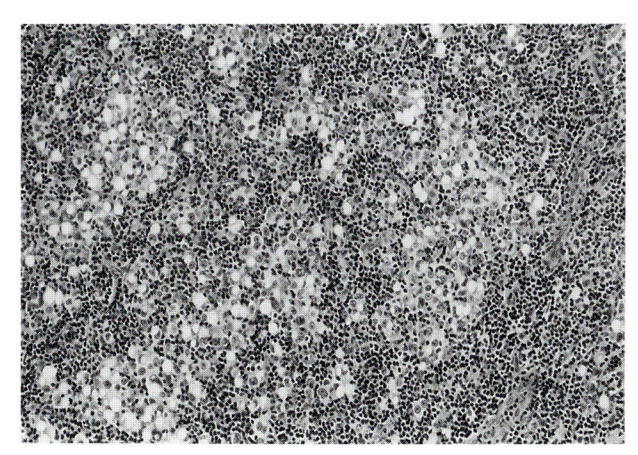

Fig. 9.12. The signet-ring-cell variant of follicular lymphoma in a lymph node showing many signet-ring tumor cells. H&E, ×250.

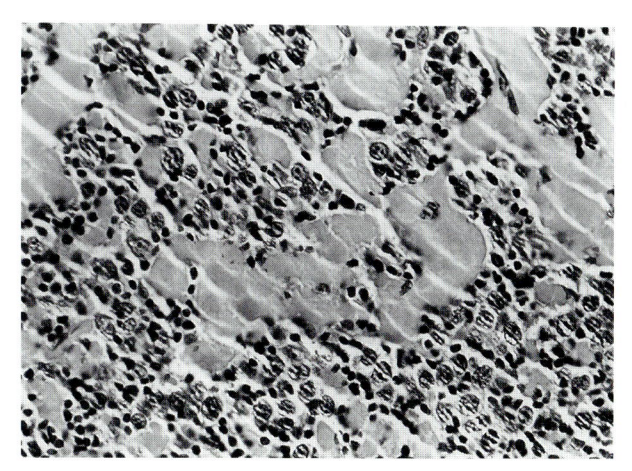

Fig. 9.14. Lymph node biopsy of follicular lymphoma showing amorphous, eosinophilic extracellular precipitate. H&E, ×500.

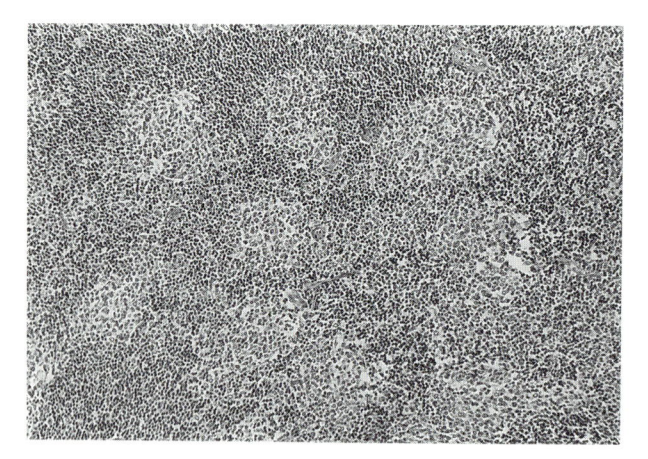

Fig. 9.15. A case of floral variant of follicular lymphoma showing the neoplastic follicles surrounded and penetrated by small lymphocytes imparting a floral appearance. H&E, ×125.

may be identical to those of the nodal tumor, but tumor cells in the bone marrow often appear more mature than those in the lymph node. Therefore, it is important to distinguish FL from benign lymphoid aggregates. Multiple, large, paratrabecular lymphoid follicles containing atypical lymphoid cells with infiltration of the surrounding normal bone marrow are features in favor of malignancy.

2. *Spleen:* Grossly, the spleen may show evenly distributed, uniform, white nodules on the cut surface in cases of FL. Microscopically, these nodules are located in the lymphoid follicles of the splenic white pulp. In the large-cell subtype, the tumor nodules may be irregular-shaped and their distribution may be uneven.[11] The distinction between FL and lymphoid hyperplasia in the spleen can be very difficult if cytologic atypia is not obvious.

3. *Liver:* FL involves primarily the portal tracts of the liver and may spread beyond the limiting plate of the lobules (Fig. 9.17). The infiltration pattern is the same in different types of lymphoma. Its distinction from lymphoid hyperplasia depends on cytologic atypia, hepatic parenchymal involvement, and the absence of plasma cells in the infiltrate.[11]

Mantle-Cell Lymphoma

MCL was initially designated by Berard and Dorfman as malignant lymphoma, lymphocytic type, intermediate differentiation for a group of lymphomas that could not be assigned to either the well-differentiated or poorly differentiated lymphoma category.[20] This group of tumors was later found to have alkaline phosphatase activity and was thus considered to originate from the mantle zone, where alkaline phosphatase is normally present.[21] This tumor was then called *mantle-zone lymphoma*. In recent years, mantle-zone lymphoma was found to be identical to centrocytic lymphoma of the Kiel classification.[3] There is no special classification for MCL in the Working Formulation. In 1992, a new name, *mantle-cell lymphoma*, was suggested by a lymphoma study group[3] and has been generally accepted.[13]

It is now clear that MCL indeed contains small lymphocytes like those of well-differentiated lymphocytic lymphoma and lymphocytes with angulated and

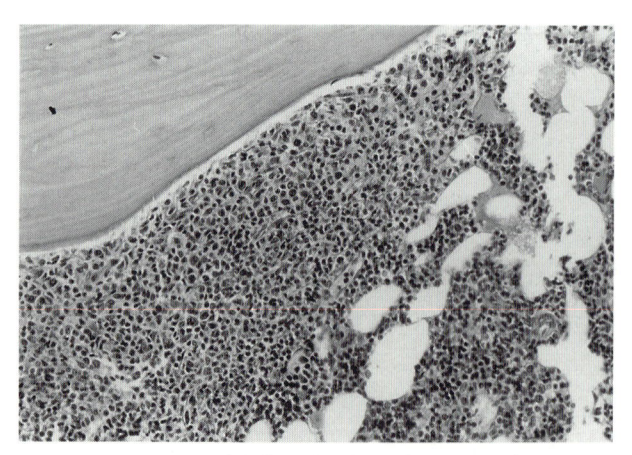

Fig. 9.16. A case of follicular lymphoma with paratrabecular infiltration of bone marrow by small cleaved cells. H&E, ×250.

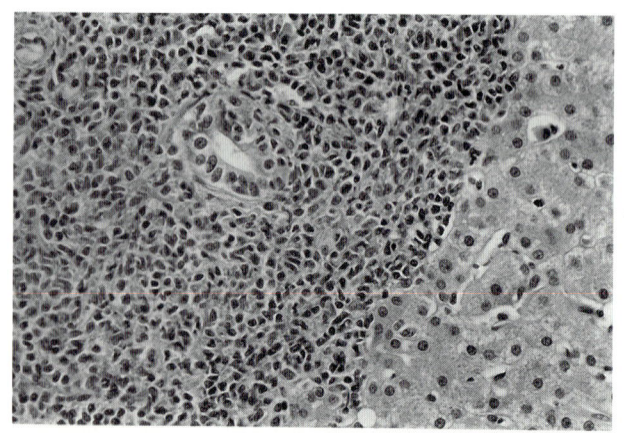

Fig. 9.17. A case of small-cleaved-cell follicular lymphoma with neoplastic infiltration in the portal area of the liver. H&E, ×250.

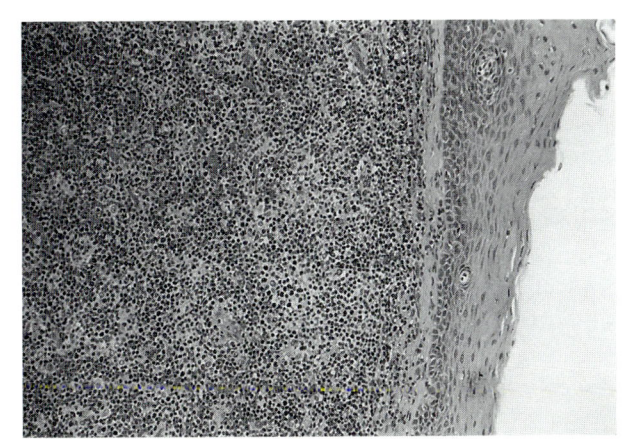

Fig. 9.18. A case of mantle-cell lymphoma involving the tonsil with the diffuse intermediate lymphocytic lymphoma pattern. H&E, ×250.

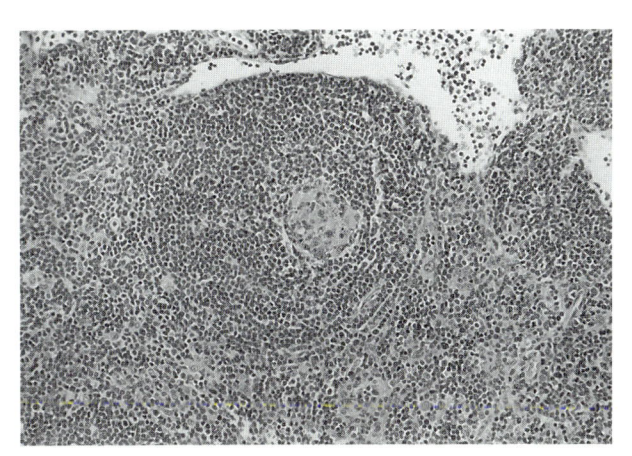

Fig. 9.20. Lymph node biopsy of mantle-cell lymphoma showing the remnant of a germinal center and the expanded mantle zone composed of tumor cells. H&E, ×250.

cleaved nuclei like those of poorly differentiated lymphocytic lymphoma. However, the tumor cells are composed primarily of small lymphoid cells having slightly irregular or indented nuclei, and each of the other two cell populations should not be more than 30% to fulfill the diagnostic criteria of MCL.[2,9] The tumor cells are also characterized by the presence of moderately coarse chromatin, inconspicuous nucleoli, and scant cytoplasm.

The lymph node architecture is usually completely effaced by a diffuse, vaguely nodular, or overtly nodular proliferation. On the basis of these patterns, MCL is further divided into diffuse intermediate lymphocytic lymphoma (Figs. 9.18, 9.19) and mantle zone lymphoma (Figs. 9.20, 9.21).[9] In the mantle-zone subtype, the neoplastic cells selectively infiltrate and expand the mantle zones surrounding the residual germinal centers. In some cases, numerous "naked" germinal centers are surrounded by neoplastic cells with a slight nodular pattern. These cases are classified as the mantle-zone subtype by the National Cancer Institute but are classified the diffuse subtype by Weisenburger's group.[20]

A rare subtype, the blastic variant, has recently been added.[22] In this variant, the tumor cells are large cells with finely dispersed chromatin pattern and inconspicuous nucleoli (Figs. 9.22, 9.23). The mitotic

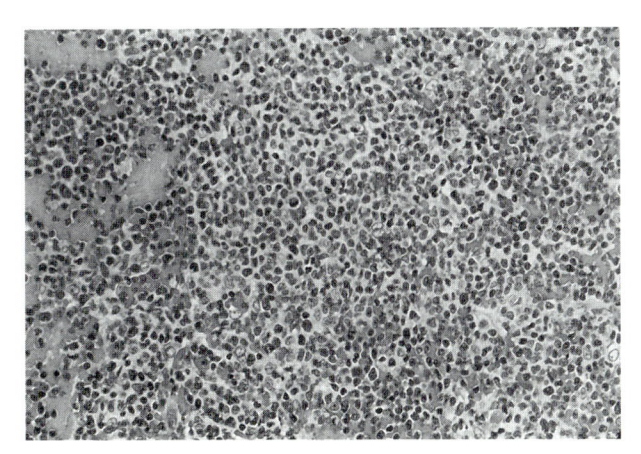

Fig. 9.19. A higher-power view of Fig. 9.18 showing diffuse infiltration of tumor cells with irregular, angulated nuclei. H&E, ×500.

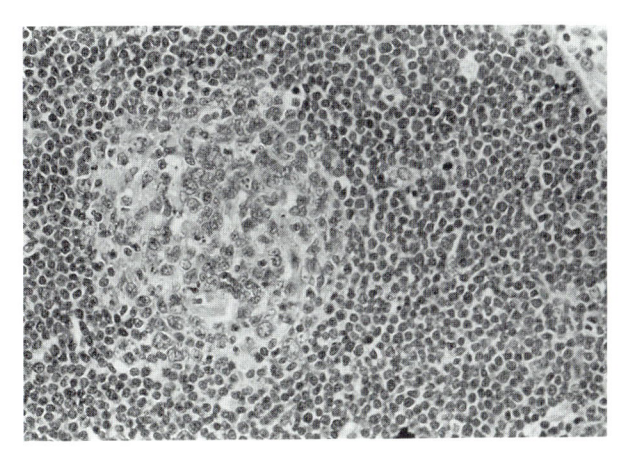

Fig. 9.21. A higher-power view of mantle-cell lymphoma showing tumor cells with slightly irregular nuclei surrounding a germinal center. H&E, ×500.

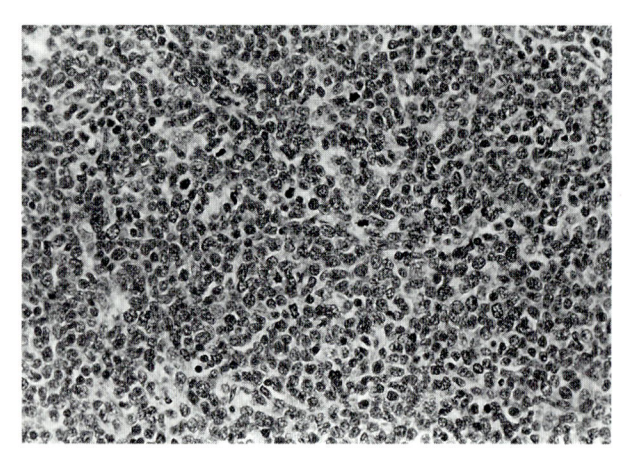

Fig. 9.22. The blastic variant of mantle-cell lymphoma showing effacement of nodal architecture by medium-sized immature lymphoid cells with a high mitotic rate. H&E, ×500.

rate is high. The histologic features are somewhat similar to lymphoblastic lymphoma.[20] Patients with this variant have an aggressive clinical course.

On the other extreme, the neoplastic cells of MCL can be very well differentiated, showing only slight nuclear irregularity. In these cases, it is difficult to distinguish from small lymphocytic lymphoma/chronic lymphocytic leukemia (SLL/CLL). However, proliferation centers and plasmacytoid differentiation, which are seen in SLL/CLL, are not demonstrated in MCL, and the presence of a "naked" germinal center is not detected in SLL/CLL.[20] Another special feature found in approximately two thirds of MCL cases is the presence of histiocytes with granular eosinophilic cytoplasm, which may give the starry-sky appearance.[20] The monotonous appearance of the MCL cells also helps distinguish it from other low-grade B-cell lymphomas, because prolymphocytes, paraimmunoblasts, and proliferation centers are present in small lymphocytic lymphoma and chronic lymphocytic leukemia, while large noncleaved lymphoid cells are seen in all types of FL.[20]

MCL frequently involves the spleen (Fig. 9.24). It may cause massive splenomegaly, and in some cases this is the primary site. MCL mainly involves the splenic white pulp showing a mantle-zone pattern. The marginal zone is often preserved.[9] The lymphoma cells may also extend into the red pulp, especially in severe cases. In the bone marrow, the infiltration is intertrabecular, but a paratrabecular pattern is occasionally seen.[20] In the liver, MCL cells usually infiltrate the portal tracts, but sinusoids may also be involved (Fig. 9.25). Lymphoma infiltration of the GI tract may lead to multiple lymphomatous polyposis, which is a distinct clinicopathologic entity considered to be caused exclusively by MCL.[23]

LABORATORY FINDINGS

Although there are still many unanswered questions concerning the evolution process and the relationship between follicular center cells and the mantle cells, the immunophenotypes of these two groups of cells are well delineated, which makes their differentiation possible. Both groups of cells carry surface im-

Fig. 9.23. A lymph node imprint showing the cytologic appearance of the blastic form of mantle-cell lymphoma. H&E, ×500.

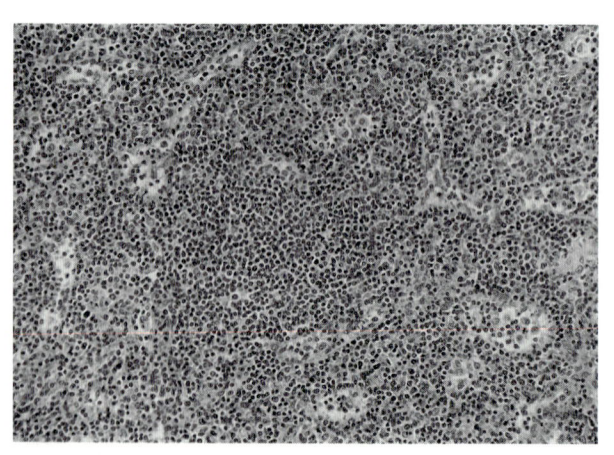

Fig. 9.24. Spleen in mantle-cell lymphoma showing neoplastic infiltration of both white and red pulp. H&E, ×250.

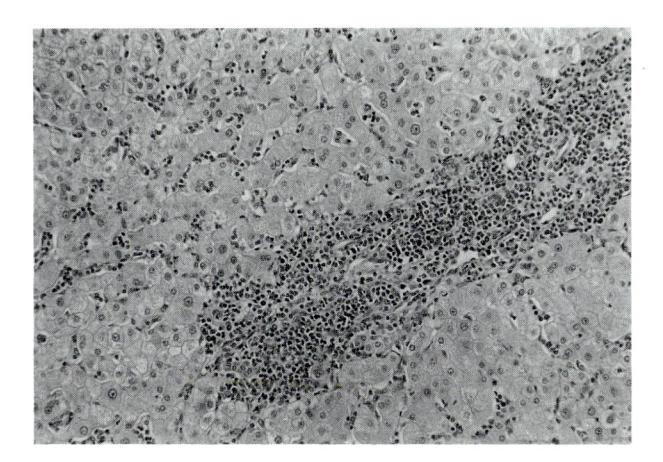

Fig. 9.25. Liver in mantle-cell lymphoma showing neoplastic infiltration in both a portal tract and sinusoids. H&E, ×250.

munoglobulin, the pan-B antigens (CD19, CD20, CD22, and CD24) and HLA-DR antigen. However, mantle cells bear both IgM and IgD, while follicular center cells carry only IgM or switch to IgG or IgA.[2,4] The characteristic marker for mantle cells is CD5, and that for follicular center cells is CD10 (Table 9.2). Leu8 is positive in MCL but negative in most cases of FL.[2,4,24,25] In paraffin sections, MCL cells also react to CD43, CD74 (LN2), and MB2 but fail to react with CDw75 (LN1).[2,9] FL cells, on the other hand, react to CD74 and CDw75 but not CD43.[2,4,9] MCL also shows

TABLE 9.2
Differentiation between FL, MCL, and SLL/CLL

	FL	MCL	SLL/CLL
CD5	−	+	+
CD10	+	−	−
CD19	+	+	+
CD20	+	+	+
CD22	+	+	±
CD23	−	−	+
CD43	−	+	+
CD45RA	+	−	−
CD74	+	+	+
CDw75	+	−	−
Leu8	±	+	+
HLA-DR	+	+	+
IgD	−	+	+
ALPase[a]	−	+	−
Cytogenetics	t(14;18)	t(11;14)	t(11;14)
Protooncogene	bcl-2	bcl-1	bcl-1

[a]ALPase = alkaline phosphatase.

alkaline phosphatase seen in normal lymphocytes in the mantle zone.[21] On the basis of the immunophenotype and a negative bcl-2 gene result, Abe et al. suggested that the diffuse small cleaved-cell lymphoma is derived from the mantle zone and not the follicular center.[24]

Phenotypically, MCL is very similar to SLL/CLL (Table 9.2). The currently available monoclonal antibody CD23 can be used to distinguish between these two entities; it is negative for MCL but positive for SLL/CLL.[26] For the distinction between FH and FL, MT-2 (CD45RA) was considered most helpful, but recent studies demonstrated that bcl-2 antibody is even more reliable for this purpose.[27]

In addition to the immunophenotypes of the tumor cells, the distribution of the dendritic reticulum cells (DRCs), as demonstrated by CD21, CD23, and S-100 protein, is also helpful in distinguishing FL from MCL. In the former, the DRCs are arranged in a nodular, spherical meshwork pattern, while DRCs in the latter form a loose meshwork pattern with ill-defined margins at the periphery of the neoplastic nodules.[28]

The molecular genetic changes in these two tumors are of particular importance, because they not only facilitate diagnosis but also provide insight into tumorigenesis. Both tumors involve the translocation of a protooncogene with the immunoglobulin heavy-chain gene. In FL, it is t(14;18)(q32;q21) translocation; bcl-2 (18q21) moves into the proximity of the Ig heavy-chain enhancer region (14q32). As a result, the protooncogene is activated and the functional bcl-2-Ig fusion protein is overexpressed. The bcl-2 gene encodes for an inner mitochondrial membrane protein that plays a role of blocking programmed cell death (apoptosis).[29] Therefore, cells with abnormal expression of this protein remain in stage G_0 in the cell cycle and become immortalized.[4,11] Since the protein does not promote proliferation, it serves to explain why most patients with FL have an indolent clinical course.

In MCL, the protooncogene bcl-1 (11q13) is juxtaposed to an Ig-enhancer sequence located on chromosome 14. Recently, a gene known as PRAD1 (parathyroid adenoma 1), was found to be linked to the bcl-1 locus.[30] This gene encodes for cyclin D1, a cell-cycle protein. When the PRAD1/bcl-1 gene is deregulated as a result of translocation, the G_1–S transition of the cell cycle is disturbed and the t(11;14)-carrying cells cannot exit from the cell cycle, resulting in an expanded B-cell department.[19,31]

Using the polymerase chain reaction, t(14;18) or

t(11;14) translocation can be detected in small numbers of tumor cells, thus greatly facilitating early diagnosis and therapeutic monitoring of these patients.[2,7,31] Furthermore, the presence of p53 gene mutation or *c-myc* gene translocation has been found to be the genetic mechanism of progression and histologic transformation of FL.[32,33]

REFERENCES

1. Utz GL, Swerdlow SH: Distinction of follicular hyperplasia from follicular lymphoma in B5-fixed tissues: Comparison of MT2 and bcl-2 antibodies. *Hum Pathol* 24:1155–1158, 1993.
2. Weisenburger DD, Chan WC: Lymphomas of follicles: Mantle cell and follicular center cell lymphomas. *Am J Clin Pathol* 99:409–420, 1993.
3. Banks PM, Chan J, Cleary ML, et al: Mantle cell lymphoma: A proposal for unification of morphologic, immunologic and molecular data. *Am J Surg Pathol* 16:637–640, 1992.
4. Harris N, Ferry JA: Follicular lymphoma and related disorders (germinal center lymphomas). In Knowles DM (ed): *Neoplastic Hematopathology*, Baltimore, Williams & Wilkins, 1992, pp 645–674.
5. Lukes RJ, Collins RD: B cell Lymphomas. In *Tumors of the Hematopoietic System*, 2nd series, Washington DC, Armed Forces Institute of Pathology, 1992, pp 97–225.
6. Lennert K, Feller AC: *Histopathology of Non-Hodgkin's Lymphomas (Based on the Updated Kiel Classification)*, 2nd ed, Berlin, Springer-Verlag, 1992, pp 80–102.
7. Lambrechts AC, Hupkes PE, Dorssers LCJ, et al: Translocation (14;18)-positive cells are present in the circulation of the majority of patients with localized (stage I and II) follicular non-Hodgkin's lymphoma. *Blood* 82:2510–2516, 1993.
8. Ioachim HL: *Lymph Node Pathology*, 2nd ed, Philadelphia, Lippincott, 1994, pp 396–401.
9. Weisenburger DD: Mantle cell lymphoma. In Knowles DM (ed): *Neoplastic Hematopathology*, Baltimore, Williams & Wilkins, 1992, pp 617–628.
10. Schnitzer B: Reactive lymphadenopathies. In Knowles DM (ed): *Neoplastic Hematopathology*, Baltimore, Williams & Wilkins, 1992, pp 427–457.
11. Mann RB: Follicular lymphomas. In Jaffe E (ed): *Surgical Pathology of the Lymph Nodes and Related Organs*, Philadelphia, Saunders, 1995, pp 252–282.
12. Nathwani BN, Winberg CD, Diamond LW, et al: Morphologic criteria for the differentiation of follicular lymphoma from florid reactive follicular hyperplasia: A study of 80 cases. *Cancer* 48:1794–1806, 1981.
13. Harris NL, Jaffe ES, Stein H, et al: A revised European–American Classification of lymphoid neoplasms: A proposal from the International Lymphoma Study Group. *Blood* 84:1361–1392, 1994.
14. Non-Hodgkin's Lymphoma Pathologic Classification Project: National Cancer Institute-sponsored study of classifications of non-Hodgkin's lymphomas; summary and description of a working formulation for clinical usage. *Cancer* 49:2112–2135, 1982.
15. Silberman S, Frisco R, Steinbecker H: Signet ring cell lymphoma: A report of a case and review of the literature. *Am J Clin Pathol* 81:358–362, 1984.
16. Schmid U, Karow J, Lennert K: Follicular malignant non-Hodgkin's lymphoma with pronounced plasmacytic differentiation: A plasmacytoma-like lymphoma. *Virchows Arch (Pathol Anat)* 405:473–481, 1986.
17. Chittal SM, Careriviere P, Voight JJ, et al: Follicular lymphoma with abundant PAS-positive extracellular material. Immunohistochemical and ultrastructural observations. *Am J Surg Pathol* 11:618–624, 1987.
18. Chan KC, Ng CS, Hui PK: An unusual morphologic variant of follicular lymphoma. Report of two cases. *Histopathology* 12:649–658, 1988.
19. Goates JJ, Kamel OW, LeBrun DP, et al: Floral variant of follicular lymphoma: Immunological and molecular studies support a neoplastic process. *Am J Surg Pathol* 18:37–47, 1994.
20. Medeiro LJ, Jaffe ES: Low-grade B-cell lymphomas not specified in the Working Formulation. In Jaffe ES (ed): *Surgical Pathology of the Lymph Nodes and Related Organs*, 2nd ed, Philadelphia, Saunders, 1995, pp 221–251.
21. Nanba K, Jaffe ES, Braylan RC, et al: Alkaline phosphatase-positive malignant lymphoma: A subtype of B-cell lymphomas. *Am J Clin Pathol* 68:535–542, 1977.
22. Lardelli P, Bookman MA, Sundeen J, et al: Lymphocytic lymphoma of intermediate differentiation: Morphologic and immunophenotypic spectrum and clinical correlations. *Am J Surg Pathol* 14:752–763, 1990.
23. O'Brian DS, Kennedy MJ, Daly PA, et al: Multiple lymphomatous polyposis of the gastrointestinal tract: A clinicopathologically distinctive form of non-Hodgkin's lymphoma of B-cell centrocytic type. *Am J Surg Pathol* 13:691–699, 1989.
24. Abe M, Ono N, Tominaga K, et al: Histogenesis of diffuse small cleaved cell lymphoma: An immunohistochemical and molecular genetic (bcl-2 gene) study with comparison to follicular small cleaved cell lymphoma and mantle zone lymphoma. *Cancer* 70:821–829, 1992.
25. Michie SA, Garcia CF, Strickler JG, et al: Expression of Leu 8 by B-cell lymphomas. *Am J Clin Pathol* 88:486–490, 1987.
26. Dorfman DM, Pinkus GS: Distinction between small lymphocytic and mantle cell lymphoma by immunoreactivity for CD23. *Mod Pathol* 7:326–331, 1994.
27. Utz GL, Swerdlow SH: Distinction of follicular hyperplasia from follicular lymphoma in B5-fixed tissues: Comparison of MT2 and bcl-2 antibodies. *Hum Pathol* 24:1155–1158, 1993.
28. Gloghini A, Carbone A: The non-lymphoid microenvironment of reactive follicles and lymphomas of follicu-

lar origin as defined by immunohistology on paraffin-embedded tissues. *Hum Pathol* 24:67–76, 1993.
29. Hockenberry D, Nunez G, Milliman C, et al: Bcl-2 is an inner-mitochondrial membrane protein that blocks programmed cell death. *Nature* 348:334–336, 1990.
30. Rosenberg CL, Wong E, Petty E, et al: PRAD1, a candidate BCL-1 oncogene: mapping and expression in centrocytic lymphoma. *Proc Natl Acad Sci* (USA) 88:9638–9642, 1991.
31. Rimokh R, Berger F, Delso G, et al: Detection of the chromosomal translocation t(11;14) by polymerase chain reaction in mantle cell lymphomas. *Blood* 83:1871–1875, 1994.
32. Sander CA, Yano T, Clark HM, et al: p53 mutation is associated with progression in follicular lymphomas. *Blood* 82:1994–2004, 1993.
33. Farrugia MM, Duan LJ, Reis MD, et al: Alterations of the p53 tumor suppressor gene in diffuse large cell lymphomas with translocations of the c-myc and BCL-2 proto-oncogenes. *Blood* 83:191–198, 1994.

10
Composite Lymphoma vs. Richter's Syndrome vs. Mixed Small- and Large-Cell Lymphoma

Composite lymphoma is defined by the Working Formulation of non-Hodgkin's lymphomas (NHL) as "two distinctly demarcated types of NHL or the rare association of Hodgkin's disease (HD) with a form of NHL within a single organ or tissue."[1] When the two neoplasms involve different sites of the same patient, it is called *discordant* lymphoma.[2] While composite lymphoma and discordant lymphoma constitute a phenomenon with the coexistence of two different types of neoplasms occurring simultaneously, the phenomenon of two types of lymphomas developing sequentially is called *secondary* lymphoma, such as an anaplastic large cell Ki-1 lymphoma secondary to a cutaneous T-cell lymphoma (see Chapter 14). However, when a large-cell lymphoma develops from a chronic lymphocytic leukemia (CLL), it is specifically designated as Richter's syndrome.[3] While the above-mentioned phenomena appear quite different from each other, in the light of phenotyping and genotyping, they all represent a common phenomenon of transformation between two types of lymphomas. Furthermore, these phenomenoan should be distinguished from the mixed small- and large-cell lymphoma in which both cell types are integral parts of the same tumor and also distinguished from small lymphocytic lymphoma with proliferation centers.

CLINICAL FEATURES

Composite Lymphoma

The incidence of composite lymphoma varies from 1% to 4.7%, while that of discordant lymphoma ranges between 9.3% and 33%.[4] The ages range widely from 3 to 85 years, and male patients are predominant.[5] The composite tumor is usually present in the lymph node but also in the liver and spleen. The prognosis is generally determined by the more malignant component. The study by Cerroni et al. showed that when mycosis fungoides transforms into a pleomorphic large-cell lymphoma, the 10-year survival rate for those patients became 11.2%, as compared to the survival rate of 46.6% in patients without transformation.[6] On the other hand, patients with a composite lymphoma, consisting of HD (nodular lymphocytic predominance subtype) and diffuse large-cell lymphoma, generally have more localized disease and a longer survival time than do those with large-cell lymphoma alone.[7,8]

Richter's Syndrome

Patients with Richter's syndrome usually have a history of CLL. The clinical manifestations of the antecedent CLL do not differ from those CLL cases not associated with Richter's syndrome. The subsequent development of a high-grade lymphoma is not necessarily related to chemotherapy or radiation therapy, because Richter's syndrome may occur in patients without any treatment for antecedent CLL.[9] Richter's syndrome usually develops 2–8 years following CLL and occurs in about 3–13% of CLL patients.[9–12] Richter's transformation is usually indicated by a sudden development of fever; asymmetric, massive lymphadenopathy; prominent splenomegaly; and moderate hepatomegaly.[11,12] Abdominal pain and weight loss can be additional warning signs.[9] Richter's transformation carries an ominous prognosis, with patients usually dying within a few months after a rapidly progressive clinical course.

PATHOLOGY

Composite Lymphoma

Composite lymphomas may be composed of various components; the most common pattern consists of two B-cell NHL. In terms of histology, the most common combination is a follicular lymphoma of the small cleaved cell and a diffuse large-cell lymphoma.[4] Monocytoid B-cell lymphoma has an unusually high incidence of forming composite lymphoma with a higher-grade lymphoma such as diffuse large-cell lymphoma (Figs. 10.1–10.3).[13–15]

Composite T-cell lymphoma is rare. The only example is the transformation of mycosis fungoides into large-cell lymphoma of T-cell lineage, and these tumors may coexist as a composite lymphoma (Figs. 10.4, 10.5).[6] A mixed T- and B-cell composite lymphoma is extremely rare. A few such cases reported

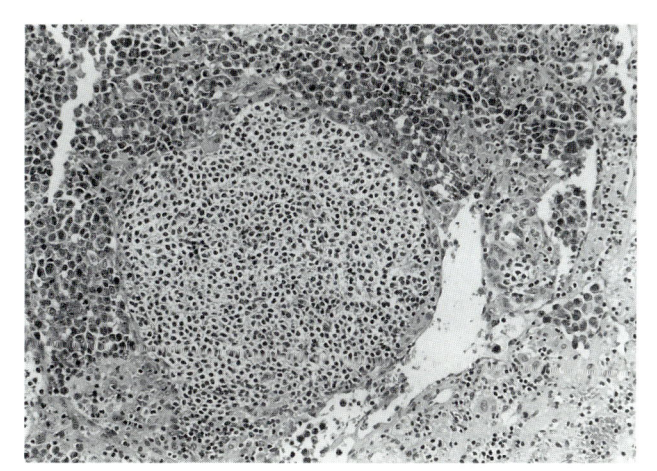

Fig. 10.1. A composite lymphoma showing a group of monocytoid B-cells in the center surrounded by large lymphoid cells. H&E, ×250.

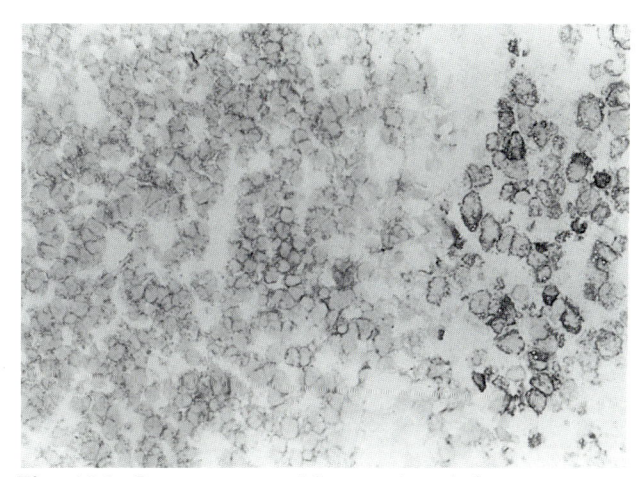

Fig. 10.3. Immunoperoxidase stain of the composite lymphoma as in Figs. 10.1 and 10.2 showing mainly λ light-chain staining; κ light-chain stain (not shown) is negative. ×250.

lacked detailed immunologic, cytogenetic, or molecular analysis.[16] Hu et al. described a case of composite lymphoma consisting of large B-lymphocytes and small T-lymphocytes.[17] However, Kim cautioned that it is sometimes difficult to determine whether both components are malignant.[4] For instance, T-cell-rich B-cell lymphoma has been frequently mistaken as T-cell lymphoma when in fact the T-cell component is reactive.[18]

Although HD and NHL may coexist in the same anatomic site of the same patient, this occurrence has been deemed coincidental because these two tumors have been considered unrelated clinicopathologic entities.[19] However, as recent studies have strongly suggested a lymphoid origin for the neoplastic cells of HD, the coexistence of Hodgkin's disease and NHL should be considered as composite lymphoma just like other combinations of NHL (Figs. 10.6–10.9).[8,19–28] The most common form of this type of composite lymphoma is a combination of nodular lymphocyte predominant HD and large-cell lymphoma. The combination of NHL and other forms of HD (nodular sclerosis or mixed cellularity) is less common but still significant.[19,21] In terms of the NHL components, most cases are of B-cell phe-

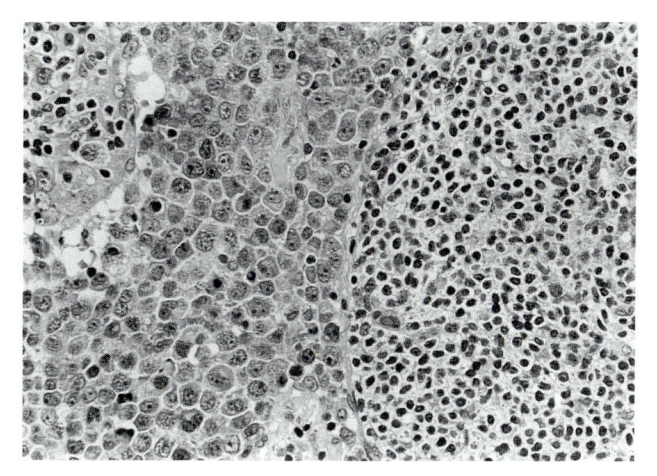

Fig. 10.2. Higher magnification showing monocytoid B-cells at right and large lymphoid cells at left. H&E, ×250.

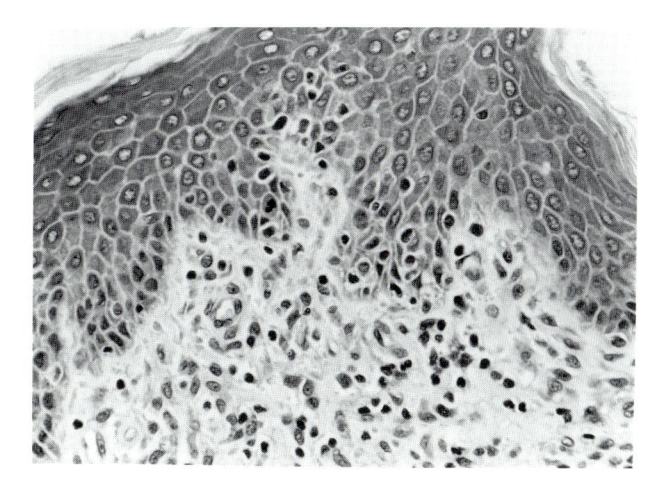

Fig. 10.4. A case of mycosis fungoides showing atypical lymphoid-cell infiltrate in the epidermis. H&E, ×500.

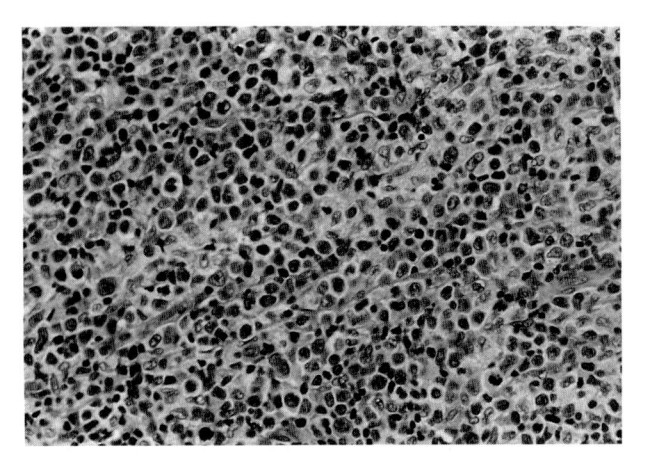

104 DIFFERENTIAL DIAGNOSIS OF LYMPHOID DISORDERS

Fig. 10.5. The same case as Fig. 10.4, which subsequently developed T-cell immunoblastic lymphoma in the lymph node. H&E, ×500.

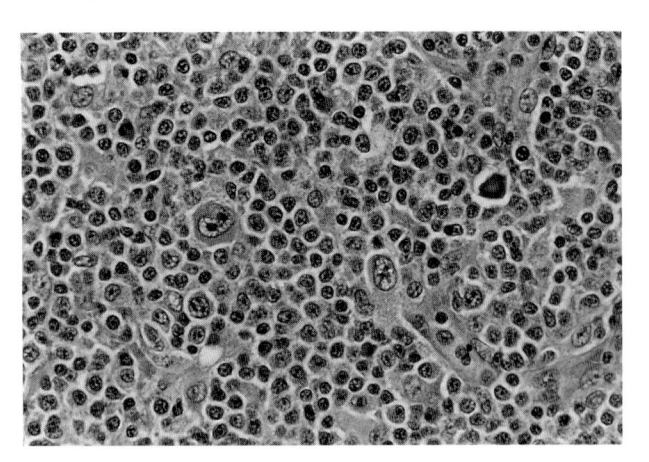

Fig. 10.7. The same case as in Fig. 10.6 showing a Reed–Sternberg cell, a few Hodgkin's cells, and a mummified cell on a background of chronic lymphocytic leukemia. H&E, ×500.

notype, and follicular lymphoma is the most common histologic pattern. However, mycosis fungoides or adult T-cell lymphoma/leukemia in combination with HD have also been reported.[19,21,24]

In addition to the simultaneous coexistence of HD and NHL, these two diseases may also develop sequentially. Travis et al. found that HD is even more common than acute leukemia as a sequela following the treatment of NHL.[20] On the other hand, the development of a high-grade NHL after patients were successfully treated for HD may represent a complication from a persistent immunodeficient state.[22]

Richter's Syndrome

This syndrome was first described by Richter in 1928 in an autopsy case of a patient with chronic lymphocytic leukemia who subsequently developed reticulum-cell sarcoma.[3] In the light of immunophenotyping, most cases of reticulum-cell sarcoma have been reported as large-cell lymphoma of B-cell lineage. The original definition has been modified and expanded by some investigators to cover loosely all high-grade non-Hodgkin's lymphoma following CLL (Fig. 10.10).[10,12] In early literature, the presence of Reed–Sternberg-like cells in

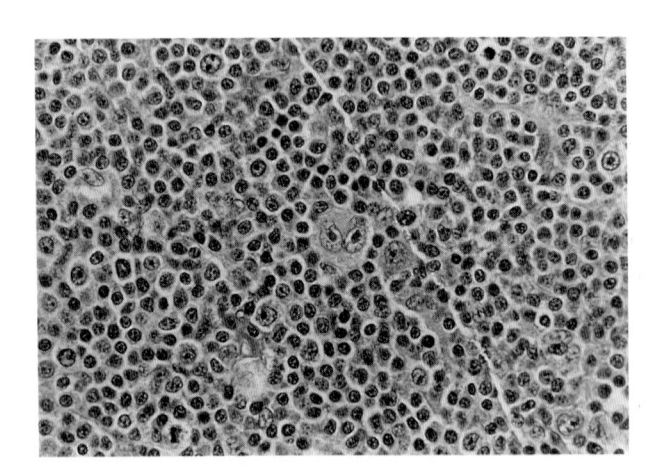

Fig. 10.6. A composite lymphoma of chronic lymphocytic leukemia and Hodgkin's disease. Note the presence of Reed–Sternberg cell in the center. The surrounding small lymphocytes show monotypic surface immunoglobulin (not shown). H&E, ×500.

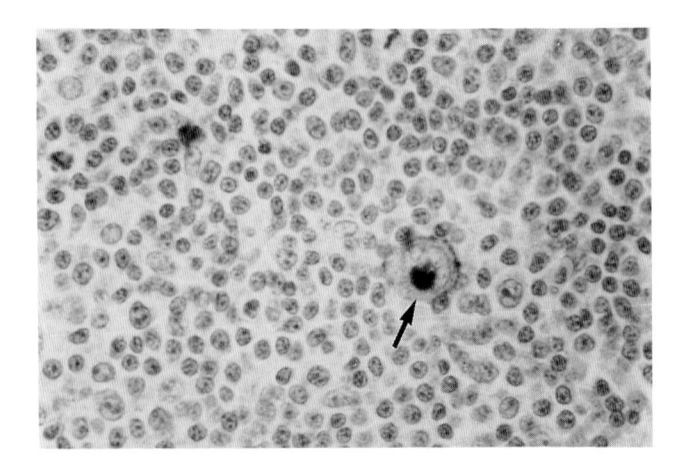

Fig. 10.8. The Reed–Sternberg cell in the case shown in Fig. 10.6 is stained for CD15 (arrow). Immunoperoxidase, ×500.

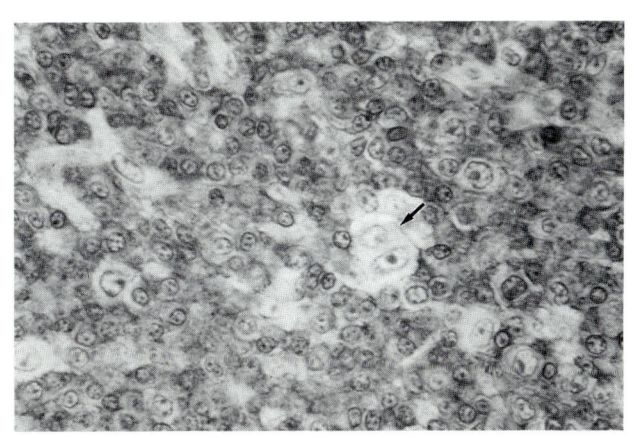

Fig. 10.9. The Reed–Sternberg cell (arrow) and other large cells (Hodgkin's cell) are negative for LCA (CD45), while the small lymphoid cells are positive. Immunoperoxidase, ×500.

Richter's syndrome was considered as probable blastic transformation of CLL.[11,25] However, current studies show that CLL can, indeed, transform into Hodgkin's disease, because full-blown Hodgkin's disease may subsequently develop in patients with this transformation.[26]

The current tendency is to further loosen up the definition of Richter's syndrome to include all transformations from a low-grade lymphoid neoplasm to a high-grade one.[4] This concept may cover large-cell lymphoma evolving from small-cell lymphoma or macroglobulinemia.[12,27,28] On the other hand, prolymphocytic and lymphoblastic (blast crisis) transformation of CLL are seldom considered in the spectrum of Richter's syndrome.[29,30]

LABORATORY FINDINGS

The diagnosis of composite lymphoma is usually made on a morphologic basis. However, with the availability of immunophenotyping techniques, increasing numbers of composite lymphoma are being diagnosed.[31] As mentioned before, the most common phenotype is B-cell/B-cell, and occasionally T-cell/T-cell or T-cell/B-cell.[4] Composite lymphoma consisting of HD/NHL has finally been established as a true clinicopathologic entity, and case reports of such an entity have become more frequent. Reed–Sternberg cells in HD stain positive for CD15 and CD30, but negative for CD45 (CLA), while Reed–Sternberg-like cells in NHL may also be positive for CD30 and/or CD15, but are frequently positive for CD45.[19,21] Besides this panel, other monoclonal antibodies do not offer much help in diagnosing HD/NHL composite lymphomas.

Immunogenotyping may help exclude HD when a prominent gene rearrangement pattern is identified. When gene rearrangement is detected in Hodgkin's disease, it shows either heavy-chain or light-chain gene alone or oligoclonal.[32] In composite lymphomas with two variants of NHL, most cases show the same phenotype and genotype.[4,19] As will be discussed later, even if biphenotype and/or bigenotype are identified in a composite lymphoma, the two variants may still arise from the same clone.[33,34] The current concept is that composite lymphoma in most cases, if not all, is the result of transformation from a low-grade lymphoma to a high-grade lymphoma.[23,31] Genomic rearrangement/translocation is probably the mechanisms of such transformation.[31,34] In the case reported by de Jong et al., chromosomal translocation activated *c-myc* oncogene and led to the development of a composite lymphoma.[34] The demonstration of Epstein–Barr virus (EBV) RNA in the Reed–Sternberg cells but not in the NHL component suggests that EBV is involved in the pathogenesis of the transformation of NHL to HD.[19]

In Richter's syndrome, a history of CLL or demonstration of CLL cells in the peripheral blood from patients who have developed a high-grade lymphoma is the basis for the diagnosis. In the involved lymph

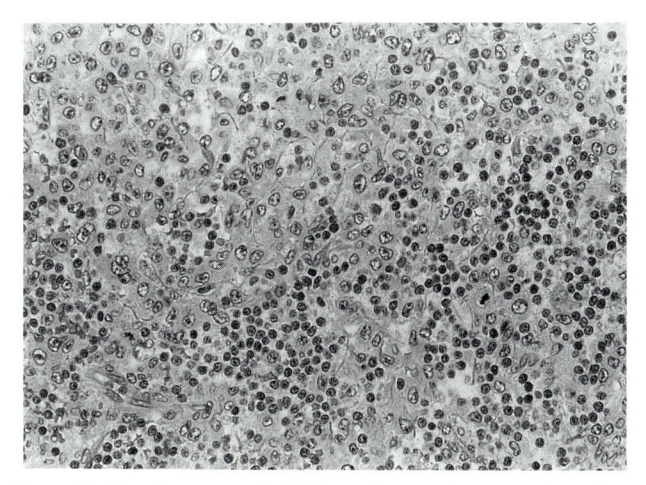

Fig. 10.10. A case of Richter's syndrome showing large lymphoma cells intermingled with cells of chronic lymphocytic leukemia. H&E, ×500.

nodes, both CLL cells and lymphoma cells can be identified in various proportions. Phenotyping may help identify two populations in the lymph node as the CLL cells express CD5 antigen and most high-grade lymphomas do not.[35] The vast majority of Richter's syndrome cases manifest transformation of CLL to a large-cell lymphoma of B-cell origin. However, at least two cases of T-CLL transforming into T-cell lymphoma have been reported.[36,37]

Current interest is focused on the clonal relationship between CLL and large-cell lymphomas.[35,38-42] Early studies were based on the surface immunoglobulin phenotyping to determine the clonal origin of the two cell populations in Richter's syndrome. Since most cases of CLL and NHL have an IgM-κ phenotype, this is obviously an oversimplified approach. Therefore, most current reports employ immunogenotyping and molecular genetic techniques to study this problem.[35,38-42] Immunogenotyping is generally reliable. However, heavy-chain gene may subject to postrearrangement deletion, point mutation, and heavy-chain switching, with resultant variation in rearranged bands. Post rearrangement changes are less frequently seen in light-chain genes; nevertheless, reiterative IgV gene rearrangements may occur in both heavy- and light-chain genes.[42] Therefore, even if the rearranged bands in both heavy- and light-chain gene representing small and large cells are not identical, the possibility still exists that both populations involved in Richter's transformation are from the same clone. Recent studies using cytogenetics,[36,39] *bcl*-2 gene analysis[41] and nuclei acid sequence analysis of the heavy- and light-chain genes[42] have proved this point. It is reasonable to assume that in most, if not all, cases of Richter's syndrome, both the CLL and lymphoma populations are from the same clone. Studies of oncogenes found that p53 tumor suppressor gene played a role in the development of lymphoma in Richter's syndrome, but *bcl*-1, *bcl*-2, and *c-myc* protooncogenes, and retinoblastoma tumor suppressor genes were not involved.[43]

DIFFERENTIAL DIAGNOSIS

Composite Lymphoma and Richter's Syndrome

Since both conditions result from transformation of a low-grade lymphoid tumor to a high-grade one, and since the definition of Richter's syndrome has been expanded, the demarcation between these two conditions becomes blurred. However, histologically, the two lymphoid variants are clearly distinguished from each other in composite lymphoma, but CLL cells are often intermingled with lymphoma cells in the lymph node from patients with Richter's syndrome. A history of CLL and sudden change in clinical symptoms favor Richter's syndrome. When the low-grade component is a lymphoid tumor other than CLL or small lymphocytic lymphoma, the diagnosis should be a composite lymphoma. Phenotyping and genotyping offer no help in the differential diagnosis.

Mixed Small- and Large-Cell Lymphoma

Mixed small- and large-cell lymphoma may mimic Richter's syndrome in histologic pattern. However, the small-cell component in the former consists of small cleaved cells in contrast to small round CLL cells in the latter (Figs. 10.11, 10.12). On the basis of the presence of CD5+ and CD5− populations, Richter's syndrome can be identified; mixed small-/large-cell lymphoma should show an identical CD5 negative phenotype in both populations. When genotyping reveals two different rearranged bands between the DNA from lymph node and that from peripheral blood, it favors Richter's syndrome. In fact, mixed-cell lymphoma may not have a leukemic phase; thus no rearranged band will be shown in samples from peripheral blood.

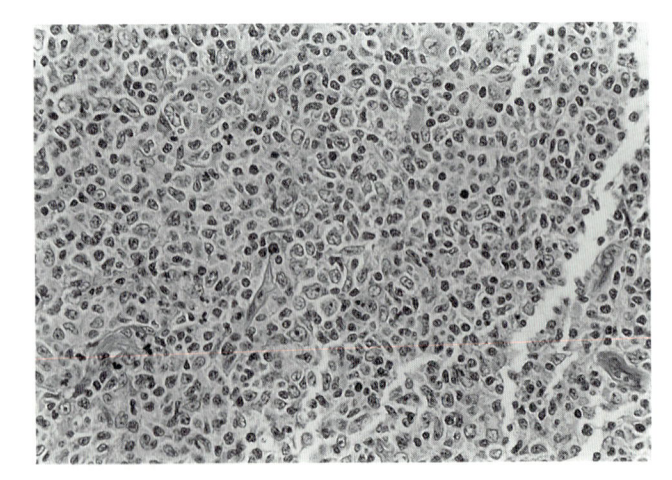

Fig. 10.11. A case of mixed small-/large-cell lymphoma showing small cleaved lymphoid cells intermixed with large lymphoma cells. H&E, ×500.

DIFFERENTIAL DIAGNOSIS OF LYMPHOID DISORDERS 107

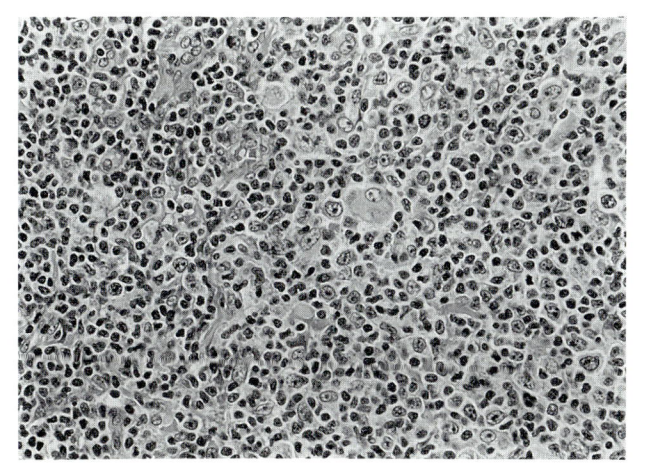

Fig. 10.12. Another case of mixed small-/large-cell lymphoma showing similar features as Fig. 10.11. H&E, ×500.

Small Lymphocytic Lymphoma with Proliferation Centers

The proliferation centers in small lymphocytic lymphoma represent aggregation of activated lymphocytes (prolymphocytes) (Fig. 10.13). This pattern may occasionally be confused with mixed small- and large-cell lymphoma or Richter's syndrome. However, the bland appearance of the activated lymphocytes may enable the pathologist to distinguish them from lymphoma cells. Small lymphocytic lymphoma is positive for CD5, and the activated lymphocytes also carry the same antigen. In Richter's syndrome, only the small-cell population is CD5 positive in most cases. The mixed small- and large-cell lymphoma does not express CD5 antigen. Genotypically, only Richter's syndrome may show different rearrangement patterns when DNA from lymphoma is compared with that from the peripheral blood.

REFERENCES

1. National Cancer Institute sponsored study of classifications of Non-Hodgkin's lymphomas: Summary and description of a Working Formulation for Clinical Usage. *Cancer* 49:2112–2135, 1982.
2. Kluin PM, van Krieken JH, Kleiverda K, et al: Discordant morphologic characteristics of B-cell lymphomas in bone marrow and lymph node biopsies. *Am J Clin Pathol* 94:59–66, 1990.
3. Richter M: Generalized reticular cell sarcoma of lymph nodes associated with lymphatic leukemia. *Am J Pathol* 4:285–292, 1928.
4. Kim H: Composite lymphoma and related disorders. *Am J Clin Pathol* 99:445–451, 1993.
5. Ioachim HL: *Lymph Node Pathology*, 2nd ed, Philadelphia, Lippincott, 1994.
6. Cerroni L, Rieger E, Kerl H: Classification and immunologic features associated with transformation of mycosis fungoides to large cell lymphoma. *Am J Surg Pathol* 16:543–552, 1992.
7. Hansmann ML, Stein H, Fellbaum C, et al: Nodular paragranuloma can transform into high-grade malignant lymphoma of B-type. *Hum Pathol* 20:1169–1175, 1989.
8. Sundeen JT, Cossman J, Jaffe ES: Lymphocytic predominant Hodgkin's disease nodular subtype with coexistent "large cell lymphoma": Histological progression or composite malignancy? *Am J Surg Pathol* 12:599–606, 1988.
9. Trump DL, Mann RB, Phelps R, et al: Richter's syndrome: Diffuse histiocytic lymphoma in patients with chronic lymphocytic leukemia: A report of five cases and review of the literature. *Am J Med* 68:539–548, 1980.
10. Armitage JO, Dick RF, Corder MP: Diffuse histiocytic lymphoma complicated chronic lymphocytic lymphoma. *Cancer* 41:422–427, 1979.
11. Foucar K, Rydell RE: Richter's syndrome in chronic lymphocytic leukemia. *Cancer* 46:118–134, 1980.
12. Harousseau JL, Flandrin G, Tricot G, et al: Malignant lymphoma supervening in chronic lymphocytic leukemia and related disorders: Richter's syndrome: A study of 25 cases. *Cancer* 48:1302–1308, 1981.
13. Ngan B, Warnke RA, Wilson M, et al: Monocytoid B-cell

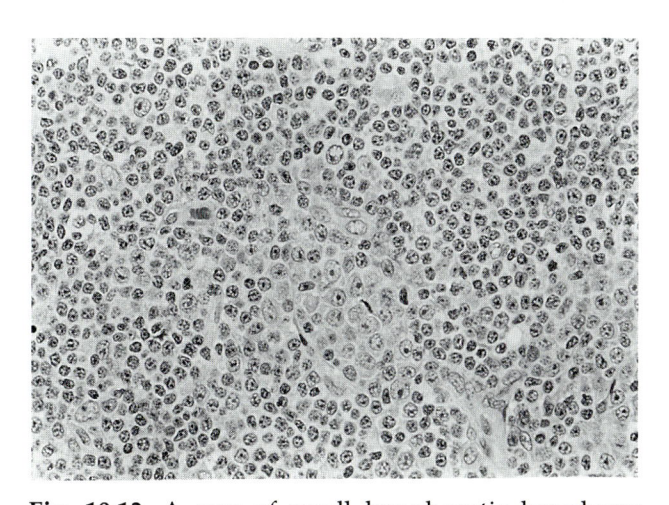

Fig. 10.13. A case of small lymphocytic lymphoma with proliferation center. Note the presence of a cluster of large, pale-stained, pro-lymphocytes in the center. H&E, ×500.

lymphoma: A study of 36 cases. *Hum Pathol* 22:409–421, 1991.
14. Sheibani K, Burke JS, Swartz WG, et al: Monocytoid B-cell lymphoma. Clinicopathologic study of 21 cases of unique type of low-grade lymphoma. *Cancer* 62:1531–1538, 1988.
15. Traweek ST, Sheibani K, Winberg CD, et al: Monocytoid B-cell lymphoma: Its evolution and relationship to other low-grade B-cell neoplasms. *Blood* 73:575–578, 1989.
16. York JC II, Cousar JB, Glick AD, et al: Morphologic and immunologic evidence of composite B- and T-cell lymphomas: A report of three cases developing in follicular center cell lymphomas. *Am J Clin Pathol* 84:35–43, 1985.
17. Hu E, Weiss LM, Warnke R, et al: Non-Hodgkin's lymphoma containing both B and T-cell clones. *Blood* 70:287–292, 1987.
18. Rodriquez J, Pugh WC, Cabanillas F: T-cell-rich B-cell lymphoma. *Blood* 1586–1589, 1993.
19. Jaffe ES, Zarate-Osorno A, Medeiros LJ: The inter-relationship of Hodgkin's disease and non-Hodgkin's lymphomas—lessons learned from composite and sequential malignancies. *Semin Diagn Pathol* 9:297–303, 1992.
20. Travis LB, Curtis RE, Boice JJ Jr, et al: Second cancers following non-Hodgkin's lymphoma. *Cancer* 67:2002–2009, 1991.
21. Zarate-Osorno A, Medeiro LJ, Kingma DW, et al: Hodgkin's disease following non-Hodgkin's lymphoma: A clinicopathologic and immunophenotypic study of nine cases. *Am J Surg Pathol* 17:123–132, 1993.
22. Zarate-Osorno A, Medeiros LJ, Longo DL, et al: Non-Hodgkin's lymphomas arising in patients successfully treated for Hodgkin's disease. A clinical, histologic, and immunophenotypic study of 14 cases. *Am J Surg Pathol* 16:885–895, 1992.
23. Gonzalez CL, Medeiros LJ, Jaffe ES: Composite lymphoma: A clinicopathologic analysis of nine patients with Hodgkin's disease and B-cell non-Hodgkin's lymphoma. *Am J Clin Pathol* 96:81–89, 1991.
24. Chan WC, Griem ML, Grozea PN, et al: Mycosis fungoides and Hodgkin's disease occurring in the same patient: Report of three cases. *Cancer* 44:1408–1413, 1979.
25. Suster S, Rywlin AM: A reappraisal of Richter's syndrome: Development of two phenotypically distinctive cell lines in a case of chronic lymphocytic leukemia. *Cancer* 59:1412–1418, 1987.
26. Williams J, Shned A, Cotelingam JD, et al: Chronic lymphocytic leukemia with coexistent Hodgkin's disease: Implication for the origin of the Reed-Sternberg cell. *Am J Surg Pathol* 15:33–42, 1991.
27. Sheibani K, Nathwani BN, Winberg CD, et al: Small lymphocytic lymphoma: Morphologic and immunologic progression. *Am J Clin Pathol* 84:237–243, 1985.
28. Chubachi A, Ohtani H, Sakuyama M, et al: Diffuse large cell lymphoma occurring in a patient with Waldenstrom's macroglobulinemia. Evidence for the two different clones in Richter's syndrome. *Cancer* 68:781–785, 1991.
29. Ghani AM, Krause JR, Brody JP: Prolymphocytic transformation of chronic lymphocytic leukemia: A report of three cases and review of the literature. *Cancer* 57:75–80, 1986.
30. Frenkel EP, Ligler FS, Graham MS, et al: Acute lymphocytic leukemia transformation of chronic lymphocytic leukemia: Substantiation by flow cytometry. *Am J Hematol* 10:391–398, 1981.
31. Sun T, Susin M, Koduru P, et al: Phenotyping and genotyping of composite lymphoma with Ki-1 component. *Hematol Pathol* 6:179–192, 1992.
32. Jaffe ES: The elusive Reed-Sternberg cell. *N Engl J Med* 320:529–531, 1989.
33. Cleary ML, Galili N, Trela M, et al: Single cell origin of bigenotypic and biphenotypic B-cell proliferations in human follicular lymphomas. *J Exp Med* 167:582–597, 1988.
34. de Jong D, Voetdijk BMH, Beuerstock GC, et al: Activation of the c-myc oncogene in a precursor B-cell blast crisis of follicular lymphoma, presenting as composite lymphoma. *N Engl J Med* 318:1373–1378, 1988.
35. Sun T, Susin M, Desner M, et al: The clonal origin of two cell populations in Richter's syndrome. *Hum Pathol* 21:722–728, 1990.
36. Norvell P, Finan J, Glover D, et al: Cytogenetic evidence for the clonal nature of Richter's syndrome. *Blood* 58:183–186, 1981.
37. Forman SJ, Nathwani BN, Woda BA, et al: Clonal evolution of T-cell prolymphocytic leukemia to a T-large-cell lymphoma: A morphologic and immunologic study. *Arch Pathol Lab Med* 109:1081–1084, 1985.
38. Schots R, Dehous MF, Jochmans K, et al: Southern blot analysis in a case of Richter's syndrome: Evidence for a postrearrangement heavy chain gene deletion associated with the altered phenotype. *Am J Clin Pathol* 95:571–577, 1991.
39. Nakamine H, Masih AS, Sanger WG, et al: Richter's syndrome with different immunoglobulin light chain types: Molecular and cytogenetic features indicate a common clonal origin. *Am J Clin Pathol* 97:656–663, 1992.
40. Koduru PRK, Lichtman SM, Smilari TF, et al: Serial phenotypic, cytogenetic and molecular genetic studies in Richter's syndrome: Demonstration of lymphoma development from the chronic lymphocytic leukemia cells. *Br J Haematol* 85:613–616, 1993.
41. Traweek ST, Liu J, Johnson RM, et al: High-grade transformation of chronic lymphocytic leukemia and low-grade non-Hodgkin's lymphoma: Genotypic confirmation of clonal identity. *Am J Clin Pathol* 100:519–526, 1993.
42. Cherepakhin V, Baird SM, Meisenholder GW, et al: Common clonal origin of chronic lymphocytic leukemia and high-grade lymphoma of Richter's syndrome. *Blood* 82:3141–3147, 1993.

43. Matolcsy A, Inghirami G, Knowles DM: Molecular genetic demonstration of the diverse evolution of Richter's syndrome (chronic lymphocytic leukemia and subsequent large cell lymphoma). *Blood* 83:1363–1372, 1994.

11
Pseudolymphoma vs. Lymphoma of Mucosa-Associated Lymphoid Tissue vs. T-Cell-Rich B-Cell Lymphoma

Small lymphocytic infiltration of the mucosa of the gastrointestinal (GI) and respiratory tracts has been a diagnostic dilemma for many years. Before the availability of some modern technologies, including immunophenotyping and immunogenotyping, most cases with this condition were diagnosed as pseudolymphoma, implying that it is either lymphoid hyperplasia or inflammatory reaction. The morphologic criteria for the diagnosis of lymphoma are monomorphic pattern, cytologic atypia, and infiltrative or destructive growth, while those of lymphoid hyperplasia, or pseudolymphoma, are polymorphous infiltrates, with or without mature plasma cells and the presence of reactive follicular centers.[1] However, the application of immunophenotyping and immunogenotyping has revealed that many of the small B-cell lymphomas may not fulfill the morphologic criteria mentioned above. For instance, they may not show cytologic atypia, and yet reactive follicular centers and mature plasma cells are frequently the integral features of this type of lymphomas.

In 1983, Isaacson and Wright first suggested that this type of lymphoma arises from the mucosa-associated lymphoid tissue (MALT).[2] This concept has gained general acceptance. The MALT-type lymphomas found in the GI[3,4] and bronchial mucosa[5] have been called the GALT (gut-associated lymphoid tissue) and BALT (bronchus-associated lymphoid tissue) type lymphomas, respectively. Since then, MALT-type lymphomas have been seen in the salivary gland,[6] thyroid,[7] ocular adnexa,[8] prostate,[9] bladder,[10] gallbladder,[9] uterine cervix,[9] thymus,[11] breast,[12] and kidney.[13] These findings suggest that the important property of these cells is homing to epithelia rather than specifically to mucosa;[14] thus, the proposal of a new terminology: GELT (glandular epithelial lymphoid tissue) lymphoma.[15]

In 1984, Jaffe et al. presented a new entity designated "pseudo-T-cell lymphoma" or diffuse B-cell lymphoma with T-cell predominance.[16] In contrast to the MALT type lymphoma, which is predominantly normal-looking B-cells, the pseudo-T-cell lymphoma is composed of predominantly T-cells, which sometimes show irregular configuration mimicking T-cell lymphoma. A diagnosis can be made only when the sparse large atypical B-cells are identified. When the large cells appear to be Reed–Sternberg-like and the background lymphocytes are normal-looking, this lymphoma is frequently mistaken as Hodgkin's disease. This type of lymphoma was later coined "T-cell-rich B-cell lymphoma (TCRBCL)" by Ramsay et al.[17] and has since become the most popular name for this entity.

CLINICAL MANIFESTATION

MALT-Type Lymphoma

Generally speaking, the MALT-type lymphomas tend to be localized at diagnosis and remain localized for long periods. They may be curable by local resection or local radiotherapy, but may recur after many years. Only a minority of these patients die of MALT-type lymphoma, probably as a result of transformation to a high-grade lymphoma. These features are in contrast to nodal low-grade lymphomas, which usually manifest widespread disease (stage III or IV) at the time of diagnosis and are unaffected by treatment.

Most of the MALT lymphomas are seen in the stomach, followed by small intestine and lungs.[1] Other glandular structures such as salivary glands, thyroid, prostate, and breast are less frequently involved. Approximately 80% of primary low-grade gastric lymphomas, 50–90% of all lung lymphomas, 40% of orbital lymphomas, and 30% of breast lymphomas belong to the MALT type.[1,10] Regardless of site, MALT lymphomas are usually associated with preexisting chronic immune system stimulation or chronic inflammation, for instance, Hashimoto's thyroiditis, Sjögren's syndrome, chronic gastric ulcer, chronic gastritis, and chronic inflammatory bowel disease (IBD).

In GALT-type lymphomas, patients may have upper-GI symptoms including abdominal pain, early satiety, vomiting, GI bleeding, and feeling of a gastric mass.[18] Gastroscopy may demonstrate ulceration, a tumor mass, and/or thickened mucosal folds. In a study of 21 patients, 2 had recurrence 15 and 17 years after resection of the primary tumor.[18]

In BALT-type lymphomas, 50% of the cases are asymptomatic and the lesions are frequently discovered during routine chest roentgenograms.[5] This is probably due to the fact that the tumor involves mainly extraalveolar pulmonary interstitium. Laboratory findings are nonspecific except that one third of the patients were found to have monoclonal gammopathies or cryoglobulinemia. BALT-type lymphomas are sometimes associated with GALT lymphomas and lymphomas of the orbit or salivary glands.[1] Most patients may be cured by surgical resection, but may recur several years after surgery.[17]

In ocular lymphomas of the MALT type, the orbit is more frequently involved than the conjunctiva or lacrimal gland.[8] Patients with ocular MALT-type lymphoma were slightly older and in one study more often had stage I disease than did those with other types of lymphomas.[8]

T-Cell-Rich B-Cell Lymphoma

Patients with TCRBCL have a broad range of age distribution, varying from 18 to 92 years in American patients[17,20-25] and from 7.5 to 94 years in Chinese patients.[26] However, most patients were in the 5th or 6th decade. Most studies showed male predominance. The clinical presentation was usually peripheral lymphadenopathy with frequent retroperitoneal and occasional mediastinal lymph node involvement in some series.[22,24] About 1/3 of the patients had splenomegaly or hepatosplenomegaly.[17,22,24] Extranodal presentation was found in 20-30% of cases.[25,26] The extranodal sites involved brain, nasopharynx, skin, liver, bone, marrow, lungs, salivary gland, tongue, and colon.[24-26] When diagnosed, the patients were usually at the late stages with tumor dissemination.[17,21-26]

Therapeutic response depends on the regiment. Most patients respond to therapy for intermediate-grade lymphomas; most cases had relapse when patients received therapy for low-grade lymphomas; and a few patients did not respond to treatment for Hodgkin's disease, and some died.[22-25] The differences in histologic type and percentage of T-cells did not show correlation to several clinical characteristics (gender, extranodal presentation, and stage distribution) or to clinical outcome, but a higher T-cell count was seen in the older age group.[25] Generally speaking, the clinical features of TCRBCL do not differ from the common diffuse large-cell lymphomas.[24,25]

PATHOLOGY

MALT-Type Lymphoma

In MALT-type lymphomas without cytologic atypia, the diagnosis is heavily dependent on immunophenotyping and occasionally, immunogenotyping. In most cases, however, some characteristic morphologic features are present and are helpful in the diagnosis.

The major diagnostic criterion for MALT lymphoma is the so-called lymphoepithelial lesions formed by lymphocytic infiltration of glandular epithelium (Figs. 11.1-11.8).[1] This feature, however, can also be seen in benign myoepithelial sialadenitis, chronic lymphocytic thyroiditis (Figs. 11.9, 11.10), and benign inflammatory infiltration (Fig. 11.11), and is thus not pathognomonic for the diagnosis.

The second characteristic feature in MALT lymphoma is the presence of reactive follicular centers (Figs. 11.12, 11.13), which may be infiltrated or colonized by the tumor cells; thus, the reactive centers may finally become monotypic, resembling follicular lymphoma.[27]

The third common feature in MALT lymphoma is the presence of plasma cells or lymphoplasmacytoid cells (Fig. 11.14). These cells may show polyclonal or monoclonal cytoplasmic immunoglobulin staining.[1,18] When a PAS-positive intranuclear inclusion (Dutcher body) is identified in this population, it is strongly suggestive of the diagnosis of MALT lymphoma.[1,8,18]

The tumor cells are usually the centrocyte-like cells,

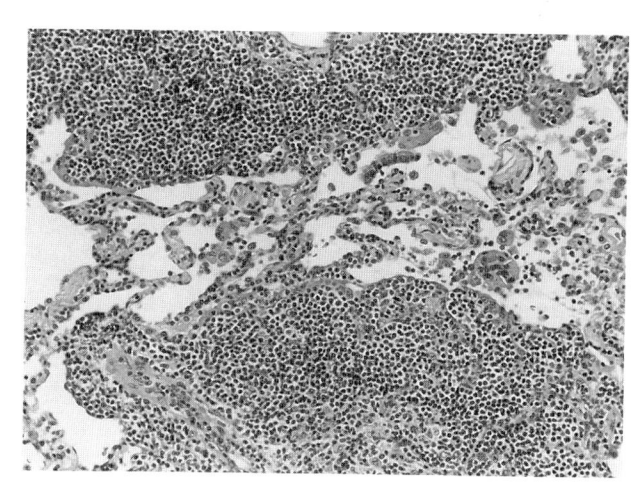

Fig. 11.1. Pulmonary lymphoma showing extensive small round-cell infiltration of the interstitium. Note presence of relatively normal alveoli in the center of the field. H&E, ×250.

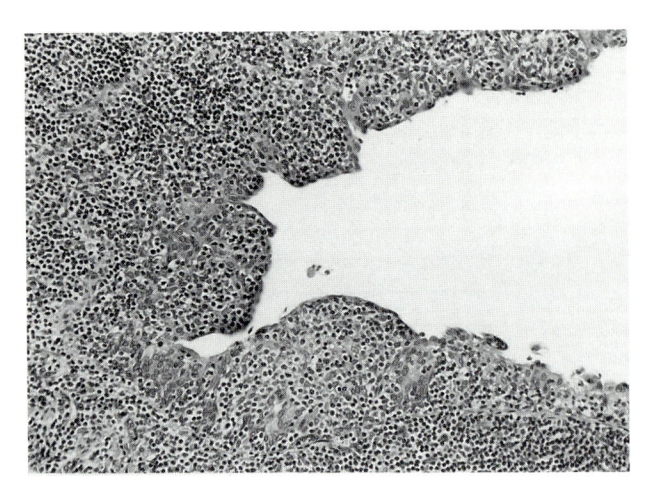

Fig. 11.2. Pulmonary lymphoma of the MALT type showing tumor-cell infiltration and destruction of the bronchial epithelium (lymphoepithelial lesion). H&E, ×250.

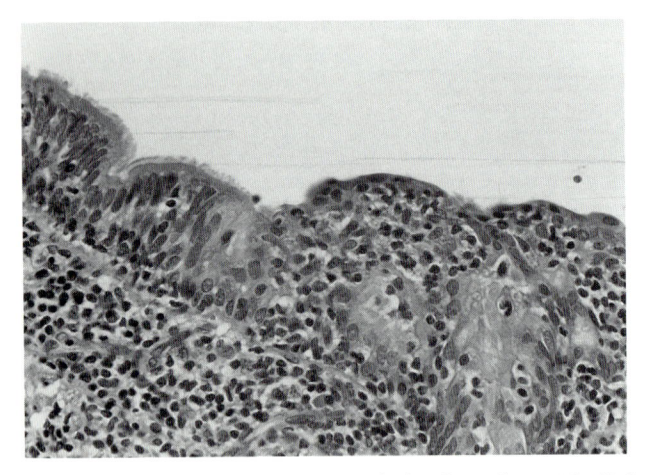

Fig. 11.3. High-power view of the lymphoepithelial lesion. H&E, ×500.

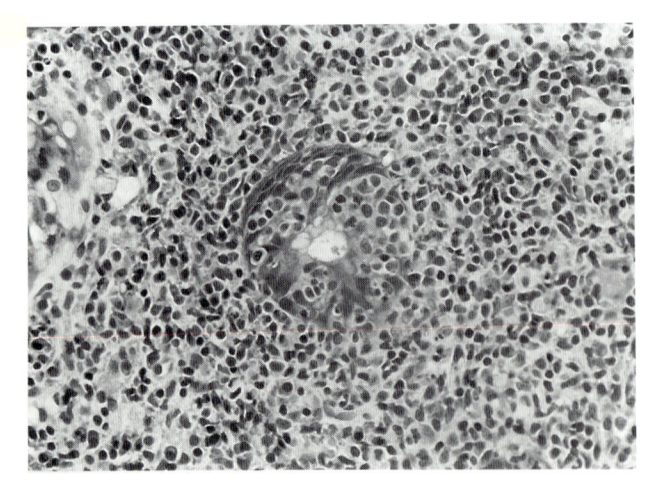

Fig. 11.4. Gastric lymphoma of the MALT type showing epithelial remnant along the tumor cells (lymphoepithelial lesion). H&E, ×500.

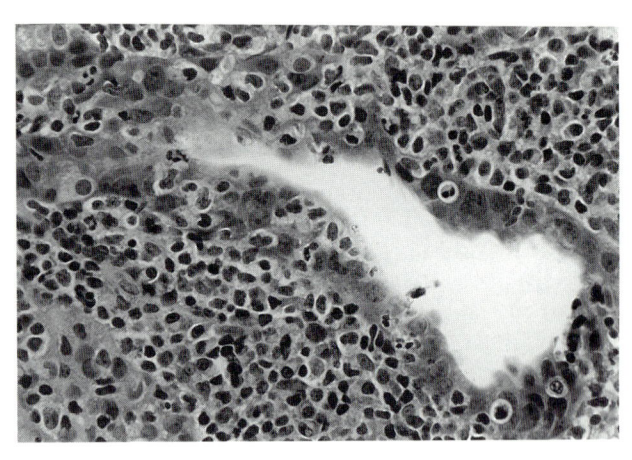

Fig. 11.5. Gastric lymphoma of the MALT type showing lymphoepithelial lesion. H&E, ×500.

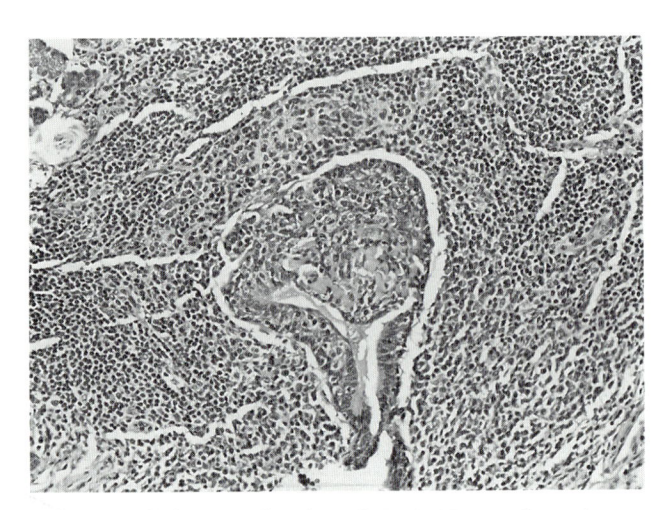

Fig. 11.6. Salivary gland with MALT-type lymphoma showing an epimyoepithelial island with lymphoepithelial lesion. H&E, ×250.

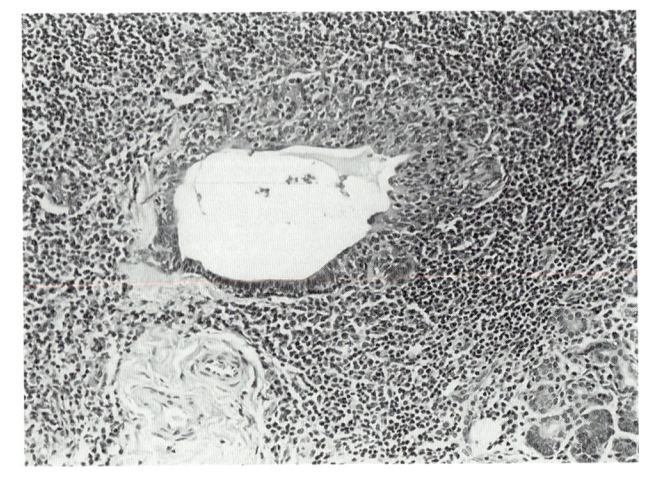

Fig. 11.7. Salivary gland with MALT-type lymphoma showing lymphoepithelial lesion. H&E, ×250.

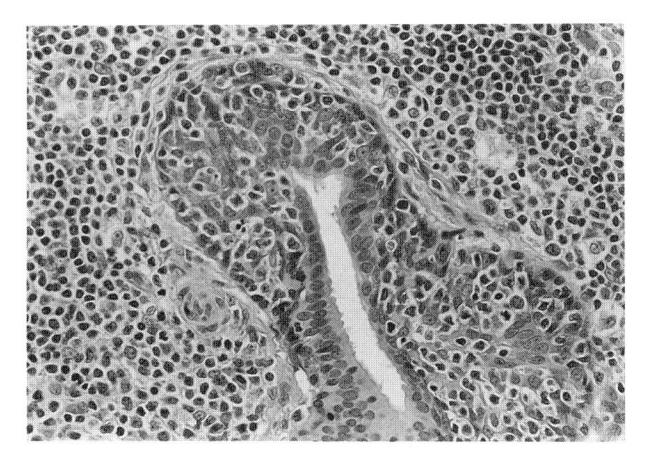

Fig. 11.8. Higher-power view of a lymphoepithelial lesion in salivary gland. H&E, ×500.

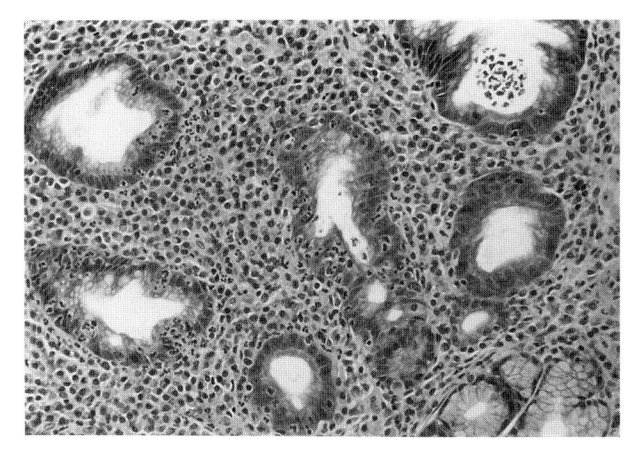

Fig. 11.11. *Helicobacter pylori* gastritis showing lymphocytic and neutrophilic infiltration of the epithelium as well as acute and chronic inflammation in the lamina propria. H&E, ×250.

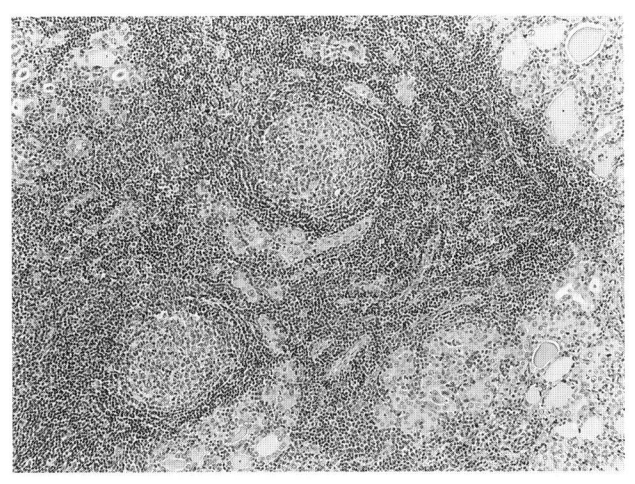

Fig. 11.9. Hashimoto thyroiditis showing entrapment of epithelia in lymphoid infiltrate. H&E, ×250.

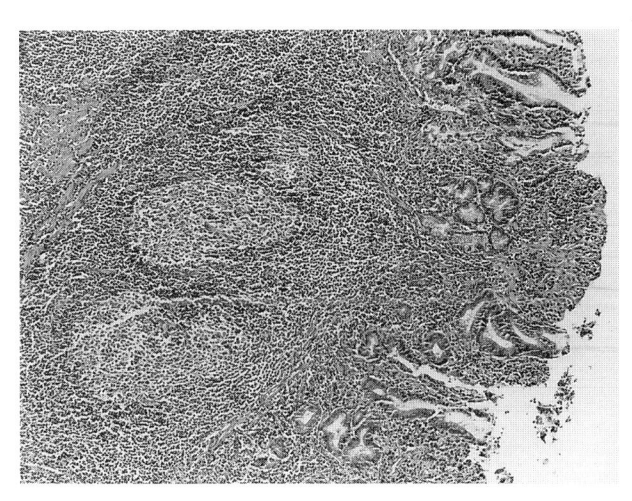

Fig. 11.12. Gastric lymphoma showing two germinal centers among the lymphoid cells. H&E, ×250.

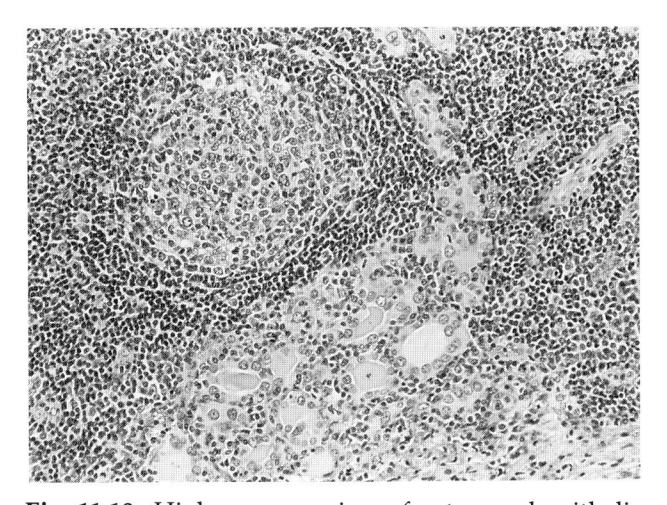

Fig. 11.10. Higher-power view of entrapped epithelia in Hashimoto's thyroiditis. H&E, ×500.

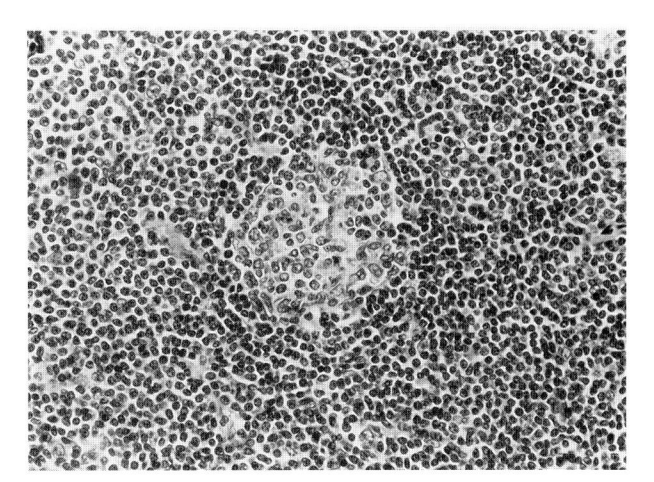

Fig. 11.13. Pulmonary lymphoma showing an atrophic germinal center. H&E, ×500.

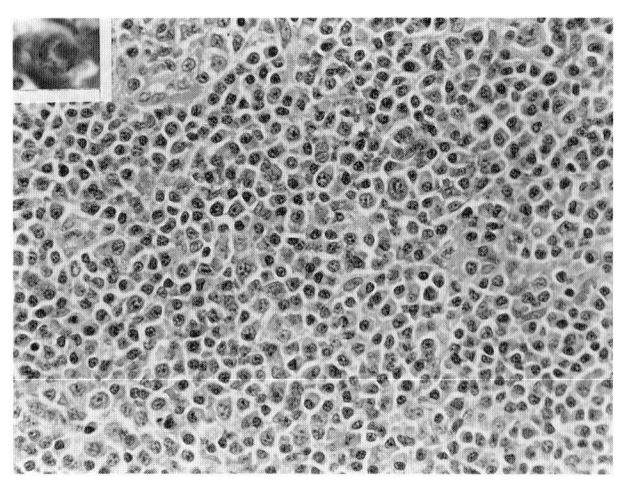

Fig. 11.14. Lymphoma of MALT type showing extensive lymphoplasmacytoid-cell infiltration. H&E, ×500. [Inset: PAS-positive intranuclear inclusion (Dutcher body), ×1250.]

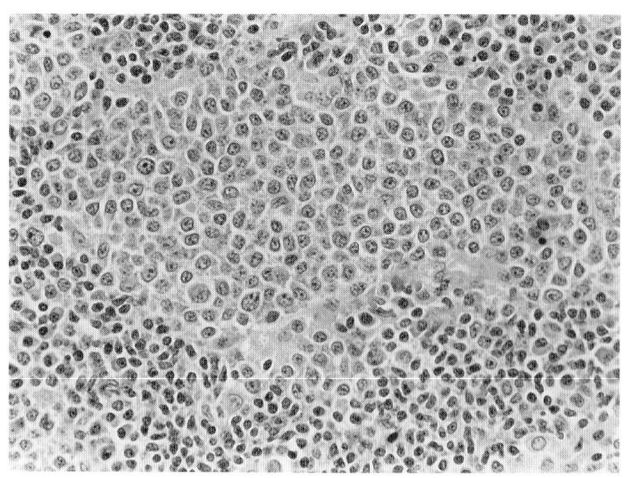

Fig. 11.16. A large sheet of monocytoid B-cells surrounded by plasmacytoid cells and small lymphocytes in a salivary lymphoma of MALT type. H&E, ×500.

which are small lymphocytes with slightly irregular to cleaved nuclei and moderate amounts of pale to clear cytoplasm. They often show moderate cytologic atypia. However, the tumor cells can also assume the form of well-differentiated small lymphocytes, monocytoid B-cells (Figs. 11.15, 11.16), or lymphoplasmacytoid cells. These cells are usually localized in the parafollicular area of the mantle/marginal zone,[10,28] but they may also infiltrate the follicles.[27]

The resemblance of the MALT lymphoma and monocytoid B-cell lymphoma in histologic pattern and cytologic morphology has drawn broad interest.

In monocytoid B-cell lymphoma, about one third of the patients simultaneously or subsequently have extranodal lymphoma in organs of the MALT.[29] On the other hand, 25% of the cases with MALT-type lymphoma exhibit morphology of monocytoid B-cell lymphoma when the tumor metastasizes to the lymph nodes.[29] However, the centrocyte-like cells in MALT lymphoma are usually small and similar to the small-cell variant of monocytoid B-cells described by Lennert and Feller[14] and Nizze et al.,[28] but not the medium-sized cell variant. Furthermore, monocytoid B-cell lymphoma disseminates more frequently than does MALT lymphoma, which is usually localized.[10] Therefore, these two lymphomas may be closely related but are not identical.[10] The current hypothesis is that the cells from MALT lymphoma arise from the marginal zone. Under certain circumstances, these lymphoid cells migrate to the parafollicular zone, become enlarged, and transform into monocytoid (parafollicular) B-cells.[10,28]

T-Cell-Rich B-Cell Lymphoma

The prototype of TCRBCL is a diffuse large-cell lymphoma with a B-cell phenotype that is hidden in a predominant T-cell population (Figs. 11.17, 11.18). However, since the range of T-cells in different studies varied greatly (from 30% to >90%), this entity has become a heterogeneous group covering multiple histopathologic types.

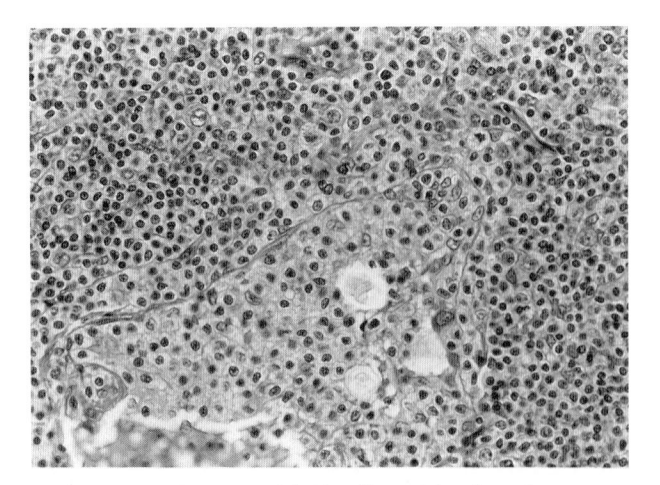

Fig. 11.15. Monocytoid B-cells with abundant cytoplasm are present among small lymphocytes in a pulmonary lymphoma of MALT type. H&E, ×500.

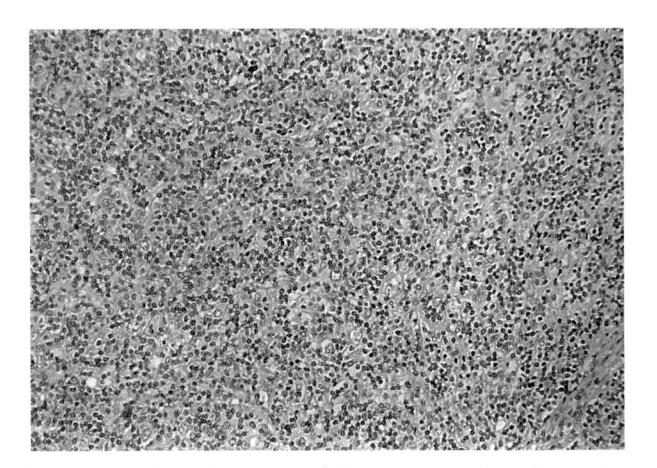

Fig. 11.17. T-cell-rich B-cell lymphoma showing a few large tumor cells surrounded by a large number of small lymphocytes. H&E, ×250.

In the report by Mirchandani et al., four cell types (convoluted cell, Lennert's lymphoma, mixed histiocytic–lymphocytic, and histiocytic) were observed.[20] In the series of Ramsay et al., four cases resembled the angioimmunoblastic lymphadenopathy-like T-cell lymphoma, and one case was a well-differentiated lymphocytic lymphoma.[17] Ng et al. described 21 cases in which the large lymphoid cells were present singly or in small aggregates on a background of many small lymphocytes.[26] The tumor cells had round irregularly folded or multilobated nuclei, vesicular chromatin, and one to multiple nucleoli. A thin or broad rim of amphophilic cytoplasm was present. The background small lymphocytes were mostly normal-looking, but some of them had slightly larger and irregularly folded nuclei with less condensed chromatin as well as occasional medium-sized blastic cells.[26] Osborned et al., on the other hand, described a mixed cellular background in their five cases showing small lymphocytes, plasma cells, epithelioid histiocyts, and a small number of eosinophils.[21] The 30 cases collected in the Armed Forces Institute of Pathology showed the patterns of follicular and diffuse mixed cell, diffuse mixed cell, and diffuse large-cell types of non-Hodgkin's lymphoma and various patterns of Hodgkin's disease.[25] In the series of Chittal et al., all 9 cases were initially diagnosed as Hodgkin's disease,[22] while in the series of Macon et al., all 14 cases resembled peripheral T-cell lymphoma.[23]

These great variations in the histopathologic pattern clearly indicate that TCRBCL is not a distinct clinicopathologic entity, but it is important to retain the concept of "T-cell-rich" for its possible prognostic implications, as emphasized by Krishnan et al.[25] Clinically, it is most significant to distinguish TCRBCL from the two most frequently misdiagnosed entities—Hodgkin's disease and peripheral T-cell lymphomas—because the treatment and prognosis differ in each entity, and patients with TCRBCL may have a fatal outcome when treated as Hodgkin's disease.[24]

In a few cases of TCRBCL, subsequent biopsy or autopsy showed a marked decrease in T-cells, while the large tumor B-cells became predominant,[17,21,24] so that the T-cell-rich phenomenon may simply represent a strong host response to tumor cells. However, diffuse large-cell lymphoma may also exist prior to TCRBCL.[23] Alternatively, the T-cell population may be a response to cytokines secreted by the neoplastic cells.[26]

LABORATORY FINDINGS

Many small B-cell lymphomas in the gastrointestinal tract, lungs, thyroid gland, and ocular adnexa were diagnosed as pseudolymphomas. It is the immunophenotyping that helps correctly identify these lesions as lymphomas of the MALT type. Immunogenotyping may further substantiate this diagnosis. The major criterion is monoclonality, and the simple way to establish the clonality is the study of surface immunoglobulin on the tumor cells by either flow cytometry or immunohistochemistry to ascertain whether light-chain restriction is present (Figs. 11.19, 11.20). Immunohistochemical stain for surface immunoglobulin should be performed on frozen sections, as staining on

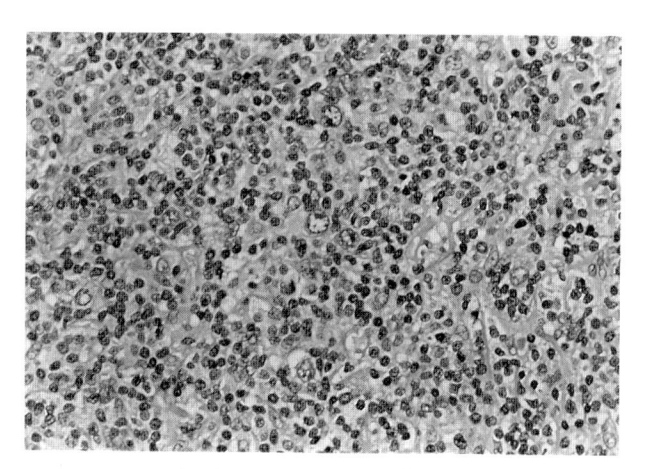

Fig. 11.18. A high-power view of Fig. 11.17 showing large tumor cells. H&E, ×500.

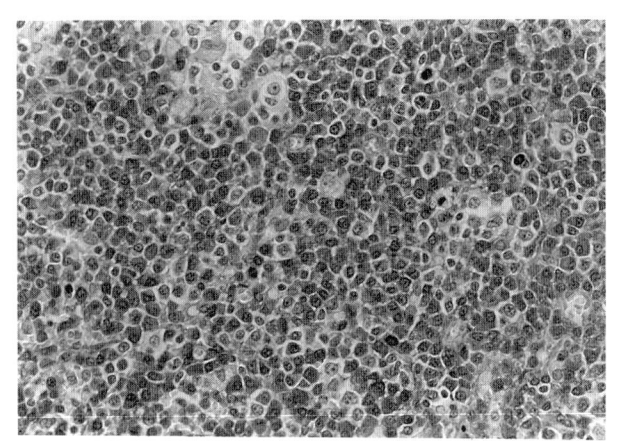

Fig. 11.19. Salivary lymphoma of MALT type showing extensive positive κ light-chain stain in plasmacytoid cells. Immunoperoxidase, ×500.

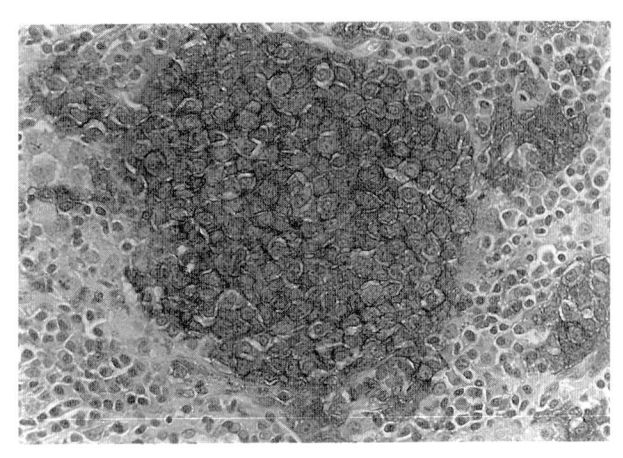

Fig. 11.21. Salivary gland lymphoma of MALT type showing CD20-positive staining. Immunoperoxidase, ×500.

paraffin sections is unsatisfactory. However, clonal proliferation in some lesions may not represent malignancy, and lack of evidence of monoclonality in other lesions can be acceptable as lymphomas. Therefore, the interpretation of immunologic data should always be correlated with morphologic and clinical data.

Monoclonality is a reliable criterion for the diagnosis of GALT- and BALT-type lymphomas, but it is not entirely dependable for the diagnosis in salivary gland lesions, because immunoglobulin gene rearrangement has been demonstrated in benign lymphoepithelial lesions.[30] Immunoproliferative small intestinal disease (IPSID) is probably of MALT origin. However, as it is associated with α heavy-chain disease, cytoplasmic α heavy chain without accompanying light-chain is frequently demonstrated in infiltrating plasma cells. Surface α-chain staining is occasionally detected on the tumor cells.[31] In ocular lymphomas, a polyclonal immunoglobulin pattern may be present in rare occasions, and gene arrangement analysis is needed to substantiate the diagnosis.[8] In addition to surface immunoglobulin stain, B-cell marker (CD19 or CD20) should be routinely used to further support the B-cell nature of the lymphoma (Fig. 11.21). CD5 and CD10 are usually negative in MALT lymphoma; thus, these two markers help exclude small lymphocytic lymphoma (SLL)/chronic lymphocytic leukemia (CLL), and mantle-cell lymphoma, which are CD5-positive, as well as follicular lymphoma, which is CD10-positive (Table 11.1).

When the reactive lymphoid follicles are colonized by the neoplastic cells, the follicles may show a monoclonal staining pattern mimicking follicular lymphoma. In addition, SLL/CLL are positive for CD23 (low-affinity receptor for IgE), CD43 (a signal transducer for cell activation), and Leu8 (lymph node homing receptor), but CD23 is consistently negative and CD43 and Leu8 are occasionally positive in MALT lymphoma.[10] Isaacson et al. advocated the use of monoclonal antibody KB61 (CDw32, Fc receptor for aggregate IgG) to distinguish mantle-zone B-cells (including marginal-zone B-cell) from follicular center B-cells.[27] This distinction is important when MALT lymphoma cells (derived from marginal zone) colonize lymph follicles mimicking follicular lymphoma (composed of follicular center cells). Two other relevant monoclonal antibodies are Ki-B3, which is positive for

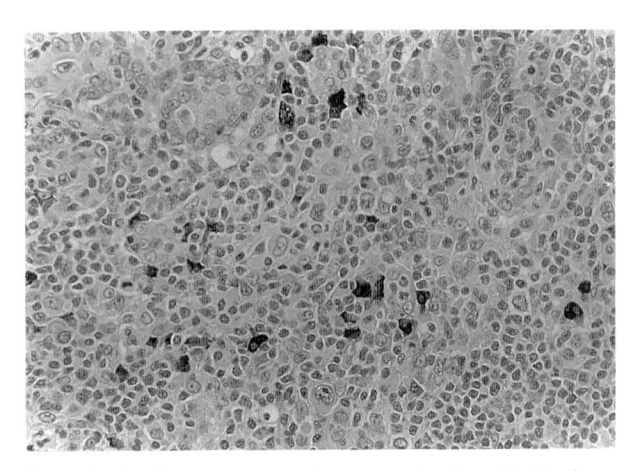

Fig. 11.20. The same specimen as in Fig. 11.19 showing λ light-chain staining in only a few cells. Immunoperoxidase, ×500.

TABLE 11.1
Comparison of Immunophenotype and Immunogenotype Among Low-Grade B-Cell Lymphomas

	MALT type	Monocytoid B-cell	WDLL/CLL	Follicular	Mantle cell
Surface immunoglobulin	Monoclonal	Monoclonal	Monoclonal	Monoclonal	Monoclonal
CD19	+	+	+	+	+
CD20	+	+	+	+	+
CD5	−	−	+	−	+
CD10	−	−	−	+	−
CD23	−	−	+	−	−
CD43	±	±	+	−	+
Leu8	±	±	+	−	+
CDw32	+	+	−	−	+
Ki-B3	−	+	NT	NT	NT
Ki-M1p	+	+	NT	NT	NT
Ig rearrangement	+	+	+	+	+
bcl-1	−	−	+	−	+
bcl-2	(+11;18)(q21;q21)	−	−	+	−

Abbreviations: CLL = chronic lymphocytic leukemia, Ig = immunoglobulin gene, NT = not tested, WDLL = well-differentiated lymphocytic lymphoma.

medium-size cell type but not small cell type in monocytoid B-cell lymphoma; and Ki-M1p, which is positive for both cell types.[28] As MALT lymphoma belongs to the small cell type, it should be theoretically positive for Ki-M1p and negative for Ki-B3. Indeed, Ki-M1p reaction has been demonstrated in the lymph node metastases of MALT-type lymphoma.[28] The immunophenotype of monocytoid B-cell lymphoma is almost identical (except for Ki-B3) to MALT lymphoma as both arise from the marginal zone.[10]

Gene rearrangement analysis may also help distinguish these low-grade B-cell lymphomas. SLL/CLL and mantle-cell lymphoma may show *bcl*-1, and follicular lymphoma may have *bcl*-2 gene rearrangement. The MALT-type lymphomas generally do not have either gene rearrangement,[1] but may have *bcl*-2 protein over expression in some cases.[32] A novel t(11;18)(q21;q21) translocation has been described in MALT lymphomas.[33]

TCRBCL can be easily distinguished from the MALT-type lymphoma by the predominance of small T-cell population and the irregular configuration of some lymphocytes in the background. When the large, abnormal tumor cells with B-cell lineage are identified, the distinction becomes apparent.

An immunohistologic pattern of B-cell antigen staining on sparse or clustered large cells in a background of small T-antigen positive cells is characteristic of TCRBCL.[25] B-cell antigens that are present in tumor cells include CD19, CD20, and CD22.[26] The tumor cells may also show a monotypic surface immunoglobulin pattern,[23] but a polyclonal pattern has also been observed.[25,26] When tumor cells are less than 10%, flow cytometry usually fails to demonstrate light-chain restriction.[34] In those cases, immunoglobulin gene rearrangement can be demonstrated by Southern blotting[21,23,25] or polymerase chain reaction.[24] *bcl*-2 rearrangement has been demonstrated in a few cases. Since TCRBCL may show a follicular pattern[25] or transform from follicular lymphoma,[16] this finding is not unexpected. In addition, Epstein–Barr virus genomic DNA has been detected in a few cases of TCRBCL.[35,36]

Peripheral T-cell lymphoma can be distinguished from TCRBCL by the atypical morphology of the T-cell population and the presence of T-cell receptor gene rearrangement. Hodgkin's disease can be diagnosed by identifying the Reed–Sternberg cells with CD15 and CD30 monoclonal antibodies, which show no reaction to the large tumor cells in TCRBCL.

REFERENCES

1. Salhany KE, Pietra GG: Extranodal lymphoid disorders. *Am J Clin Pathol* 99:472–485, 1993.
2. Isaacson PG, Wright DH: Malignant lymphoma of mucosa-associated lymphoid tissue: A distinctive B-cell lymphoma. *Cancer* 52:1410–1416, 1983.
3. Hall PA, Levison DA: Malignant lymphoma in the gastrointestinal tract. *Semin Diagn Pathol* 8:163–177, 1991.

4. Radaszkiewicz T, Dragosics B, Bauer P: Gastrointestinal malignant lymphomas of the mucosa-associated lymphoid tissue: Factors relevant to prognosis. *Gastroenterology* 102:1628–1638, 1992.
5. Li G, Hausmann ML, Zwingers T, et al: Primary lymphomas of the lung: Morphological, immunohistochemical and clinical features. *Histopathology* 519–531, 1990.
6. Hyjek E, Smith WJ, Isaacson PG: Primary B-cell lymphoma of salivary glands and its relationship to myoepithelial sialadenitis. *Hum Pathol* 19:766–776, 1988.
7. Hyjek E, Isaacson PG: Primary B-cell lymphoma of the thyroid and its relationship to Hashimoto's thyroiditis. *Hum Pathol* 19:1315–1326, 1988.
8. Medeiro LJ, Harris LN: Lymphoid infiltrates of the orbit and conjunctiva: A morphologic and immunophenotypic study of 99 cases. *Am J Surg Pathol* 13:459–471, 1989.
9. Pelstring RJ, Essell JH, Kurtin PJ, et al: Diversity of organ site involvement among malignant lymphomas of mucosa-associated tissues. *Am J Clin Pathol* 96:738–745, 1991.
10. Harris NL: Low-grade B-cell lymphoma of mucosa-associated lymphoid tissue and monocytoid B-cell lymphoma: Related entities that are distinct from other low-grade B-cell lymphomas. *Arch Pathol Lab Med* 117:771–775, 1993.
11. Isaacson PG, Chan JKC, Tang C, et al: Low grade B-cell lymphoma of mucosa-associated lymphoid tissue arising in the thymus: A thymic lymphoma mimicking myoepithelial sialoadenitis. *Am J Surg Pathol* 14:342–351, 1990.
12. Aozasa K, Ohsawa M, Sacki K, et al: Malignant lymphoma of the breast: Immunologic type and association with lymphocytic mastopathy. *Am J Clin Pathol* 97:699–704, 1992.
13. Parveen T, Navarro-Roman L, Medeiros LJ, et al: Low-grade B-cell lymphoma of mucosa-associated lymphoid tissue, arising in the kidney. *Arch Pathol Lab Med* 117:780–783, 1993.
14. Lennert K, Feller A: *Histopathology of Non-Hodgkin's Lymphomas*, 2nd ed, New York, Springer Verlag, 1992.
15. Harris NL: Extranodal lymphoid infiltrates and mucosa-associated lymphoid tissue (MALT): A unifying concept. *Am J Surg Pathol* 15:879–884, 1991.
16. Jaffe ES, Longo DL, Cossman J, et al: Diffuse B-cell lymphomas with T-cell predominance in patients with follicular lymphoma or "pseudo T cell lymphoma." *Lab Invest* 50:27A–28A, 1984.
17. Ramsay AD, Smith WJ, Isaacson PG: T-cell-rich B-cell lymphoma. *Am J Surg Pathol* 12:433–443, 1988.
18. Zukerberg LR, Ferry JA, Souther JF, et al: Lymphoid infiltrates of the stomach: Evaluation of histologic criteria for the diagnosis of low grade gastric lymphoma on endoscopic biopsy specimens. *Am J Surg Pathol* 14:1087–1099, 1990.
19. Kennedy JL, Nathwani BN, Burke JS, et al: Pulmonary lymphomas and other pulmonary lymphoid lesions: A clinicopathologic and immunologic study of 64 patients. *Cancer* 56:539–552, 1985.
20. Mirchandani I, Palitke M, Tabaczka P, et al: B-cell lymphoma morphologically resembling T-cell lymphomas. *Cancer* 56:1578–1583, 1985.
21. Osborne BM, Butler JJ, Pugh WC: The value of immunophenotyping on paraffin sections in the identification of T-cell rich B-cell lymphomas: Lineage confirmation by JH rearrangement. *Am J Surg Pathol* 14:933–938, 1990.
22. Chittal SM, Brousset P, Voigt JJ, et al: Large B-cell lymphoma rich in T-cells and simulating Hodgkin's disease. *Histopathology* 19:211–220, 1991.
23. Macon WR, Williams ME, Greer JP, et al: T-cell-rich B-cell lymphomas: A clinicopathologic study of 19 cases. *Am J Surg Pathol* 16:351–363, 1992.
24. Rodriquez J, Pugh WC, Cabanillas F: T-cell-rich B-cell lymphoma. *Blood* 82:1586–1589, 1993.
25. Krishnan J, Wellberg K, Frizzera G: T-cell-rich large B-cell lymphoma: A study of 30 cases, supporting its histologic heterogeneity and lack of clinical distinctiveness. *Am J Surg Pathol* 18:455–465, 1994.
26. Ng CS, Chan JKC, Hui PK, et al: Large B-cell lymphomas with a high content of reactive T-cells. *Hum Pathol* 20:1145–1154, 1989.
27. Isaacson PG, Wotherspoon AC, Diss T, et al: Follicular colonization in B-cell lymphoma of mucosa-associated lymphoid tissue. *Am J Surg Pathol* 819–828, 1991.
28. Nizze H, Cogliatti SB, von Schilling C, et al: Monocytoid B-cell lymphoma: Morphological variants and relationship to low-grade B-cell lymphoma of the mucosa-associated lymphoid tissue. *Histopathology* 18:403–414, 1991.
29. Tabrizchi H, Hansmann M-L, Parwaresch MR, et al: Distribution pattern of follicular dendritic cells in low-grade B-cell lymphomas of the gastrointestinal tract immunostained by Ki-FDC1p, a new paraffin resistant monoclonal antibody. *Mod Pathol* 3:470–478, 1990.
30. Fishleder A, Tubbs R, Hesse B, et al: Uniform detection of immunoglobulin-gene rearrangement in benign lymphoepithelial lesions. *N Engl J Med* 316:1118–1121, 1987.
31. Price SK: Immunoproliferative small intestinal disease: A study of 13 cases with alpha heavy chain disease. *Histopathology* 17:7–17, 1990.
32. Pezella F, Tse AGD, Cordell JL, et al: Expression of the bcl-2 oncogene protein is not specific for the 14;18 chromosomal translocation. *Am J Pathol* 137:225–232, 1990.
33. Horsman D, Gascoyne R, Klasa R, et al: t(11;18)(q21;q21.1): A recurring translocation in lymphomas of mucosa-associated lymphoid tissue (MALT). *Genes chromosome Cancer* 4:183–187, 1992.
34. Sun T: *Color Atlas/Text of Flow Cytometric Analysis of Hematologic Neoplasms*, New York, Igaku-Shoin, 1993, pp 67–69.
35. Dolcetti R, Carbone A, Zagonel V, et al: Type 2 Epstein–Barr virus genome and latent membrane pro-

tein-1 expression in a T-cell-rich lymphoma of probable B-cell lineage. *Am J Clin Pathol* 100:541–549, 1993.
36. Baddoura F, Chan WC, Masih AS, et al: T-cell-rich B-cell lymphoma: A clinicopathologic study of eight cases. *Am J Clin Pathol* 103:65–75, 1995.
37. Schmid C, Sargent C, Isaacson PG: L and H cells of nodular lymphocytic predominant Hodgkin's disease show immunoglobulin light-chain restriction. *Am J Pathol* 139:1281–1289, 1991.

12
Hairy-Cell Leukemia vs. Monocytoid B-Cell Lymphoma vs. Splenic Lymphoma with Villous Lymphocytes

The diagnosis of hairy-cell leukemia (HCL) often requires a multiparameter approach for the exclusion of many similar lymphoproliferative disorders. The most important differential diagnoses include several low-grade lymphomas and leukemias, such as chronic lymphocytic leukemia (CLL), prolymphocytic leukemia (PLL), monocytoid B-cell lymphoma (MBCL), and splenic lymphoma with villous lymphocytes (SLVL). In addition, there are HCL variants and hybrid forms, which pose a dilemma in diagnosis of HCL. In this chapter, the emphasis is placed on the distinction between HCL, MBCL, and SLVL, because their immunophenotypes are very similar and their morphology is almost indistinguishable in either tissue section (HCL vs. MBCL) or peripheral blood (HCL vs. SLVL).

CLINICAL FEATURES
Hairy Cell Leukemia

HCL accounts for about 2% of all leukemias and is seen mainly in male patients with a mean age about 51.[1] HCL is a chronic leukemia with an indolent clinical course. As splenomegaly is present in 80% of patients, clinical symptoms are usually related to hypersplenism (pancytopenia), fatigue, or secondary infections.[1] Hepatomegaly is seen in about 33% of patients, but lymphadenopathy is an unusual feature in HCL and occurs mainly in HCL variants.[2] Most patients at the time of diagnosis have normochromic, normocytic anemia, neutropenia, thrombocytopenia, and monocytopenia. Monocytopenia is a constant feature in most patients with HCL. In fact, if a patient has normal or an increase in monocytes in the peripheral blood, the diagnosis of HCL should be questioned.[1] Dry tap of bone marrow due to reticulin fibrosis is characteristic of HCL, but bone marrow biopsy often demonstrates the neoplastic cells and helps establish the diagnosis of HCL. The currently available therapeutic agents (α-interferon and Pentostatin) are extremely effective in controlling or possibly curing this disorder.[1]

Monocytoid B-Cell Lymphoma

MBCL is a newly discovered lymphoma with about 125 cases registered in the City of Hope.[3] It is seen mainly in female patients with a median age of 64 years.[4] In contrast to HCL, MBCL primarily involves lymph nodes, presenting localized or, less frequently, generalized lymphadenopathy.[3,4] Extranodal lymphoma is seen in about 20% of all cases, and similar percentages of cases have splenomegaly and/or hepatomegaly. The extranodal sites include the salivary gland, spleen, stomach, pharynx, tonsil, breast, thyroid, chest wall, and ovary.[4] Peripheral blood and bone marrow involvement is relatively infrequent. Unusual numbers of patients have coexistent autoimmune disease, such as Sjögren's syndrome, systemic lupus erythematosus and Raynaud's phenomenon.[5,6] In the MBCL registry at City of Hope, 52 patients were followed; 35 were alive and free of disease, 9 were alive with disease, 5 died of lymphoma, and 3 died of other causes.[3] A German study emphasized relapse as a common feature.[7]

Splenic Lymphoma with Villous Lymphocytes

Although SLVL is a relatively new entity, as Melo et al. coined this term in 1987[8], and less than 200 cases have been reported[9], it is probably not a rare disease. Its incidence is estimated to be similar to that of hairy-cell leukemia, more common than prolymphocytic leukemia and hairy-cell leukemia variants, but 10-fold less common than chronic lymphocytic leukemia of B-cell origin.[10] The sex preponderance differed in various series, and the mean age ranged from 54 to 72 years in these series. SLVL is generally considered as a low-grade non-Hodgkin's lymphoma with a stable or slowly progressive clinical course. The presenting symptoms are usually limited to mild weakness, fatigue, and abdominal discomfort caused by the enlarged spleen.[8] Splenomegaly and lymphocytosis are an integral part of SLVL. Lymphadenopathy was seen in 5 patients and hepatomegaly in 15 from a series of 22 patients.[8] Some patients do not require any treatment for long periods, and most patients do well and do not require further treatment after splenectomy.[9-11] In a series of 50 cases, 24% expired 1 month to 8 years from time of diagnosis, and one-third of the deaths were directly related to the progression of SLVL.[10]

PATHOLOGY

Hairy Cell Leukemia

The histologic features of HCL in the bone marrow and spleen are highly characteristic and are frequently diagnostic.[1,2] As the leukemic hairy cells possess abundant cytoplasm that does not take up the stain in H&E-stained preparations, the nuclei of the tumor cells appear to be widely separated from each other, forming a characteristic pattern. This pattern is easily recognizable even under low magnification and designated variably as "fried-egg," "honeycomb," or "sponge-like" appearance. Because the tumor cells themselves are closely packed, the cell borders appear interlocking. These features are invariably demonstrated in the bone marrow biopsy (Figs. 12.1, 12.2), provided that sufficient tissue is obtained. A reticulin stain may demonstrate increased reticulin in the neoplastic area, but collagen fibrosis is typically absent in HCL. Reticulin fibrosis and interlocking pattern of tumor cells may explain the high frequency of dry taps in HCL patients.

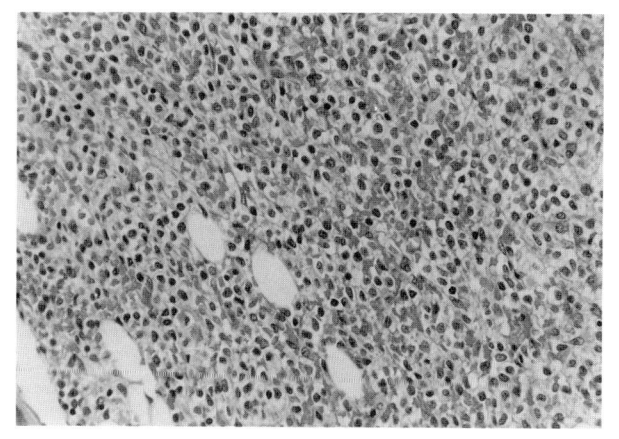

Fig. 12.2. A higher magnification showing the fried-egg pattern. H&E, ×500.

The spleen may show a honeycomb pattern similar to that in the bone marrow (Fig. 12.3). The leukemia infiltration is characteristically confined to the red pulp; the white pulp usually becomes atrophied. These tumor cells probably damage the sinus wall with resultant "blood lake" formation. The blood lakes are usually lined by hairy cells and form the so-called "pseudosinuses" (Figs. 12.4, 12.5).[12] Although this pattern may be found in other conditions, such as chronic lymphocytic leukemia, chronic myeloid leukemia, and multiple myeloma[13], in an appropriate clinicopathology setting, it is diagnostic of HCL.

The changes in the liver have not drawn as much attention as the marrow and spleen, but the hepatic

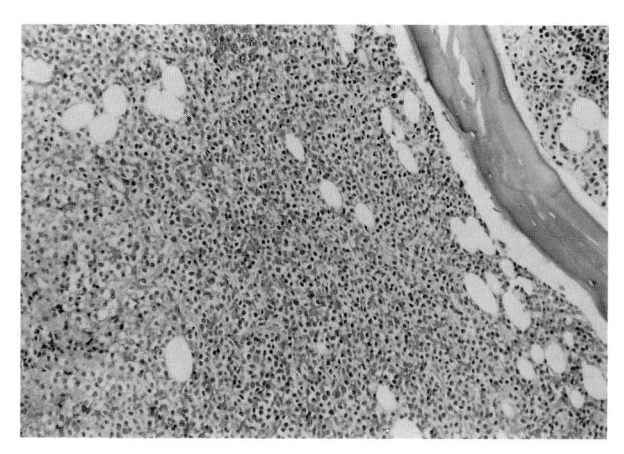

Fig. 12.1. Bone marrow biopsy in a case of hairy-cell leukemia showing the widely spaced and interlocking tumor cells (fried-egg pattern). H&E, ×250.

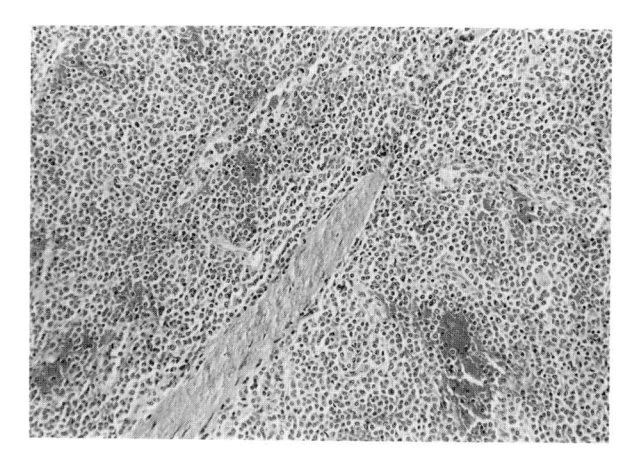

Fig. 12.3. The fried-egg pattern and a few blood lakes are seen in the accessory spleen in a case of hairy-cell leukemia. H&E, ×250.

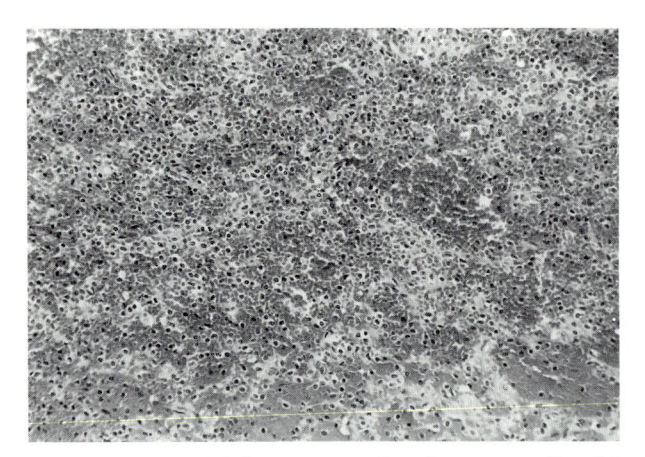

Fig. 12.4. Blood lakes or pseudoesinuses are lined by hairy cells in the spleen. H&E, ×250.

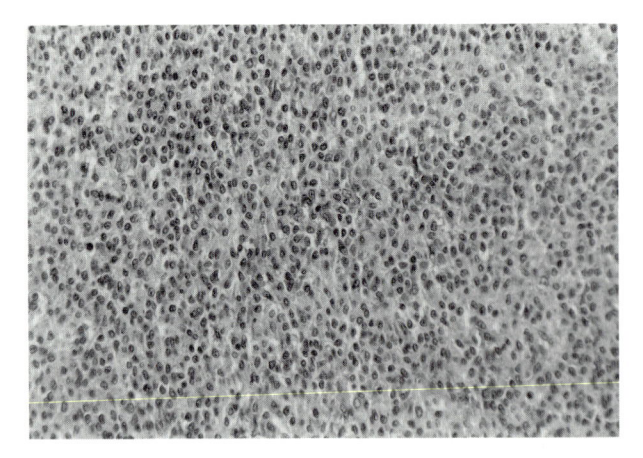

Fig. 12.6. A case of hairy-cell leukemia showing hairy-cell infiltration in a lymph node. A fried-egg pattern is not apparent. H&E, ×500.

lesions are also characteristic. Both portal areas and sinuses are involved by hairy cells. Similar to the mechanism of pseudosinus formation in the spleen, leukemic infiltration of sinusoid wall produces angiomatoid lesions that can be distributed randomly within the lobules.[14]

Peripheral lymphadenopathy is observed in only 5–10% of patients, but abdominal and mediastinal adenopathies are frequently found at autopsy.[1] The normal architecture is partially or completely replaced by leukemic cells, which often surround the lymph follicles (Fig. 12.6).

Tumor cells of HCL may also infiltrate skin, lungs, kidneys, colon, stomach, myocardium, meninges, adrenals, and pancreas, but the histologic pattern is not specific and the infiltrates seldom cause clinical symptoms.

Monocytoid B-Cell Lymphoma

In tissue sections, the cytologic morphology of MBCL is indistinguishable from that of HCL; it shows a honeycomb pattern consisting of tumor cells with bland nuclei and abundant clear cytoplasm. The differences between these two entities are mainly on their tissue distribution and the frequent presence of composite lymphoma in MBCL.[3-5] In contrast to HCL, MBCL is primarily a node-based lymphoma and seldom involves peripheral blood and bone marrow. If tumor cells are found in blood or bone marrow, an advanced-stage disease and a poor prognosis are indicated.[15] MBCL frequently coexists with lymphoma of mucosa-associated lymphoid tissue (MALT), and monocytoid B-cells are present in splenic marginal-zone lymphoma.[3-5,7,16] These three neoplasms are hypothesized to derive from the same cells of the splenic marginal zone.[16] Recent studies also suggested that splenic marginal-zone lymphoma is identical to SLVL.[17] MBCL also has a propensity to transform into large-cell lymphoma (Fig. 12.7).[3-5,7]

The tumor cells are characteristically located in the interfollicular area between the mantle zones of adjacent follicles. On comparison with reactive monocytoid B-cells (Fig. 12.8), the tumor cells of MBCL show more predominant, confluent infiltration in the tissue, more nuclear irregularity, higher mitotic rate, and more large transformed cells coexistent.[18] Neutrophils and plasma cells are also frequently seen among the tumor cells of MBCL.

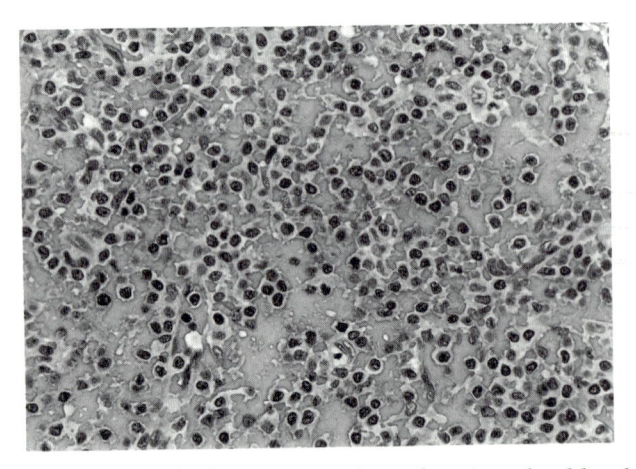

Fig. 12.5. A higher-power view showing the blood lakes and lining hairy cells. H&E, ×500.

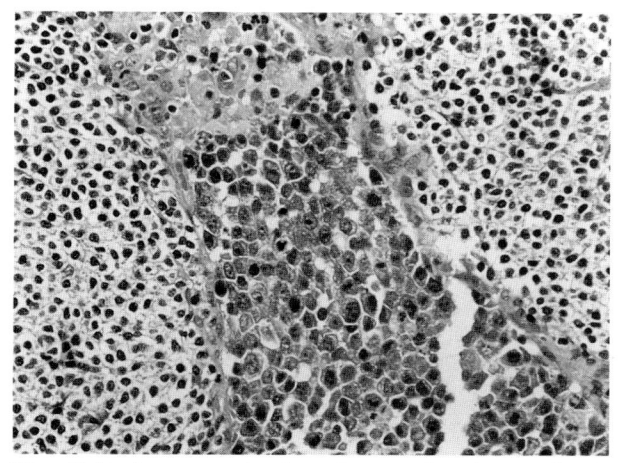

Fig. 12.7. A composite lymphoma showing a cluster of large lymphoma cells in between two groups of monocytoid B-cell lymphoma. H&E, ×500.

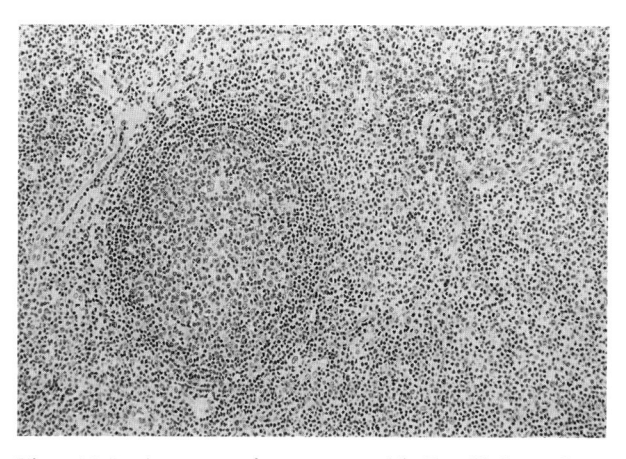

Fig. 12.9. A case of monocytoid B-cell lymphoma showing interfollicular/mantle-zone-like pattern. H&E, ×250.

There are three distinct histologic patterns when MBCL is seen in the lymph nodes[3]:

1. *Interfollicular/mantle-zone-like pattern* (Fig. 12.9), showing tumor cells in the interfollicular region. The tumor cells may invade the follicles, and, although they may be in direct contact with the germinal center, they are usually separated by a band of mantle-zone cells from the germinal center.

2. *Sinusoidal pattern* (Fig. 12.10), showing the tumor cells in the sinuses. The expanded sinuses may, however, create a nodular appearance. The lymph node architecture is basically preserved.

3. *Diffuse pattern* (Fig. 12.11), showing diffuse tumor-cell infiltration. The lymph node architecture is effaced. This is an uncommon pattern and is seen in longstanding cases.

In the extranodal sites, the parotid gland is most frequently involved in MBCL. The salivary gland is usually diffusely infiltrated by the tumor cells. The glandular structure is usually obliterated by tumor infiltration, but neoplastic cells may also be around or within the ductal structure or epimyoepithelial islands.

In the spleen, which is occasionally infiltrated by the tumor cells, the white pulp is mainly involved, whereas red pulp involvement is seen only in advanced cases. The histologic pattern is that of mantle-

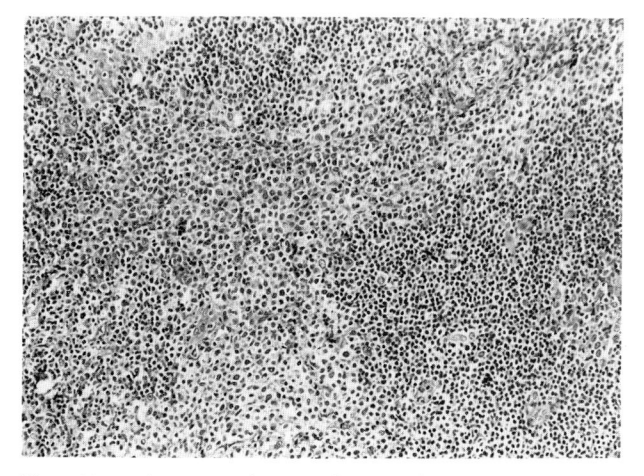

Fig. 12.8. A case of toxoplasmic lymphadenopathy showing monocytoid B-cells in the sinuses. H&E, ×250.

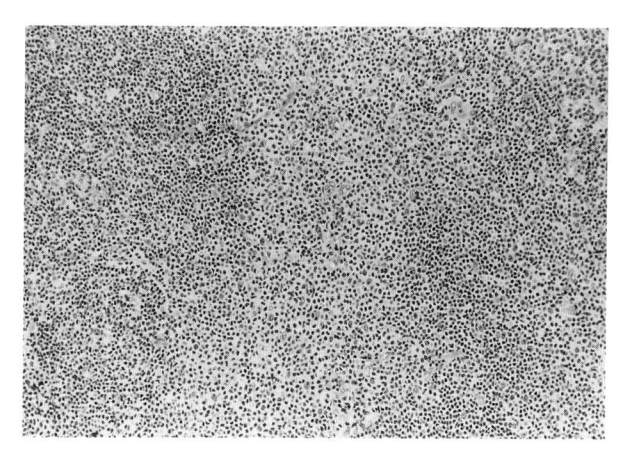

Fig. 12.10. A case of monocytoid B-cell lymphoma showing sinusoidal pattern. H&E, ×250.

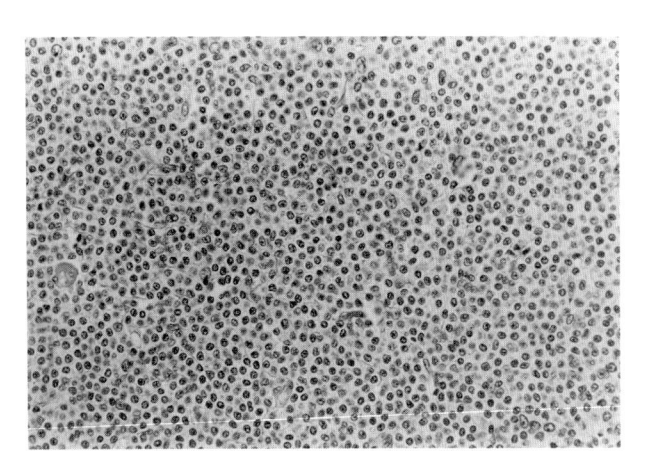

Fig. 12.11. A case of monocytoid B-cell lymphoma showing diffuse pattern. H&E, ×500.

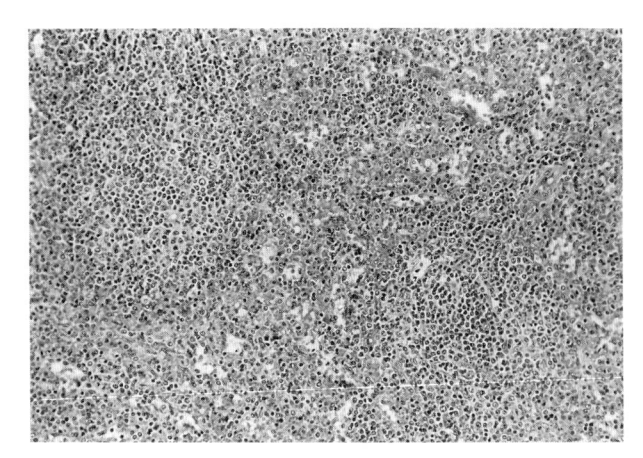

Fig. 12.12. A case of splenic lymphoma with villous lymphocytes showing tumor-cell infiltration of both white and red pulp. H&E, ×250.

zone-like appearance. Bone marrow infiltration is as rare as spleen and shows a focal, predominantly paratrabecular pattern. In the GI tract, there is transmural infiltration and the gastric and intestinal glands are generally obliterated. Hepatic involvement is usually confined to the sinuses.

Splenic Lymphoma with Villous Lymphocytes

The histologic pattern in SLVL is markedly different from that of HCL and MBCL. The major similarity between SLVL and HCL is that splenomegaly is a prominent feature in both diseases and that the circulating villous lymphocytes in SLVL simulates the leukemic hairy cells. The tumor cells in tissues are usually small to intermediate lymphoid cells with round nuclei, clumped chromatin, scanty cytoplasm, and low mitotic rate. Small numbers of plasma cells are frequently present. In the spleen, the neoplastic cells involve both white and red pulp (Fig. 12.12), but the infiltration in the white pulp is usually more prominent than that in the red pulp.[8,9,11,17,19-25] Blood lakes or pseudosinus formation are not seen in the spleen of SLVL cases. In the lymph nodes, neoplastic infiltration is seen mainly in the cortical and paracortical areas,[11,19] but diffuse effacement can be seen in later stages.[9,11,23] In the liver, the portal area is mainly involved.[9,11,19,22] The bone marrow shows a nodular and paratrabecular infiltration of tumor cells, but diffuse infiltration is also seen in severe cases (Figs. 12.13, 12.14).[8,9,11,19,22,25]

Systematic Mast-Cell Disease

In the spleen and bone marrow biopsy, mast cell disease may show a honeycomb pattern mimicking HCL and MBCL. However, mast cells tend to aggregate around trabeculae in the bone marrow (Figs. 12.15, 12.16), and spleen, and myelofibrosis is frequently encountered. Giemsa stain demonstrates cytoplasmic granules in mast cells, thus distinguishing them from HCL and MBCL (Fig. 12.17). Their morphology in tissue imprints is quite different from that of tumor cells of other two diseases. In case of doubt, a toluidine blue stain may help demonstrate the metachromatic cytoplasmic granules in mast cells.

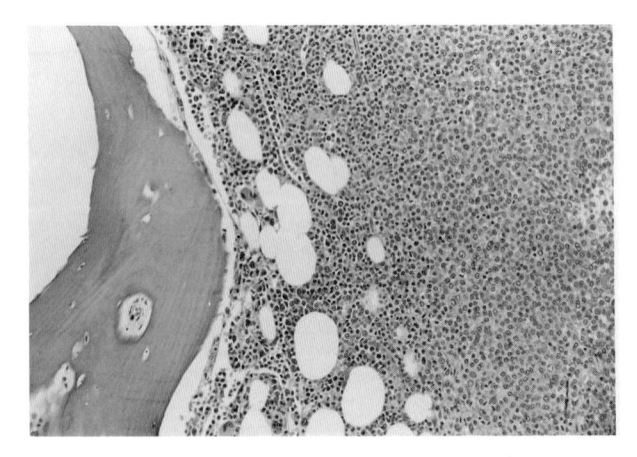

Fig. 12.13. A case of splenic lymphoma with villous lymphocytes showing diffuse bone marrow infiltration by small and medium-sized lymphoid cells. H&E, ×250.

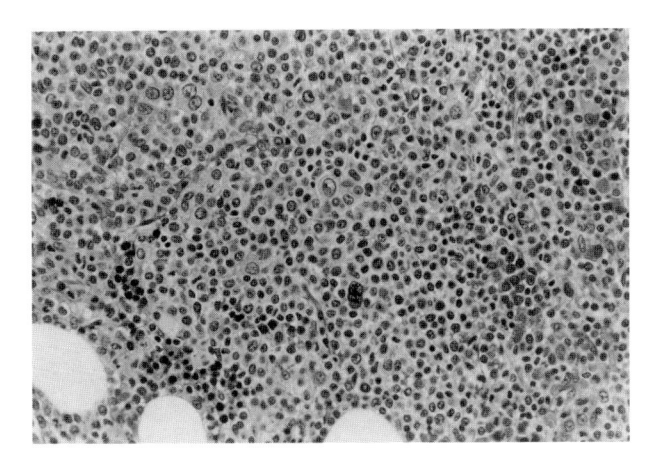

Fig. 12.14. Higher magnification shows the mixed small and large cell population in the bone marrow of the same case as in Fig. 12.13. H&E, ×500.

LABORATORY FINDINGS

Peripheral Blood

HCL is a B-cell leukemia with a splenomegaly in most patients. From this point of view, several B-cell leukemias, including CLL and PLL, in addition to SLVL, should be considered in the differential diagnosis (Table 12.1). SLVL more closely resembles HCL than other entities because of the presence of circulating villous lymphocytes. However, in aged blood specimens, artifactual cytoplasmic projections can be demonstrated in other leukemic cells, particularly those of CLL. A leukocyte count may facilitate a pre-

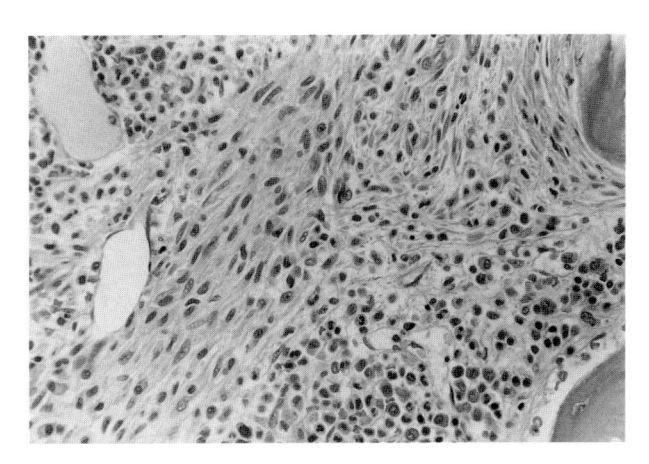

Fig. 12.16. Another case of mast-cell disease showing spindle tumor cells with elongated nuclei that can be readily differentiated from hairy-cell leukemia. H&E, ×500.

liminary distinction among these closely related disorders. HCL is characterized by pancytopenia, although leukocytosis can be seen in its variants. SLVL usually shows mild peripheral lymphocytosis with a leukocyte count of 3–38 × 10^9/L. The leukocyte count in CLL usually ranges within 10–150 × 10^9/L. PLL is typical for its extremely high leukocyte count, usually > 100 × 10^9/L.

The morphology of various leukemic cells may be very similar with some subtle differences. The leukemic hairy cells are comparable in size to a large lymphocyte. They have round, reniform, or convoluted nuclei, which contain uniformly distributed

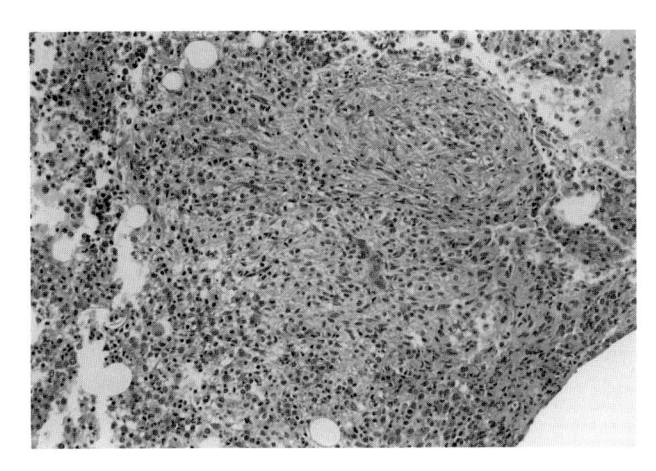

Fig. 12.15. A case of mast cell disease showing tumor-cell infiltration in the bone marrow, mimicking the fried-egg pattern of hairy-cell leukemia. H&E, ×250.

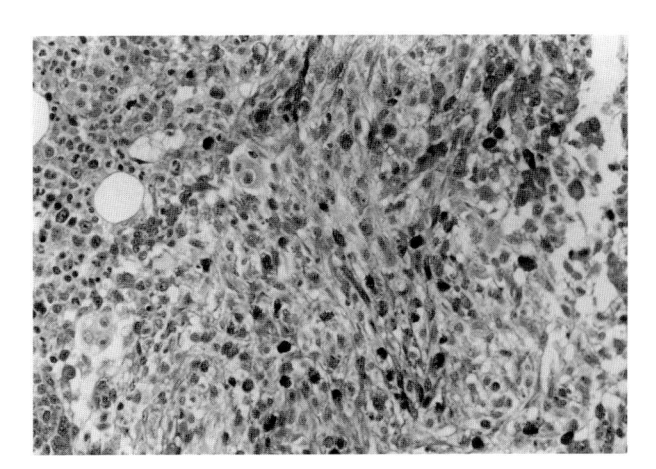

Fig. 12.17. Mast cells with dark cytoplasmic staining in Giemsa stain in the bone marrow of a case of mast-cell disease. ×500.

TABLE 12.1
Comparison of Five Low-Grade B-Cell Neoplasms

	HCL	CLL	PL	SLVL	MCBL
Circulating cells	Hairy cells	Small lymphocytes	Prolymphocytes	Villous lymphocytes	Rare
Leukocytosis	Leukopenia	Moderate	Marked	Moderate	Rare
Splenomegaly	+	+	++	+	−
Major pulp involved	Red	White	White	White	Rare
Hepatomegaly	+	+	+	+	−
Lymphadenopathy	−	+	−	−	+
Marrow infiltrate	+	+	+	+	Rare
CD5	−	⊕	±	−	−
CD11c	+	−	−	±	±
CD19	+	+	+	+	+
CD20	+	+	+	+	+
CD22	+	±	±	+	+
CD25	+	−	−	−	−
TRAP	+	−	−	±	−
Monoclonal protein	Rare	Rare	Relatively common	Most common	Relatively common

Modified from Sun T: *Color Atlas/Text of Flow Cytometric Analysis of Hematologic Neoplasms*, New York, Igaku-Shoin, 1993, p 129; reproduced with permission.

chromatin and inconspicuous nucleoli. There is a moderate amount of cytoplasm with numerous slender cytoplasmic villi (hairy projections) (Fig. 12.18). A typical villous lymphocyte is larger than the small lymphocytes found in CLL, is close in size to a prolymphocyte, has a round or ovoid nucleus with clumped chromatin, and, in 50% of the cases, has a small but distinct nucleolus. The cytoplasm is usually basophilic and moderate in amount. The striking features of the SLVL cells, however, is the presence of thin and short cytoplasmic villi with uneven or polar distribution (Fig. 12.19). The cells in PLL may mimic those of SLVL, but the absence of cytoplasmic projection and basophilia and the presence of prominant nucleoli in PLL cells may help distinguish these two cells types. The CLL cells usually appear like the small mature lymphocytes with a clumped chromatin pattern and scant cytoplasm, but mixed small and

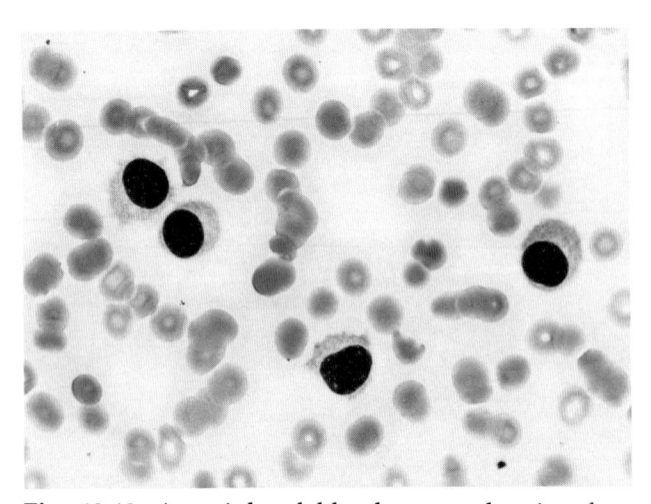

Fig. 12.18. A peripheral blood smear showing four hairy cells with abundant cytoplasm and multiple hairy cytoplasmic projections covering entire cell surface. Wright–Giemsa, ×1250.

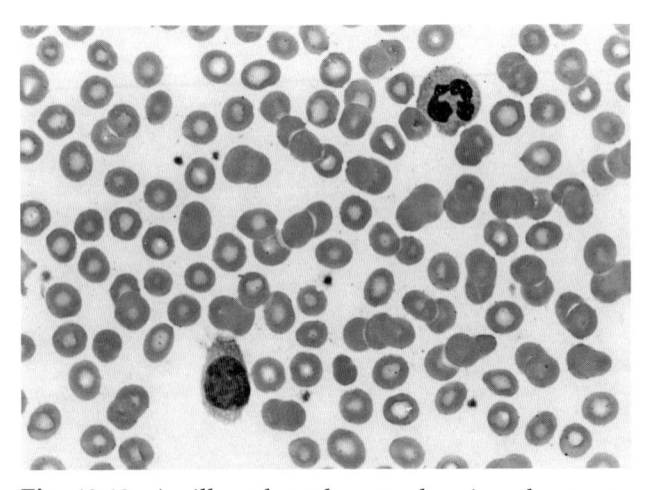

Fig. 12.19. A villous lymphocyte showing short cytoplasmic villi with polar distribution from a case of splenic lymphoma with villous lymphocytes. Wright–Giemsa, ×1250.

large lymphocytes or even prolymphocytes can be seen in the peripheral blood of CLL cases.

In addition, 3–12% of plasma cells or plasmacytoid cells may be found in the peripheral blood in SLVL cases. Monoclonal gammopathy is a frequent finding both in SLVL and MBCL. These features are helpful in differential diagnosis but are by no means specific.

Electron-microscopic examination is helpful in distinguishing between HCL and SLVL. The HCL cells have numerous longer and evenly distributed cytoplasmic projections (Fig. 12.20), but the villi on SLVL cells are less numerous, shorter, and frequently localized to one pole (Fig. 12.21). The presence of the ribosome–lamella complex in 50% of HCL cases is useful in distinguishing HCL from SLVL cells. The ribosome–lamella complex can now be detected in plastic embedded tissue[26] and the hairy projections on hairy cells can be demonstrated with a monoclonal antibody DBA-44 (Fig. 12.22).[27]

Immunophenotyping

When morphologic diagnosis is not conclusive, immunophenotyping becomes very helpful. In fact, as this group of low-grade B-cell neoplasms are so closely related to each other, immunophenotyping

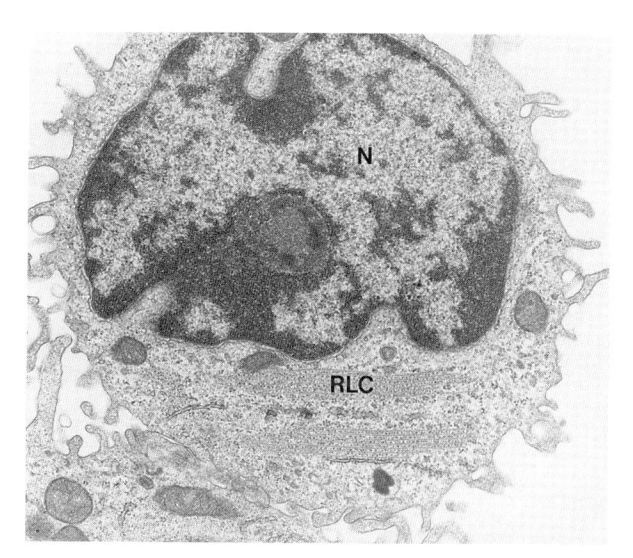

Fig. 12.20. A hairy cell showing many fairly uniformly distributed long and slender surface projections and two ribosome–lamella complexes (RLCs). ×25,000 (From Sun T: *Color Atlas/Text of Flow Cytometric Analysis of Hematologic Neoplasms*, New York, Igaku-Shoin, 1993.)

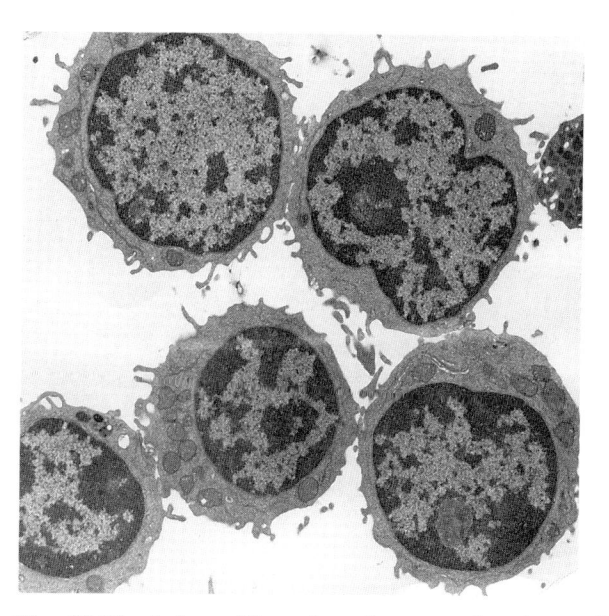

Fig. 12.21. A few villous lymphocytes showing polar distribution of a few short villi. ×11,6000 (Courtesy of Dr. Saul Teichberg and Beth Roberts.)

should be included in the routine diagnostic procedure to make sure a diagnosis is accurate.

Hairy Cell Leukemia

The cell lineage of HCL was considered to be a hybrid of B-cell and monocytes, because hairy cells have the characteristic features of monocytes (weak phagocytic capability, ability to adhere to glass, and bearing a receptor for the Fc portion of IgG) as well as those of B-lymphocytes (presence of surface immunoglobulin and B-cell antigens). However, as immunoglobulin gene rearrangement has been demonstrated in HCL, it is now established as a B-cell leukemia.

Most pan-B-cell antigens, such as CD19, CD20, and CD22, are present in HCL (Fig. 12.23).[1,2] The plasma-cell-associated antigen PCA-1 is also positive. However, another plasma-cell-associated antigen PC-1 and other early-appearing B-cell antigens, such as CD10, CD21, and CD24, are usually negative in HCL, although one report showed CD10 positivity in HCL.[1,2] The demonstration of both a B-cell antigen (CD22) and a monocyte antigen (CD11c) in a monoclonal B-cell population was considered highly specific for the diagnosis of HCL as both monoclonal antibodies were raised in mice using hairy cells as the immunogen.[28] However, the coexistence of these antigens has been found in other leukemias and lymphomas, such as MBCL, SLVL, and occasionally CLL, but a negative

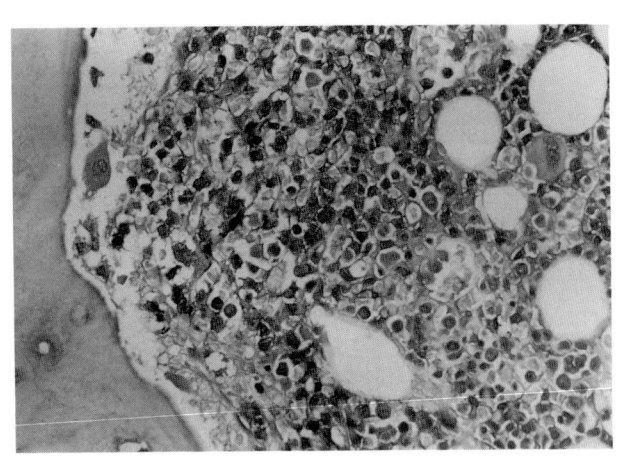

Fig. 12.22. A bone marrow biopsy showing positive DBA-44 staining on hairy cells. Immunoperoxidase, ×500.

CD11c can practically rule out HCL. When these markers are positive, the presence of CD25 (IL-2 receptor) is decisive in making the diagnosis, but CD25 is negative in some cases of HCL. While CD25 is very helpful in distinguishing HCL from other low-grade B-cell neoplasms by flow cytometry, one should be cautioned in interpreting CD25 positivity by immunohistochemistry, because many lymphomas can be stained with CD25 antibody, probably due to cross-reactivity.[29] On the other hand, serum IL-2R levels can be used for therapeutic monitoring in HCL.[30]

There are three monoclonal antibodies specific for HCL but not available commercially. Anti-HC1 is positive in 40–70% of HCL cases but is also positive in some epithelial and endothelial cells.[31] Anti-HC2 is positive in 80–100% of HCL cases but is also reactive with other B-cell lymphoproliferative disorders and myeloid leukemias.[31] The third antibody, B-ly7, seems to be relatively restricted to HCL.[32]

Other positive but nonspecific markers for HCL include CD45 (leukocyte common antigen), HLA-DR, FMC-7, and S-100 protein.[1] Other antigens, such as CD38, CD45RO (Fig. 12.24), CD23, CD15, CD4, CD5, and CD10, can be occasionally demonstrated in decreasing order in HCL.[33] In paraffin sections, hairy cells are positive for CD45, CD45RA(MT2), CD20(L26), CDw75(LN1), CD74(LN2), LN3, and MB2.[34]

Monocytoid B-Cell Lymphoma

The immunophenotype of MBCL is very similar to that of HCL, except that MBCL is negative for CD25.[3,4] Among nonhematopoietic antigens, muscle-specific actin and epithelial membrane antigen (EMA) are detected in some cases of MBCL but not in cases of HCL.[34]

Splenic Lymphoma with Villous Lymphocytes

According to most studies, the major difference between the immunophenotypes of HCL and SLVL is the absence of CD25 in the latter.[1] However, a recent study demonstrated CD25 in 25% of SLVL cases.[35] The same study also showed positive reaction to CD22, CD11c, CD24, FMC7, CD10, CD23, and CD38 in SLVL cases.[35] These authors suggested that only HC2 and B-ly7 were specific for HCL, but even these two antigens were positive in a few cases of SLVL.[35]

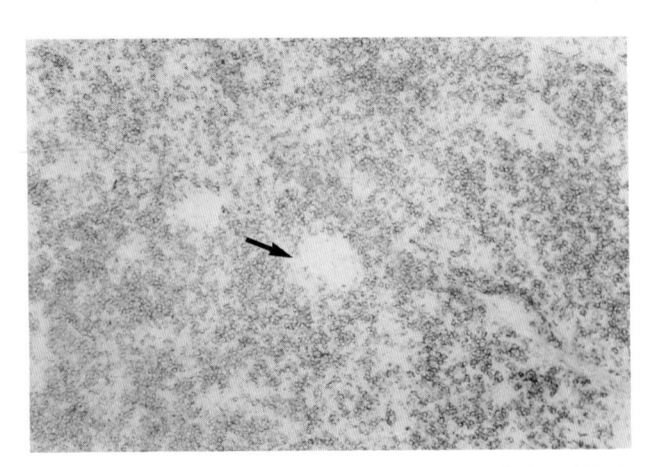

Fig. 12.23. Splenectomy specimen stained for CD22 showing large unstained blood lakes (arrow) in a case of hairy-cell leukemia. Immunoperoxidase, ×250.

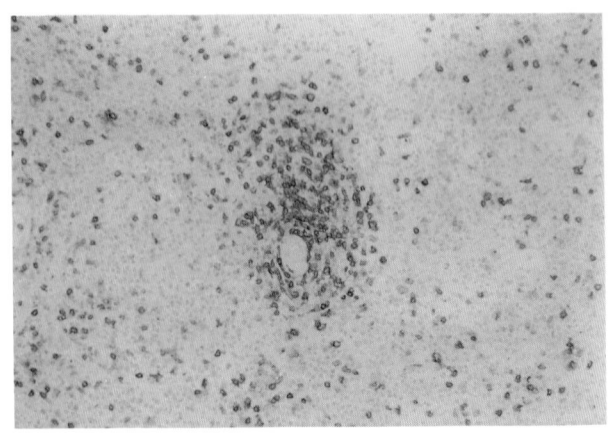

Fig. 12.24. The same specimen as in Fig. 12.23 showing CD45RO stain for T-cells in the white pulp that is not involved by hairy cells. Immunoperoxidase, ×250.

Chronic Lymphocytic Leukemia

The presence of CD5 and the absence of CD11c and CD25 in most CLL cases distinguish CLL from HCL. However, some chronic lymphoproliferative disorder with neoplastic cells similar to those of CLL may also express CD11c.[36]

Prolymphocytic Leukemia

In addition to the B-cell markers, PLL also shares a special marker, FMC-7, with HCL. However, PLL is negative for CD11c and CD25, and one-third of PLL is CD5 positive.

HCL Variants and Hybrid Forms

HCL variants have been reported with increasing frequency. The most common form is the hybrid form of HCL and CLL, which shows a mixed clinical and phenotypic feature of both disorders.[36-38] The second one is the hybrid form of HCL and PLL, which is also known as type II HCL.[39] In addition, there are a blastic variant, which shows blast morphology of tumor cells and prominent lymphadenopathy[40], and a Japanese variant, which expresses CD5 and CD10 antigens.[41] As Melo et al. suggested, HCL, HCL variant, SLVL, and PLL represent a spectrum of cell type frozen at slightly different stages during late B-cell maturation.[8] This statement has been supported by several *in vitro* experiments that show induction of CLL and PLL into HCL by TPA (tetradecanoyl phorbal acetate).[42]

HCL of T-Cell Phenotype

Two cases of HCL of T-cell lineage have been reported.[43,44] Both cases were believed to be associated with infections by the retrovirus HTLV-II. Reexamination of one of the two cases revealed that the case was actually composed of B-cell HCL and a CD8-positive T-cell leukemia.[41] The HTLV-II genome was found in the DNA of the leukemic T-cells, but not in the hairy cells.[45]

Cytochemistry

Positive cytochemical staining for tartrate-resistant acid phosphatase (TRAP) is the first specific marker and still one of the most reliable parameters for the diagnosis of HCL. Although many studies claimed to find positive TRAP stain in other lymphoproliferative disorders, most of these reports did not adhere to the strict definition of real TRAP positivity. In HCL, the TRAP staining is heavy (> 40 granules) and diffuse (not focal), and the staining intensity before and after tartrate treatment should be comparable (not markedly different) (Fig. 12.25). The most commonly encountered misinterpretation is probably classifying a focal acid phosphatase stain in the Golgi region as TRAP positivity.[1] This punctate staining pattern is consistently demonstrated in T-lymphocytes. By summarizing their 15 years' experience, Yam et al. have concluded that false-positive or false-negative TRAP results are usually due to either technical or interpretive errors.[46] Besides HCL, only SLVL shows real TRAP staining with considerable frequency.[9,23] TRAP staining is preferred for buffy-coat preparations, bone marrow aspirates, and tissue imprints; however, a few reports have demonstrated TRAP staining in HCL cells in paraffin-embedded tissue sections.[47]

Other cytochemical stains positive in HCL include β-glucuronidase, α-naphthyl acetate esterase and α-naphthyl butyrate esterase[1], but these results are not specific and are thus not of diagnostic importance.

Molecular-Genetic Studies

Immunoglobulin gene rearrangement but not T-cell receptor gene rearrangement has been demonstrated in HCL. Gene rearrangement does not help in differential diagnosis between HCL and other low-grade B-cell neoplasms. However, HCL may have more than one neoplastic clone; while one clone is sensitive to chemotherapy, the other one may be refractory.[48] Therefore, it may be occasionally useful in evaluating

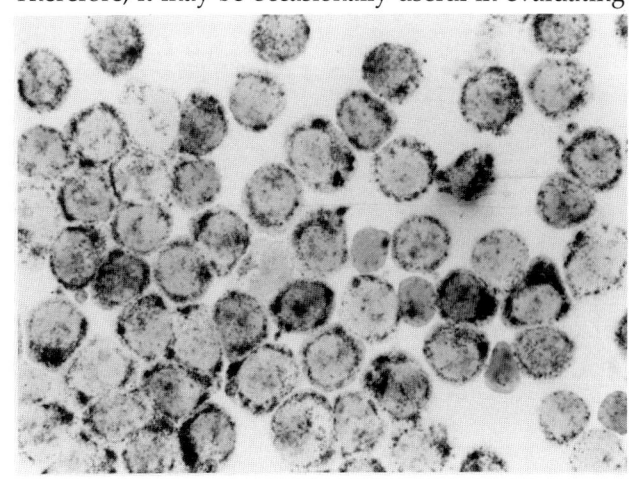

Fig. 12.25. A cytopreparation from the peripheral blood of a HCL case showing strong tartrate-resistant acid phosphatase stain. ×1250.

therapeutic problems. Cytogenetic studies have demonstrated numeric and structural abnormalities in HCL.[1,2] Recurrent chromosomal aberrations have been found in chromosomes 1, 2, 5, 6, 11, 19, and 20.[49] The abnormalities are mostly deletions and inversions. The expression of c-fos protooncogene in HCL was reported in one study.[49]

Cytogenetic studies in SLVL showed chromosomal abnormalities in 87% of cases.[50] Four recurrent abnormalities were demonstrated: t(11;14) (q13;q32), translocations or deletions in 7q; iso 17q; and translocation involving 2p11.[50] In cases with t(11;14), bcl-1 rearrangement and cyclin D1 gene were demonstrated.[51]

REFERENCES

1. Bitter MA: Hairy-cell leukemia. In Knowles DM (ed): *Neoplastic Hematopathology*. Baltimore, Williams & Wilkins, 1992, pp 1209–1234.
2. Chang KL, Stroup R, Weiss LM: Hairy cell leukemia: Current status. *Am J Clin Pathol* 97:719–738, 1992.
3. Sheibani K: Monocytoid B-cell lymphoma. In Knowles DM (ed): *Neoplastic Hematopathology*, Baltimore, Williams & Wilkins, 1992, pp 629–644.
4. Shin SS, Sheibani K: Monocytoid B-cell lymphoma. *Am J Clin Pathol* 99:421–425, 1993.
5. Ngan BY, Warnke RA, Wilson M, et al: Monocytoid B-cell lymphoma: A study of 36 cases. *Hum Pathol* 22:409–421, 1991.
6. Shin SS, Sheibani X, Fishleder A, et al: Monocytoid B-cell lymphoma in patients with Sjögren's syndrome: A clinicopathologic study of 13 patients. *Hum Pathol* 22:422–430, 1991.
7. Cogliatti SB, Lennert K, Hansmann ML, Zwingers TL: Monocytoid B-cell lymphoma: Clinical and prognostic features of 21 patients. *J Clin Pathol* 43:619–625, 1990.
8. Melo JV, Hedge V, Parreira A, et al: Splenic B-cell lymphoma with circulating villous lymphocytes: Differential diagnosis of B-cell leukemia with large spleens. *J Clin Pathol* 40:642–651, 1987.
9. Sun T, Susin M, Brody J, et al: Splenic lymphoma with circulating villous lymphocytes: Report of seven cases and review of the literature. *Am J Hematol* 45:39–50, 1994.
10. Mulligan SP, Matutes E, Dearden C, et al: Splenic lymphoma with villous lymphocytes: Natural history and response to therapy in 50 cases. *Br J Haematol* 78:206–209, 1991.
11. Spriano P, Barosi G, Invernizzi R, et al: Splenomegalic immunocytoma with circulating hairy cells: Report of eight cases and review of the literature. *Haematologica* 71:25–33, 1986.
12. Namba K, Soban EJ, Bowling MC, et al: Splenic pseudosinuses and hepatic angiomatous lesions: Distinctive features of hairy cell leukemia. *Am J Clin Pathol* 67:415–426, 1977.
13. Burke JS, Rappaport H: The diagnosis and differential diagnosis of hairy cell leukemia in bone marrow and spleen. *Semin Oncol* 11:334–336, 1984.
14. Roquet ML, Zafrani E, Farcet JP, et al: Histopathological lesions of the liver in hairy cell leukemia: A report of 14 cases. *Hepatology* 5:496–500, 1985.
15. Traweek ST, Sheibani K: Monocytoid B-cell lymphoma: The biologic and clinical implication of peripheral blood involvement. *Am J Clin Pathol* 97:591–598, 1992.
16. Mollejo M, Menarquez J, Cristobal E, et al: Monocytoid B-cells: A comparative clinical pathological study of their distribution in different types of low-grade lymphomas. *Am J Surg Pathol* 18:1131–1139, 1994.
17. Issacson P, Matutes E, Burke M, et al: The histopathology of splenic lymphoma with villous lymphocytes. *Blood* 84:3826–3834, 1994.
18. Nathwani BN, Mohrmann RL, Brynes RK, et al: Monocytoid B-cell lymphomas: An assessment of diagnostic criteria and a perspective on histogenesis. *Hum Pathol* 23:1061–1071, 1992.
19. Neiman RS, Sullivan AL, Jaffe R: Malignant lymphoma simulating leukemic reticuloendotheliosis: A clinicopathologic study of ten cases. *Cancer* 43:329–342, 1979.
20. Melo JV, Robinson DSF, Gregory C, et al: Splenic B-cell lymphoma with villous lymphocytes in the peripheral blood: A disorder distinct from hairy cell leukemia. *Leukemia* 1:294–299, 1987.
21. Lampert IA, Thompson I: The spleen in chronic lymphocytic leukemia and related disorders. In Polliack A, Catovsky D (eds): *Chronic Lymphocytic Leukemia*, Chur (Switzerland), Harwood Academic Publishers, 1988, pp 193–208.
22. Valensi F, Durand V, Bastenaire B, et al: Splenic B-cell lymphoma with villous lymphocytes (SLVL): A lymphocytic lymphoma simulating hairy cell leukemia. *Nouv Rev Fr Hematol* 32:409–414, 1990.
23. Kettle P, Morris TCM, Markey GM, et al: Tartrate resistant acid phosphatase positive splenic lymphoma: A relative benign condition occurring in a time–space cluster? *J Clin Pathol* 43:714–718, 1990.
24. Robeiro I, Costa MM, Fernandes BA, et al: Splenic lymphoma with villous lymphocytes in two sisters. *J Clin Pathol* 45:1111–1113, 1992.
25. Rousselet MC, Gardenbas-pain M, Reinier CT, et al: Splenic lymphoma with circulating villous lymphocytes: Report of a case with immunologic and ultrastructural studies. *Am J Clin Pathol* 97:147–152, 1992.
26. Lazzaro B, Munger R, Flick J, et al: Visualization of the ribosome–lamella complex in plastic embedded biopsy specimens as an aid to diagnosis of hairy cell leukemia. *Arch Pathol Lab Med* 115:1259–1262, 1991.

27. Hounieu H, Chittal SM, Saati TA, et al: Hairy cell leukemia: Diagnosis of bone marrow involvement in paraffin embedded section with monoclonal antibody DBA-44. *Am J Clin Pathol* 98:26–33, 1992.
28. Schwarting R, Stein H, Wang CY: The monoclonal antibodies αS-HCL1 (αLeu-14) and αS-HCL3 (αLeu-M5) allow the diagnosis of hairy cell leukemia. *Blood* 65:974–983, 1985.
29. Weiss LM, Michie SA, Medeiros LJ, et al: Expression of Tac antigen by non-Hodgkin's lymphomas. *Am J Clin Pathol* 88:483–485, 1987.
30. Richards JM, Mick R, Latta JM, et al: Serum soluble interleukin-2 receptor is associated with clinical and pathologic disease status in hairy cell leukemia. *Blood* 76:1941–1945, 1990.
31. Posnett DN, Chiorazzi N, Kunkel HG: Monoclonal antibodies with specificity for hairy cell leukemia cells. *J Clin Invest* 70:254–251, 1982.
32. Visser L, Shaw A, Slupsky J, et al: Monoclonal antibodies reactive with hairy cell leukemia. *Blood* 74:320–325, 1989.
33. Juliusson G, Lenkei R, Lilliemark J: Flow cytometry of blood and bone marrow cells from patients with hairy cell leukemia: Phenotype of hairy cells and lymphocyte subsets after treatment with 2-chlorodeoxyadenosine. *Blood* 83:3672–3681, 1994.
34. Stroup R, Sheibani K: Antigenic phenotypes of hairy cell leukemia and monocytoid B-cell lymphoma: An immunohistochemical evaluation of 66 cases. *Hum Pathol* 23:172–177, 1992.
35. Matutes E, Morilla R, Owusu-Ankomah K, et al: The immunophenotype of splenic lymphoma with villous lymphocytes and its relevance to the differential diagnosis with other B-cell disorders. *Blood* 83:1558–1562, 1994.
36. Hanson CA, Gribbin TE, Schnitzer B, et al: CD11c (Leu M5) expression characterizes a B-cell chronic lymphoproliferative disorder with features of both chronic lymphocytic leukemia and hairy cell leukemia. *Blood* 76:2360–2367, 1990.
37. Sun T, Susin M, Shevde N, et al: Hybrid form of hairy cell leukemia and chronic lymphocytic leukemia. *Hematol Oncol* 8:283–294, 1990.
38. Wormsley SB, Baird SM, Gadal N, et al: Characteristics of CD11c+ CD5+ chronic B-cell leukemias and the identification of novel peripheral B-cell subsets with chronic lymphoid leukemia immunophenotypes. *Blood* 76:123–130, 1990.
39. Sainati L, Matules E, Mulligan S, et al: A variant form of hairy cell leukemia resistant to -interferon: Clinical and phenotypic characteristics of 17 patients. *Blood* 76:157–162, 1990.
40. Diez Martin JL, Li CY, Banks PM: Blastic variant of hairy cell leukemia. *Am J Clin Pathol* 87:576–583, 1987.
41. Katayama I, Hirashima K, Maruyama K, et al: Hairy cell leukemia in Japanese patients: A study with monoclonal antibodies. *Leukemia* 1:301–305, 1987.
42. Ziegler-Heitbrock HWL, Munker R, Dorken BM, et al: Induction of features characteristic of hairy cell leukemia in chronic lymphocytic leukemia and prolymphocytic leukemia cells. *Cancer Res* 46:2172–2178, 1986.
43. Saxon A, Stevens RH, Golde DW: T-lymphocyte variant of hairy cell leukemia. *Ann Intern Med* 88:323–326, 1978.
44. Rosenblatt JD, Golde DW, Wachsman W, et al: A second isolate of HTLV-II associated with atypical hairy cell leukemia. *N Engl J Med* 315:372–377, 1986.
45. Rosenblatt JD, Giorgi JV, Golde DW, et al: Integrated human T-cell leukemia virus II genome in CD8+ T-cells from a patient with "atypical" hairy cell leukemia: Evidence for distinct T and B cell lymphoproliferative disorders. *Blood* 71:363–369, 1988.
46. Yam LT, Janckila AJ, Li CY, et al: Cytochemistry of tartrate-resistant acid phosphatase: Fifteen years' experience. *Leukemia* 1:285–288, 1987.
47. Janckila AJ, Cardwell EM, Yam LT, et al: Hairy cell identification by imunohistochemistry of tartrate-resistant acid phosphatase. *Blood* 85:2839–2844, 1995.
48. Raghavachar A, Bartram CR, Porzsolt F: Eradication by alpha-interferon of one clone in biclonal hairy cell leukemia. *Lancet* 2:516, 1986.
49. Lehn P, Sigaux F, Grausz D, et al: c-myc and c-fos expression during interferon therapy for hairy cell leukemia. *Blood* 68:967–970, 1986.
50. Oscier DG, Matutes E, Gardiner A, et al: Cytogenetic studies in splenic lymphoma with villous lymphocytes. *Br J Haematol* 85:487–491, 1993.
51. Jadayel D, Matutes E, Dyer MJS, et al: Splenic lymphoma with villous lymphocytes: Analysis of BCL-1 rearrangements and expression of the cyclin D1 gene. *Blood* 83:3664–3671, 1994.

13
Lymphoblastic Lymphoma vs. Burkitt's Lymphoma vs. Acute Lymphoblastic Leukemia

Lymphoblastic lymphoma and Burkitt's lymphoma were both classified under lymphoblastic lymphoma in the original Kiel classification. However, they are now treated as separate, independent entities in the updated Kiel classification, because they can be clearly defined morphologically and show no immunohistochemical relationship.[1] Lymphoblastic lymphoma is called *convoluted lymphocytic lymphoma* in the Lukes–Collins classification. Burkitt's lymphoma is designated *small noncleaved follicular center-cell lymphoma* in the same scheme and *small non-cleaved-cell lymphoma* in the Working Formulation.

Although both lymphomas are high-grade malignancy seen predominantly in childhood, their clinical presentations are quite different: lymphoblastic lymphoma involves mainly the mediastinum, and Burkitt's lymphoma is seen in the jaw (endemic type) or the abdominal organs (sporadic type). The need for distinguishing these two neoplasms is due to their histologic similarity. Furthermore, both lymphomas have their leukemic counterparts, thus requiring further distinction from each other.

CLINICAL FEATURES

Lymphoblastic Lymphoma and Acute Lymphoblastic Leukemia

Lymphoblastic lymphoma accounts for one third to one half of all non-Hodgkin's lymphomas in childhood, but only 3–5% of those in adults.[2] About half of the pediatric patients are ≥ 10 years of age. Adult patients are mostly < 30 years old, but a second peak incidence is demonstrated in patients in the 7th decade.[3] The male:female ratio in lymphoblastic lymphoma varies from 2:1 to 10:1 in different reports.

The major clinical presentation is the presence of a mediastinal mass and/or peripheral lymphadenopathy in pediatric patients. The supradiaphragmatic (cervical, supraclavicular, or axillary) lymph nodes are most frequently involved. Patients with mediastinal involvement may have airway obstruction, pleural effusion, pericardial effusion, dysphagia, and/or superior vena cava syndrome. In adult patients, however, the presentation is frequently extramediastinal, mainly abdominal and cutaneous lesions.[4] A small number of pediatric patients may also show primary cutaneous lesions without mediastinal involvement. These patients are usually very young (6 months to 6 years), and the tumor cells are usually of the pre-B lymphocyte phenotype.[5]

About 20% of patients with lymphoblastic lymphoma have involvement of the central nervous system (CNS), an incidence higher than that of any other non-Hodgkin's lymphomas.[6] About 60% of patients may have bone marrow or peripheral blood involvement, and about 90% of pediatric patients have a mediastinal mass. When the bone marrow is heavily involved, the clinical features of lymphoblastic lymphoma are indistinguishable from those of acute lymphoblastic leukemia. However, acute lymphoblastic leukemia usually has more prominent peripheral blood and bone marrow involvement, more severe anemia and thrombocytopenia and more often splenomegaly than lymphoblastic lymphoma does.[2] The cutoff point of 25% lymphoblasts in the bone marrow is generally accepted for the distinction between these two entities.[7] The presence of convoluted lymphoblasts in the peripheral blood is also in favor of a leukemic phase of lymphoblastic lymphoma.[8]

Burkitt's Lymphoma

Burkitt's lymphoma was first found in the jaws of children in Equatorial Africa. Subsequently, neoplasms of similar morphology were reported from countries outside Africa. Since these two groups of patients differ in epidemiology, clinical features, and serologic aspects, they are divided into endemic (African) type and sporadic (non-African) type (Table 13.1).[10] The annual incidence of the endemic type is about 20–40 times higher than that of the sporadic type.[9]

In Africa, Burkitt's lymphoma is seen mainly in boys; but a bimodal age distribution (children and elderly) is seen in the sporadic type. The initial presentation is either a jaw or orbital tumor in 60% of African patients, but intraabdominal lesions in 90% of American patients.[9,11,12] Bone marrow involvement is rarer, but CNS involvement is more common in the endemic type than in the sporadic type.[9,11,12] A leukemic phase of Burkitt's lymphoma

DIFFERENTIAL DIAGNOSIS OF LYMPHOID DISORDERS

TABLE 13.1
Comparison of Endemic and Sporadic
Burkitt's Lymphoma

	Endemic Type	Sporadic Type
Annual incidence per 100,000 population	2.3–3.8	0.1–0.3
Age group with high incidence	4–8 years	Bimodal
Male:female ratio	2:1–3:1	2.3:1–3.7:1
Initial presentation	Jaw lesion	Abdominal tumor
Bone marrow involvement (%)	~8	16–20
CNS involvement (%)	~30	5–20
Leukemic form	Absent	Present
Positive serologic test for EBV (%)	88–97	20
EBV receptor on tumor cells	Common	Rare
EBV genome in tumor cells (%)	95	11–20

From Sun T: *Color Atlas/Text of Flow Cytometric Analysis of Hematologic Neoplasms*, New York, Igaku-Shoin, 1993.

is seen only in the sporadic type.[9] Pleura, breast, kidneys, testes, and ovaries can also be involved at presentation.[11]

The clinical manifestation of Burkitt's leukemia differs from that of acute lymphoblastic leukemia in the absence of mediastinal but presence of extranodal involvement. However, Burkitt's lymphoma may occasionally be found in mediastinum,[11] in which case it requires immunophenotyping to distinguish from lymphoblastic lymphoma. Recently, Burkitt's lymphoma, mostly involving the brain, has been frequently found in patients with the acquired immunodeficiency syndrome (AIDS).[13–15] It accounts for 35–40% of all lymphomas in AIDS patients, compared with the 1–2% in the general population. The tumors in AIDS patients do not differ from those in other patients in terms of morphology and chromosomal characteristics.

PATHOLOGY

Lymphoblastic Lymphoma

Lymphoblastic lymphoma was called *convoluted lymphocytic lymphoma* in both Lukes–Collins and the old Kiel classifications. Although most (85%) lym-

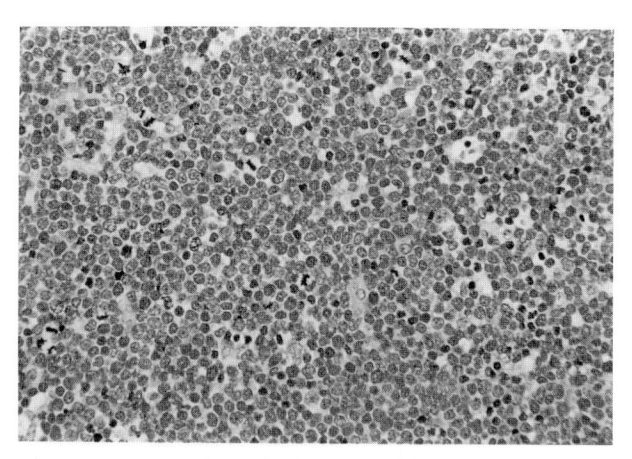

Fig. 13.1. Lymph node biopsy of lymphoblastic lymphoma showing convoluted and nonconvoluted nuclei, dust-like chromatin, inconspicuous nucleoli, scanty cytoplasm, and ill-defined cell borders. A starry-sky pattern and many mitotic figures are present. H&E, ×500.

phoblastic lymphomas are of the convoluted type, small percentages may show nonconvoluted or atypical pleomorphic patterns.[2,16,17] A convoluted subtype is defined as the presence convoluted tumor cells (even in a small percentage), which show deep clefts or infoldings in the nuclei (Figs. 13.1–13.5).[2] Besides the nuclei, the nonconvoluted subtype shares the same morphologic features as the convoluted subtype in showing scanty cytoplasm, ill-defined cell border, evenly distributed dust-like chromatin, and inconspicuous nucleoli (Table 13.2). In tissue imprints, the lymphoblasts assume the L1 morphology

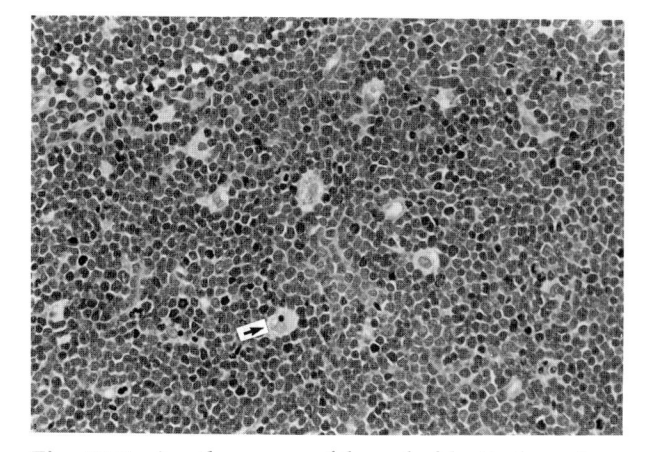

Fig. 13.2. Another case of lymphoblastic lymphoma showing tingible-body macrophages (arrow). H&E, ×500.

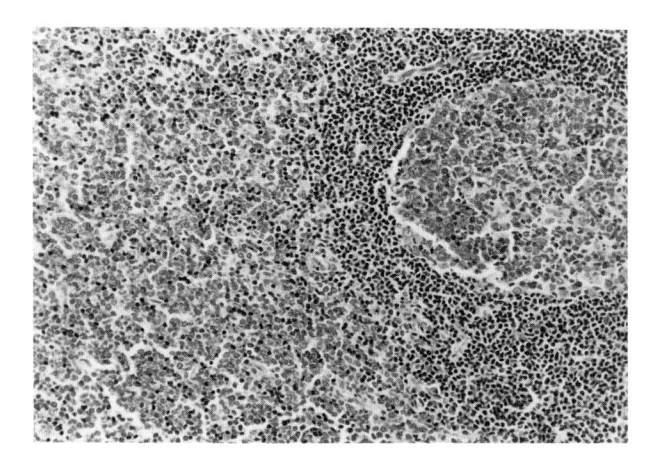

Fig. 13.3. Lymph node biopsy showing a paracortical lymphoblastic lymphoma of T-cell lineage. H&E, ×250.

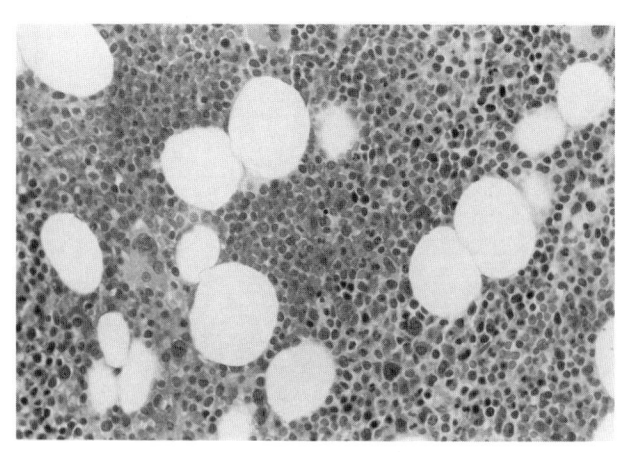

Fig. 13.5. Bone marrow biopsy of lymphoblastic lymphoma showing focal infiltration of neoplastic cells. H&E, ×500.

(Fig. 13.6) according to the French–American–British (FAB) classification of acute lymphoblastic leukemia.[17] The atypical pleomorphic subtype is composed of 10% of lymphoblastic lymphoma.[16] The lymphoblasts in this subtype usually vary in size and shape but are usually larger than tumor cells in other subtypes and have one or two relatively prominent nucleoli; thus it is sometimes very difficult to distinguish this subtype from non-Burkitt's lymphoma. Tissue imprints can be very helpful in the differential diagnosis. The atypical lymphoblastic lymphoma is morphologically similar to L2 lymphoblastic leukemia, whereas non-Burkitt's lymphoma belongs to the L3 category. The most important criterion for differential diagnosis is the chromatin pattern, which is quite different between these two types of neoplasms: the chromatin is delicate in lymphoblasts but clumped in Burkitt's lymphoma.

TABLE 13.2
Comparison of Lymphoblastic Lymphoma and Burkitt's Lymphoma

	Lymphoblastic lymphoma	Burkitt's lymphoma
High-incidence group	Children	Children
Clinical presentation	Mediastinal mass	Jaw or abdominal lesion
Mitotic rate	High	High
Starry-sky background	Less prominent	More prominent
Cell size	Small to intermediate	Intermediate to large
Cytoplasm	Scanty	Abundant with vacuoles
Nuclear shape	Usually convoluted	Round or ovoid
Chromatin pattern	Finely speckled	Clumped
Nucleoli	Inconspicuous	Multiple, distinct
Phenotype	Predominantly T-cell	B-cell
Cytogenetic abormality	Not specific	t(8;14), t(8;22), or t(2;8)
EBV-related[a]	No	Yes

EBV = Epstein Barr virus
From Sun T: *Color Atlas/Text of Flow Cytometric Analysis of Hematologic Neoplasms*, New York, Igaku-Shoin, 1993.

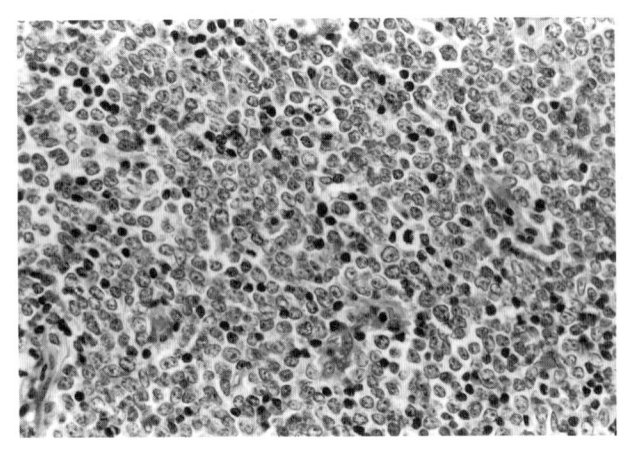

Fig. 13.4. A higher-power view of Fig. 13.3 showing nonconvoluted lymphoblasts and multiple mitoses. H&E, ×500.

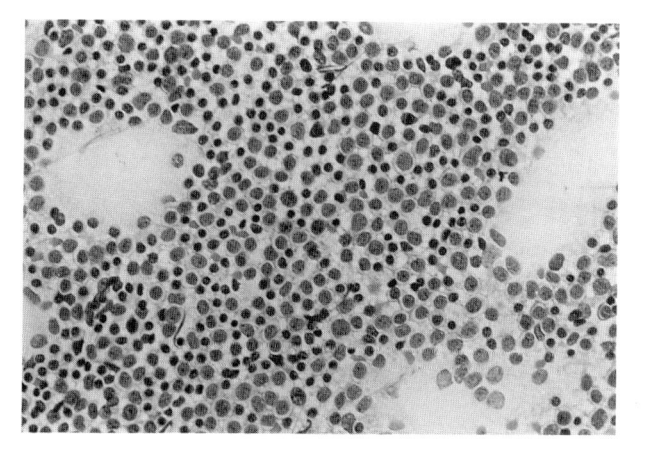

Fig. 13.6. Lymph node imprint of lymphoblastic lymphoma showing dust-like chromatin pattern and inconspicuous nucleoli. The small, uniform-sized neoplastic cells are consistent with L1 morphology. H&E, ×500.

The histologic pattern of lymphoblastic lymphoma usually shows diffuse infiltration, which obliterates the normal architecture of the lymph node and invades the lymph node capsule and the perinodal fibroadipose tissue. The neoplastic cells are frequently interspersed with tingible-body macrophages with the resultant starry-sky appearance. However, this pattern is not as frequently seen and not as prominent in lymphoblastic lymphoma as in Burkitt's lymphoma. Mitotic rate is usually high in both tumors.

Acute Lymphoblastic Leukemia

According to the FAB classification, acute lymphoblastic leukemia can be divided into L1, L2, and L3 (Table 13.3).[18] The leukemic cells in L1 are uniformly small with scanty cytoplasm. Their nuclei are regular in shape, and the nucleoli, if present, are inconspicuous. This form is usually seen in pediatric cases. The neoplastic cells in L2 are generally large, but their size is variable, as is the cytoplasm. Their nuclei also vary in shape, and the nucleoli are prominent. This form appears more frequently in adults than in children. The tumor cells in L3 are uniformly large with moderate amounts of deep basophilic cytoplasm, which contain many vacuoles. The nuclei are round and regular with prominent nucleoli (Figs. 13.7–13.9). This form is rare in comparison with L1 and L2 and is more frequently seen in adults. It can also be seen in the leukemic form of Burkitt's lymphoma.

As mentioned before, the convoluted and nonconvoluted subtypes of lymphoblastic lymphoma usually assume the morphology of L1, while the atypical subtype resembles L2.

Acute lymphoblastic leukemia must be distinguished from acute myeloblastic leukemia (see Chapter 23). By the same token, lymphoblastic lymphoma should be distinguished from granulocytic sarcoma (see Chapter 23). Sometimes it is difficult to distinguish between these two entities by morphology, but cytochemistry usually provides a clearcut answer. Lymphoblasts are negative for myeloperoxidase (Fig. 13.10), specific and nonspecific esterases, but are positive for periodic-acid Schiff (PAS) staining in 80–90% of cases. For very immature blasts, all cytochemical stains can be negative. Monoclonal antibodies of the lymphoid and myeloid lineages should then be used for definitive identification.

Burkitt's Lymphoma

Burkitt's lymphoma is designated as small non-cleaved-cell lymphoma in the Working Formulation, as the tumor cells are compared with the size of macrophages. In fact, Burkitt's lymphoma cells are usually intermediate in size between large-cell lym-

TABLE 13.3
The FAB Classification for Acute Lymphoblastic Leukemia

	L1	L2	L3
Cell size	Small, uniform	Large, variable	Large, uniform
Cytoplasm	Scanty, moderate basophilia	Variable in amount and degree of basophilia	Moderately abundant; deep basophilia with vacuoles
Nucleus	Regular shape	Irregular shape	Regular shape
Nucleolus	0–1, inconspicuous	≥1, prominent	2–5, prominent
Nuclear/cytoplasmic ratio	High	Low	Low

From Sun T: *Color Atlas/Text of Flow Cytometric Analysis of Hematologic Neoplasms*, New York, Igaku-Shoin, 1993.

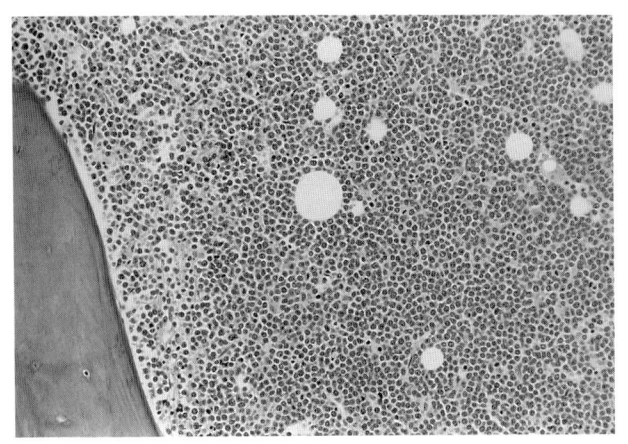

136 DIFFERENTIAL DIAGNOSIS OF LYMPHOID DISORDERS

Fig. 13.7. Bone marrow biopsy of acute lymphoblastic leukemia (L3) showing diffuse infiltration of lymphoblasts completely replacing the normal elements. H&E, ×250.

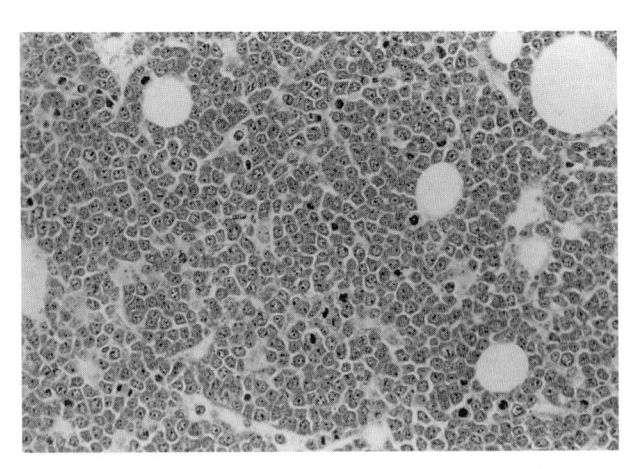

Fig. 13.9. A Giemsa-stained preparation of the same case as in Fig. 13.8 showing uniform-sized neoplastic cells with prominent nucleoli and high mitotic rate. ×500.

phoma cells and small lymphocytic lymphoma cells. The major cytologic feature is the clumped nuclear chromatin pattern and clear parachromatin with 2–5 prominent basophilic nucleoli.[11] There is a moderate amount of cytoplasm. The characteristics of cytoplasm, which can be appreciated only in tissue imprints (Figs. 13.11, 13.12) or smears from the bone marrow (Fig. 13.13) or blood, are its deep basophilic stain and the presence of multiple cytoplasmic vacuoles. The cytoplasmic basophilia represents a high content of polyribosomes, which can be demonstrated with methyl green pyronin (Fig. 13.14). The cytoplasmic vacuoles contain a lipid substance that is demonstrable by lipid stains such as oil red O, but not by

PAS. Since the tumor cells are frequently interspersed with tingible-body macrophages, a starry-sky appearance is usually demonstrated (Figs. 13.15–13.17) and is more prominent than is seen in lymphoblastic lymphoma. The tumor cells usually cause complete effacement of the normal architecture of the lymph node and infiltrate the surrounding tissues.

The morphology of Burkitt's lymphoma in the endemic and sporadic types appear the same. However,

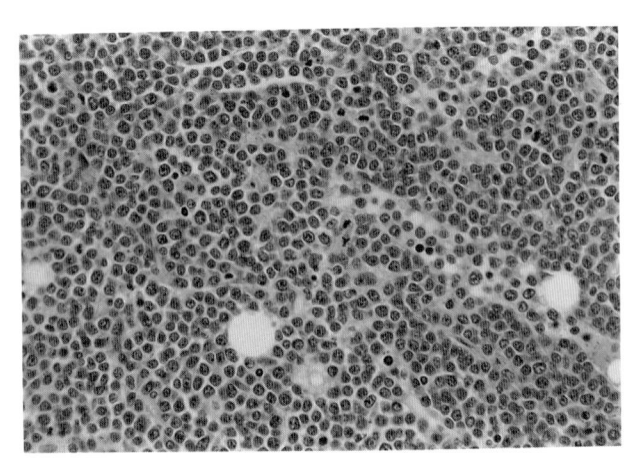

Fig. 13.8. A higher-power view of Fig. 13.7 showing uniform-sized neoplastic cells. H&E, ×500.

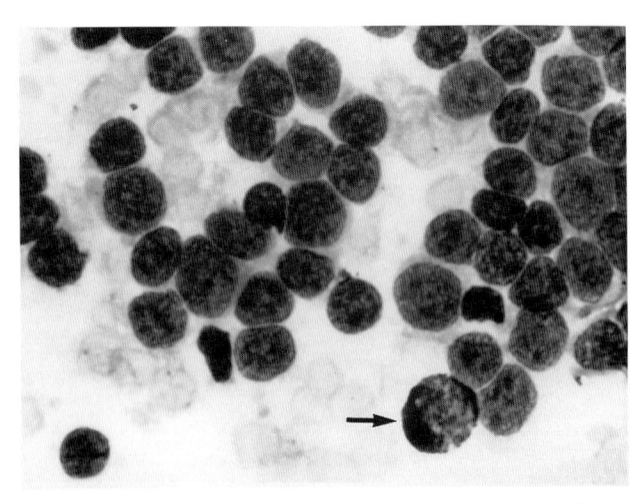

Fig. 13.10. Bone marrow aspirate of acute lymphoblastic leukemia showing negative myeloperoxidase staining. Only a myelocyte (arrow) is positive for this stain. Note the clumped chromatin pattern and inconspicuous nucleoli in blasts. Myeloperoxidase/Wright–Giemsa, ×1,250.

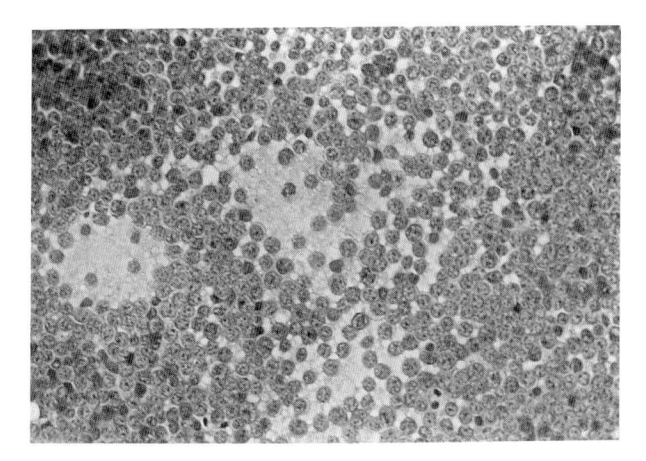

Fig. 13.11. Lymph node imprint of Burkitt's lymphoma showing uniform neoplastic cells with prominent nucleoli. H&E, ×500.

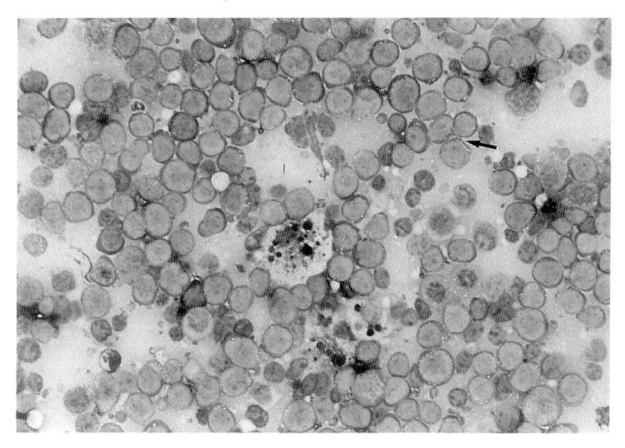

Fig. 13.12. Lymph node imprint of Burkitt's lymphoma with Wright–Giemsa stain showing uniformly large tumor cells with basophilic cytoplasm containing vacuoles (arrow). Tingible-body macrophages are seen in the center of the field. ×500.

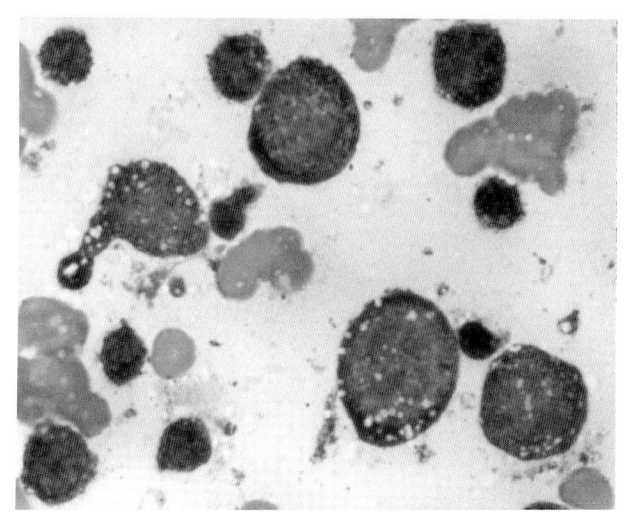

Fig. 13.13. Bone marrow aspirate of Burkitt's lymphoma showing uniformly large tumor cells with deep basophilic cytoplasm containing multiple vacuoles. Wright–Giemsa, ×1250.

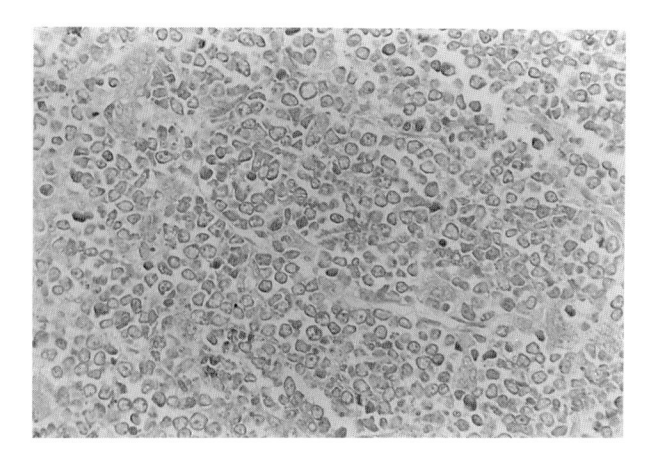

Fig. 13.14. Lymph node biopsy of Burkitt's lymphoma showing positive methyl-green pyronin stain. ×500.

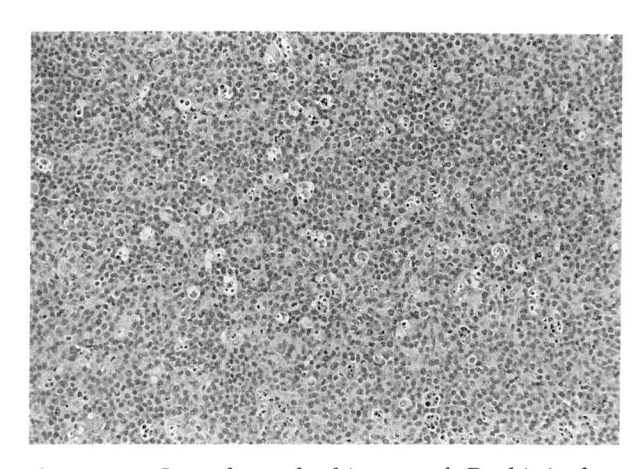

Fig. 13.15. Lymph node biopsy of Burkitt's lymphoma showing many tingible-body macrophages with a starry-sky pattern. H&E, ×250.

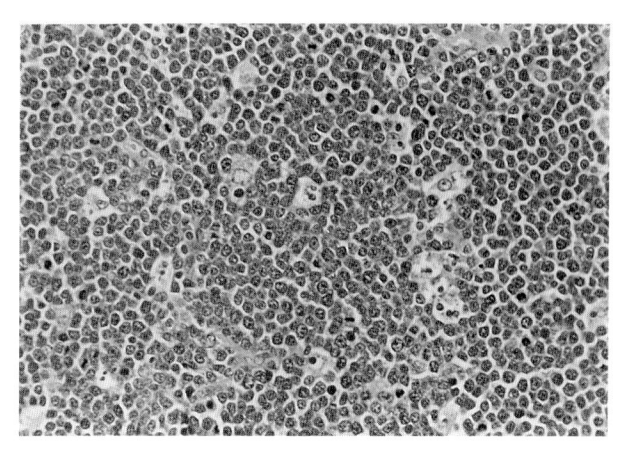

Fig. 13.16. A higher-power view of Fig. 13.15 showing tingible-body macrophages, prominent nucleoli in tumor cells, and multiple mitosis. H&E, ×520.

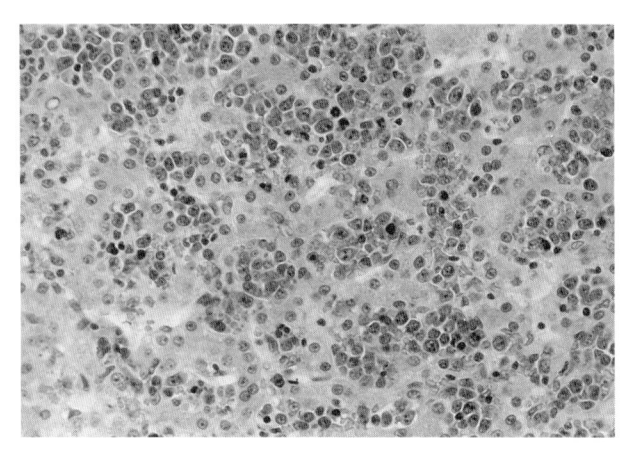

138 DIFFERENTIAL DIAGNOSIS OF LYMPHOID DISORDERS

Fig. 13.17. A case of Burkitt's lymphoma showing pleomorphic tumor cells infiltrating the liver sinusoids. H&E, ×500.

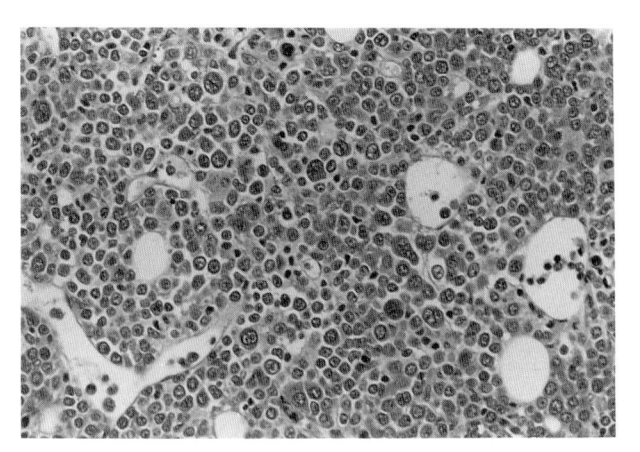

Fig. 13.19. Bone marrow biopsy of non-Burkitt's lymphoma showing marked variation in size and shape of tumor cells. A few binucleated tumor cells are present. H&E, ×500.

there is a morphologic variant of Burkitt's lymphoma in the nonendemic areas designated as non-Burkitt's lymphoma.[19,20] In non-Burkitt's lymphoma, the nuclear size and shape are variable, as compared with the monotonous morphology of Burkitt's lymphoma (Figs. 13.18–13.20, Table 13.4). In addition, non-Burkitt's lymphoma has 1–2 large eosinophilic nucleoli, while Burkitt's lymphoma contains 2–5 small but distinct basophilic nucleoli. Non-Burkitt's lymphoma is more frequently seen in adults with no sexual predilection, is less frequently extranodal, and involves the bone marrow more often than Burkitt's lymphoma. The 5-year survival rate in non-Burkitt's is lower than that in Burkitt's lymphoma according to most studies.[19,20]

As mentioned before, the sporadic subtype of Burkitt's lymphoma may have a leukemic phase and bone marrow involvement. The tumor cells in the blood and bone marrow are indistinguishable from those of L3 acute lymphoblastic leukemia. In most cases, there are no differences in immunophenotype, cytogenetics, therapeutic response, and survival rate between these two groups of patients.[11,21] Their distinction is somewhat arbitrary. For instance, Burkitt's lymphoma is considered if < 25% of bone marrow is involved, while > 25% of bone marrow involvement is designated L3 acute lymphoblastic leukemia.[22] Burkitt's lymphoma is probably best defined by Magrath et al. as a small non-cleaved-cell lymphoma with a B-cell phenotype and a

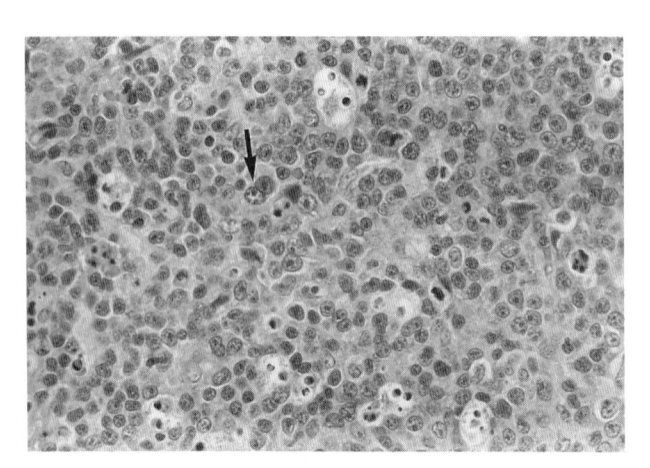

Fig. 13.18. Lymph node biopsy of non-Burkitt's lymphoma showing variation in size, many apoptotic cells, and tingible-body macrophages. A binucleated cell (arrow) is present. H&E, ×500.

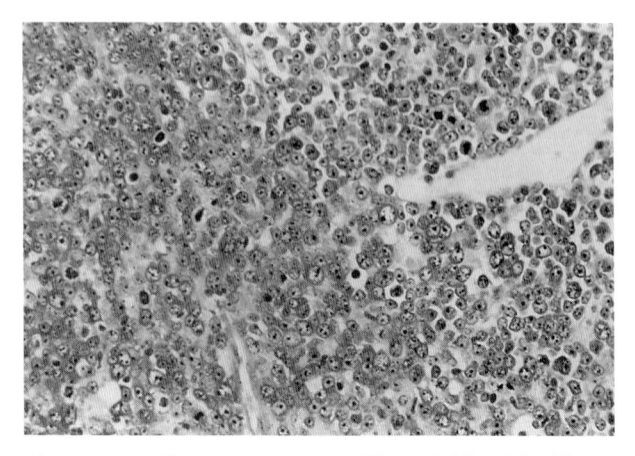

Fig. 13.20. The same case as Fig. 13.19 with Giemsa stain, demonstrating prominent nucleoli in neoplastic cells. ×500.

TABLE 13.4
Comparison of BL and NBL

	BL	NBL
Nuclei	Uniform, round	Variable size, irregular sharp
Multinucleation	Absent	Present
Nucleoli	Small, 2–5, basophilic	Larger, 1–2, eosinophilic
Cytoplasm	Deep basophilic with vacuoles	Light basophilic with vacuoles
Age	Mainly in children	Mainly in adults
Sex ratio	Male-predominant	Nearly equal
Extranodal presentation	Frequent	Less frequent
Abdominal involvement	Frequent	Frequent
Bone marrow involvement	Rare	More frequent
Oncogene involved	c-*myc*	*bcl*-2
Stages III and IV	About 2/3 patients	About 4/5 patients
Median survival	<1 year	<1 year
Five-year survival (%)	42	11

From Sun T: *Color Atlas/Text of Flow Cytometric Analysis of Hematologic Neoplasms*, New York, Igaku-Shoin, 1993.

chromosomal translocation that results in c-*myc* and immunoglobulin genes being juxtaposed on the same chromosome.[11] Therefore, only those leukemic cases with a T-cell phenotype or expression of terminal deoxynucleotidyl transferase (TdT), but no characteristic chromosomal translocation should be considered as an entity separate from Burkitt's lymphoma.[23,24]

LABORATORY FINDINGS

For lymphomas composed of lymphoblasts, the two most important markers for differential diagnosis are TdT and surface immunoglobulin. A positive TdT denotes lymphoblastic lymphoma, while a monoclonal surface immunoglobulin pattern identifies Burkitt's lymphoma. Among T-cell lymphomas, only lymphoblastic lymphoma is positive for TdT. Although many B-cell lymphomas express surface immunoglobulins, immature B-cell tumors (pre-pre-B-cell or pre-B-cell stage) do not show surface immunoglobulins until the early B-cell stage, which is represented by Burkitt's lymphoma.

Lymphoblastic Lymphoma and Acute Lymphoblastic Leukemia

A complete immunophenotyping may divide lymphoblastic lymphoma into five major types (Table 13.5). The major phenotype is T-cell lymphoblastic lymphoma, which is further divided into early thymocyte, common thymocyte, and late (mature) thymocyte subtypes.[25,26] All T-cell phenotypes are positive for TdT, CD2, CD5, and CD7 with variable expression of CD1, CD3, CD4, and CD8 depending on the developmental stage (Fig. 13.21). A small percentage of T-cell lymphoblastic lymphomas may carry the common ALL antigen (CD10), and have higher frequency of skin involvement than CD10 negative T-cell type.[25] Another small group of T-cell lymphoblastic lymphoma bearing natural-killer-cell antigens is seen predominantly in nonwhite female patients with an aggressive clinical course.[25,26] In the pre-B-cell and B-cell lymphoblastic lymphomas, mediastinal mass is usually absent. Skin and bone lesions occur more often in the pre-B-cell phenotype.[27–29]

For activated T-cell antigens, most cases of lymphoblastic lymphomas express CD38, about two thirds of cases carry CD71, but none of the cases studied shows CD25 (α subunit of the interleukin-2 receptor).[25,29] However, the β subunit of IL-2 is widely expressed among T-lymphoblastic lymphomas.[30]

Cases of acute lymphoblastic leukemia may have immunophenotypes identical to those of lymphoblastic lymphoma. However, the former usually express a more immature T-cell phenotype than do the latter.[7,31] This finding may also explain the fact that TCR (an early T-cell receptor) is more frequently expressed in acute lymphoblastic leukemia than in lymphoblastic lymphoma.[32] In addition, most (80%) lymphoblastic leukemia cases are of B-cell lineage, while most (80%) lymphoblastic lymphoma cases are derived from precursor T-cells.[2]

Gene rearrangement analysis in lymphoblastic lymphoma/leukemia is usually consistent with the phe-

TABLE 13.5
Immunophenotypes of Lymphoblastic Lymphoma

Immunophenotype	Special Features
I. T cell lymphoblastic lymphoma	Mediastinal mass (86%)
1. Early thymocytes	
TdT + CD1 − CD2 + CD3 − CD4 − CD5 + CD7 + CD8 −	
2. Common thymocytes	
TdT + CD1 + CD2 + CD3 − CD4 + CD5 + CD7 + CD8 +	
3. Late thymocytes	
TdT + CD1 − CD2 + CD3 + CD4 ± CD5 + CD7 + CD8 ±	
II. T-cell lymphoblastic lymphoma with CALLA	Skin involvement
Thymocyte phenotype with positive CALLA	
III. T-cell lymphoblastic lymphoma with NK antigens	Nonwhite-female-predominant,
Thymocyte phenotype with positive CD16 and/or CD57	aggressive course
IV. Pre-B cell lymphoblastic lymphoma	Bone or skin lesions
TdT + CALLA + HLA-DR + Cμ + CD9 + CD24 + T-antigen-negative	No mediastinal mass
V. B-cell lymphoblastic lymphoma	No mediastinal mass
TdT − HLA-DR + SIg + T-antigen-negative	

From Sun T: *Color Atlas/Text of Flow Cytometric Analysis of Hematologic Neoplasms*, New York, Igaku-Shoin, 1993.

notype, specifically, immunoglobulin gene rearrangement in B-cell neoplasms and T-cell receptor (TCR) gene rearrangement in T-cell tumors. However, in prethymic lymphoblastic lymphomas, the TCR gene may show a germline configuration.[33] In a small subset of precursor B-cell lymphoma/leukemia, immunoglobulin genes are not rearranged, although phenotyping shows positive CD19 and HLA-DR.[34] The major problem in gene rearrangement studies is "lineage promiscuity." TCR gene rearrangement can be demonstrated in as high as 80% of precursor B-cell lymphoblastic lymphoma/leukemia. On the other hand, immunoglobulin gene rearrangement may be demonstrated in 10–25% of precursor T-cell lymphoblastic lymphoma/leukemia.[2]

Burkitt's lymphoma

The immunophenotype of Burkitt's and non-Burkitt's lymphomas is similar to that of other lymphomas of the mature B-cell stage (such as presence of monoclonal surface immunoglobulin, various percentages of other B-cell antigens, including CD19, CD20, CD21, CD22, CD23, CD37, and FMC1, and HLA-DR).[35] CD10 is demonstrated in most cases of Burkitt's lymphoma and helps distinguish it from other B-cell lymphomas except for follicular lymphomas, which are also CD10 positive. There are minor differences in the phenotypes between the endemic and sporadic subtypes. The former expresses more CD23 and less CD10 antigen than the latter.[11] In addition, sporadic tumors may secrete IgM and be accompanied by a monoclonal IgM gammopathy, whereas monoclonal gammopathy is not seen in the endemic form.[36]

The most characteristic finding in Burkitt's lymphoma is its association with a nonrandom cytogenetic abnormality, t(8;14) (q24;q32), which is found in 70% of cases.[9] Two other translocations, t(8;22) (q24;q11) and t(2;8) (p12;q24), were found in 25% of cases.[9] The breakpoint on chromosome 8 corresponds

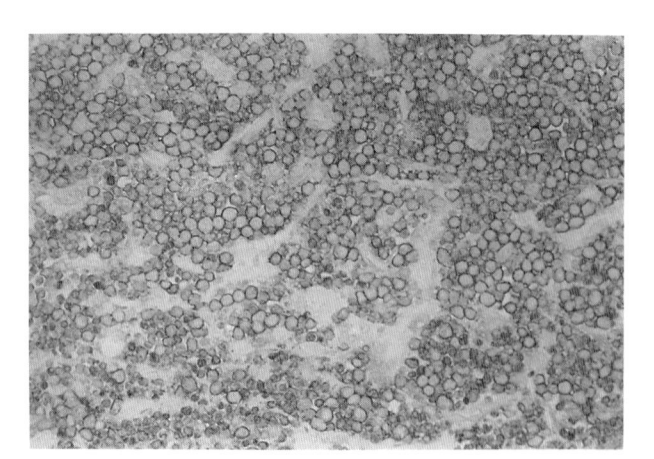

Fig. 13.21. Lymph node biopsy of lymphoblastic lymphoma showing T-cell marker (MT-1) staining. Immunoperoxidase, ×500.

to the *c-myc* oncogene, and those on chromosomes 14, 2, and 22 correspond to heavy-chain κ and λ light-chain genes, respectively. Therefore, the translocations in Burkitt's lymphoma are always between the *c-myc* oncogene and an immunoglobulin gene. This translocation results in deregulation of the *c-myc* oncogene, and this is considered the mechanism of tumorigenesis.[11] Although the translocation pattern [e.g., t(8;14), t(8;22) or t(2;8)] may be the same, the breakpoints on tumor chromosomes differ in cases from different geographic areas (e.g., Africa, United States, and tropical and temperate South America).

Another characteristic finding in Burkitt's lymphoma is its association with Epstein-Barr virus (EBV), which has been isolated from virtually all tumor samples from Africa.[11] Serologic tests demonstrate EBV antibodies in 88-97% of patients in the endemic area, but only 20% of patients in nonendemic areas.[9] Similar results have been obtained by the identification of EBV genomes: 95% in endemic tumors, 20% in sporadic tumors, and 40% in HIV-associated lymphomas.[11] EBV receptors have also been found on cultured tumor cells from Africa but seldom found on tumor cells from nonendemic areas.[9]

The roles that *c-myc* oncogene and EBV play in the oncogenesis of Burkitt's lymphoma are complicated. The deregulation of *c-myc* oncogene may prevent the cells from entering a resting phase or programmed cell death (apoptosis), leading to continuing cell proliferation.[11] However, when a transgene that consists of *c-myc* coupled to the immunoglobulin heavy-chain enhancer is introduced into the murine genome, the mouse first shows polyclonal proliferation of pre-B cells before a lymphoma is developed.[37] Therefore, it appears that an additional genetic event must take place after t(8;14) translocation, leading to final development of a monoclonal neoplasm. This second genetic change may well be induced by EBV-latent genes.[11] A current study of 11 non-Burkitt's lymphomas demonstrated no *c-myc* rearrangements, but 3 cases manifested *bcl-2* rearrangements.[38] These findings suggest that the mechanism of oncogenesis in Burkitt's and non-Burkitt's lymphoma may be different and that the distinction of these two types of tumor has biologic significance.

REFERENCES

1. Lennert K, Feller AC: Histopathology of Non-Hodgkin's Lymphomas (based on the updated Kiel classification), Berlin, Springer-Verlag, 1992, pp 12-18.
2. Knowles DM: Lymphoblastic lymphoma. In Knowles DM (ed): *Neoplastic Hematopathology*, Baltimore, Williams & Wilkins, 1992, pp 715-747.
3. Nathwani BN, Diamond LW, Winberg CD, et al: Lymphoblastic lymphoma: A clinicopathologic study of 95 patients. *Cancer* 48:2347-2357, 1981.
4. Mazza P, Bertini M, Macchi S, et al: Lymphoblastic lymphoma in adolescents and adults. Clinical, pathological and prognostic evaluation. *Eur J Cancer Clin Oncol* 22:1503-1510, 1986.
5. Link MP, Roper M, Dorfman RF, et al: Cutaneous lymphoblastic lymphoma with pre-B markers. *Blood* 61:838-841, 1983.
6. Herman TS, Hammond N, Jones SE, et al: Involvement of the central nervous system by non-Hodgkin's lymphoma: The Southwest Oncology Group Experience. *Cancer* 943:390-397, 1979.
7. Bernard A, Boumsell L, Reinherz EL, et al: Cell surface characterization of malignant T-cells from lymphoblastic lymphoma using monoclonal antibodies: Evidence for phenotypic differences between malignant T-cells from patients with acute lymphoblastic leukemia and lymphoblastic lymphoma. *Blood* 57:1105-1110, 1981.
8. Lukes RJ, Parker JW, Taylor CR, et al: Immunologic approach to non-Hodgkin's lymphomas and related leukemias. Analysis of the results of multiparameter studies of 425 cases. *Semin Hematol* 15:322-356, 1978.
9. Bouffet E, Frappaz D, Pinkerton R, et al: Burkitt's lymphoma: A model for clinical oncology. *Eur J Cancer* 27:504-509, 1991.
10. Sun T: *Color Atlas/Text of Flow Cytometric Analysis of Hematologic Neoplasms*, New York, Igaku-Shoin, 1993, pp 62-66.
11. Magrath IT, Jain V, Jaffe ES: Small noncleaved cell lymphoma. In Knowles DM (ed): *Neoplastic Hematopathology*, Baltimore, Williams & Wilkins, pp 749-772, 1992.
12. Ostronoff M, Soussain C, Sambon E, et al: Burkitt's lymphoma in adults: A retrospective study of 46 cases. *Nouv Rev Fr Hematol* 34:389-397, 1992.
13. Knowles DM, Chamulak GA, Subar M, et al: Clinicopathologic, immunophenotypic and molecular genetic analysis of AIDS-associated lymphoid neoplasia: Clinical and biologic implications. *Pathol Annu* 23(pt 2): 33-67, 1988.
14. Levine AM: AIDS-associated malignant lymphoma. *Med Clin N Am* 76:253-267, 1992.
15. Vital C, Merlio JP, Rivel J, et al: Three cases of primary cerebral lymphoma in AIDS patients: Detection of Epstein-Barr virus by in situ hybridization and Southern blot technique. *Acta Neuropathol* 84:331-334, 1992.
16. Griffith RC, Kelly DR, Nathwani BN, et al: A morphologic study of childhood lymphoma of the lymphoblastic type: The pediatric oncology group experience. *Cancer* 59:1602-1607, 1987.
17. Kjeldsberg CR, Wilson JF, Berard CW: Non-Hodgkin's lymphoma in children. *Hum Pathol* 14:612-627, 1983.

18. Bennett JM, Catovsky D, Daniel MT, et al: Proposals for the classification of acute leukemias. *Br J Haematol* 33:451–458, 1976.
19. Wilson JF, Kjeldsberg CR, Sporto R, et al: The pathology of non-Hodgkin's lymphoma of childhood: 2. Reproducibility and relevance of the histologic classification of "undifferentiated" lymphomas (Burkitt's versus non-Burkitt's). *Hum Pathol* 18:1008–1014, 1987.
20. Hutchinson RE, Murphy SB, Fairclough DL, et al: Diffuse small non-cleaved cell lymphoma in children, Burkitt's versus non-Burkitt's types: Results from the pediatric oncology group and St. Jude Children's Research Hospital. *Cancer* 64:23–28, 1989.
21. Dayton VD, Arthur DC, Gajl-Peczalska KJ, et al: L3 acute lymphoblastic leukemia: Comparison with small noncleaved cell lymphoma involving the bone marrow. *Am J Clin Pathol* 101:130–139, 1994.
22. Murphy SB, Magrath IT: Workshop on pediatric lymphomas: Current results and prospects. *Am Oncol* 2 (suppl 2):219–223, 1991.
23. Mangran KF, Rauch AE, Bishop M, et al: Acute lymphoblastic leukemia of Burkitt's type (L3ALL) lacking surface immunoglobulin and the 8;14 translocation. *Am J Clin Pathol* 83:121–126, 1985.
24. Michiels JJ, Adriaansen HJ, Hagemeiger A, et al: TdT positive B-cell acute lymphoblastic leukemia (B-ALL) without Burkitt characteristics. *Br J Haematol* 68:423–426, 1988.
25. Sheibani K, Nathwani BN, Winberg CD, et al: Antigenically defined subgroups of lymphoblastic lymphoma: Relationship to clinical presentation and biologic behavior. *Cancer* 60:183–190, 1987.
26. Swerdlow JH, Habeshaw JA, Richard MA, et al: T-lymphoblastic lymphoma with Leu 7 positive phenotype and unusual clinical course: A multiparameter study. *Leu Res* 9:167–173, 1985.
27. Grogan T, Spier C, Wirt DP, et al: Immunologic complexity of lymphoblastic lymphoma. *Diagn Immunol* 4:81–88, 1986.
28. Link MP, Ropper M, Dorfman RF, et al: Cutaneous lymphoblastic lymphoma with pre-B markers. *Blood* 61:838–841, 1983.
29. Cossman J, Chused TM, Fisher RI, et al: Diversity of immunological phenotype of lymphoblastic lymphoma. *Cancer Res* 43:4486–4490, 1983.
30. Rosolen A, Nakanishi M, Poplack DG, et al: Expression of interleukin-2 receptor β subunit in hematopoietic malignancies. *Blood* 73:1968–1972, 1989.
31. Weiss L, Bindl J, Picozzi V, et al: Lymphoblastic lymphoma: An immunophenotype study of 26 cases with comparison of T-cell acute lymphoblastic leukemia. *Blood* 67:474–478, 1986.
32. Gouttefangeus C, Bensursan A, Boumsell L: Study of the CD-3 associated T-cell receptors reveals further differences between T-cell acute lymphoblastic lymphoma and leukemia. *Blood* 75:931–934, 1990.
33. Quintanilla-Martinez L, Zukerberg LR, Harris NL: Prethymic adult lymphoblastic lymphoma: A clinicopathologic and immunohistochemical analysis. *Am J Surg Pathol* 16:1075–1084, 1992.
34. Felix CA, Reaman GH, Korsmeyer SJ, et al: Immunoglobulin and T-cell receptor gene configuration in acute lymphoblastic leukemia in infancy. *Blood* 70:536–541, 1987.
35. Aiello A, Delia D, Fontanella E, et al: Expression of differentiation and adhesion molecules in sporadic Burkitt's lymphoma. *Hematol Oncol* 8:229–238, 1990.
36. Magrath I, Benjamin D, Papadopoulos N: Serum monoclonal immunoglobulin bands in undifferentiated lymphomas of Burkitt and non-Burkitt types. *Blood* 61:726–731, 1983.
37. Lory S, Adams JM: Transgenic mice and oncogenesis. *Annu Rev Immunol* 6:25–48, 1986.
38. Yano T, van Krieken JHJM, Magrath IT, et al: Histogenetic correlations between subcategories of small noncleaved cell lymphomas. *Blood* 79:1282–1290, 1992.

14
Anaplastic Large-Cell Ki-1 Lymphoma vs. Hodgkin's Disease, Metastatic Carcinoma, and Malignant Histiocytosis

In 1982, Schwab et al. described a monoclonal antibody, Ki-1, which was considered to be specific for Reed–Sternberg cells.[1] Subsequently, Stein et al. found strong Ki-1 antigen expression in a group of anaplastic large-cell lymphomas that showed distinct morphologic features such as sinus and paracortical distribution and a cohesive pattern.[2] This tumor has now been established as a distinct clinicopathologic entity, designated large-cell anaplastic (Ki-1+) lymphoma or anaplastic large-cell Ki-1 lymphoma (Ki-1 lymphoma), and is included in the updated Kiel classification.[3] In the International Working Formulation, this lymphoma corresponds to a large-cell immunoblastic lymphoma (polymorphous type).[4] In 1986, a similar lymphoma was described in the skin and lymph nodes of children by Kadin et al.[4,5] Ki-1 lymphoma is estimated to represent 1–8% of non-Hodgkin's lymphoma.[6] Because of its morphologic similarity to metastatic carcinoma, malignant histiocytosis, melanoma, Hodgkin's disease, and other lymphoid diseases, it is important to know how to recognize Ki-1 lymphoma to avoid misdiagnoses.

CLINICAL FEATURES

Initially, Ki-1 lymphoma was considered a highly aggressive lymphoma and is still classified as high-grade malignant lymphomas in the updated Kiel classification. Subsequently, it has been found that Ki-1 lymphoma is a heterogeneous group of lymphomas, and its cutaneous subtype is a low-grade lymphoma with frequent spontaneous regression.[6–8] While patients with nodal involvement usually have a rapidly progressive clinical course, complete remission is easily achieved with radiation therapy, although the overall relapse rate is very high (75%).[7,9] Combined chemotherapy appears to be the treatment of choice. A few exceptional cases with long survival (e.g., 10 years) have been reported.[7,10] The prognosis in patients younger than 40 years or patients in early stages (I and II) at presentation is often better than in those older than 40 years and presented at stages III and IV.[7,10] Children usually have a high rate of complete remission and a lower rate of relapse. In one study, patients who presented at stage I or II had an actuarial 2-year disease-free survival and overall survival of 54% and 75%, respectively, compared to 25% and 48% for those who presented at stage III or IV.[5]

The most common initial presentation in patients with Ki-1 lymphoma includes constitutional symptoms (42–59%) and peripheral lymphadenopathy (56–84%) (7–10). The supradiaphragmatic (cervical or axillary) lymph nodes are involved in 70% of cases as compared to 50% involvement in infradiaphragmatic (inguinal, iliac, or paraaortic) lymph nodes.[9] Mediastinal lymphadenopathy is relatively rare (16%).[5] Splenomegaly is seen in 20% of patients.[7] Hepatic involvement is unusual.[7,10,11] Bone marrow infiltration is exceptional in primary Ki-1 lymphoma but frequent in secondary Ki-1 lymphoma.[9,12] Extranodal involvement is frequent with skin, the most common extranodal site.[7,10] Involvement of gastrointestinal tract, bone, lung, kidney, placenta, and central nervous system (CNS) has also been reported.[4,11–16]

In various studies, a bimodal age distribution is demonstrated in patients with Ki-1 lymphoma, with one peak between 10 and 30 years and another beyond age 60.[10,17] The male:female ratio of patients varies from 1.3:1 to 2.2:1.[7,9,10,17]

PATHOLOGY

The tumor cells of Ki-1 lymphoma vary in size (10–50 μm) and shape (round, oval, or polyclonal), but they are usually large and pleomorphic.[9] Their cytoplasm is often abundant, and nuclei are bizarre with one or more, small or large nucleoli. A paranuclear hof is frequently present. Multinucleated tumor cells may be present in various numbers. The mitotic rate is high. The lymph node architecture is usually partially effaced by tumor cell infiltration in the sinuses from the subcapsular to the paracortical region. The neoplastic infiltration in skin is primary dermal but may extend into the subcutaneous tissue. The lymphoma cells seldom involve the epidermis.

Two studies have divided the tumor cells in two morphologic categories.[10,17] Group A is composed of large pleomorphic tumor cells with prominent nucleoli and frequent paranuclear hof. Multinucleated giant cells sometimes with wreath-like and embryo-like nuclei are frequently observed. Some of the tumor cells appear like Reed–Sternberg cells. Group B consists of relatively monomorphic tumor cells, usually without a prominent nucleolus or a paranuclear hof. Multinucleated giant cells and Reed–Sternberg-like cells are seldom detected. Patients with Ki-1 lymphoma of group B morphology more frequently presented with advanced stage of disease and bone marrow involvement and shorter survival time than did patients with a tumor of group A morphology. However, the differences were not statistically significant.[10] A small-cell-predominant variant of Ki-1 lymphoma in which the large anaplastic lymphoma cells are scarce has recently been reported.[18] Patients with this variant appear to have a prognosis worse than that of previously reported groups of Ki-1 lymphoma.

Stein et al. categorized Ki-1 lymphoma into four morphologic types.[9] The first type is the most commonly encountered variant and is designated "common type" (Figs. 14.1–14.3). The tumor cells of this type are relatively uniform in size and show a cohesive growth pattern, manifested either as solid sheets or intrasinusoidal growth. The second type is called the Hodgkin-related type because of the often presence of Hodgkin or Reed–Sternberg-like tumor cells (Figs. 14.4, 14.5). The tumor cells may show a cohesive growth pattern or sclerosis or may intermingle with numerous macrophages. Type 3 is the giant-cell variant, which is composed of many multinucleated tumor cells or is dominated by very large, bizarre, often multinucleated tumor cells (Figs. 14.6–14.8). The last type is the lymphohistiocytic variant, which contains mainly histiocytes with varying numbers of large anaplastic lymphoid cells, small lymphocytes, and plasma cells (Figs. 14.9, 14.10).

Ki-1 lymphoma can also be "secondary," meaning transforming from other lymphomas. The German Lymphoma Group divides the secondary Ki-1 lymphoma into simultaneous and subsequent categories using 3 months as the cutoff point.[9] Secondary Ki-1 lymphoma of the T-cell or null-cell type has been reported to arise from pleomorphic T-cell lymphoma, angioimmunoblastic lymphadenopathy-like T-cell lymphoma, T-zone lymphoma, lymphoepithelioid lymphoma, mycosis fungoides, and cutaneous T-cell lymphoma.[9] The B-cell type of Ki-1 lymphoma has been most frequently reported as secondary to

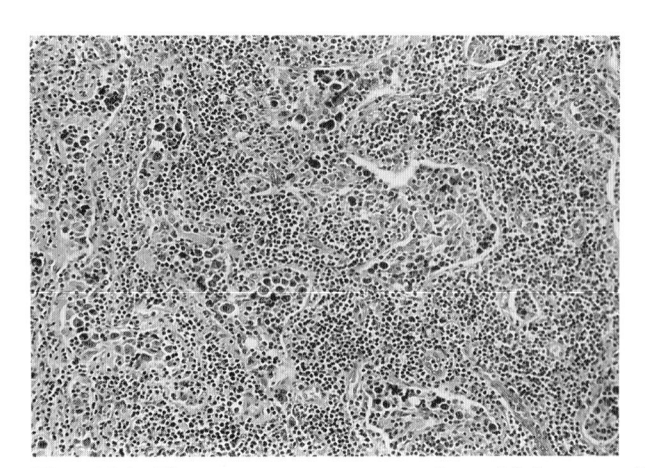

Fig. 14.1. The common type or sinusoidal type of Ki-1 lymphoma showing sinusoidal infiltrate pattern by sheets of relatively uniform-sized anaplastic large tumor cells. H&E, ×250.

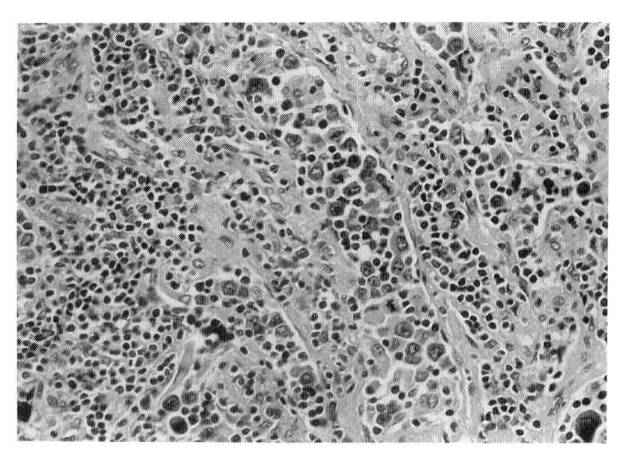

Fig. 14.2. A high-power view of Fig. 14.1 showing sinusoidal tumor infiltration. H&E, ×500.

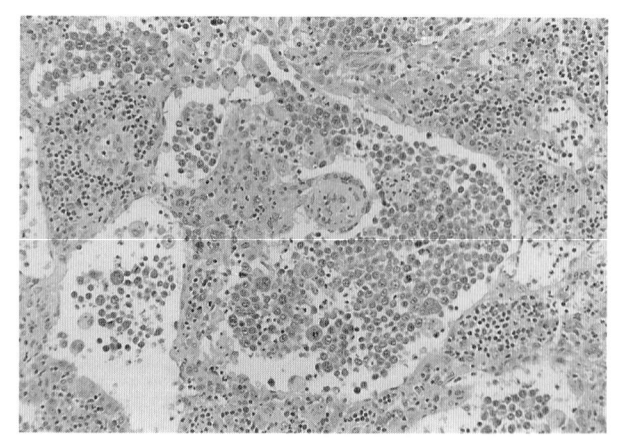

Fig. 14.3. Another case of common type of Ki-1 lymphoma showing uniform tumor cells in sinuses. H&E, ×250.

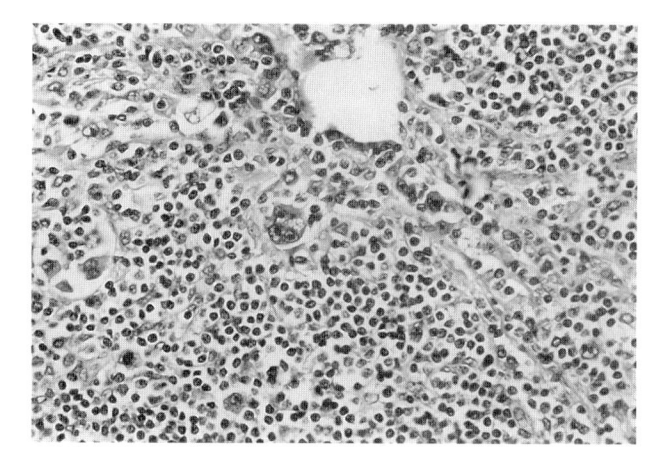

Fig. 14.4. The Hodgkin-related type of Ki-1 lymphoma showing a Reed–Sternberg-like cell in the center. H&E, ×500.

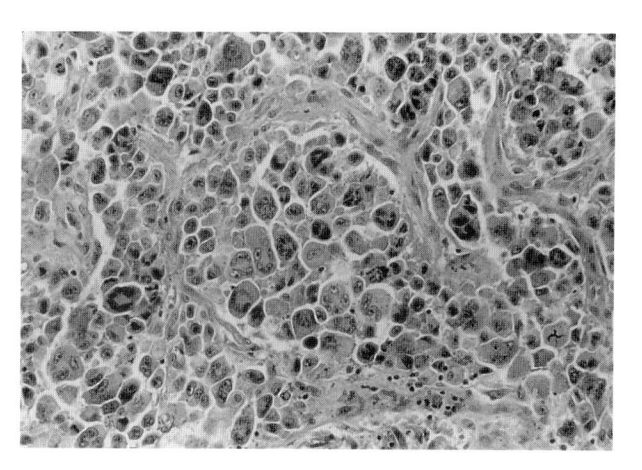

Fig. 14.7. The same case as in Fig. 14.6. H&E, ×250.

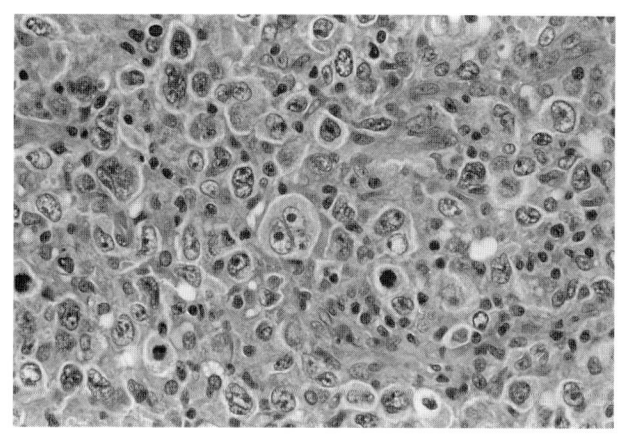

Fig. 14.5. A higher-power view of the same case as in Fig. 14.4 showing a Reed–Sternberg-like cell in the center, accompanied by many large anaplastic tumor cells. H&E, ×500.

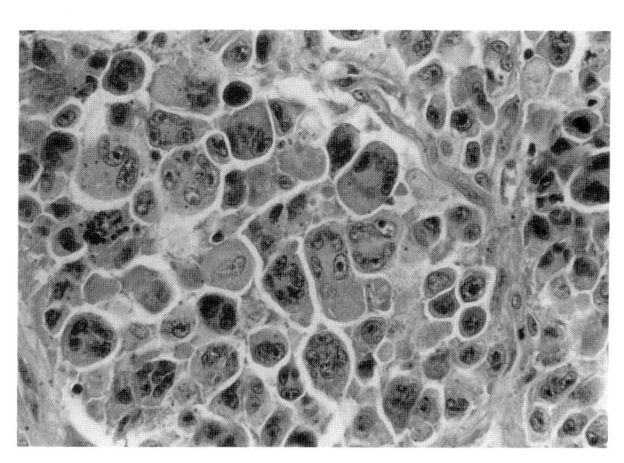

Fig. 14.8. The same case as in Fig. 14.6. H&E, ×500.

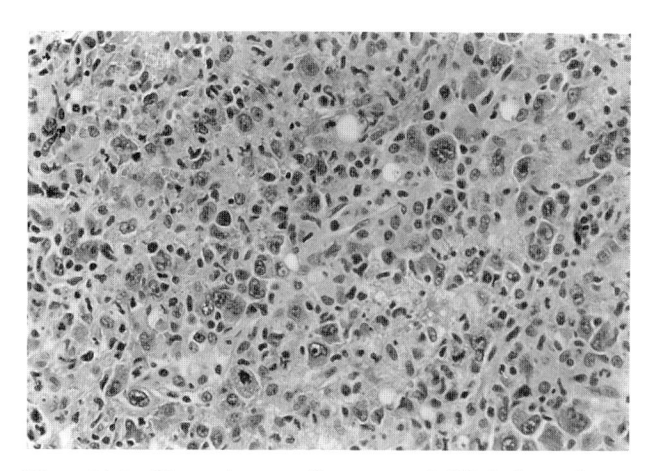

Fig. 14.6. The giant cell type of Ki-1 lymphoma showing multinucleated giant tumor cells and pleomorphism among tumor cells. H&E, ×250. (Case contributed by Dr. Daniel Filippa.)

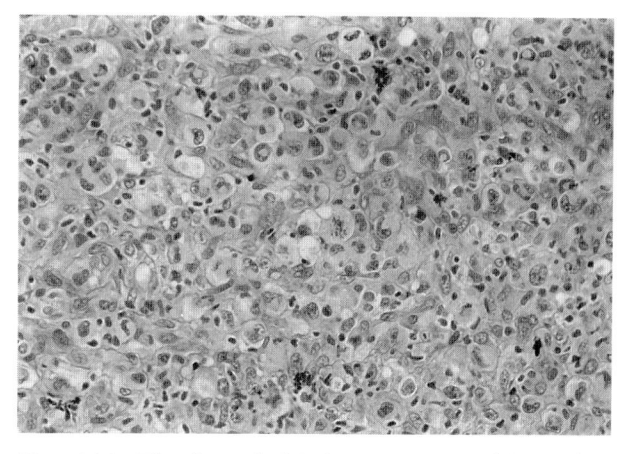

Fig. 14.9. The lymphohistiocytic type of Ki-1 lymphoma showing lymphohistiocytic infiltration among neoplastic cells. H&E, ×500. (Case contributed by Dr. Daniel Filippa.)

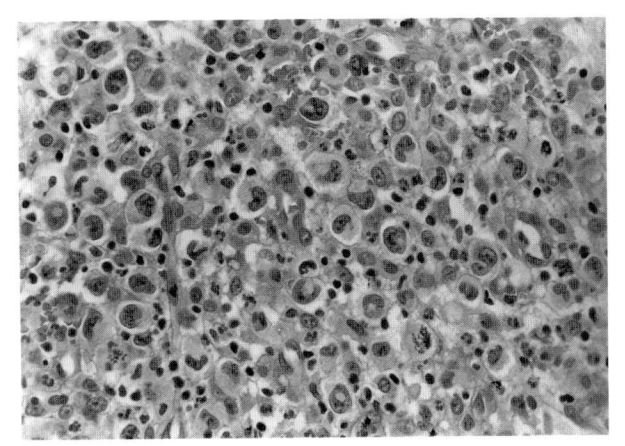

Fig. 14.10. The same case as in Fig. 14.9. H&E, ×500.

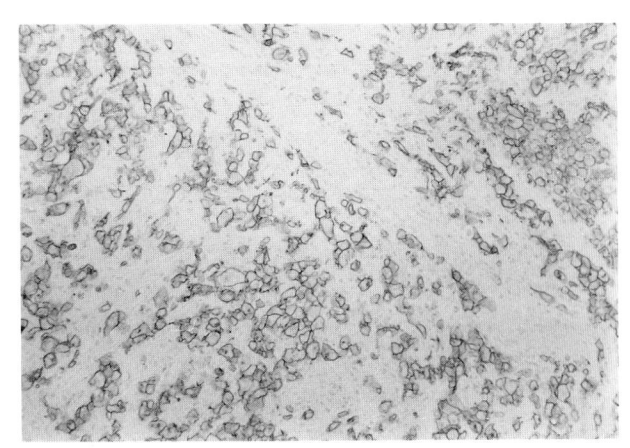

Fig. 14.11. Strongly positive staining for Ki-1 antigen in a Ki-1 lymphoma. H&E, ×250.

Hodgkin's lymphoma of the lymphocytic predominance type[9] and occasionally to follicular lymphoma.[19] Secondary Ki-1 lymphoma is usually seen in older age group (median 5th decade) and presents more frequently at advanced stage than does its primary counterpart. Bone marrow and skin infiltration are also more common in the secondary than the primary type.[9]

LABORATORY FINDINGS

Although the morphology of Ki-1 lymphoma varies, the requirement of immunophenotypic markers is absolute; Ki-1 antigen (CD30) must be expressed strongly in most tumor cells (Fig. 14.11). For paraffin sections, monoclonal antibody against Ber-H2 (a Ki-1 equivalent) should be used. A typical immunohistologic staining pattern for CD30 is shown on the cell membrane and in the Golgi region. Cytoplasmic staining pattern can be seen in plasma cells, some carcinomas, and melanoma and should not be considered positive.[20] However, one should be cautioned that cytoplasmic staining for CD30 can also be encountered in Ki-1 lymphoma of B-cell lineage.[9]

In normal lymph nodes, scattered Ki-1 positive large lymphocytes are localized mainly around the follicles.[2] The number of Ki-1-positive cells increase considerably in certain reactive conditions, such as toxoplasma lymphadenitis, infectious mononucleosis, and Kikuchi's lymphadenitis.[2,21] Stein et al. consider Ki-1-positive cells as extrafollicular T- and B-blasts.[9] Many types of non-Hodgkin's lymphoma may also express Ki-1 antigen in some cases, and the number of positive cells may be few, moderate, or extensive.[3,22] These lymphomas include immunoblastic lymphoma, centroblastic lymphoma, pleomorphic T-cell lymphoma, small cleaved-cell follicular lymphoma, small lymphocytic lymphoma, and peripheral T-cell lymphoma.

Another characteristic marker for Ki-1 lymphoma is epithelial membrane antigen (EMA). EMA is usually present in carcinomas and not in lymphomas; thus its presence on lymphoma cells facilitates the diagnosis of Ki-1 lymphomas. In some studies, all cases of Ki-1 lymphoma tested for EMA showed strong membrane and cytoplasmic staining of the tumor.[23,24] However, most studies showed only 30–60% positive cases. Because the positive EMA staining may cause confusion as to whether the tumor is a carcinoma or lymphoma, the leukocyte common antigen (CD45) should be routinely tested. Unfortunately, CD45 is absent in about 50% of Ki-1 lymphoma cases when paraffin sections are stained, whereas studies on frozen sections may provide better results.[9,10]

Most of Ki-1 lymphomas are of T-cell lineage, and the rest are either of B-cell lineage or lack T- and B-cell antigens. In the original study by Stein et al.[2], 57.8% were definitely of T-cell type, 26.7% were probably of T-cell type, and 5.6% were of B-cell type. In another study of 41 cases, 68% were classified as T-cell, 10% as B-cell, and 22% as non-T, non-B cell (null-cell) lymphomas.[10] Because of the frequent random loss of cell lineage markers in Ki-1 lymphoma, a larger panel of cell lineage markers should be studied to avoid misclassification of cases as non-T, non-B phenotype. In terms of helper/suppressor subsets, CD4 is frequently present, while CD8 is often absent.[10,25]

The coexistence of a series of activation antigens

(HLA-DR, CD25, CD71) and a nuclear proliferative antigen (Ki-67) as well as the marked loss of differentiation antigens (T-cell or B-cell) suggest that Ki-1 lymphoma is a dedifferentiated neoplasm of activated lymphoid cells.[5,10]

The negative reactions to some antigens are helpful in differential diagnosis for Ki-1 lymphoma. The absence of histiocytic antigens, such as lysozyme, KP-1, PG-M1, and Ber-MAC3, is important for distinguishing Ki-1 lymphoma from malignant histiocytosis. Lack of CD15 may be helpful in ruling out Hodgkin's disease; negative cytokeratin, in ruling out carcinoma; and negative S100, in excluding melanoma.

Genotyping of Ki-1 lymphoma shows T-cell receptor (TCR) gene rearrangement in the majority of cases and immunoglobulin (Ig) gene rearrangement in the minority of cases.[26,27] Some cases revealed both TCR and Ig gene rearrangements, but about one third of cases did not show gene arrangement in spite of a lymphoid phenotype.

A nonrandom cytogenetic abnormality, t(2;5) (p23;q35), has been identified in most cases of Ki-1 lymphoma studied.[28,29] It is interesting to note that this chromosomal pattern was initially considered characteristic for malignant histiocytosis, but further studies proved that all cases with t(2;5) translocation expressed CD30 and were morphologically consistent with Ki-1 lymphoma.[28,29] As N-*myc* is located on the short arm of chromosome 2 and many hematopoietic/lymphoid growth factors and growth factor receptor genes are on the long arm of chromosome 5, it is possible that dysregulation of these gene products may be involved in the pathogenesis of Ki-1 lymphoma.[5] On the other hand, patients with Ki-1 lymphoma bearing no t(2;5) responded poorly to chemotherapy.[4]

There is evidence that a virus may be the etiologic agent of Ki-1 lymphoma. Its association with Epstein–Barr virus (EBV) has been supported by the demonstration of EBV-specific DNA sequences with the polymerase chain reaction, EBV-encoded RNA with *in situ* hybridization, as well as the EBV-encoded latent membrane protein, and EBV nuclear antigen 2 with antibody staining of the tumor cells.[9,30] In a study of 10 cutaneous T-cell lymphomas using Southern blot hybridization and polymerase chain reaction, HTLV-1 specific sequences were demonstrated in all 6 cutaneous Ki-1 lymphomas but in none of the 4 cases of mycosis fungoides.[9]

DIFFERENTIAL DIAGNOSES

1. *Hodgkin's disease:* Morphologically, Ki-1 lymphoma may mimic Hodgkin's disease, especially the Hodgkin-related subtype that shows conspicuous Reed–Sternberg-like cells. Nevertheless, the sinus growth pattern is unusual for Hodgkin's disease. In Hodgkin's disease, Reed–Sternberg and Hodgkin's cells also show Ki-1 antigen, but they are positive for CD15 (LeuM1) and negative for CD45 (LCA), EMA, and T- or B-cell associated antigens, which may help distinguish from Ki-1 lymphoma (Table 14.1). A monoclonality demonstrated by phenotyping or genotyping favors Ki-1 lymphoma. However, Stein and Dallenbach cautioned that Hodgkin's disease can coexist with or transform into Ki-1 lymphoma.[9]

2. *Malignant histiocytosis:* The cytology of tumor cells, the sinusoidal infiltrating pattern, the occasional feature of hemophagocytosis, and the positive staining for α-1-antitrypsin in Ki-1 lymphoma[2] may sometimes cause confusion between this lymphoma and a

TABLE 14.1
Immunophenotypic Differences Between Ki-1 Lymphoma and Related Neoplasms[a]

Neoplasm	CD30	CD15	CD45	EMA	Keratin	T-antigen	B-antigen	S100
Ki-1 lymphoma	+	−	+	+	−	±	±	−
Hodgkin's disease[b]	+	⊕	−	−	−	−	−	−
Malignant histiocytosis	−	+	−	−	−	−	−	−
Metastatic carcinoma	−	−	−	+	+	−	−	−
Malignant melanoma	−	−	−	−	−	−	−	+
Microvillous lymphoma	−	−	+	−	−	−	+	−

[a] This table includes only the major phenotypes of each tumor.
[b] The nodular lymphocytic predominance subtype of Hodgkin's disease is not included.

histiocytic tumor. However, none of the histiocytic antigens (lysozyme, KP-1, PG-M1, Ber-MAC3) is positive for Ki-1 lymphoma. A few reports that claimed to demonstrate histiocytic antigens in Ki-1 lymphoma turned out to be staining the reactive macrophages.[9] Histiocytic tumors are generally negative for CD30, EMA, and T- or B-cell antigens. However, CD45, CD4, CD25, HLA-DR, and EMA can be demonstrated occasionally in histiocytic disorders.[5] Under these circumstances, ultrastructural confirmation, genotyping, or cytogenetic studies can be helpful.

3. *Metastatic carcinoma:* Ki-1 lymphoma shows many features similar to carcinoma, such as the sinus growth pattern, cohesive appearance and positive staining for EMA (Figs. 14.12, 14.13). Unlike carcinoma, Ki-1 lymphoma is generally negative for cytokeratin but positive for CD30, CD45, and T-cell or B-cell antigens. Occasionally, Ki-1 lymphoma cells may show dot-like reactivity to cytokeratin antibodies, and carcinoma may express cytoplasmic CD30 antigen.[9] In controversial cases, electron microscopy, cytogenetics, and genotyping may help.

4. *Malignant melanoma:* Melanoma can mimic Ki-1 lymphoma morphologically and may show diffuse cytoplasmic staining for BerH2.[20] However, this tumor is positive for S100 and HMB45, but negative for CD45, EMA, and T- and B-cell antigens.

5. *Lymphomatoid papulosis:* This clinically benign disease may show dermal infiltration of medium-sized and large atypical lymphoid cells, some of which are Reed–Sternberg-like and express CD30 antigen.[9] These cells are clonal T-cells as proved by phenotyping and genotyping. To make the matter more complicated is the fact that lymphomatoid papulosis may coexist with or develop into Ki-1 lymphoma.[5] Therefore, it is difficult to distinguish lymphomatoid papulosis from Ki-1 lymphoma, and, in fact, it may be a variant of primary cutaneous Ki-1 lymphoma.[9]

6. *Regressing atypical histiocytosis:* This disease overlaps with lymphomatoid papulosis in the clinicopathologic spectrum. It shows anaplastic large lymphoma cells that are monoclonal T-cells expressing Ki-1 antigen.[31] Some authors consider that regressing atypical histiocytosis may in fact be a Ki-1 lymphoma.[5,17,31]

7. *Microvillous lymphoma:* This lymphoma shows polymorphic infiltrate with a prominent sinus growth pattern similar to Ki-1 lymphoma.[32] Ultrastructurally, Ki-1 lymphoma may also have microvilli on the surface. However, microvillous lymphoma is a B-cell tumor and is negative for CD30 and EMA. Therefore, these two tumors can be distinguished easily by immunophenotyping.

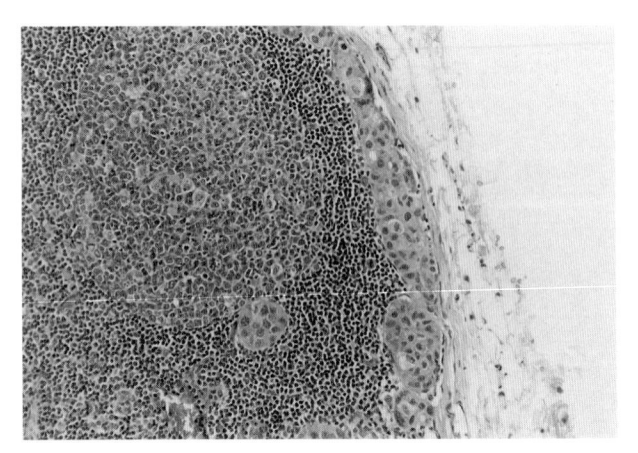

Fig. 14.12. A case of metastatic breast carcinoma showing carcinoma cells in a subcapsular sinus and the cortex of a lymph node. H&E, ×250.

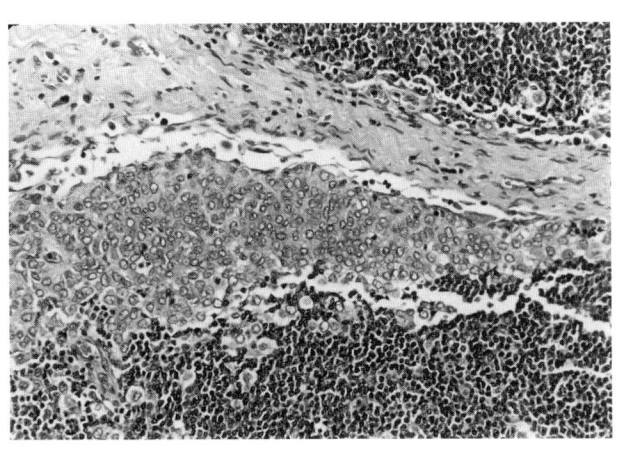

Fig. 14.13. Another case of metastatic carcinoma showing carcinoma cells in trabecular sinus. The cohesiveness of the tumor cells distinguishes carcinoma from lymphoma. H&E, ×500.

REFERENCES

1. Schwab U, Stein H, Gerdes J, et al: Production of a monoclonal antibody specific for Hodgkin and Sternberg–Reed cells of Hodgkin's disease and a subset of normal lymphoid cells. *Nature* 299:65–67, 1982.
2. Stein H, Mason DY, Gerdes J, et al: The expression of the Hodgkin's disease associated antigen Ki-1 in reactive and neoplastic lymphoid tissue: Evidence that Reed–Sternberg cells and histiocytic malignancies are

derived from activated lymphoid cells. *Blood* 66: 848–858, 1985.
3. Lennert K, Feller AC: *Histopathology of Hodgkin's Lymphomas* (based on the updated Kiel classification), 2nd ed, Berlin, Springer-Verlag, 1992.
4. Kadin ME: Ki-1 positive anaplastic large-cell lymphoma: A clinicopathologic entity? *J Clin Oncol* 9: 533–536, 1991.
5. Kinney MC, Greer JP, Glick AD, et al: Anaplastic large-cell Ki-1 malignant lymphomas. Recognition, biological and clinical implications. *Pathol Annu* 26 (pt 1):1–24, 1991.
6. Lindhold JS, Barron DR, Williams ME, et al: Ki-1-positive cutaneous large cell lymphoma of T-cell type: Report of an indolent subtype. *J Am Acad Dermatol* 20: 342–348, 1989.
7. Greer JP, Kinney MC, Collins RD, et al: Clinical features of 31 patients with Ki-1 anaplastic large-cell lymphoma. *J Clin Oncol* 9:539–547, 1991.
8. Beljaards RC, Kaudewitz P, Berti E, et al: Primary cutaneous CD30-positive large cell lymphoma: Definition of a new type of cutaneous lymphoma with a favorable prognosis. *Cancer* 71:2097–2104, 1993.
9. Stein, Dallenbach F: Diffuse large cell lymphomas of B and T cell type. In Knowles D. (ed): *Neoplastic Hematology*; Baltimore, Williams & Wilkins, 1992; pp 675–714.
10. Chott A, Kaserer K, Augustin I, et al: Ki-1 positive large cell lymphoma: A clinicopathologic study of 41 cases. *Am J Surg Pathol* 14:439–448, 1990.
11. Perkins PL, Ross CW, Schnitzer B: CD 30-positive anaplastic large-cell lymphomas that express CD15 but lack CD45: A possible diagnostic pitfall. *Arch Pathol Lab Med* 116:1192–1196, 1992.
12. Wong KF, Chan JKC, Ng CS, et al: Anaplastic large cell Ki-1 lymphoma involving bone marrow: Marrow findings and association with reactive hemophagocytosis. *Am J Hematol* 37:112–119, 1991.
13. Chan JKC, Ng CS, Hui PK, et al: Anaplastic large cell Ki-1 lymphoma of bone. *Cancer* 68:2186–2191, 1991.
14. Ross CW, Hanson CA, Schnitzer B: CD30 (Ki-1)-positive, anaplastic large cell lymphoma mimicking gastrointestinal carcinoma. *Cancer* 70:2517–2523, 1992.
15. Tsukamoto N, Mortia K, Maehara I, et al: Ki-1 positive large cell anaplastic lymphoma with protean manifestations including central nervous system involvement. *Acta Haematol* 88:147–150, 1992.
16. Close PM, Macrae MB, Hammond JM, et al: Anaplastic large-cell Ki-1 lymphoma: Pulmonary presentation mimicking miliary tuberculosis. *Am J Clin Pathol* 99:631–636, 1993.
17. Chan JKC, Ng CS, Hui PK, et al: Anaplastic large cell lymphoma. Delineation of two morphological types. *Histopathology* 15:11–34, 1989.
18. Kinney MC, Collins RD, Greer JP, et al: A small-cell-predominant variant of primary Ki-1 (CD30)+ T-cell lymphoma. *Am J Surg Pathol* 17:859–868, 1993.
19. Hugh J, Poppema S: Ki-1 (CD30) antigen expression on transformed follicular lymphoma. *Lab Invest* 62:46A, 1990.
20. Schwarting R, Gerdes J, Durkop H, et al: Ber-H2: A new anti-Ki (CD30) monoclonal antibody directed at a formalin resistant epitope. *Blood* 74:1678–1689, 1989.
21. Rivano MT, Falini B, Stein H, et al: Histiocytic necrotizing lymphadenitis without granulocytic infiltration. (Kikuchi's lymphadenitis): Morphological and immunohistochemical study of 8 cases. *Histopathology* 11: 1013–1027, 1987.
22. Miettinem M: CD30 distribution: Immunohistochemical study on formaldehyde-fixed paraffin-embedded Hodgkin's and non-Hodgkin's lymphomas. *Arch Pathol Lab Med* 116:1197–1201, 1992.
23. Delsol G, Saati TA, Gatter KC, et al: Coexpression of epithelial membrane antigen (EMA), Ki-1 and interleukin-2 receptor by anaplastic large cell lymphomas. Diagnostic value in so-called malignant histiocytosis. *Am J Pathol* 30:59–70, 1988.
24. Fujimoto J, Hata JI, Ishii E, et al: Ki-1 lymphomas in childhood; immunohistochemical analysis and the significance of epithelial membrane antigen (EMA) as a new marker. *Virchows Archiv A Pathol Anat Histopathol* 412:307–314, 1988.
25. Reinhold U, Abken H, Kukel, S, et al: Tumor infiltrating lymphocytes isolated from a Ki-1 positive large cell lymphoma of the skin. *Cancer* 68:2155–2160, 1991.
26. O'Connor NTJ, Stein H, Gatter KC, et al: Genotypic analysis of large cell lymphomas which express the Ki-1 antigen. *Histopathology* 11:733–740, 1987.
27. Herbst H, Tippelmann G, Anagnostopoulos I, et al: Immunoglobulin and T-cell receptor gene rearrangements in Hodgkin's disease and Ki-1 positive anaplastic large cell lymphoma: Dissociation between phenotype and genotype. *Leu Res* 13:103–116, 1989.
28. Bitter MA, Franklin WA, Larson Ra, et al: Morphology in Ki-1 (CD30)-positive non-Hodgkin's lymphoma is correlated with clinical features and the presence of a unique chromosomal abnormality, t (2;5) (p23;q35). *Am J Surg Pathol* 14:305–316, 1990.
29. Mason DY, Bastard C, Rimokh R, et al: CD30-positive large cell lymphoma (Ki-1 lymphoma) are associated with a chromosomal translocation involving 5q35. *Br J Haematol* 74:161–168, 1990.
30. Herbst H, Dallenbach F, Hummel M, et al: Epstein–Barr virus DNA and latent gene products in Ki-1 (CD30)-positive anaplastic large cell lymphomas. *Blood* 78:1–10, 1991.
31. Headington JT, Roth MS, Schnitzer B: Regressing atypical histiocytosis: A review and critical appraisal. *Semin Diagn Pathol* 4:28–37, 1987.
32. Kinney MC, Glick AD, Stein H, et al: Comparison of anaplastic large cell Ki-1 lymphomas and microvillous lymphomas in their immunologic and ultrastructural features. *Am J Surg Pathol* 14:1047–1060, 1990.

15
Thymoma vs. Malignant Lymphoma vs. Hodgkin's Disease

Thymoma is a neoplasm of the thymic epithelium. However, varying proportions of lymphocytes are always present and intermingled with the tumor cells. Although a predominantly epithelial thymoma with a conspicuous lobular pattern is seldom a problem in diagnosis, a predominantly lymphocytic thymoma can be confused with non-Hodgkin's lymphomas and occasionally Hodgkin's disease.[1,2] The immunophenotype of thymoma is especially similar to that of a T-lymphoblastic lymphoma. Therefore, when a mediastinal mass is examined, a T-cell panel cannot be useful in distinguishing between these two entities. Furthermore, lymphocyte aggregates may be demonstrated in the bone marrow, and peripheral lymphocytosis may be occasionally present in the case of thymoma.[3] In one reported case of invasive thymoma, the bone marrow biopsy, peripheral blood smear, and a lung biopsy of the metastatic tumor were all interpreted as a T-cell lymphoma.[3] It is apparent that thymoma is an important entity to be distinguished from a mediastinal lymphoma or Hodgkin's disease. In addition, T-lymphoblastic malignancies may coexist with thymoma.[4]

CLINICAL FEATURES

Thymoma

Most cases of thymoma are diagnosed incidentally by chest roentgenogram and in those cases, the patient may remain asymptomatic for many years; for instance, 2–23 years was reported in one series.[1,5] Clinical symptoms are usually attributed to direct compression of neighboring structures by the tumor, metastasis to other organs, and/or to an associated systemic syndrome (paraneoplastic syndrome).[1,5]

Direct compression of adjacent structures may cause cough, chest pain, dysphagia, dyspnea, hoarseness, respiratory infection, and superior vena cava syndrome. Even in the invasive thymoma, metastasis is extremely rare. Invasion usually involves direct extension of tumor; in unusual cases it can extend as far as the peritoneum. The paraneoplastic syndrome includes myasthenia gravis, anemia due to erythroid hypoplasia, and hypogammaglobulinemia.

Other systemic disorders that have been associated with thymomas include systemic lupus erythematosus (SLE), rheumatoid arthritis, polymyositis, and myocarditis.[1,5]

The prognosis of a thymoma depends on its invasiveness and the presence or absence of a paraneoplastic syndrome. The incidence of invasion is about 25–35%.[5] In patients with noninvasive thymoma, their death is usually associated with myasthenia gravis or anemia.[5]

Non-Hodgkin's Lymphoma and Hodgkin's Disease

The clinical symptoms of these two entities are caused by compression of neighboring structures or tumor spread. Lymphoblastic lymphoma of T-cell lineage is the most frequently seen non-Hodgkin's lymphoma in the mediastinum with a predilection for pediatric patients[6] (see Chapter 13). The nonlymphoblastic lymphoma of the mediastinum or the so-called primary mediastinal lymphoma is usually a B-cell lymphoma.[7] It is frequently seen in young females with prominent local compression symptoms and may metastasize to the kidney, adrenals, liver, thyroid, abdominal lymph nodes, and central nervous system (CNS).[8] Both lymphoblastic lymphoma and primary mediastinal B-cell lymphoma are aggressive neoplasms, carrying an ominous prognosis. Hodgkin's disease is also frequently found in the mediastinum. Its clinical manifestations are described in Chapter 7. The paraneoplastic syndrome mentioned above is not associated with lymphomas; therefore, its presence may help exclude the diagnosis of lymphomas.

PATHOLOGY

Thymoma

Most thymomas show a lobular pattern with broad fibrous bands separating cellular masses.[1,2,5] The tumor cells are epithelial cells that can be polygonal (round or oval) (Fig. 15.1) or spindle-shaped (Figs. 15.2, 15.3). Rosai and Levine have found that 82% of thymomas

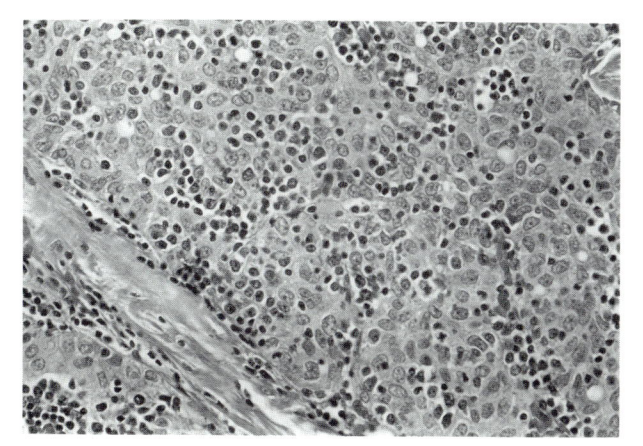

Fig. 15.1. A case of thymoma showing polygonal thymic epithelial cells intermingled with small lymphocytes. A fibrous band is present at the lower left corner. H&E, ×500.

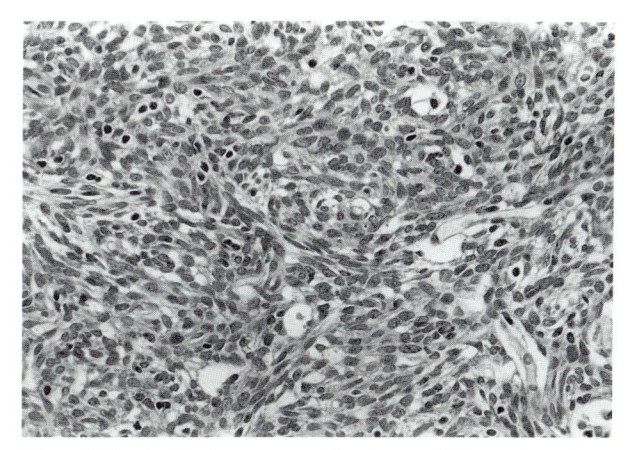

Fig. 15.3. A higher magnification of Fig. 15.2. H&E, ×500.

are composed of polygonal cells, 12% of spindle cells, and 18% of a mixture of both types.[1] They consider that these two cell types represent a continuous morphologic spectrum rather than two clearly separable entities. However, other studies revealed that tumors with polygonal cells are commonly associated with myasthenia gravis, and those with spindle cells are associated with anemia.[5] The nuclei of the tumor cells are usually vesicular with a small, inconspicuous nucleolus. The cytoplasm is of variable amount and pale acidophilic. In 96% of cases, the tumor cells are admixed with varying proportions of lymphocytes (Figs. 15.4–15.6). The remaining cases may show no lymphocytes. The diagnosis of a thymoma depends on the identification of the epithelial tumor cells. When no epithelial cells are found, the diagnosis of thymoma should be excluded.

In addition to this basic pattern, there are several histologic features that may help in the diagnosis of thymoma, although their presence varies in different thymomas. When the tumor is composed of spindle cells, it may grow in parallel bundles, whorls, and in a cartwheel or storiform pattern that mimics fibrous histiocytoma. When the spindle cells grow along blood vessels, the tumor may be indistinguishable from hemangiopericytoma.[1] In 20% of thymomas, rosette formation is present and is confused with neuroepithelioma.[1] In thymomas with lymphocytic predominance, it may show scattered well-defined, pale-stained, round areas composed of loosely packed

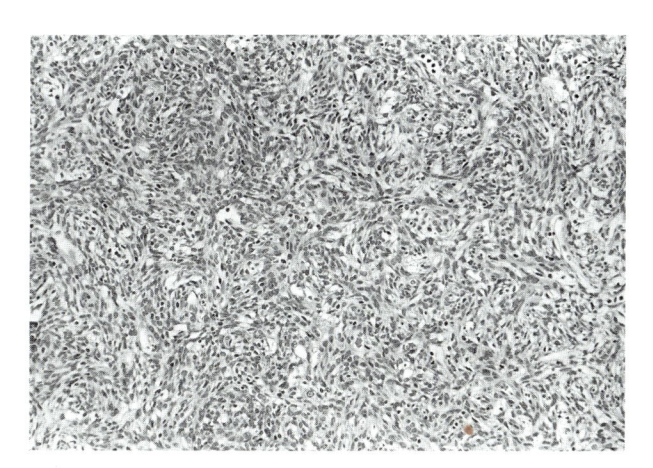

Fig. 15.2. A case of thymoma showing spindle cells in whorls that may mimic a fibrous histiocytoma or hemangiopericytoma. H&E, ×250.

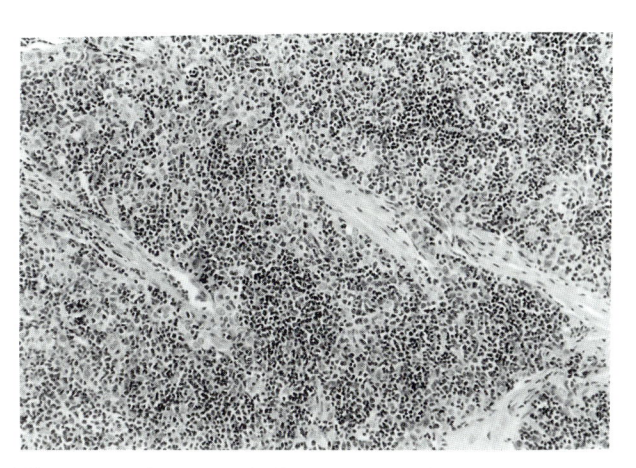

Fig. 15.4. A case of thymoma with predominantly lymphocytes. H&E, ×250.

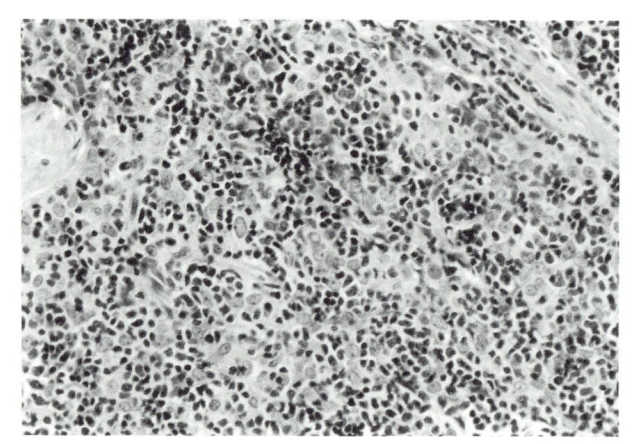

Fig. 15.5. A higher-power view of Fig. 15.4. H&E, ×500.

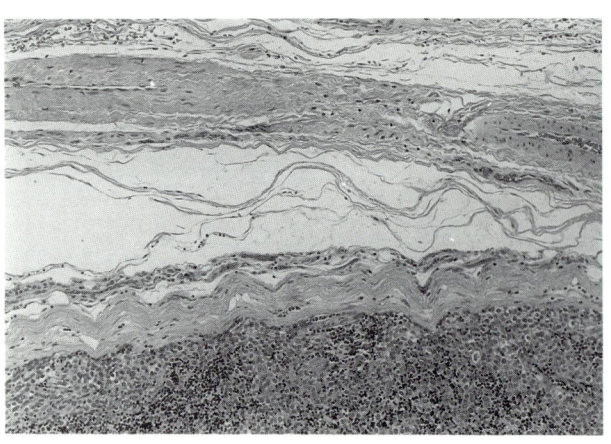

Fig. 15.7. An encapsulated thymoma extending into the pericardium. H&E, ×125.

lymphocytes. These areas appear like the medulla of a normal thymus and, in fact, may represent the neoplastic counterpart of the medulla; hence this feature has been designated medullary differentiation.

In 56% of thymomas, there are multiple perivascular spaces.[1] These spaces contain capillaries or postcapillary venules. In addition, coagulated proteinaceous material, lymphocytes, mast cells, foam cells, and erythrocytes may fill these spaces. In 16% of thymomas, the empty spaces may represent microcystic degeneration, and in 20% of thymomas, the spaces are lined by cuboidal or flattened cells and are called *gland-like formations*.[1] Furthermore, thymomas may also contain germinal centers, foam cells and Hassall's corpuscles.

About 60–80% of thymomas are well encapsulated and grow slowly, thus being regarded as benign.[2] The remaining cases may show microscopic invasion of the capsule (minimally invasive or microinvasive thymoma) or invasion of the adjacent structures (grossly invasive or macroinvasive thymoma) (Figs. 15.7, 15.8). These invasive thymomas usually show no cytologic atypica. When cytologic atypica is obvious, the tumor is designated thymic carcinoma.[9–11] There are several types of thymic carcinoma reported, including keratinizing squamous-cell carcinoma, nonkeratinizing squamous carcinoma, mucoepidermoid carcinoma, basaloid carcinoma, clear-cell carcinoma, and sarcomatoid carcinoma (carcinosarcoma).[2]

There are at least 15 different systems for the classification of thymoma.[1] The most commonly used classification is probably that of Bernatz et al., which divides thymomas into predominantly lymphocytic,

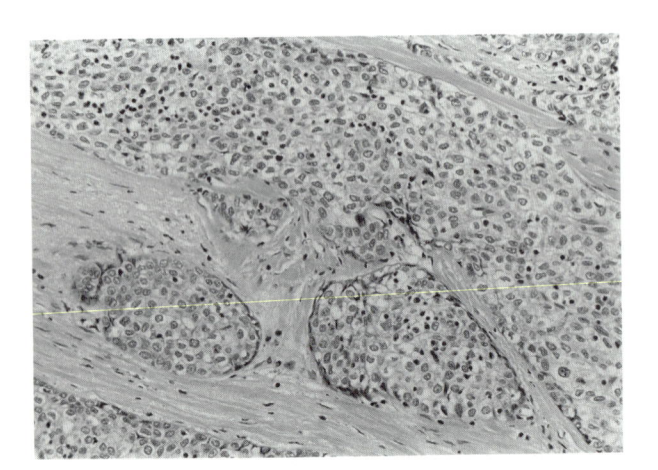

Fig. 15.6. A case of thymoma with polygonal thymic epithelial cells and lobulated pattern. Only a few lymphocytes are present. H&E, ×500.

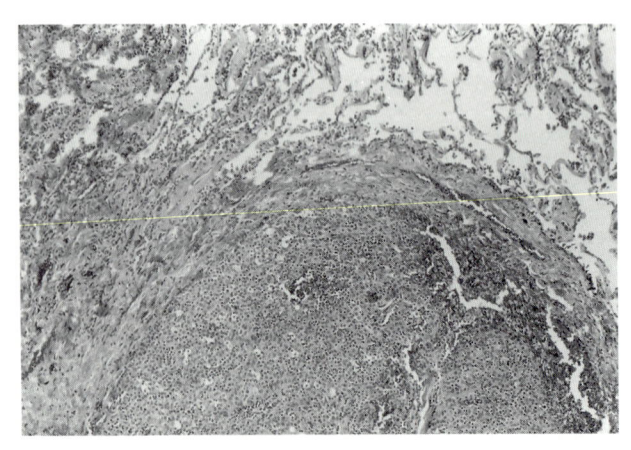

Fig. 15.8. A case of invasive thymoma invading the pulmonary tissue. H&E, ×125.

predominantly epithelial, mixed lymphocytic and epithelial, and predominantly spindle cells.[1,12] However, this classification shows no clinical correlation, particularly for prognostic significance. Other systems are simply based on the morphology of the tumor cells and/or the proportions of tumor cells and lymphocytes; these factors are now deemed to have no clinical significance. Therefore, Rosai advocated the use of a descriptive diagnosis (shape of epithelial cells, amount of lymphocytic population, and special histologic features) and staging/grading (encapsulated, invasive, metastatic and cytologically malignant) to replace other classifications.[2]

Recently, Muller-Hermelink and associates proposed a new classification system of thymoma based on the proportion of two epithelial-cell populations in the normal thymus—the cortex and the medulla.[13] Accordingly, thymomas can be classified as cortical, predominantly cortical, mixed, and medullary types. Kuo and Lo found that this new system is superior to the traditional system in clinical correlation.[12] Their study showed that cortical thymomas correlate with both microinvasive and macroinvasive thymomas, while none of the medullary thymomas showed such correlation. Cortical thymoma was also associated with myasthenia gravis, an association that was statistically significant.[12] Quintanilla-Martinez et al. also demonstrated a good clinical correlation with this new system.[14] They found that cortical and predominantly cortical types were associated with an intermediate degree of invasiveness, but that medullary and mixed type had only microscopic invasion in 36% of cases.[14] In addition, there was an increased association of myasthenia gravis and the cortical and predominantly cortical types.[14] Kornstein et al., however, found the Muller-Hermelink system to be no more advantageous than the traditional classification.[15]

Hodgkin's Disease

Hodgkin's disease can be found in the thymus and may be confused with a thymoma (Figs. 15.9, 15.10). The subtype of Hodgkin's disease in the thymus is nearly always nodular sclerosis[2], and the nodular appearance may be mistaken for a lobular pattern. In addition, residual foci of thymic epithelium may be entrapped in Hodgkin's disease. On the other hand, the so-called granulomatous thymoma may contain many Reed–Sternberg-like cells. However, this type of thymoma has been reclassified as Hodgkin's disease.[5] The distinction between thymoma and

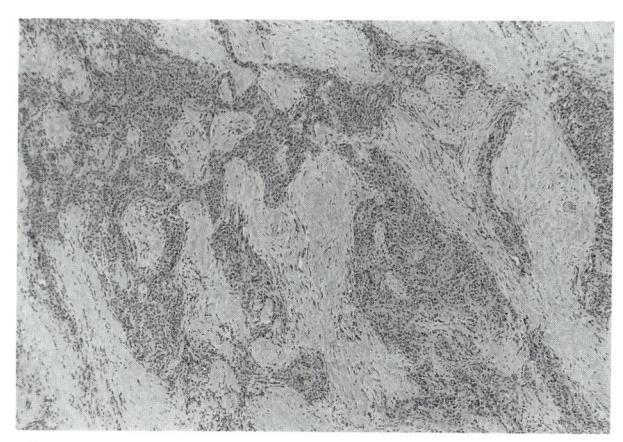

Fig. 15.9. A case of thymoma with nodular sclerosis pattern mimicking Hodgkin's disease. H&E, ×125.

Hodgkin's disease hinges on the identification of the epithelial tumor cells by either immunoperoxidase stain, or electron microscopy.

Non-Hodgkin's Lymphoma

The two types of non-Hodgkin's lymphomas that frequently involve the thymus or mediastinal lymph nodes are lymphoblastic lymphoma and large-cell lymphoma with sclerosis (primary mediastinal large B-cell lymphoma).[2] Both neoplasms may contain entrapped epithelial cells and Hassall's corpuscles of the normal thymus leading to misdiagnosis. Thymoma of the predominantly lymphocytic subtype may simulate non-Hodgkin's lymphomas. Occasionally, a

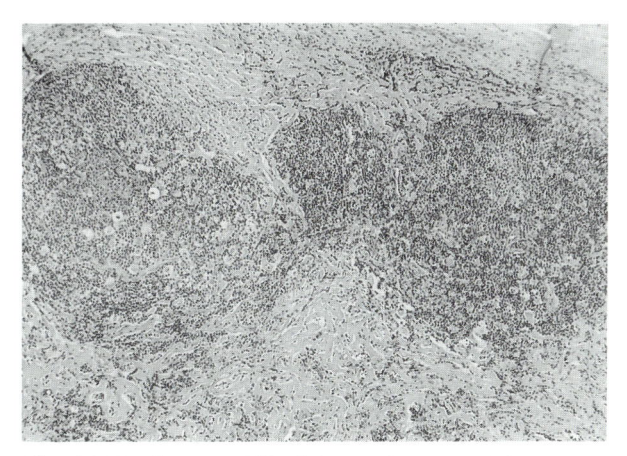

Fig. 15.10. A case of Hodgkin's disease of the nodular sclerosis type mimicking the lobular pattern in thymoma. H&E, ×125.

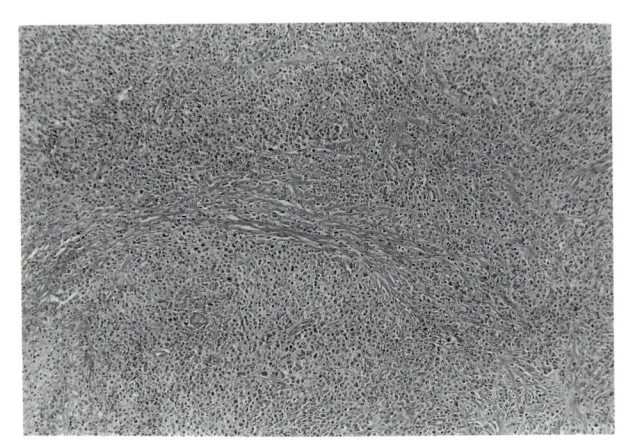

Fig. 15.11. A case of mediastinal large-cell lymphoma with sclerosis shows fibrous bands separating large tumor cells simulating thymoma. H&E, ×125.

thymoma may show a scattering of tingible-body macrophages among the epithelial tumor cells and lymphocytes forming the starry-sky pattern that is characteristic of lymphoblastic lymphoma. However, the thymocytes in thymoma show a clumped chromatic pattern with low mitotic rate, as compared with the dust-like chromatin and high mitotic rate in lymphoblastic lymphoma.[6] Lymphoblastic lymphoma also invades the mediastinal fat and the wall of blood vessels, a phenomenon that is not seen in benign thymomas.[2] The mediastinal large-cell lymphoma with sclerosis frequently shows fibrous bands that separate the tumor cells, mimicking thymoma (Figs. 15.11, 15.12).[2] Electron microscopy and immunophenotyping can readily distinguish between these neoplasms (Fig. 15.13).

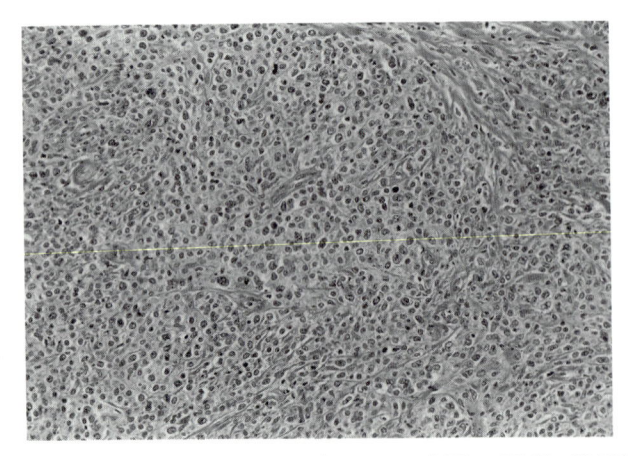

Fig. 15.12. Higher magnification of Fig. 15.11. H&E, ×250.

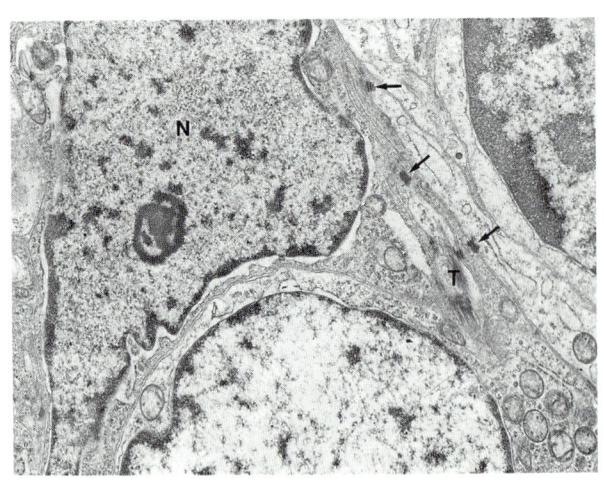

Fig. 15.13. Electron micrograph of thymoma showing desmosomes (arrows) and bundles of tonofilaments (T) (N = nucleus) ×23,000. (From Sun T: *Color Atlas/Text of Flow Cytometric Analysis of Hematologic Neoplasms,* New York, Igaku-Shoin, 1993.)

LABORATORY FINDINGS

Immunophenotyping of thymoma by flow cytometry usually shows the phenotype of cortical thymocytes, which is also the major phenotype of lymphoblastic lymphoma; thus these two entities are indistinguishable immunophenotypically (Table 15.1). Cortical thymocytes are CD1+, CD3−, while the mature thymocytes are CD1−, CD3+.[16–18] The presence of CD1-positive cells in a carcinoma at the site of the thymus denotes thymic carcinoma and distinguishes it from metastatic carcinoma to the thymus.[9] It should be clarified that the negative CD3 reaction is based on the results by flow cytometry, which detects only surface membrane CD3. When frozen sections are examined by immunohistochemical techniques, about 80% of cases of thymoma show cytoplasmic CD3.[6]

Alternatively, study with CD4/CD8 antibodies may divide thymocytes into early thymocyte (CD4−, CD8−), common (cortical) thymocyte (CD4+, CD8+), and late thymocyte (CD4+, CD8− or CD4−, CD8+). The immature lymphoid nuclear marker, terminal deoxynucleotidyl transferase, is positive for lymphoid cells in both thymoma and lymphoblastic lymphoma. However, another immature lymphoid marker, CD10 (CALLA), is demonstrated in a small percentage of lymphoblastic lymphoma but not in thymoma.[19] Although CD20+ B-lymphocytes and asteroid cells are frequently found in the medulla of the normal thymus and in areas of medullary differentiation in thy-

TABLE 15.1
Comparison Between Thymoma, Lymphoblastic Lymphoma, and Hodgkin's Disease[a]

	Thymoma	Lymphoblastic lymphoma	Hodgkin's disease
CD1	+	+	−
CD2	+	+	−
CD3[b]	−	−	−
CD4	+	+	−
CD5	+	+	−
CD7	+	+	−
CD8	+	+	−
CD10	−	±	−
CD15	−	−	+
CD25	−	−	+
CD30	−	−	+
CD38	+	+	−
CD45	+	+	−
CD57	±	±	−
CD71	+	+	+
HLA-DR	±	±	+
TdT	+	+	−
Cytokeratin	+	−	−
EMA	+	−	−
NSE	±	−	−
TCR gene	−	+	−

[a] Based on the major phenotype of respective disease.
[b] Surface membrane CD3−, cytoplasmic CD3+.

Abbreviations: TdT = terminal deoxynucleotidyl transferase; EMA = epithelial membrane antigen; NSE = neuron-specific enolase; TCR gene = T-cell receptor gene rearrangement.

momas by immunohistochemical techniques[20,21], flow cytometric studies often show fewer than 10% of B-cells in thymomas and a higher percentage of B-cells in lymphoblastic lymphoma.[19] The primary mediastinal large-cell lymphoma is usually of B-cell origin and is thus easily distinguishable from lymphoblastic lymphoma and thymoma.

Although the lymphoid markers frequently offer equivocal results for the distinction between thymoma and lymphoblastic lymphoma, epithelial markers as identified by immunohistochemical techniques are most useful in distinguishing these two entities. The most important marker for the differential diagnosis is cytokeratin, which usually leads to a definitive diagnosis; only thymoma shows cytokeratins (Figs. 15.14, 15.15) but not Hodgkin's disease or non-Hodgkin's lymphoma. An attempt at using different sets of cytokeratins to distinguish the various morphologic subsets of thymoma was, however, unsuccessful.[22] A study of epithelial membrane antigen

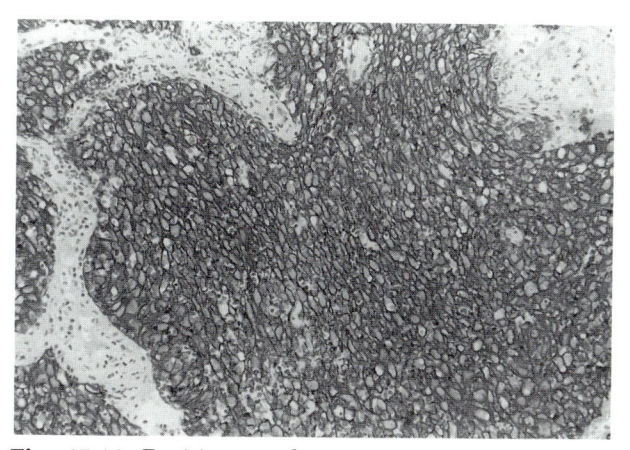

Fig. 15.14. Positive cytokeratin staining in a case of thymoma. H&E, ×250.

(EMA) demonstrated a quantitative difference between thymic carcinoma, invasive thymoma, and noninvasive thymoma; a higher concentration was exhibited in the higher-grade malignancy.[23] An extensive immunohistochemical study of thymomas showed that cytokeratin was positive in 94% of cases, EMA 75%, neuron specific enolase (NSE), 11%, CD57 (Leu7) 80%, and HLA-DR 58%, but it was essentially negative for chromogranin and carcinoembyonic antigen.

Thymic germ-cell tumors may mimic high-grade lymphomas. This possibility is usually ruled out by demonstration of lymphoid antigens. When lymphoid antigens are not present, cytokeratin, α-fetoprotein, placental alkaline phosphatase, and β-human chorionic gonadotropin may help establish the diagnosis.[24]

The evaluation of malignant grade can be facilitated

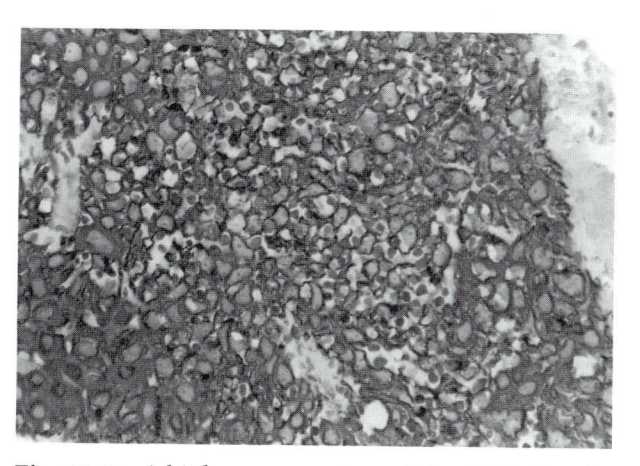

Fig. 15.15. A higher-power view of Fig. 15.14 showing strong cytokeratin staining. H&E, ×500.

by quantification of proliferating-cell nuclear antigen (PCNA) and argyrophilic nucleolar organizer regions (AgNORs). In one study, the differences in PCNA and AgNORs were statistically significant between thymic carcinoma and thymoma, but not significant between invasive and noninvasive thymomas.[25]

Immunoglobulin and T-cell receptor (TCR) gene analyses in thymomas usually show a germline configuration but germline deletion of TCR genes may be occasionally encountered.[19,26] T-cell lymphoblastic lymphoma often shows a TCR gene rearrangement, and Hodgkin's disease usually reveals a germline configuration for TCR genes. Primary mediastinal large-cell lymphoma may have immunoglobulin gene but not TCR gene rearrangement. Recently, two cases of thymoma were reported to show TCR gene rearrangement for lymphocytes in pleural effusion; whether this phenomenon represents the malignant nature of these "metastasized" lymphocytes or an aberrant immunologic response to the thymoma is not clear.[27]

REFERENCES

1. Rosai J, Levine GD: *Tumors of the Thymus. Atlas of Tumor Pathology*, 2nd series, Fascicle 13, Washington DC, Armed Forces Institute of Pathology, 1976.
2. Rosai J: The pathology of thymic neoplasia. In Berard CW, Dorfman RF, Kaufman, N (eds): *Malignant Lymphoma*, Baltimore, Williams & Wilkins, 1986, pp 161–183.
3. Medeiros LJ, Bhagat SKM, Naylor P, et al: Malignant thymoma associated with T-cell lymphocytosis: A case report with immunophenotypic and gene rearrangement analysis. *Arch Pathol Lab Med* 117:279–283, 1993.
4. Macon WR, Rynalski TH, Swerdlow SH, et al: T-cell lymphoblastic leukemia/lymphoma presenting in a recurrent thymoma. *Mod Pathol* 4:525–528, 1991.
5. Gray GF, Gutowski WT, III: Thymoma: A clinicopathologic study of 54 cases. *Am J Surg Pathol* 3:235–249, 1979.
6. Knowles DM: Lymphoblastic lymphoma. In Knowles DM (ed): *Neoplastic Hematopathology*, Baltimore, Williams & Wilkins, 1992, pp 715–747.
7. Lamarre L, Jacobson JV, Aisenberg AC, et al: Primary large cell lymphoma of the mediastinum. A histologic and immunophenotypic study of 29 cases. *Am J Surg Pathol* 13:730–739, 1989.
8. Menestrina F, Chidosi M, Bonetti F, et al: Mediastinal large cell lymphoma of B-cell type with sclerosis: Histopathological and immunohistochemical study of eight cases. *Histopathology* 10:589–600, 1986.
9. Kirchner T, Schalke B, Buchwald J, et al: Well-differentiated thymic carcinoma: An organotypical low-grade carcinoma with relationship to cortical thymoma. *Am J Surg Pathol* 16:1153–1169, 1992.
10. Weide LG, Ulbright TM, Loehrer PJ Sr, et al: Thymic carcinoma: A distinct clinical entity responsive to chemotherapy. *Cancer* 71:1219–1223, 1993.
11. Vilela DS, Valien JSS, Moran MAG, et al: Thymic carcinosarcoma associated with a spindle cell thymoma: An immunohistochemical study. *Histopathology* 21:263–268, 1992.
12. Kuo TT, Lo SK: Thymoma: A study of the pathologic classification of 71 cases with evaluation of the Muller–Hermelink system. *Hum Pathol* 24:766–771, 1993.
13. Kirchner T, Muller-Hermelink HK: New approaches to the diagnosis of thymic epithelial tumors. *Prog Surg Pathol* 10:167–189, 1989.
14. Quintanilla-Martinez L, Wilkins EW Jr, Ferry JA, et al: Thymoma-morphologic subclassification correlates with invasiveness and immunohistologic features: A study of 122 cases. *Hum Pathol* 24:958–969, 1993.
15. Kornstein MJ, Curran WJ Jr, Turrisi AT III, et al: Cortical versus medullary thymomas: A useful morphologic distinction? *Hum Pathol* 19:1335–1339, 1988.
16. Woda BA, Brain K, Saln TV: The phenotype of lymphocytes in a thymoma as studied with monoclonal antibody. *Clin Immunol Immunopathol* 30:197–201, 1984.
17. Ichikawa Y, Shimizu H, Yoshida M, et al: Two color flow cytometric analysis of thymic lymphocytes from patients with myasthenia gravis and/or thymus. *Clin Immunol Immunopathol* 62:91–96, 1992.
18. Fujii Y, Hayakawa M, Nakahara K: Thymus cells in myasthenia gravis: A two color flow cytometric analysis of lymphocytes in the thymus and thymoma. *J Neurol* 239:82–88, 1992.
19. Sun T: *Color Atlas/Text of Flow Cytometric Analysis of Hematologic Neoplasms*, New York, Igaku-Shoin, 1993, pp 88–92, 98–105.
20. Taubenberger JK, Jaffe ES, Medeiro J: Thymoma with abundant L26 positive "Asteroid" cells: A case report with an analysis of normal thymus and thymoma specimens. *Arch Pathol Lab Med* 115:1254–1257, 1991.
21. Chilosi M, Castelli P, Mantignoni G, et al: Neoplastic epithelial cells in a subset of human thymomas express the B-cell associated CD20 antigen. *Am J Surg Pathol* 16:988–997, 1992.
22. Fukai I, Masaoka A, Hashimoto T, et al: Cytokeratin in normal thymus and thymic epithelial tumors. *Cancer* 71:99–105, 1993.
23. Fukai I, Masaoka A, Hashimoto T, et al: The distribution of epithelial membrane antigen in thymic epithelial neoplasms. *Cancer* 70:2077–2081, 1992.
24. Kaut JA, Hicks DG: Interpretation of non-lymphoid elements in lymph node biopsy specimens. In Jaffe ES (ed): *Surgical Pathology of the Lymph Nodes and Related Organs*, 2nd ed, Philadelphia, Saunders, 1995, pp 594–623.

25. Tateyama H, Mizuno T, Tada T, et al: Thymic epithelial tumors: Evaluation of malignant grade by quantification of proliferating cell nuclear antigen and nucleolar organizer regions. *Virchow Archiv A Pathol Anat* 422:265–269, 1993.
26. Katzin WE, Fishleder AJ, Linden MD, et al: Immunoglobulin and T-cell receptor genes in thymomas: Genotypic evidence supporting the non-neoplastic nature of the lymphocytic component. *Hum Pathol* 19:323–328, 1988.
27. Delannoy A, Philippe M, Hamels J, et al: Clonal rearrangement of the T-cell receptor beta-chain gene in the pleural fluid of a patient with thymoma. *Nouv Rev Fr Hematol* 35:121–124, 1993.

16
Angioimmunoblastic Lymphadenopathy vs. Immunoblastic Lymphadenopathy-Like T-Cell Lymphoma

Angioimmunoblastic lymphadenopathy with dysproteinemia (AILD) was first described by Frizzera et al. in 1974.[1] The same entity was described by Lukes and Tindle[2] as immunoblastic lymphadenopathy (IBL) and by Lennert as lymphogranulomatosis X(Lgx)[3] This disease was considered to be an abnormal hyperimmune reaction with severe impairment of cell-mediated immune surveillance.[2-4] However, its frequent evolution into malignant lymphoma led it to the designation as a prelymphomatous lesion.[5] Shimoyama et al. first proposed the term "IBL-like T-cell lymphoma" to describe lymphomas similar to or arising from IBL or AILD.[6] Nevertheless, Frizzera et al. suggested AILD to be a continuum ranging from purely reactive (hyperplastic) to a frankly neoplastic disorder.[7] This group proposed dividing angioimmunoblastic lymphadenopathy (AIL) into AIL, AIL-like lymphoma, and AIL-like dysplasia.[7] However, this concept was challenged because it is almost impossible to distinguish these three entities on a morphologic basis.[8]

CLINICAL FEATURES

AILD is usually seen in adults between 60 and 70 years of age, but it has been reported in all age groups, including a few children,[9] and with almost equal incidence in males and females. AILD usually has a sudden onset, with full-blown clinical features appearing within days or weeks.[1-3] The constitutional symptoms include fever, weight loss, and general malaise. Physical examination may reveal general lymphadenopathy, hepatosplenomegaly, and skin rash. Some patients may have local or generalized edema, pleural effusion, ascites, pulmonary infiltrates, or enlargement of parotid glands.[9] About 30% of cases are associated with drug-related hypersensitivity. Withdrawal of the offending drug may occasionally lead to resolution of the clinical symptoms and signs.[10] In the minority of patients, the onset of disease may be insidious, presenting with lymphadenopathy and anorexia for up to 2 years before diagnosis.[9]

Dysproteinemia is a constant finding in AILD.[1] It is usually presented as marked polyclonal gammopathy, but monoclonal gammopathy has also been reported occasionally.[1] Hematologic abnormalities are also common, including Coombs' positive hemolytic anemia, thrombocytopenia, and lymphocytopenia. A rather unusual finding in AILD is the presence of autoantibodies specific for vimentin.[11]

In about 10% of cases, the disease may have spontaneous remission in the first weeks or months that last for more than 5 years.[9] Most patients, however, have a progressive clinical course and require prompt treatment, such as prednisone or chemotherapy. The median overall survival of AILD patients varies from 11, 19, and 30 months, respectively, in three studies.[9] The complete responders to chemotherapy may achieve long-term (>5 years) survival and account for 20% of patients. The malignant transformation rate in AILD is 5–20%.[8,12] Malignant lymphoma may involve multiple lymph nodes or extranodal organs, including kidneys, gastrointestinal (GI) tract, and lungs.[5,9,13] AILD may also be associated with carcinoma and human immunodeficiency virus (HIV)-negative Kaposi's sarcoma.[7,14] However, the most common cause of death in AILD patients is overwhelming opportunistic infections, and not malignancy.

PATHOLOGY

AILD, IBL, and LgX are grouped together as a single entity because they have similar clinical manifestations, a high incidence of malignant transformation, high susceptibility to infections, and short survival rates.[9] However, they have subtle differences histologically.

The essential histologic features are (1) total effacement of lymph node architecture, which is replaced by diffuse polymorphic cellular infiltration with lymphoid depletion (Figs. 16.1, 16.2); (2) marked proliferation of arborizing, small blood vessels (postcapillary venules) lined by tall endothelial cells (Fig. 16.3); and (3) interstitial deposition of periodic-acid Schiff (PAS)-positive, granular, eosinophilic proteinaceous material (Figs. 16.4, 16.5).[1-3] The cellular components consist of immunoblasts, small lymphocytes, and plasma cells

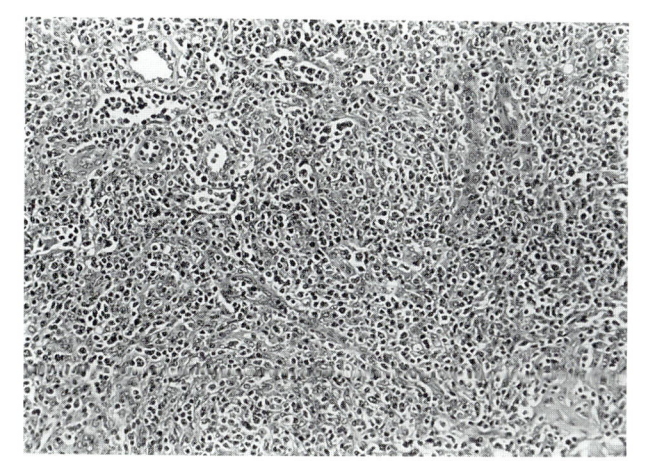

DIFFERENTIAL DIAGNOSIS OF LYMPHOID DISORDERS 159

Fig. 16.1. Lymph node biopsy of AILD showing total effacement of nodal architecture by diffuse polymorphic cellular infiltration with lymphoid depletion and increase in vascularity. H&E, ×250.

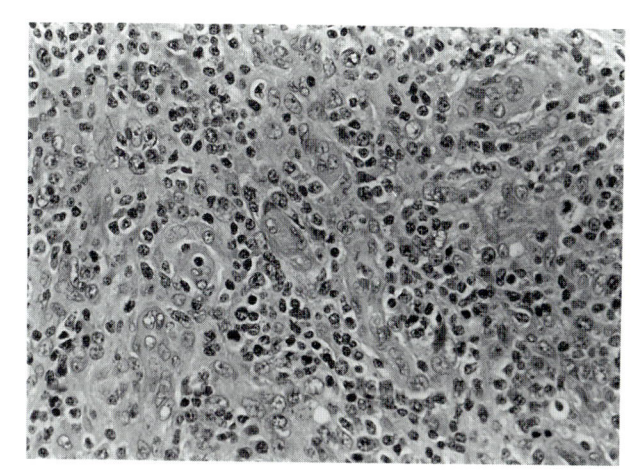

Fig. 16.3 A higher-power view of Fig. 16.2 showing marked proliferation of arborizing small blood vessels lined by tall endothelial cells. H&E, ×500.

(Figs. 16.6, 16.7). In some cases, eosinophils and epithelioid histiocytes are also present. The hallmark component is the immunoblasts (large transformed lymphoid cells), which are about 3 times the size of small lymphocytes, with a thin rim of cytoplasm and a large vesicular nucleus containing one or more prominent nucleoli. Some large immunoblasts may show polylobate nuclei simulating Reed–Sternberg cells. Mitotic rate is usually high. Lennert and Feller emphasized the accumulation of follicular dendritic cells outside the preexistent follicles as a special feature for AILD.[3] However, when an AIL-like pattern is accompanied by follicular hyperplasia, this condition

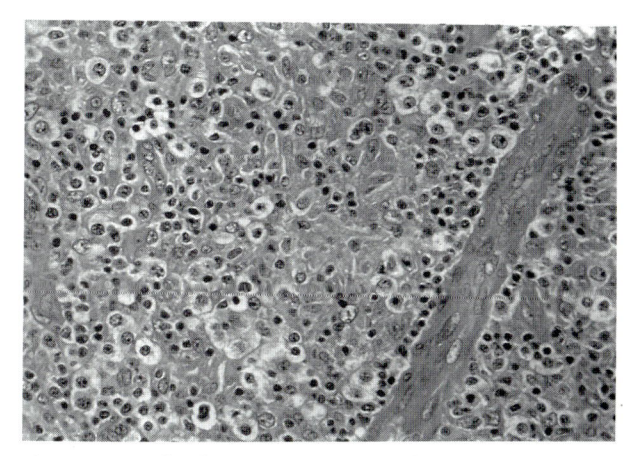

Fig. 16.4. A higher-power view of Fig. 16.2 showing interstitial deposition of eosinophilic proteinaceous material. H&E, ×500.

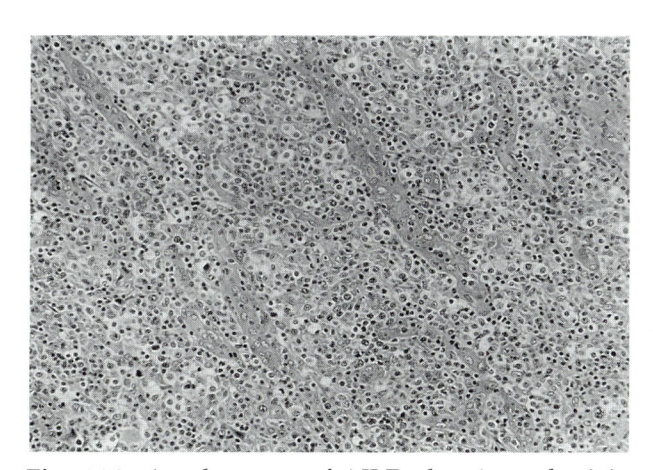

Fig. 16.2. Another case of AILD showing arborizing blood vessels on a polymorphic cellular infiltration background. H&E, ×250.

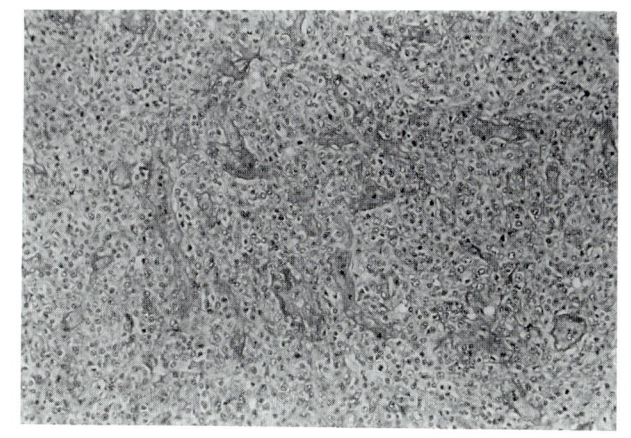

Fig. 16.5. The eosinophilic proteinaceous material shown in Fig. 16.4 is positive for PAS stain. ×250.

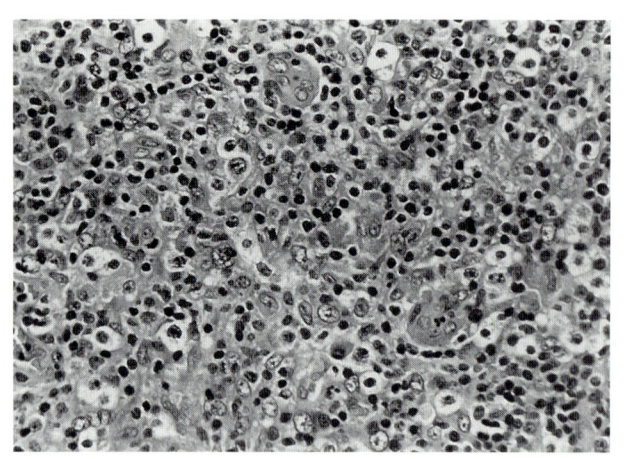

Fig. 16.6. A higher-power view of an AILD case showing a polymorphic cellular infiltration by small lymphocytes, immunoblasts, histiocytes, and plasma cells. H&E, ×500.

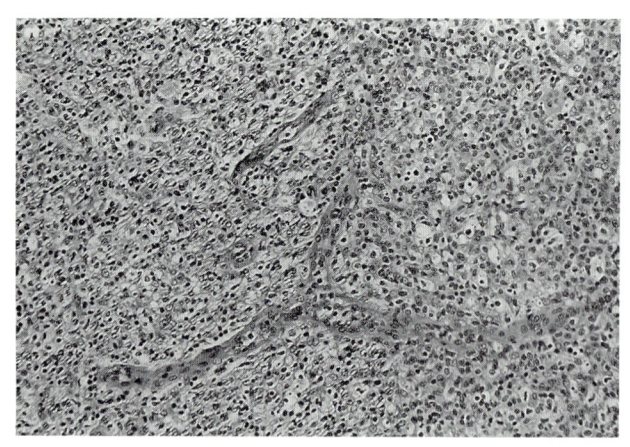

Fig. 16-8. IBL-like T-cell lymphoma in lymph node showing diffuse infiltration of abnormal lymphoid cells with pale-stained cytoplasm (pale cells or clear cells). H&E, ×250.

should be diagnosed as hyperimmune reaction, which has different clinical features and better prognosis than AILD.[15]

The subtle morphologic differences between AILD, IBL, and LgX is reviewed by Frizzera et al.[7] In AILD, burned-out and fibrosed germinal centers are part of the integral histologic feature, but the presence of PAS-positive proteinaceous material is not essential.[1] However, the diagnosis of IBL requires the absence of residual follicles, presence of PAS-positive material, and lymphocyte depletion.[2] LgX, on the other hand, covers a broader spectrum, including a subtype with predominance of lymphocytes.[3]

The histologic pattern in the earliest phase of malignant transformation is the presence of a monomorphic infiltrate of large lymphoid cells in clusters.[8] The proliferation of abnormal lymphoid cells with pale cytoplasm (pale cells or clear cells) is another special feature of the IBL-like T-cell lymphoma (Figs. 16.8–16.12).[6,16,17] Tobinai et al. further divided the IBL-like T-cell lymphoma into inconspicuous type, patchy type, and diffuse type on the basis of pale-cell distribution.[18] However, they found no obvious differences in T-cell receptor gene rearrangement between the inconspicuous and the diffuse type, but genotyping was not performed in the cases of the patchy type.[18]

Nevertheless, histopathologic difference between benign and malignant conditions is not clearcut in

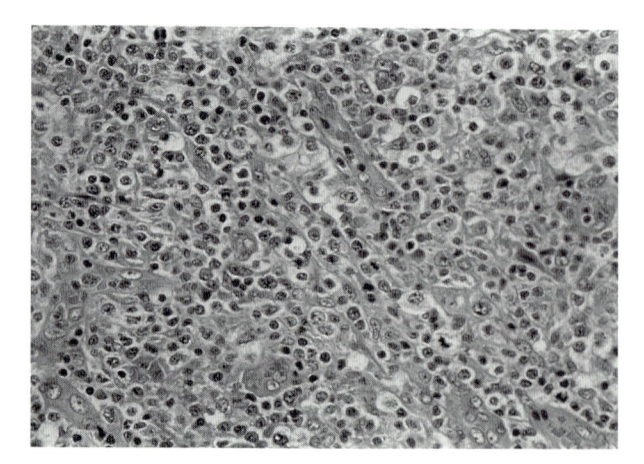

Fig. 16.7. A case of AILD in lymph node showing polymorphic cellular infiltration. H&E, ×500.

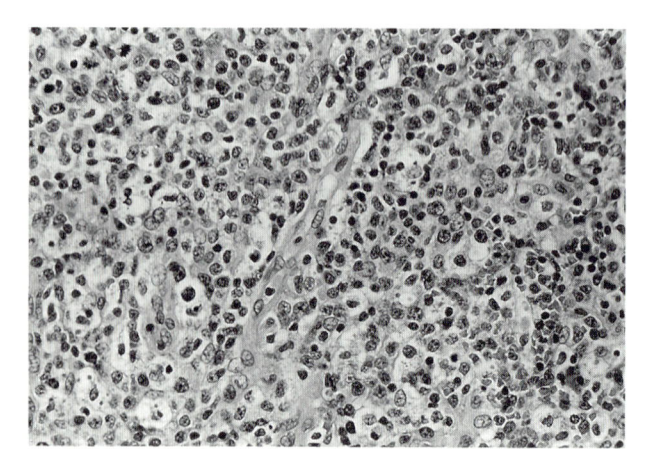

Fig. 16.9. A higher-power view of Fig. 16.8 showing atypical lymphoid cells. H&E, ×500.

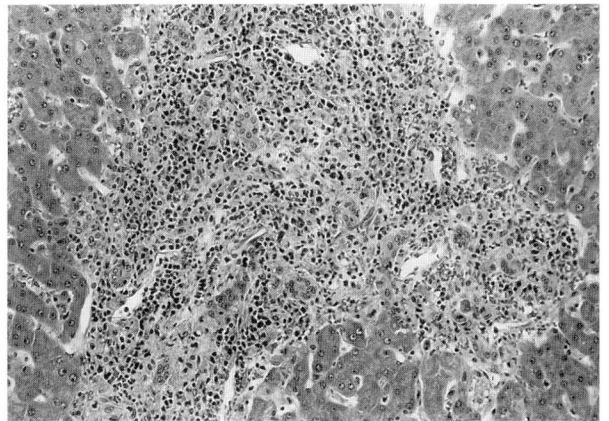

Fig. 16.10. IBL-like T-cell lymphoma in the liver showing atypical neoplastic cell infiltration in the portal area. H&E, ×500.

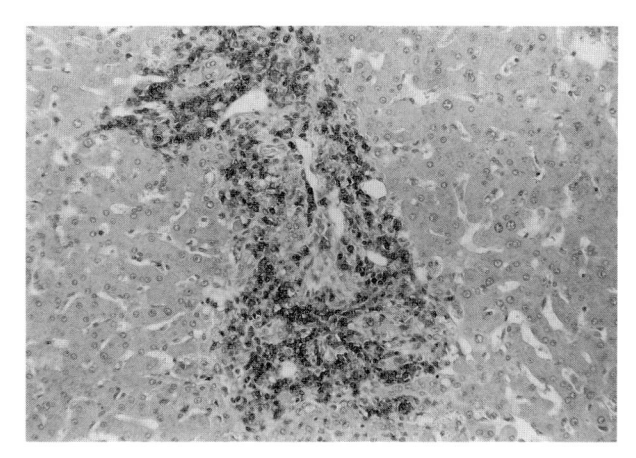

Fig. 16.13. IBL-like T-cell lymphoma in the portal area of liver showing positive T-cell antigen (CD43 or MT-1) staining. Immunoperoxidase, ×250.

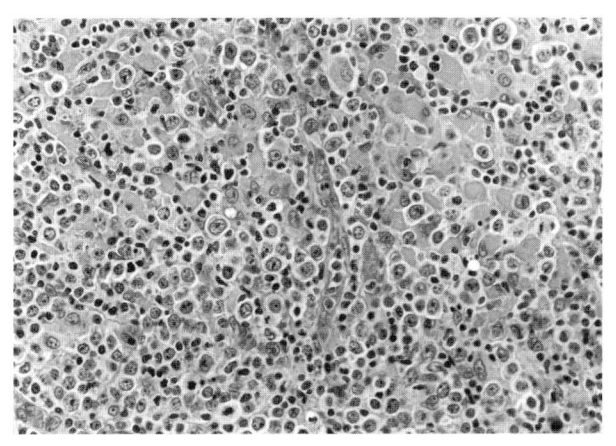

Fig. 16.11. IBL-like B-cell lymphoma in lymph node showing atypical lymphoid cells. Some have clear cytoplasm. H&E, ×500.

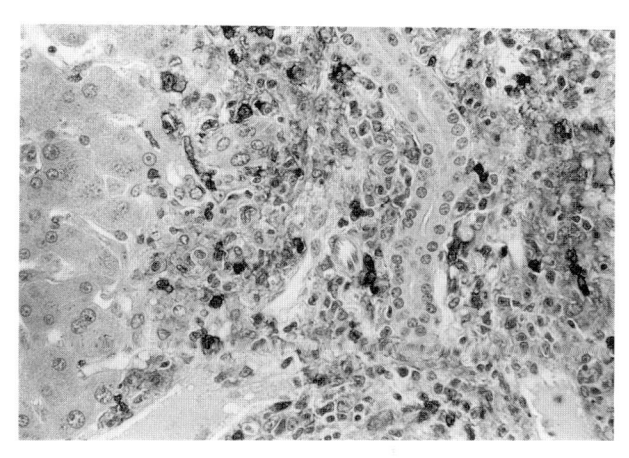

Fig. 16.14. IBL-like T-cell lymphoma in the portal area of liver showing positive T-cell antigen (CD45RO or UCHL-1) staining. Immunoperoxidase, ×500.

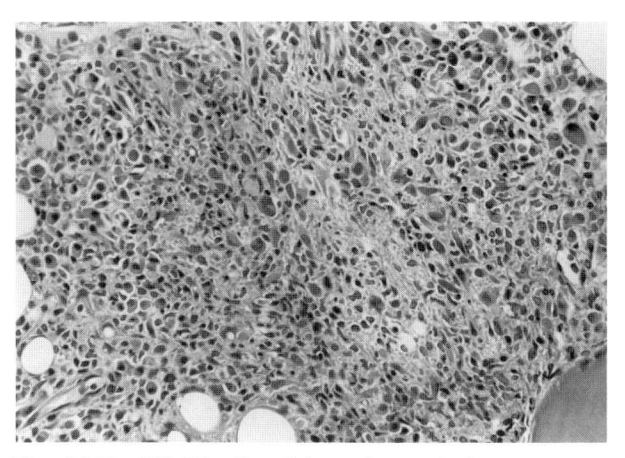

Fig. 16.12. IBL-like B-cell lymphoma in bone marrow showing atypical lymphoreticular-cell infiltration. H&E, ×500.

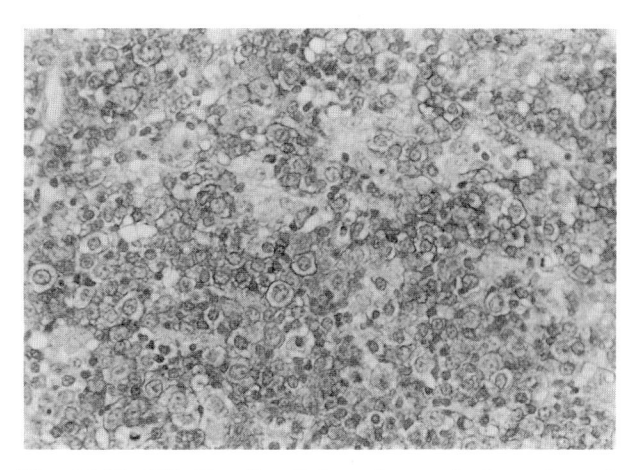

Fig. 16.15. IBL-like B-cell lymphoma in lymph node showing positive B-cell antigen (CD20 or L26) staining of the large lymphoid cells (clear cells). Immunoperoxidase, ×500.

many cases.[8,16] Lennert and Feller emphasize that they are unable to separate these conditions by morphology.[3] Furthermore, as a systemic disease, AILD may involve the blood, bone marrow, and other organs (spleen, liver, lungs, and skin) in addition to lymph nodes.[19,20] Therefore, Frizzera et al.[7] and Watanabe et al.[16] consider AILD as a spectrum of diseases from T-cell dysplasia to peripheral T-cell lymphoma. Since they are frequently indistinguishable morphologically, immunophenotyping, immunogenotyping, and cytogenetic analysis are required for their distinction. Most cases of malignant transformation develop into T-cell lymphoma (Figs. 16.13, 16.14), but B-cell immunoblastic lymphoma (Fig. 16.15) and Hodgkin's disease have also been reported.[3,14,19,21]

LABORATORY FINDINGS

In immunophenotyping, the benign lesions usually show mixed T- and B-cell proliferation, mixed population of CD4+ and CD8+ lymphocytes, and no loss of T-cell antigen.[19] In ILB-like T-cell lymphoma, aberrant T-cell phenotypes, including selective loss of CD3, CD5, and/or CD7, are frequently demonstrated.[7,19,22] Predominant CD4+ or CD8+ phenotypes have been demonstrated in IBL-like T-cell lymphoma,[15,16,23] but in at least three study series, CD4+ phenotype is much more common than CD8+ phenotype.[8,13,18]

Clonal rearrangement of T-cell receptor (TCR) β-chain gene has been successfully demonstrated in most cases of ILB-like T-cell lymphoma, but it has also been shown in some morphologically benign lesions.[15,18,23,24] In the study conducted by Feller et al., immunoglobulin heavy-chain gene was rearranged in addition to TCR gene rearrangement in 7 cases.[15] These cases showed a predominant CD8+ phenotype and were more often presented with hemolytic anemia. In the same study, those cases with only TCR gene rearrangement showed a predominant CD4+ phenotype and had a longer survival time than did the previous group.[15]

Cytogenetic studies in AILD and related lesions may show a normal karyotype, unrelated abnormal clonal karyotype, and nonclonal abnormalities.[25,26] The most common abnormalities are trisomy of chromosome 3 and chromosome 5.[25,26] The possible correlation with oncogenes was demonstrated in one AILD patient who had significantly increased levels of *c-myb* RNA in bone marrow cells, and N-*ras* messenger RNA was detected in the blood mononuclear cells of four AILD patients.[9]

In terms of pathogenesis, the finding of interleukin-6 (IL-6) production by T-cell lymphoma of the AILD type is most interesting.[27] In the case with a IL-6-producing lymphoma, the tumor is accompanied by a marked plasmacytic tissue response and hypergammaglobulinemia. In 3 cases with no IL-6 production by the tumors, no hypergammaglobulinemia and only minimal plasma cell infiltration were demonstrated.[27]

The latest interest seems to concentrate on the relationship between Epstein–Barr virus (EBV) and AILD.[28-30] The existence of EBV infection can be established in three levels: the EBV-DNA by Southern blotting or polymerase chain reaction, EBV-encoded small nuclear RNAs by *in situ* hybridization, and EBV-encoded latent membrane protein by immunohistochemistry. Since EBV infects both T-cell and B-cell in clinical specimens, and only a small amount of EBV protein is demonstrated in some cases, the role EBV plays is still controversial. One school considers it as a consequence of the disease (secondary infection),[30] while another school feels that EBV, in conjunction with genetic abnormalities and selective defects of the immune system, may play a primary role in the pathogenesis of AILD.[29]

REFERENCES

1. Frizzera G, Moran EM, Rappaport H: Angio-immunoblastic lymphadenopathy with dysproteinemia. *Lancet* 1:1070–1073, 1974.
2. Lukes RJ, Tindle BH: Immunoblastic lymphadenopathy: A hyperimmune entity resembling Hodgkin's disease. *N Engl J Med* 292:1–8, 1975.
3. Lennert K, Feller AC: *Histopathology of Non-Hodgkin's Lymphomas* (based on the updated Kiel classification), Berlin, Springer-Verlag, 1992.
4. Skibin A, Yeremiyahu T, Keynan A, et al: Immunological studies in angioimmunoblastic lymphadenopathy. *Clin Exp Immunol* 39:386–394, 1980.
5. Nathwani BN, Rappaport H, Moran EM, et al: Malignant lymphoma arising in angio-immunoblastic lymphadenopathy. *Cancer* 41:578–606, 1978.
6. Shimoyama M, Minato K, Saito H, et al: Immunoblastic lymphadenopathy (IBL-) like T-cell lymphoma. *Jpn J Clin Oncol* 9 (suppl 1):347–356, 1979.
7. Frizzera G, Kaneko Y, Sakurai M: Angioimmunoblastic lymphadenopathy and related disorders: A retrospective look in search of definitions. *Leukemia* 3:1–5, 1989.
8. Ohsaka A, Saito K, Sakai T, et al: Clinicopathologic and therapeutic aspects of angioimmunoblastic lymphadenopathy-related lesions. *Cancer* 69:1259–1287, 1992.
9. Knecht H: Angioimmunoblastic lymphadenopathy: Ten

years' experience and state of current knowledge. *Semin Hematol* 26:208–215, 1989.
10. Ganesan TS, Dhaliwal HS, Doreen MS, et al: Angioimmunoblastic lymphadenopathy: A clinical immunological and molecular study. *Br J Cancer* 55:437–442, 1987.
11. Dellagi K, Brouet JC, Seligmann M: Antivimentin autoantibodies in angioimmunoblastic lymphadenopathy. *N Engl J Med* 310:215–218, 1984.
12. Pangalis GA, Morgan EM, Nathwani BN, et al: Angioimmunoblastic lymphadenopathy. Long-term follow-up study. *Cancer* 52:318–321, 1983.
13. Nakamura S, Takagi N, Kitoh K, et al: Peripheral T-cell lymphoma of AILD (Angioimmunoblastic lymphadenopathy with dysproteinemia) type involving gastrointestinal tract: A morphologic, phenotypic and genotypic study. *Acta Pathol Jpn* 42:141–149, 1992.
14. Steinberg AD, Seldin MF, Jaffe ES, et al: Angioimmunoblastic lymphadenopathy with dysproteinemia. *Ann Intern Med* 108:575–584, 1988.
15. Feller AC, Griesser H, Schilling CV, et al: Clonal gene rearrangement patterns correlate with immunophenotype and clinical parameters in patients with angioimmunoblastic lymphadenopathy. *Am J Pathol* 133:549–556, 1988.
16. Watanabe S, Sato Y, Shimoyama M, et al: Immunoblastic lymphadenopathy (IBL)-like T-cell lymphoma: A spectrum of T-cell neoplastia. *Cancer* 58:2224–2232, 1986.
17. Suchi T, Lennert K, Tu LY, et al: Histopathology and immunohistochemistry of peripheral T-cell lymphomas: A proposal for their classification. *J Clin Pathol* 40:995–1015, 1987.
18. Tobinai K, Minato K, Ohtsu T, et al: Clinicopathologic, immunophenotypic and immunogenotypic analysis of immunoblastic lymphadenopathy-like T-cell lymphoma. *Blood* 72:1000–1006, 1988.
19. Pinkus GS, Said JW: Peripheral T-cell lymphomas. In Knowles DM (ed): *Neoplastic Hematopathology*, Baltimore, Williams & Wilkins, 1992, pp 837–866.
20. Ishiyama T, Watanabe K, Akimoto Y, et al: Circulating abnormal cells detected in a patient with immunoblastic lymphadenopathy. *Intern Med* 32:455–458, 1993.
21. Yataganas X, Papadimitrious C, Pangalis G, et al: Angioimmunoblastic lymphadenopathy terminating as Hodgkin's disease. *Cancer* 39:2183–2189, 1977.
22. Doi S, Nasu K, Arita Y, et al: Immunohistochemical analysis of peripheral T-cell lymphoma in Japanese patients. *Am J Clin Pathol* 91:152–158, 1989.
23. Takagi N, Nakamura S, Veda R, et al: A phenotypic and genotypic study of three node-based, low-grade peripheral T-cell lymphomas: Angioimmunoblastic lymphoma, T-zone lymphoma and lymphoepithelial lymphoma. *Cancer* 69:2571–2582, 1992.
24. Weiss LM, Strickler JG, Dorfman RF, et al: Clonal T-cell populations in angioimmunoblastic lymphadenopathy and angioimmunoblastic lymphadenopathy-like lymphoma. *Am J Pathol* 122:393–397, 1986.
25. Godde-Salz E, Feller AC, Lennert K: Chromosomal abnormalities in lymphogranulomatosis X(LgX)/angioimmunoblastic lymphadenopathy (AILD). *Leuk Res* 11:181–190, 1987.
26. Kaneko Y, Maseki N, Sakurai M, et al: Characteristic karyotypic pattern in T-cell lymphoproliferative disorders with reactive "angioimmunoblastic lymphadenopathy with dysproteinemia-type" features. *Blood* 72:413–421, 1988.
27. Hsu SM, Waldron JA, Fink L, et al: Pathogenic significance of interleukin-6 in angioimmunoblastic lymphadenopathy-type T-cell lymphoma. *Hum Pathol* 24:126–131, 1993.
28. Su IJ, Hsieh HC: Clinicopathological spectrum of Epstein–Barr virus-associated T-cell malignancies. *Leuk Lymphoma* 7:47–53, 1992.
29. Anagnostopoulos I, Hummel M, Finn T, et al: Heterogeneous Epstein–Barr virus infection patterns in peripheral T-cell lymphoma of angioimmunoblastic lymph-. adenopathy type. *Blood* 80:1804–1812, 1992.
30. Khan G, Norton AJ, Slavin G: Epstein–Barr virus in angioimmunoblastic T-cell lymphoma. *Histopathology* 72:145–149, 1993.

17
T-Cell Lymphoma vs. Malignant and Benign Histiocytosis

In the light of current studies, most cases that were diagnosed previously as malignant histiocytosis are probably lymphomas of T-cell lineage or the virus-associated hemophagocytic syndrome.[1,2] Some of these T-cell lymphomas have clinical symptoms similar to those of malignant histiocytosis, such as fever, hepatosplenomegaly, and pancytopenia. Histologically, there is sinusoidal infiltration of lymphoma cells with or without associated hemophagocytosis in the liver, spleen, and bone marrow.[3-7] This group of lymphoma was first designated by Kadin et al. as erythrophagocytic T-gamma lymphoma.[3] However, the term "hepatosplenic γδ T-cell lymphoma" as suggested by Farcet et al. seems to be more appropriate to describe this situation.[4] The second group of lymphomas that mimicks malignant histiocytosis is also of T-cell lineage, occurring in the nasal/nasopharyngeal areas, and is associated with hemophagocytosis.[8-10] These cases are mainly confined to Asian countries. The third group of lymphomas showing a sinusoidal infiltrating pattern is the anaplastic large-cell Ki-1 lymphoma, which is mostly of T-cell lineage and involves mainly the lymph nodes and skin.[11,12] This group of lymphomas, however, is easier to distinguish from malignant histiocytosis because of the anaplastic large-cell morphology[13] (see Chapter 14). The fourth group of T-cell lymphomas mimicking malignant histiocytosis is confined to the intestine in patients with celiac sprue.[14,15] The last group of T-cell lymphoma, which is associated with hemophagocytosis and has been included in the Revised European–American Classification of lymphoid neoplasms, is subcutaneous panniculitic T-cell lymphoma.[16]

Many benign conditions may also simulate malignant histiocytosis with or without coexistence of the hemophagocytic syndrome. The differential diagnoses should include virus and other infection-associated disorders, Langerhans' cell histiocytosis, familial or gene-related diseases (e.g., familial erythrophagocytic lymphohistiocytosis and X-linked lymphoproliferative syndrome), sinus histiocytosis with massive lymphadenopathy (Rosai–Dorfman disease), congenital immunodeficiency, drug-induced histiocytosis, lipid-rich hyperalimentation, and systemic lupus erythematosus (SLE).[17-20] The list of malignant and benign histiocytic disorders and lymphomas that simulate histiocytosis are presented in Table 17.1. Storage histiocyte disorders are included separately in Chapter 6. True histiocytic lymphoma and monocytic leukemia are discussed in Chapter 23. Dendritic reticulum-cell sarcoma and interdigitating reticulum cell sarcoma are very rare and will not be discussed in this chapter. For a more comprehensive classification of histiocytic diseases, the reader is referred to a recent review by Cline.[21]

CLINICAL FEATURES

Malignant Histiocytosis

Malignant histiocytosis is the leukemic counterpart of true histiocytic lymphoma (see Chapter 23), showing systemic dissemination in the bone marrow, peripheral blood, and other organs.[2,21-25] The clinical features include fever, progressive wasting, generalized lymphadenopathy, and hepatosplenomegaly. The onset of the disease is usually abrupt and the clinical course fulminant. Pleural effusions, jaundice, purpura, anemia, thrombocytopenia and leukopenia may occur in the final stages.[2,21-25] Malignant histiocytosis can be found in a wide-range age group, but it is seen predominantly in younger age group with a male preponderance.

Infection-Associated Hemophagocytic Syndrome

Most cases of hemophagocytic syndrome have been reported from patients with viral infection. Most reports emphasized the role played by Epstein–Barr virus, but several other viruses, such as cytomegalovirus, *Herpes simplex* virus, *Varicella zoster* virus, adenovirus, ECHO virus, and parovirus B19, may also induce hemophagocytosis.[18] In addition, this syndrome may also be triggered by fungal (*Histoplasma capsulatum*, *Candida albicans*, and *Cryptococcus neoformans*), parasitic (*Leishmania donovani* and *Babesia microti*), richettsial (*Coxiella burnetii*), mycobacterial, several bacterial (gram-negative enteric bacilli, *Hemophilus influenzae*, *Streptococcus pneumoniae*, *Staphyloc-*

TABLE 17.1
Malignant and Benign Histiocytic Disorders and Lymphomas Mimicking Histiocytosis

I. *Malignant histiocytic disorders:*
  Malignant histiocytosis
  True histiocytic lymphoma
  Monocytic leukemia
  Dendritic reticulum-cell sarcoma
  Interdigitating reticulum-cell sarcoma
II. *Benign histiocytic disorder:*
  Infection-associated hemophagocytic syndrome
  Langerhans' cell histiocytosis
  Familial erythrophagocytic lymphohistiocytosis
  X-linked lymphoproliferative syndrome
  Rosai–Dorfman disease (sinus histiocytosis with massive lymphadenopathy)
III. *Lymphomas mimicking histiocytosis:*
  Hepatosplenic lymphoma γδ T-cell (erythrophagocytic T-gamma lymphoma)
  Nasal/nasopharyngeal lymphoma
  Anaplastic large-cell Ki-1 lymphoma
  Intestinal lymphoma with celiac sprue
  Subcutaneous panniculitic T-cell lymphoma

cus aureus), and other agents.[18] These patients may have fever, constitutional symptoms (e.g., myalgias, malaise), hepatosplenomegaly, generalized lymphadenopathy, and additional symptoms caused by the underlying infection.[17,18,23]

Langerhans' Cell Histiocytosis

This disease is a proliferation of benign-appearing histiocytes containing Langerhans (Birbeck) granules.[2,23,25,26] It includes three entities: eosinophilic granuloma, Hand–Schuller–Christian syndrome, and Letterer–Siwe disease. Eosinophilic granuloma may be monostotic or polyostotic and involves bones, skin, lymph nodes, and lungs. It is most common in the first decade of life. The Hand–Schuller–Christian syndrome, now considered by many as the polyostotic form of eosinophilic granuloma, is characterized by a triad of bony lesions, exophthalmos, and diabetes insipidus. Letterer–Siwe disease, the disseminated form of Langerhans' cell histiocytosis, usually seen in infants less than 3 years old, is manifested with hepatosplenomegaly and a generalized skin lesion, most prominently in axillary and inguinal areas. Recently, Ben-Ezra et al. described a new entity designated malignant histiocytosis X, in which the Langerhans' cells appeared malignant and the clinical course aggressive.[27]

Familial or Gene-Related Diseases

Familial erythrophagocytic (hemophagocytic) lymphohistiocytosis is an uncommon familial disease (probably autosomal recessive) of infants and children.[17,18,23,28] Its incidence is about 1.2 cases per 1,000,000 children.[5] The major clinical symptoms are fever, failure to thrive, hepatosplenomegaly, and anemia. Lymph nodes, lungs, central nervous system (CNS), pericardium, bone, and gastrointestinal (GI) tract may be involved. The patient may also have leukopenia, coagulopathy, hypofibrinogenemia, hypertransferrinemia, hypertriglyceridemia, and/or hypercholesterolemia.

X-linked lymphoproliferative syndrome (XLP) is a systemic histiocytic proliferation caused by the Epstein–Barr virus in children carrying the XLP gene.[18,19,28] In 75% of cases, the patient expires due to a fatal infectious mononucleosis. These patients may have high fever, leukocytosis, lymphocytosis, and maculopapular skin rash, but the major clinical manifestation is progressive liver damage resulting in liver failure. Other causes of death include coagulopathy, thrombocytopenia, bacterial sepsis, and a fulminating lymphoma-like disease.

Rosai–Dorfman Disease

This is a benign, chronic disorder characterized by painless, bilateral, massive enlargement of cervical lymph nodes, which are filled with histiocytes in the sinuses.[20,29,30] Although it can be seen in all age groups, the disease is seen mainly in young males. In addition to lymphadenopathy, patients frequently have fever, leukocytosis, elevated erythrocyte sedimentation rate, and polyclonal gammopathy. Extranodal involvement and autoimmune phenomenon are increasingly seen in these patients.

T-Cell Lymphomas with Sinusoidal Infiltration and/or Hemophagocytosis

As mentioned before, five groups of T-cell lymphomas may mimic histiocytosis. The clinical symptoms in patients with hepatosplenic γδ T-cell lymphoma may include fever, hepatosplenomegaly, anemia, and thrombocytopenia, mimicking malignant histiocytosis.[3–7,31] Lymphadenopathy, skin rash, and erythrophagocytosis may be encountered in some patients, but they are not a constant feature as hepatosplenomegaly is. The other four groups of lymphomas may simulate malignant histiocytosis histologically but not necessarily clinically.

PATHOLOGY

Malignant Histiocytosis

In the lymph nodes, the malignant histiocytes mainly infiltrate the subcapsular and medullary sinuses in the early phase.[2,22–25] In a later phase, the cortex is gradually involved. The tumor cells are noncohesive and pleomorphic (Fig. 17.1) with the presence of at least three types of of histiocytes: prohistiocytes or immunoblast-like cells, histiocytes with polypoid features (Reed–Sternberg-like cells), and normal histiocytes.[25] Phagocytosis of erythrocytes, lymphocytes, platelets, and hemosiderin is frequently encountered, especially in mature normal histiocytes. The mitotic rate is high. The neoplastic cells are often intermingled with inflammatory cells, especially plasma cells. In the spleen, malignant histiocytes primarily infiltrate the red pulp sinus and cord. In the liver, both sinuses and portal areas are involved.

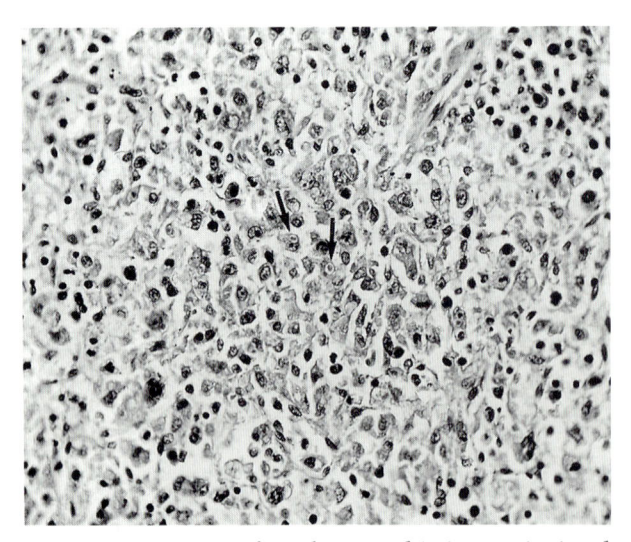

Fig. 17.1. A case of malignant histiocytosis in the spleen showing a diffuse infiltration of atypical histiocytes in the red pulp cords and sinuses with erythrophagocytosis (arrows). H&E, ×500. (AFIP 219932-200.)

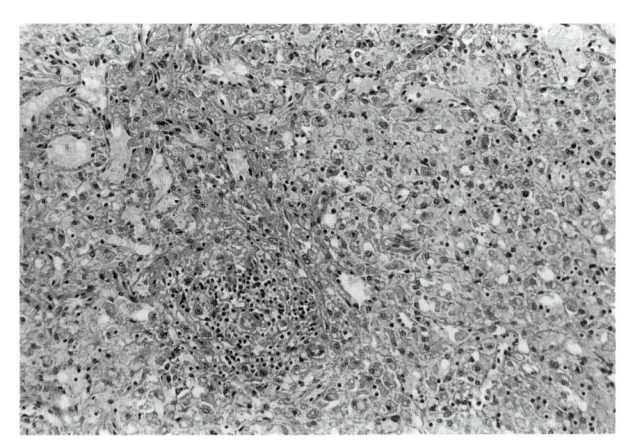

Fig. 17.2. A case of virus-associated hemophagocytic syndrome showing replacement of normal splenic tissue by numerous foamy macrophages. H&E, ×250. (Case provided by Dr. I. J. Su.)

Infection-Associated Hemophagocytic Syndrome

The major difference between this entity and malignant histiocytosis is the morphology of the histiocytes. In infection-associated hemophagocytic syndrome, all histiocytes with or without hemophagocytosis are benign-appearing (Figs. 17.2, 17.3). The bone marrow may be hypercellular with few infiltrating histiocytes in the early phase, but shows diminished hemopoiesis and increasing numbers of infiltrating histiocytes in the late phase.[17,18,23] Similarly, the lymph node shows immunoblastic proliferation ini-

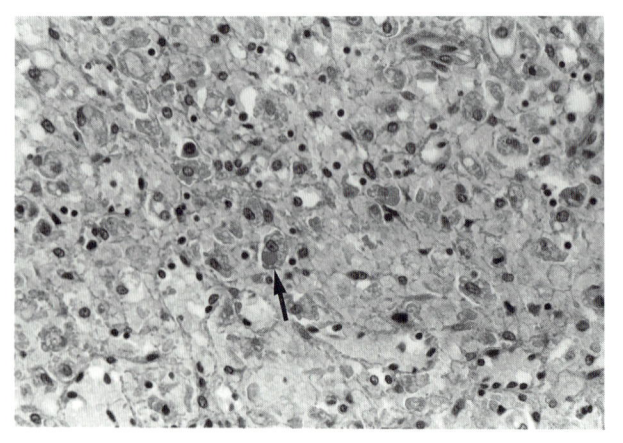

Fig. 17.3. The same case as in Fig. 17.2 showing erythrophagocytosis (arrow) and focal necrosis. H&E, ×500.

tially, and becomes lymphoid depleted with massive histiocytosis in the late stage. The liver biopsy may reveal histiocytic infiltration in both liver sinusoids and portal areas. Erythrophagocytosis may be visible in lymph nodes, liver, and bone marrow aspirates, but is difficult to identify in marrow biopsies. It is believed that immunodeficiency or underlying immunosuppression may play a role in the hemophagocytic syndrome.[17] Infective agents may activate T-lymphocytes, which, in turn, secrete cytokines to stimulate histiocytic proliferation. When this normal immune mechanisms is not under appropriate control, excess histiocytosis with hemophagocytic syndrome may result.

Langerhans' Cell Histiocytosis

The major diagnostic feature in this disease is the present of masses of Langerhans' histiocytes (Figs. 17.4, 17.5).[2,23,25,26] This histiocyte is characterized by its longitudinal nuclear grooves (Fig. 17.6), which can be visualized on tissue sections or touch imprints, and Langerhans' (Birbeck) granules, which can be demonstrated by electron microscopy as a rod- or flask-shaped structure with a central zipper-like component (Fig. 17.7). In eosinophilic granuloma, Langerhans' histiocytes are admixed with variable numbers of eosinophils as well as mononucleated and multinucleated macrophages, giving the appearance of a granuloma. Plasma cells, lymphocytes, and osteoclast-like giant cells are also present. In lymph nodes, the histiocytes usually infiltrate the markedly distended sinuses. The infiltration may extend to the capsule and surrounding soft tissue of the lymph node. Eosinophilic microabscess and coagulation necrosis are also seen in some cases. In Letterer–Siwe disease, the infiltrate of histiocytes is more monomorphous, and eosinophils are fewer than in eosinophilic granuloma (Figs. 17.8, 17.9).

Familial Erythrophagocytic Lymphohistiocytosis

This entity is characterized by generalized lymphoid depletion and histiocytic infiltration of all lymphoreticular organs, including lymph nodes, spleen,

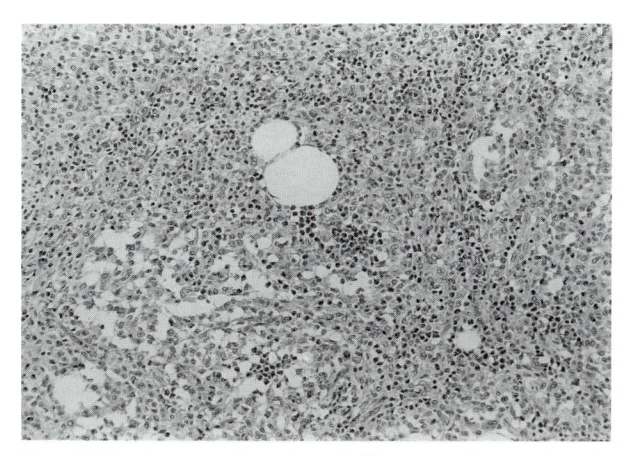

Fig. 17.5. A case of eosinophilic granuloma showing pale-stained Langerhans' cells intermingled with darkly stained eosinophils. H&E, ×250.

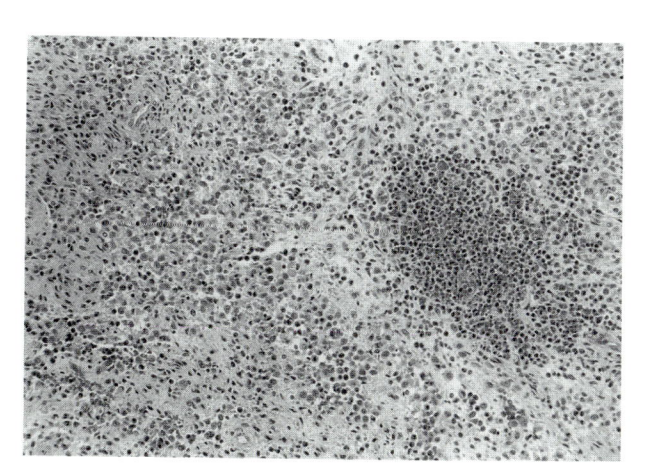

Fig. 17.4. A case of eosinophilic granuloma showing an eosinophilic abscess at right surrounded by many pale-stained Langerhans' cells. H&E, ×250.

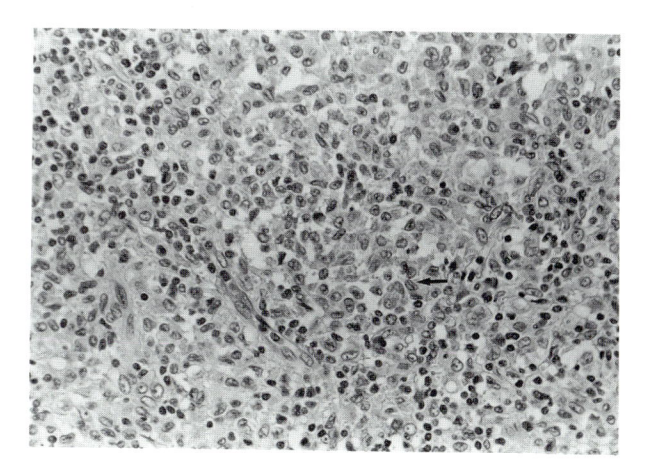

Fig. 17.6. A higher-power view of the case in Fig. 17.5 showing the longitudinal nuclear grooves in some Langerhans' cells (arrow). H&E, ×500.

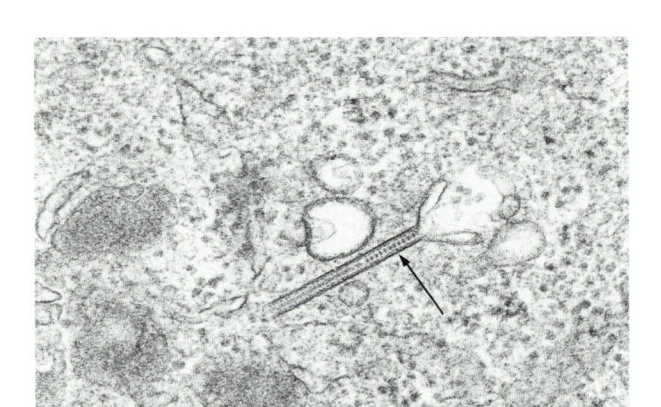

168 DIFFERENTIAL DIAGNOSIS OF LYMPHOID DISORDERS

Fig. 17.7. Langerhans' granule (arrow) with an internal paracrystalline lattice in a Langerhans' cell from a patient with eosinophilic granuloma. ×132,000 (Courtesy of Dr. Saul Teichberg and Beth Roberts.)

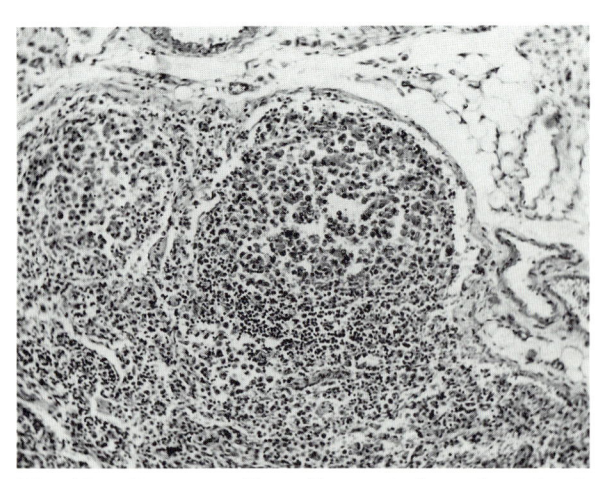

Fig. 17.8. Letterer–Siwe disease in lymph node showing extensive replacement of lymphoid tissue by monomorphous histiocytes. No eosinophils are noted. H&E, ×250. (AFIP 219932-186.)

liver, and bone marrow.[18,23,28] The histiocytes are well differentiated with bland nuclei and abundant eosinophilic cytoplasm. Erythrophagocytosis and leukophagocytosis are also characteristic. The thymus may also show lymphoid depletion.

X-Linked Lymphoproliferative Syndrome

The pathologic findings are similar to those of virus-associated syndrome.[18,19,28] The sinuses of lymph nodes and the splenic red pulp may show histiocytic infiltration. Areas of necrosis can be found in the lymph nodes and spleen. In addition, the normal architecture of the lymph node may be effaced with proliferation of immunoblasts. Progressive hepatic damage is also characteristic of this disease. The liver may show widespread necrosis and periportal infiltration by small lymphocytes and immunoblasts.

Rosai–Dorfman Disease

The typical feature in this entity is filling of the lymph node sinuses by numerous distinctive histiocytes (Fig. 17.10).[20,29,30] The histiocytes have abundant pink cytoplasm and oval or round vesicular nuclei. Although most histiocytes appear benign, their nuclei contain one to multiple nucleoli. Multilobulated nuclei or nuclear atypia may be encountered occasionally. The mitotic rate is usually low. The most characteristic finding is phagocytosis of lymphocytes by many of the histiocytes, which is referred to as *lymphophagocytosis* or *emperipolesis* (Fig. 17.11). In reactive sinus histiocy-

tosis, emperipolesis is rare or absent. Phagocytosis of plasma cells, neutrophils, or erythrocytes are often seen in small numbers of histiocytes. The distended sinuses and medullary cords may contain numerous plasma cells. Microabscesses and reactive germinal centers may be seen infrequently. In extranodal sites, the histologic features are similar to those seen in lymph nodes, with dilated lymphatics mimicking dis-

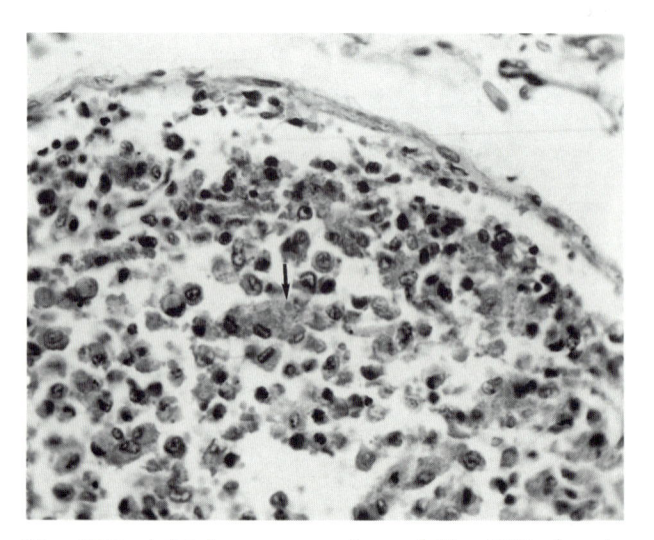

Fig. 17.9. A higher-power view of Fig. 17.8 showing proliferating histiocytes with abundant cytoplasm and moderate nuclear variations. Note a phagocytized red blood cell in the large histiocyte (arrow). H&E, ×1000. (AFIP 219932-177)

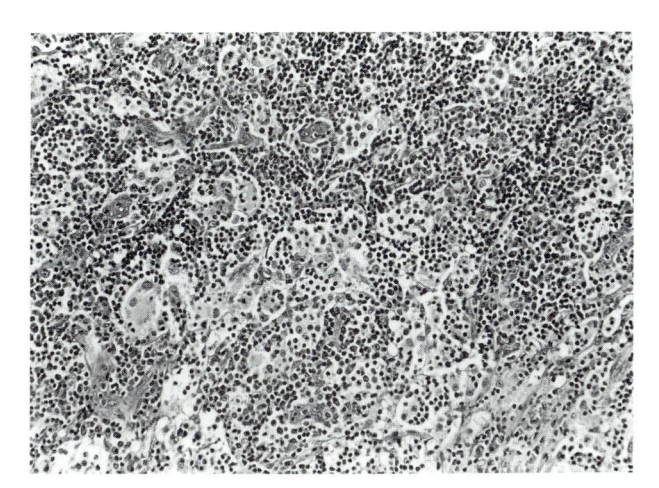

Fig. 17.10. A case of Rosai–Dorfman disease showing many distinctive histiocytes filling the sinuses of the lymph node. H&E, ×250.

tended sinuses and aggregates of lymphocytes simulating reactive germinal centers.

Lymphomas

The hepatosplenic γδ T-cell lymphoma shows sinusoidal infiltrate of lymphoma cells in the liver (Figs. 17.12, 17.13), spleen (Figs. 17.14, 17.15), and bone marrow (Figs. 17.16, 17.17).[3–7,31] Lymph nodes are less frequently involved, but this lymphoma shows a sinusoidal infiltrating pattern in lymph node similar to those in the liver and spleen. Erythrophagocy-

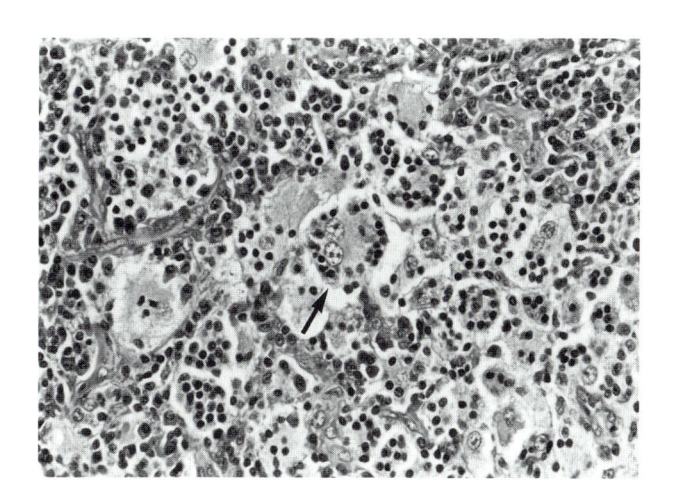

Fig. 17.11. A higher-power view of the case in Fig. 17.10 showing prominent emperipolesis (arrow). H&E, ×500.

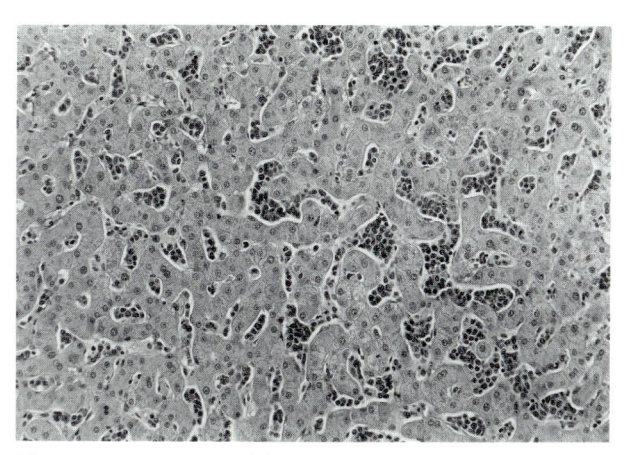

Fig. 17.12. A case of hepatosplenic T-cell lymphoma showing tumor-cell infiltrate of the liver sinusoids. H&E, ×250.

tosis may be demonstrated in either lymphoma cells[3] or normal histiocytes.[31] Jaffe et al postulated that a lymphokine (macrophage-activating factor) released by lymphoma cells might induce benign histiocytosis,[32] a theory later proved by culture of tumor cells.[33]

The nasal T-cell lymphoma may also involve focally the liver and spleen, namely, the hepatic portal zone, and splenic white pulp, but only the erythrophagocytic histiocytes infiltrate the sinuses of liver, spleen, lymph nodes, and bone marrow.[8–10] The anaplastic large-cell Ki-1 lymphoma infiltrates the sinuses accompanied by a large number of reactive histiocytes that may be confused with malignant histiocytosis,[11,12] but the striking feature of the anaplastic large

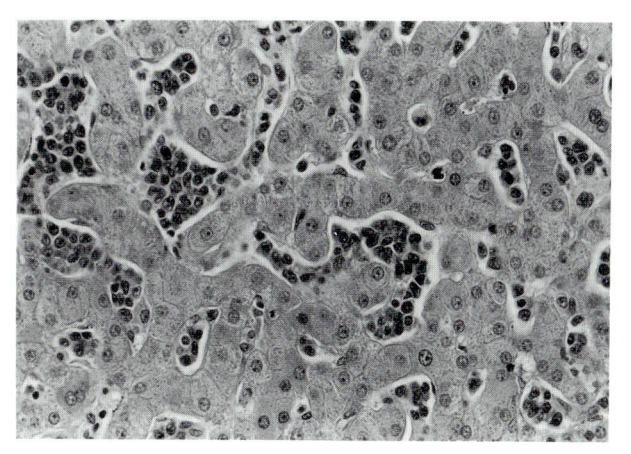

Fig. 17.13. A higher-power view of the case in Fig. 17.12 showing the irregular-shaped tumor cells in hepatic sinusoids. H&E, ×500.

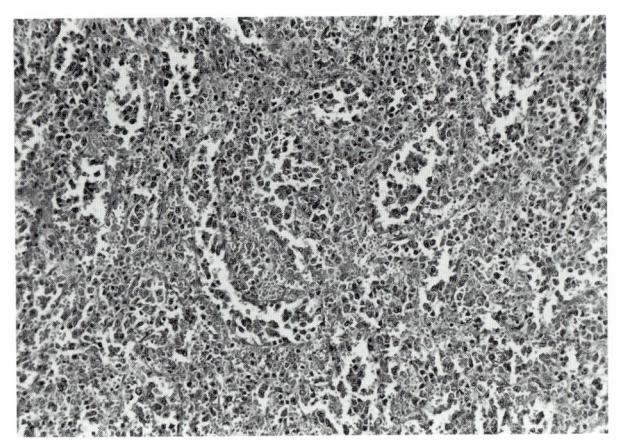

Fig. 17.14. The same case as in Fig. 17.12 showing tumor-cell infiltrate of both the sinuses and the red pulp cords of the spleen. H&E, ×250.

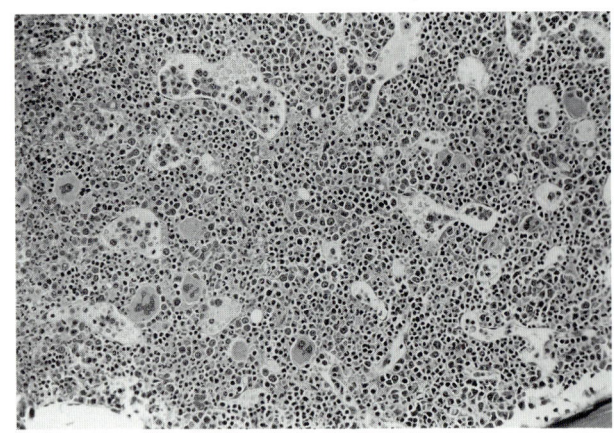

Fig. 17.16. The same case as in Fig. 17.12 showing sinusoidal infiltrate of the tumor cells in the bone marrow. H&E, ×250.

lymphoma cells facilitates a correct diagnosis of lymphoma and distinguishes it from a histiocytic lesion.[13] The intestinal T-cell lymphoma in patients with celiac sprue and the subcutaneous paniculitic T-cell lymphoma (Figs. 17.18, 17.19) may also mimic malignant histiocytosis.[14,16] The distinction between these three entities relies on morphologic and immunologic recognition of lymphoma cells versus malignant histiocytes on a cytologic basis.

LABORATORY FINDINGS

Histiocytosis, regardless of whether it is malignant or benign in nature, is characterized by hemophagocytosis. This phenomenon is frequently triggered by viral infection. Early literature emphasized virus-associated hemophagocytic syndrome as a distinct clinicopathologic entity. However, recent studies have detected viruses in varying categories of histiocytosis. An *in situ* hybridization study revealed Epstein–Barr virus RNA in 3 of 4 cases of infection-related hemophagocytic syndrome, 1 of 3 cases of familial hemophagocytic syndrome, and 3 of 5 cases of secondary hemophagocytosis associated with malignant T-cell lymphoma.[34] The role of Epstein–Barr virus in hemophagocytosis secondary to lymphomas has been substantiated in several studies.[13,31] Evidence of viral infections, including Epstein–Barr virus, cytomegalovirus, and human paraovirus was demonstrated in 22

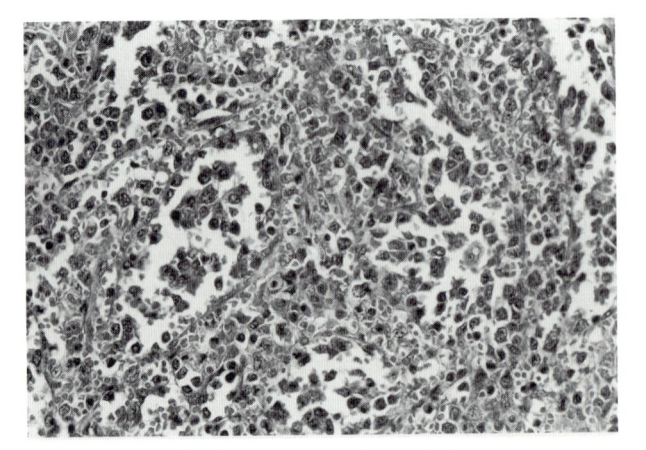

Fig. 17.15. A higher-power view of the same case as in Fig. 17.14. H&E, ×500.

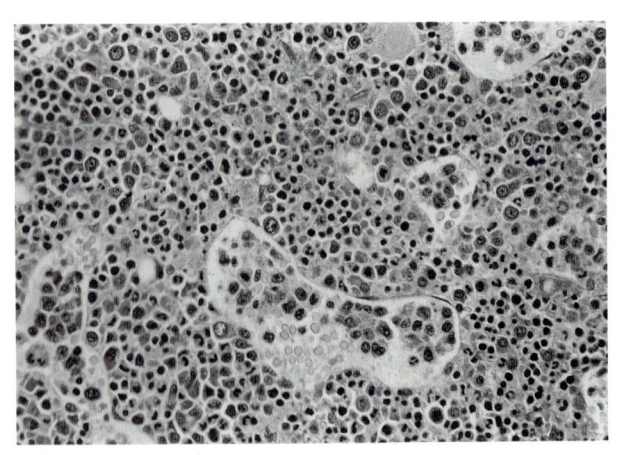

Fig. 17.17. A higher-power view of Fig. 17.16. H&E, ×500.

of 32 children with hemophagocytic lymphohistiocytosis.[28] Of the 22 positive cases, 13 were familial. The authors concluded that viral infection cannot serve as the sole criterion for distinguishing a virus-associated hemophagocytic syndrome from familial hemophagocytic lymphohistiocytosis. Rather, the virus may stimulate hemophagocytosis in genetically predisposed individuals. This mechanism of pathogenesis is also applicable to X-linked lymphoproliferative syndrome.[18,19] On the other hand, if hemophagocytic syndrome develops in seemingly immunocompetent adults after viral infection, an underlying immune deficiency should by sought, as virus alone may not be sufficient to cause the syndrome.[34]

Besides viral infections, cytokines also play an important role in the pathogenesis of hemophagocytosis.[17,18,32,33] This mechanism is especially important in familial erythrophagocytic lymphohistiocytosis, infection-associated hemophagocytic syndrome, and histiocytosis secondary to lymphoma. A virus or other infectious agent may activate T-lymphocytes, which, in turn, may release a lymphokine or macrophage-activating factor, resulting in histiocytosis. In patients with immunoregulatory deficiency, persistent, uncontrollable proliferation of histiocytes occurs.[18,35] Lymphomas may also release a lymphokine without a predisposing infection. Many cytokines have been incriminated in this process, including interleukin (IL)-1, IL-2, IL-6, soluble IL-2 receptor, interferon gamma(δ), and tumor necrosis factor.[17,28]

In terms of markers, almost all cases of lymphoma-related hemophagocytosis occur in T-cell lymphomas.[1-16] However, concomitant histiocytosis has also been reported in a few cases of B-cell lymphoma.[36] A pan-leukocyte marker (CD45) plus some selected T-cell (CD3, CD5, CD7) and B-cell (CD19, CD20) markers should be helpful to distinguish lymphoma cells from malignant histiocytes in which only T-cell markers are occasionally demonstrated (Table 17-2). Even in those cases, biphenotypic nature is suspected.[24]

As malignant histiocytosis is currently a rare disease, there are not many studies using monoclonal antibodies. In cytochemical studies, cases of malignant histiocytosis are positive for α-naphthyl butyrate esterase (or α-naphthyl acetate esterase with sodium fluoride inhibition), tartrate-sensitive acid phosphatase, and β-glucuronidase.[2,23] Immunocytochemical studies may demonstrate positive lysozyme, α-1 antitrypsin, α-1 antichymotrypsin, and peanut agglutinin. Receptors for complement, as well as Fc receptors for IgM and IgG, are also present.[2] For monoclonal antibodies, malignant histiocytes react to CD11b, CD11c, CD14, CD15, CD45, CD68, CD71, HLA-DR, and Mac 387.[2,23,24,37,38] They react to CD4 and S-100 variably.[2,23,37] Hsu et al. found that cases of malignant histiocytosis frequently expressed monocytic markers, such as CD11b, CD11c, and CD14, suggestive of monocytic or free histiocytic origin, while cases of true histiocytic lymphoma often expressed CD30, CD25, 2H9, and 1A2, similar to cases of Hodgkin's disease and Ki-positive lymphoma; thus they may arise from fixed histiocytes.[38]

In infection-associated and congenital hema-

TABLE 17.2
Comparison Between Histiocytic Disorders and T-Cell Lymphomas

	Malignant histiocytosis	Langerhans'–cell histiocytosis	Rosai–Dorfman disease	T-lymphomas
CD1	−	+	±	−
CD4	±	+	+	±
CD11c	+	+	+	−
CD14	+	+	+	−
CD25	−	+	+	±
CD30	−	−	−	±
CD68	+	−	+	−
S-100	−	+	+	−
Nonspecific esterase	+	−	ND[a]	+
Acid phosphatase	+	−	ND	+
Lysozyme	+	−	+	−
α-antitrypsin	+	−	+	−
α-antichymotrypsin	+	−	+	−

[a]ND = not done.

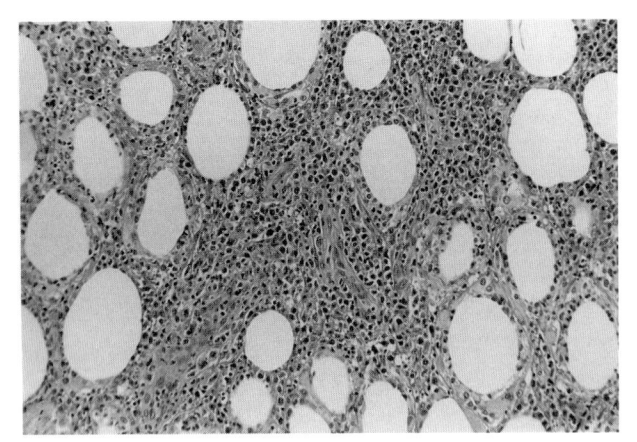

Fig. 17.18. A case of subcutaneous panniculitic T-cell lymphoma showing tumor-cell infiltrate of the adipose tissue. H&E, ×250. (Case contributed by Dr. I. J. Su.)

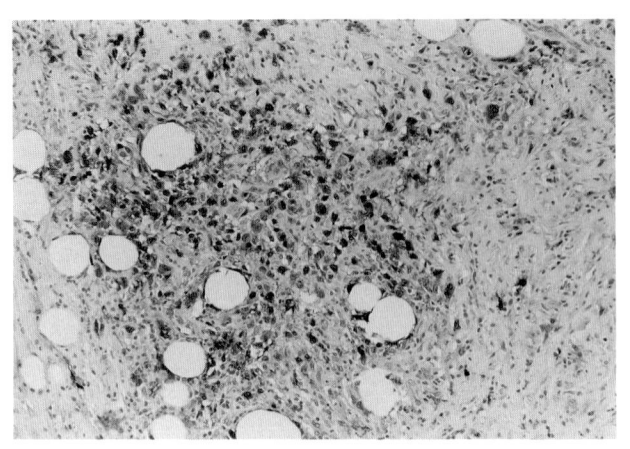

Fig. 17.20. A case of eosinophilic granuloma showing positive S-100 staining in Langerhans' cells. ×250.

tophagocytic syndromes, the histiocytes exhibit the phenotype of macrophages with negative reactions to S-100 protein and peanut agglutinin.[23]

In Langerhans' cell histiocytosis, the abnormal Langerhans' cells are characterized by their positive reactions to CD1 and S100 (Figs. 17.20–17.21).[2,23,37] Since CD1 is negative in other histiocytic lesions and S-100 is only occasionally positive in other similar conditions, the presence of these two markers is diagnostic for Langerhans' cell histiocytosis. Other markers that are positive in Langerhans' cell histiocytosis include CD4, CD11c, CD14, CD15, CD25, CD74, HLA-DR, and vimentin.[2] CD4, CD11, and CD14 are not expressed in normal Langerhans' cells.[2,23,37] Besides the above mentioned monoclonal antibodies, Langerhans' cells are also positive for ATPase, α-mannosidase, and peanut agglutinin.[23] Their reactions to CD13, CD33, and CD71 are variable.[37] The important negative markers in Langerhans' cell histiocytosis are CD30 and CD45 for distinction from lymphomas.[2] A recent study using X-linked polymorphic DNA probes has found Langerhans' cell histiocytosis a clonal proliferative disease.[39]

In Rosai–Dorfman disease, the histiocytes reacted to all 20 pan-macrophage antibodies in one study.[40] Among the more commonly used pan-macrophage antibodies are CD11b (Mo-1, OKM-1, Mac-1), CD14 (LeuM3, Mo-2), CD68 (EBM-11), Mac-387, and HAM 56.[23,37,40] These histiocytes also react to some macrophage-associated antibodies, such as CD11c

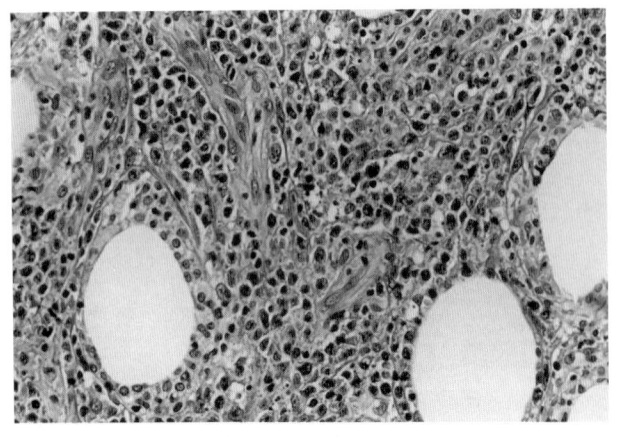

Fig. 17.19. Higher magnification of Fig. 17.18 showing tumor-cell infiltrate and focal necrosis. Hemophagocytosis is not shown in this field. H&E, ×500.

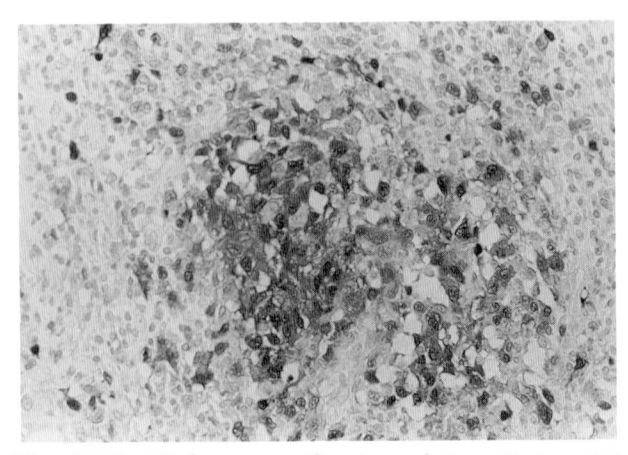

Fig. 17.21. Higher magnification of Fig. 17.20. ×500.

(LeuM5), CD15 (LeuM1), lysozyme, α_1-antitrypsin, and α_1-antichymotrypsin. In the study by Eisen et al.,[40] three CD1a antibodies were used: NA1-34 reacted to 2 of 2 cases; OKT6, to 1 of 2 cases; and Leu6, to none of 2 cases of Rosai-Dorfman disease. Although histiocytes in this entity react positively to S100, their variable reactivity to CD1a and the consistently negative reactions to several macrophage antibodies (CD68, Mac-387, lysozyme, α_1-antitrypsin, and α_1-antichymotrypsin) by Langerhans' cells distinguish Rosai-Dorfman disease from Langerhans'-cell histiocytosis.[23,40]

Histiocytes in Rosai-Dorfman disease also react to some lymphoid markers, including CD43 (Leu22), CDw75 (LN-1), and CD4 (Leu3). Their reactive to CD74 (LN-2) and CD45RO (UCHL-1) are variable,[40] and their reaction to L-26 (CD20) is consistently negative. These histiocytes are positive for several activation antigens: CD25 (IL2-R), CD30 (Ki-1, Berh2), and CD71 (transferrin receptor). According to Rosai's group, these histiocytes are functionally activated macrophages, perhaps recently derived from monocytes, although the etiology of this disease is still unknown.[40]

In summary, this group of histiocytosis are very similar clinically, and pathologically, and among the benign histiocytosis, they are also similar in pathogenesis. Distinction between these entities can be made only on a multiparameter basis. Lymphomas may mimic histiocytosis morphologically and clinically, but marker studies may help distinguish them easily. In controversial cases, the T-cell receptor gene analysis should be helpful, T-cell lymphomas are frequently positive, but histiocytosis is consistently negative in this analysis.

REFERENCES

1. Wilson MS, Weiss LM, Gatter KC, et al: Malignant histiocytosis: A reassessment of cases previously reported in 1975 based on paraffin section immunophenotyping studies. *Cancer* 66:530-536, 1990.
2. Ben-Ezra JM, Koo CH: Langerhans' cell histiocytosis and malignancies of the M-PIRE system. *Am J Clin Pathol* 99:464-471, 1993.
3. Kadin ME, Kamoun M, Lamberg J: Erythrophagocytic T-gamma lymphoma: A clinicopathologic entity resembling malignant histiocytosis. *N Engl J Med* 304:648-653, 1981.
4. Farcet JP, Gaulard P, Marolleau JP, et al: Hepatosplenic T-cell lymphoma: Sinusal/sinusoidal localization of malignant cells expressing the T-cell receptor $\gamma\delta$. *Blood* 75:2213-2219, 1990.
5. Sun T, Brody J, Susin M, et al: Extranodal T-cell lymphoma mimicking malignant histiocytosis. *Am J Hematol* 35:269-274, 1990.
6. Lin MT, Shen MC, Su IJ, et al: Peripheral T-gamma/delta lymphoma representing with idiopathic thrombocytopenic purpura-like picture. *Br J Haematol* 78:280-282, 1991.
7. Mastovich S, Ratech H, Ware RE, et al: Hepatosplenic T-cell lymphoma: An unusual case of a $\gamma\delta$ T-cell lymphoma with a blast-like terminal transformation. *Hum Pathol* 25:102-108, 1994.
8. Ng Cs, Chan JKC, Cheng PNM, et al: Nasal T-cell lymphoma associated with hemophagocytic syndrome. *Cancer* 58:67-71, 1986.
9. Kadokura N, Shinmyouzu K, Moritoyo H, et al: T-cell malignant lymphoma with hemophagocytic histiocytosis, hyperferritinemia and disseminated intravascular coagulation syndrome. *Jpn J Clin Hematol* 31:1826-1830, 1990.
10. Chubachi A, Hirokazu I, Nishimura S, et al: Nasal T-cell lymphoma associated with hemophagocytic syndrome: Immunohistochemical and genotypic studies. *Arch Pathol Lab Med* 116:1209-1212.
11. Kadin ME, Sako D, Berliner N, et al: Childhood Ki-1 lymphoma presenting with skin lesions and peripheral lymphoadenopathy. *Blood* 1042-1049, 1986.
12. Kinney MC, Greer JP, Glick AD, et al: Anaplastic large-cell Ki-1 malignant lymphomas. Recognition, biological and clinical implications. *Pathol Annu* 26 (pt 1): 1-24, 1991.
13. Craig FE, Clare CN, Sklar JL, et al: T-cell lymphoma and the virus-associated hemophagocytic syndrome. *Am J Clin Pathol* 97:189-194, 1992.
14. Isaacson PG, Spencer J, Connally CE, et al: Malignant histiocytosis of the intestine: A T-cell lymphoma. *Lancet* 2:688-691, 1985.
15. Loughran TP, Kadin ME, Diez HJ: T-cell intestinal lymphoma associated with celiac sprue. *Ann Intern Med* 104:44-50, 1986.
16. Gonzalez C, Medeiros L, Braziel R, et al: T-cell lymphoma involving subcutaneous tissue: A clinicopathologic entity commonly associated with hemophagocytic syndrome. *Am J Surg Pathol* 15:17-27, 1991.
17. Favara BE: Hemophagocytic lymphohistiocytosis: A hemophagocytic syndrome. *Semin Diagn Pathol* 9:63-74, 1992.
18. Woda BA, Sullivan JL: Reactive histiocytic disorders. *Am J Clin Pathol* 99:459-463, 1993.
19. Krishnan J, Danon AD, Frizzera G: Reactive lymphadenopathies and atypical lymphoproliferative disorders. *Am J Clin Pathol* 99:385-396, 1993.
20. Foucar E, Rosai J, Dorfman R: Sinus histiocytosis with massive lymphadenopathy (Rosai-Dorfman Disease): Review of the entity. *Semin Diagn Pathol* 7:19-73, 1990.
21. Cline MJ: Histiocytes and histiocytosis. *Blood* 84:2840-2853, 1994.

22. Ioachim HL: *Lymph Node Pathology*, 2nd ed, Philadelphia, Lippincott, 1994, pp 566–572.
23. Malone M: The histiocytosis of childhood. *Histopathology* 19:105–119, 1991.
24. Oka L, Mori N, Yatabe Y, et al: Malignant histiocytosis: A report of three cases. *Arch Pathol Lab Med* 116:1228–1233, 1992.
25. Lukes RJ, Collins RD: *Atlas of Tumor Pathology*, 2nd series: *Tumors of the Hematopoietic System*, Washington DC, Armed Forces Institute of Pathology, 1992, pp 316–400.
26. Swerdlow SH: *Biopsy Interpretation of Lymph Nodes*, New York, Raven Press, 1992, pp 347–351.
27. Ben-Ezra J, Bailey A, Azumi N, et al: Malignant histiocytosis X: A distinct clinicopathologic entity. *Cancer* 68:1050–1060, 1991.
28. Henter JI, Ehrnst A, Andersson J, et al: Familial hemophagocytic lymphohistiocytosis and viral infection. *Acta Paediatr* 82:369–372, 1993.
29. Wenig BM, Abbondanzo SL, Childers EL, et al: Extranodal sinus histiocytosis with massive lymphadenopathy (Rosai–Dorfman disease) of the head and neck. *Hum Pathol* 24:483–492, 1993.
30. Perrin C, Michiels JF, Lacour JP, et al: Sinus histiocytosis (Rosai–Dorfman disease) clinically limited to skin. *J Cutan Pathol* 20:368–374, 1993.
31. Su IJ, Hsu YH, Lin MT, et al: Epstein–Barr virus-containing T-cell lymphoma presents with hemophagocytic syndrome mimicking malignant histiocytosis. *Cancer* 72:2019–2027, 1993.
32. Jaffe ES, Costa J, Fauci AS, et al: Malignant lymphoma and erythrophagocytosis simulating malignant histiocytosis. *Am J Med* 75:741–749, 1983.
33. Simrell CR, Margolick JB, Grabtree GR, et al: Lymphokin-induced phagocytosis in angiocentric immunoproliferative lesions (AIL) and malignant lymphoma arising in AIL. *Blood* 65:1469–1476, 1985.
34. Gaffey MJ, Frierson HF Jr, Medeiros LJ, et al: The relationship of Epstein–Barr virus to infection-related (sporadic) and familial hemophagocytic syndrome and secondary (lymphoma-related) hemophagocytosis: An in situ hybridization study. *Hum Pathol* 24:657–667, 1993.
35. Bujan W, Schangene L, Ferster A, et al: Abnormal T-cell phenotype in familial erythrophagocytic lymphohistiocytosis. *Lancet* 342:1296, 1993.
36. Kuratsume H, Machii T, Aozasa K, et al: B-cell lymphoma showing clinicopathological features of malignant histiocytosis. *Acta Haematol* 79:94–98, 1988.
37. Jaffe ES: Histiocytosis and true histiocytic lymphoma. In Jaffe ES (ed): *Surgical Pathology of the Lymph Nodes and Related Organs*, 2nd ed, Philadelphia, Saunders, 1995, pp 560–593.
38. Hsu SM, Ho YS, Hsu PL: Lymphomas of true histiocytic origin. Expression of different phenotypes in so-called true histiocytic lymphoma and malignant histiocytosis. *Am J Pathol* 138:1389–1404, 1991.
39. Willman CL, Busque L, Griffith BB, et al: Langerhans' cell histiocytosis (Histiocytosis X)—a clonal proliferative disease. 331:154–160, 1994.
40. Eisen RN, Buckley PJ, Rosai J: Immunophenotypic characterization of sinus histiocytosis with massive lymphadenopathy (Rosai–Dorfman disease). *Semin Diagn Pathol* 7:74–82, 1990.

18
True Natural-Killer-Cell Lymphoma vs. Natural-Killer-Like T-Cell Lymphoma

Natural-killer (NK) cells are a group of lymphocytes which possess a distinct form of natural cytotoxicity that differs from the cell-mediated immunity associated with cytotoxic T-lymphocytes.[1] This natural cytotoxicity occurs without previous exposure to the target cells and is independent of major histocompatibility antigen expression by the target cells. Another function of the NK cells is antibody-dependent cellular cytotoxicity (ADCC), which is associated with a functional receptor for the Fc portion of IgG molecules, designated as CD16.

The NK-cell classification was controversial. Because it shares CD11b, CD11c, and CD16 antigens with myelomonocytic cells, some authors considered the NK cell to be of myeloid lineage.[2] However, it also carries variably many T-cell antigens, such as CD2, CD4, CD5, CD7, and CD8. Thus, most believed the NK cell to be a T-cell until it was separated from T-cells recently by the absence of CD3. The so-called CD3+ NK cell is now called NK-like T-cell, and the T-cells that are induced by IL-2 to express NK activity are referred to an *lymphokine-activated killer* (LAK) cells. However, T-cells and NK cells are ontogenically related, sharing the same progenitor cell.[3] The current definition of NK cells is restricted to CD56+, CD3-lymphocytes with neither rearrangement of T-cell receptor (TCR) genes nor expression of TCR heterodimers.[2]

Most NK cells assume the morphology of large granular lymphocytes (LGLs), which are larger than the small lymphocytes and smaller than monocytes (Fig. 18.1). Their characteristics are a high cytoplasmic:nuclear ratio and the presence of abundant azurophilic cytoplasmic granules, although more than 3 granules is sufficient to define a large granular lymphocytes.[4] However, NK markers may occasionally be demonstrated in cells other than large granular lymphocytes, and large granular lymphocytes do not invariably process NK activities.[1]

CLINICAL FEATURES

A wide spectrum of clinical manifestations has been demonstrated in large granular lymphoproliferative disorders. This was particularly obvious in the early literature when NK cells and NK-like T-cells were not clearly separated. There are at least four clinical types (Table 18.1).[5] The most frequently encountered type is that of chronic lymphocytic leukemia (CLL), which is often referred to as *large granular lymphoproliferative disorder* and is held accountable for most cases reported in the literature. This group of patients usually have a chronic indolent course,[6] although most patients may eventually require treatment.[7] The most constant findings in these cases are neutropenia and relative large granular lymphocytosis with positive NK-cell markers.[6] Immunophenotyping, however, usually indicates a NK-like T-cell phenotype (T-LGL leukemia).[6,7] This group of patients frequently have spenomegaly and rheumatoid arthritis but not lymphadenopathy. The presence of rheumatoid factor, antinuclear antibodies, and antineutrophil and/or antiplatelet antibodies is often reported but is not a constant feature in certain phenotypes.[6] This type of leukemia usually has a good prognosis. Death is often caused by recurrent infections secondary to neutropenia.

On the other hand, the true NK-cell leukemia or NK-LGL leukemia usually has an acute clinical course, which can be classified into the acute lymphocytic leukemia category.[7] This category may also include some overt cases of acute lymphoblastic leukemia, the tumor cells of which may or may not contain cytoplasmic granules.[8,9]

The third category, lymphoma of LGL, is a heterogeneous group consisting of either NK cells or NK-like T-cells.[10] Most of the cases have an aggressive clinical course. Those LGL lymphomas with a NK-cell phenotype usually have a leukemic phase; thus, Imamura et al. coined this entity as "aggressive natural-killer-cell leukemia/lymphoma".[11] This group of patients frequently have fever, hepatosplenomegaly, lymphadenopathy, and bone marrow involvement.[10] All patients died within a few months except for a few who had a chronic course preceding the acute one.[10]

Finally, lymphoblasts with NK markers can be demonstrated in chronic myelogenous leukemia (CML) with blast crisis.[12] Warzynski et al. emphasized that because of morphologic resemblance, LGL in CML might have been mistaken as basophils or mast cells; thus, this entity could have been underreported.[12]

It has been suggested that patients from Asia have

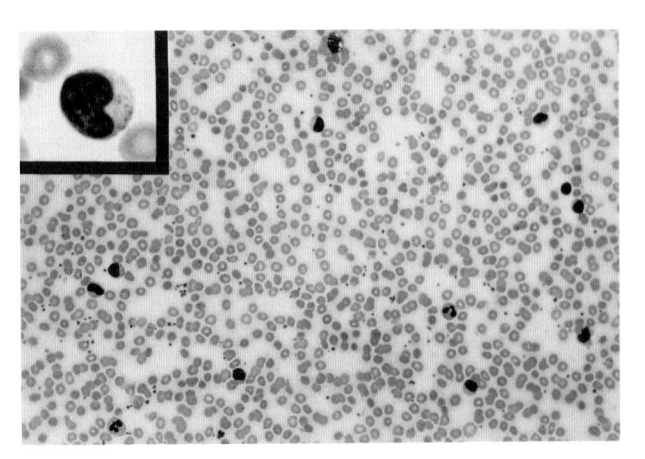

Fig. 18.1. Peripheral blood smear from a case of large granular lymphoproliferative disorder showing multiple large granular lymphocytes. Wright–Giemsa, ×125. (*Inset*: a large granular lymphocyte with abundant granular cytoplasm, ×1250.) (From Sun T et al: *Am J Hematol* 37:173–178, 1991.)

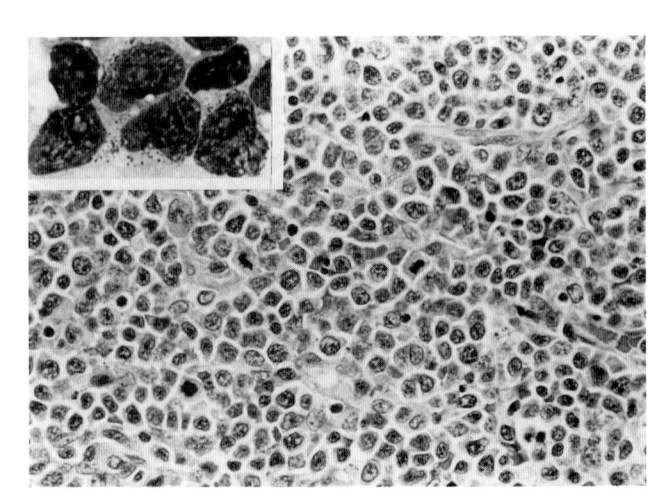

Fig. 18.2. Lymph node biopsy of natural-killer-cell lymphoma showing large lymphoma cells. H&E, ×500. (*Inset*: tissue imprint from lymph node showing azurophilic granules in the cytoplasm of lymphoma cells. H&E, ×1250. (From Sun T et al: *Am J Hematol* 40:135–145, 1992.)

more clinical manifestations and severe clinical symptoms than do those seen in the West; these differences may be contributed by environmental factors, such as viral infections.[13,14] In fact, Epstein–Barr virus DNA has been isolated from NK lymphomas in Hong Kong.[15]

Large granular lymphocytosis can also be reactive.

TABLE 18.1
Classification of Large Granular Lymphoproliferative Disorder

Category	Major phenotype
Primary or neoplastic	
Chronic lymphocytic leukemia type	NK-like T-cell
Acute lymphocytic leukemia type	NK cell
Lymphoma type	NK cell, NK-like T-cell
Chronic myelogenous leukemia with blast crisis	NK cell
Secondary or reactive	
Viral infections (e.g., HIV, HTLV-I)	NK cell, NK-like T-cell
Neoplastic diseases	NK cell, NK-like T-cell
Rheumatoid arthritis	NK cell, NK-like T-cell
Postsplenectomy	NK cell
Chronic infections (e.g., tuberculosis, hepatitis)	NK cell, NK-like T-cell
Nephrotic syndrome	NK cell
Others	

It has been demonstrated in viral infections (e.g., HIV, HTLV-I), neoplastic diseases, rheumatoid arthritis, postsplenectomy, chronic infections (e.g., tuberculosis, hepatitis), nephrotic syndrome and others.[5]

PATHOLOGY

Lymphoma of LGL may assume many different histologic patterns, varying from well-differentiated small-cell, small-cleaved-cell, large-cell, immunoblastic, lymphoblastic, to mixed small-/large-cell lymphomas (Fig. 18.2).[5,10,16–26] Therefore, a diagnosis of LGL lymphoma cannot be made histologically. In lymphoma patients with an acute clinical course showing fever, splenomegaly, and/or a leukemic phase, tissue imprints (Fig. 18.3), bone marrow (Fig. 18.4), or peripheral blood (Fig. 18.5) smears stained with Wright–Giemsa should be examined for cytoplasmic granules. Alternatively, electron microscopy may demonstrate the cytoplasmic granules as a structure with parallel tubular arrays (Fig. 18.6). However, one study shows that this structure is demonstrated in NK-like T-cells but not NK cells.[27] Furthermore, a few cases of NK-cell or NK-like T-cell lymphomas showed no cytoplasmic granules in tumor cells[13,28] Nevertheless, when cytoplasmic granules are detected, immunophenotyping and TCR gene analysis should be performed to confirm the diagnosis.

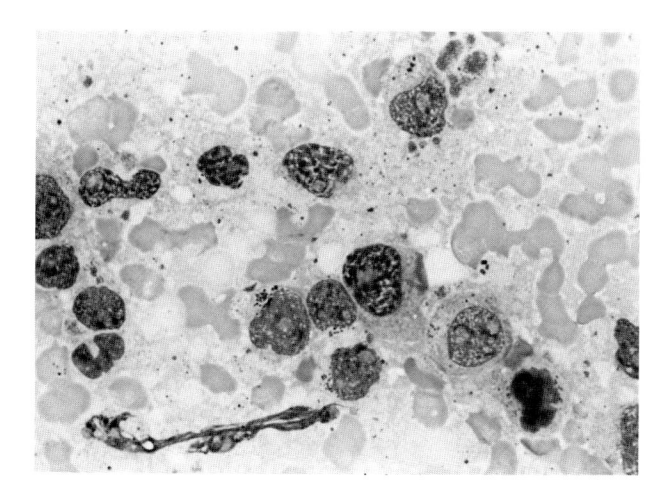

Fig. 18.3. Splenic imprint of NK-cell lymphoma showing lymphoma cells with cytoplasmic granules. Wright–Giemsa, ×1250. (Courtesy of Dr. Judith Brody.)

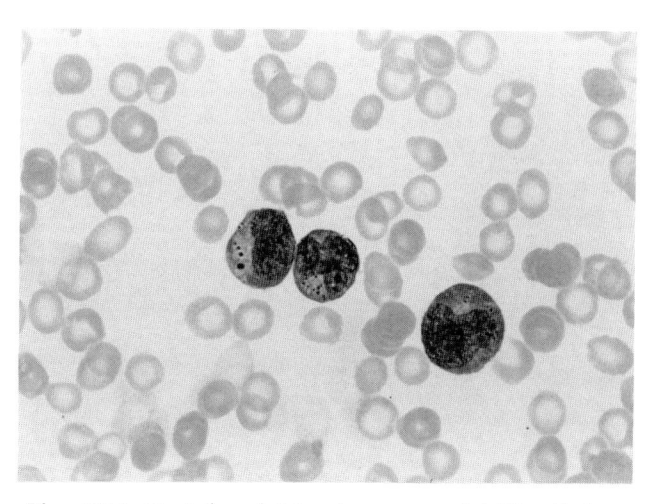

Fig. 18.5. Peripheral blood smear of NK-cell lymphoma showing three lymphoma cells with cytoplasmic granules. Wright–Giemsa, ×1250. (Courtesy of Dr. Judith Brody.)

Lymphoma of LGL is frequently seen in nasal/paranasal tumors in patients from Hong Kong.[21,25] In a study of lymphoblastic lymphomas, 6 out of 36 (17%) carried NK antigens (CD16 and/or CD57).[19] A study of 7 cases of CD8+ immunoblastic lymphoma showed CD57+ in 3 cases.[18] Bone marrow (Fig. 18.7), spleen (Fig. 18.8), liver (Fig. 18.9), and skin are frequently involved by LGL lymphoma, regardless of the phenotype. Gastrointestinal (GI) tract, lung, brain, kidney, and testis (Fig. 18.10) are also involved in a lower frequency.[10] Kern et al. suggested that since

CD56 is a neural-cell adhesion molecule; it may be associated with tumor dissemination to unusual sites, especially the central nervous system (CNS).[26]

LABORATORY FINDINGS

A definitive diagnosis of NK-cell and NK-like T-cell lymphomas depends on immunophenotyping and

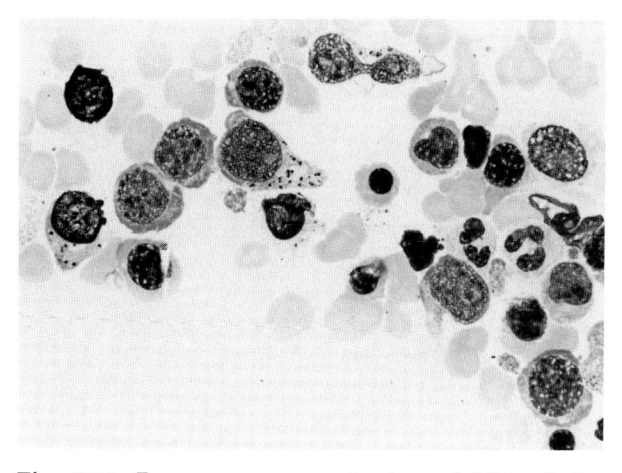

Fig. 18.4. Bone marrow aspiration of NK-cell lymphoma showing cytoplasmic granules in lymphoma cells. Wright–Giemsa, ×1250. (Courtesy of Dr. Judith Brody.)

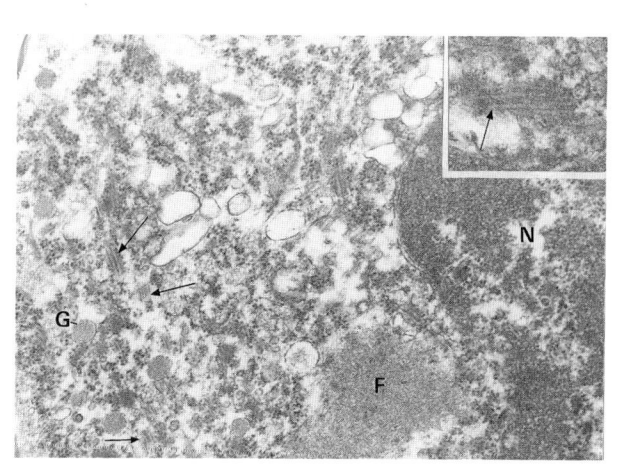

Fig. 18.6. Electron micrograph of lymph node from NK-cell lymphoma case showing bundles of parallel tubular arrays (arrows) in the cytoplasm of a tumor cell (G = membrane-bound granule; F = a filament bundle; N = nucleus). ×43,500. [*Inset:* higher magnification of the parallel tubular arrays (arrow), ×78,300.] (From Sun T et al: *Am J Clin Pathol* 40:135–145, 1992.)

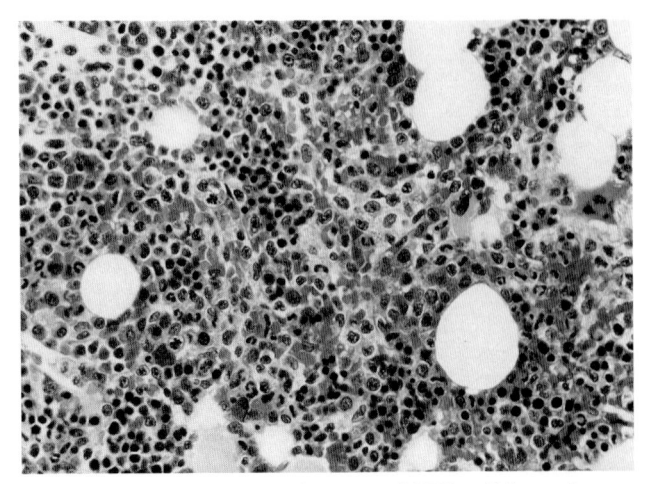

178 DIFFERENTIAL DIAGNOSIS OF LYMPHOID DISORDERS

Fig. 18.7. Bone marrow biopsy of NK-cell lymphoma showing interstitial infiltration by large lymphoma cells. H&E, ×500. (Courtesy of Dr. Judith Brody.)

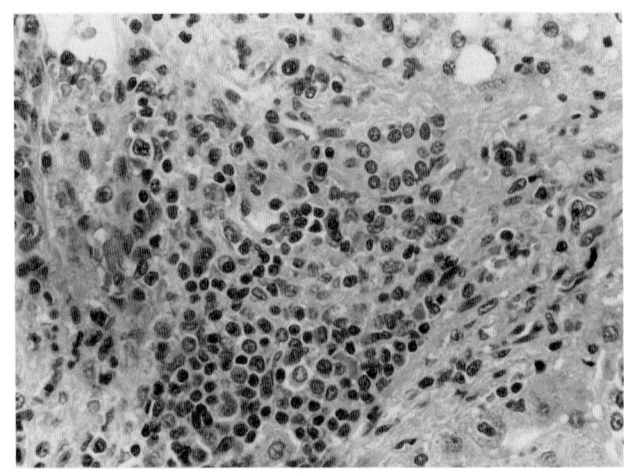

Fig. 18.9. Liver of NK-cell lymphoma showing large-lymphoma-cell infiltration of portal area. (B = bile duct).

genotyping. As mentioned before, the minimal requirement of identifying NK cells is CD3−, CD56+, and TCR− and absence of TCR gene rearrangement (Table 18.2). The fetal NK cells may express cytoplasmic CD3, which is demonstrated in some cases of NK lymphomas.[29] Nk-like T-cells, on the other hand, are defined as CD3+ NK antigen+ TCR+ with rearrangement of TCR genes. Although several monoclonal antibodies react consistently with NK cells, only those reacting to CD16, CD56, and CD57 are considered specific for NK cells. CD16 is usually expressed in both NK cells and NK-like T-cells. CD56 is consistently present on NK cells but is uncommon on NK-like T-cells.[7] CD57 is frequently demonstrated on NK-like T-cells but rarely on NK cells.[7]

In addition to NK markers, T-cell markers are also frequently expressed on these two groups of cells; CD2 and CD7 are the most consistent findings.[2] T-suppressor type (CD8+) is more frequently seen than T-helper type (CD4+), but CD4+, CD8+; CD4+, CD8−; and CD4−, CD8− phenotypes are encountered infrequently.[1,7] CD5 is also demonstrated occasionally on these two groups of cells. For myeloid

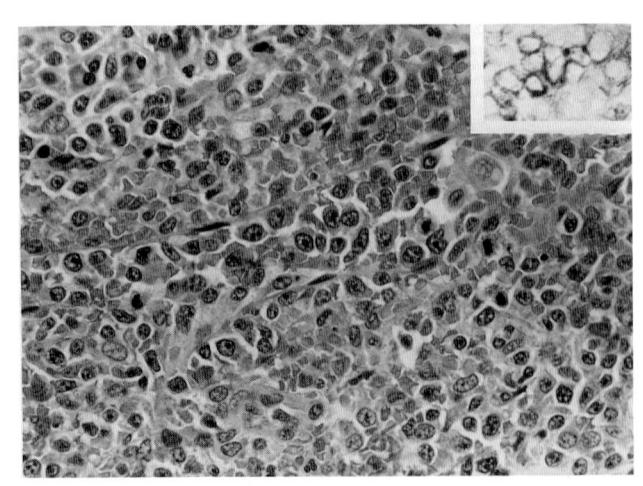

Fig. 18.8. Spleen of NK-cell lymphoma showing large-lymphoma-cell infiltration in the sinuses and cord of red pulp. H&E, ×500. (*Inset*: CD56-stain-positive lymphoma cells; immunoperoxidase, ×500.

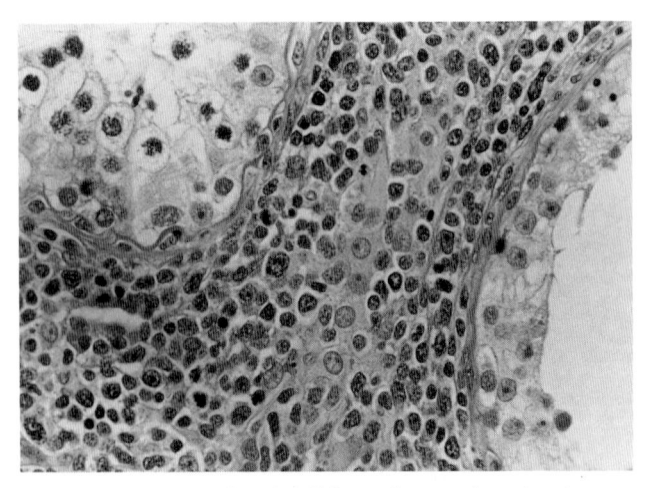

Fig. 18.10. Testis of NK-cell lymphoma showing interstitial infiltrate of lymphoma cells between seminiferous tubules. H&E, ×500.

TABLE 18.2
Differences between NK Cells
and NK-Like T-Cells

	NK-cells	NK-like T-cells
CD3	−	+
cCD3	+	±
TCR	−	+
TCR gene rearrangement	−	+
CD56	+	±
CD57	±	+
CD16	+	+
Clinical types	Acute leukemia, lymphoma, reactive	Chronic leukemia, lymphoma, reactive

Abbreviations: TCR = T-cell receptor, cCD3 = cytoplasmic CD3.

antigens, CD11b and CD11c are present on 80–90% and 30–60% of LGL cells, respectively.[2]

An intriguing question is whether markers are helpful in identifying the aggressive nature of this tumor. Kern et al. and Wong et al. suggested that CD56, a neural-cell adhesion molecule, may contribute to the poor prognosis.[25,26] This assumption is supported by a few recent case reports.[13,3] McDaniel et al. suggested that the absence of CD57 may predict the aggressive behavior of the tumor.[31] Most authors agreed that the activation antigens, such as HLA-DR, CD25, CD38, and proliferation-associated antigen ki-67, may be associated with poor prognosis.[11,22,32]

However, increase of NK cells does not indicate a lymphoproliferative disorder. The minimal requirements for the diagnosis of a primary large granular lymphocytosis are the presence of >2000/μL of large granular lymphocytes in the peripheral blood for more than 6 months, and all possible causes, as listed in Table 18.1, for reactive lymphocytosis should be excluded.[4] Obviously, these criteria are not applicable to lymphomas without a leukemic phase. The second step is to determine whether there is clonal proliferation by TCR gene rearrangement analysis. In most cases of NK–T-cell proliferative disorder, TCRβ gene rearrangement is identified. When the phenotype is CD3+, CD4−, and CD8−, the genotype is TCRδ indicating that proliferation takes place at a more primitive stage.[33,34] For lymphoma of NK-cell origin, the pleomorphic morphology of the tumor cells usually gives a clue to its clonal nature. Otherwise, a sex-linked DNA analysis should be performed to determine the clonality.[35]

REFERENCES

1. Richard SJ, Scott CS: Human NK cells in health and disease: Clinical, functional, phenotypic and DNA genotypic characteristics. *Leuk Lymphoma* 7:377–399, 1992.
2. Robertson MJ, Ritz J: Biology and clinical relevance of human natural killer cells. *Blood* 76:2421–2438, 1990.
3. Lanier LL, Spits H, Phillips JH: The developmental relationship between NK cells and T cells. *Immunol Today* 13:392–395, 1992.
4. Oshimi K: Granular lymphocyte proliferative disorders: Report of 12 cases and review of the literature. *Leukemia* 2:617–627, 1988.
5. Sun T, Schulman P, Kolitz J, et al: A study of lymphoma of large granular lymphocytes with modern modalities: Report of two cases and review of the literature. *Am J Hematol* 40:135–145, 1992.
6. Sun T, Brody J, Koduru P, et al: Study of the major phenotype of large granular T-cell lymphoproliferative disorder. *Am J Clin Pathol* 98:516–521, 1992.
7. Loughran TP Jr: Clonal diseases of large granular lymphocytes. *Blood* 82:1–14, 1993.
8. Kaplan J, Ravindranath Y, Inone S: T-cell acute lymphoblastic leukemia with natural killer cell phenotype. *Am J Hematol* 22:355–364, 1986.
9. Pirruccello SJ, Bicak MS, Gordon BG, et al: Acute lymphoblastic leukemia of NK-cell lineage: Response to IL-2. *Leuk Res* 13:735–743, 1989.
10. Sun T, Brody J, Susin M, et al: Aggressive natural killer cell lymphoma/leukemia: A recently recognized clinicopathologic entity. *Am J Surg Pathol* 17:1289–1299, 1993.
11. Imamura N, Kusunoki Y, Kawa-Ha K, et al: Aggressive natural killer cell leukemia/lymphoma: Report of four cases and review of the literature. *Br J Haematol* 75:49–59, 1990.
12. Warzynski J, White C, Golightly R, et al: Natural killer lymphocyte blast crisis of chronic myelogenous leukemia. *Am J Hematol* 32:279–286, 1989.
13. Abenoza P, Parkin J. Bowers S, et al: Lymphoproliferative process with natural killer cell phenotype: Histopathologic, ultrastructural and surface marker observations. *Arch Pathol Lab Med* 117:851–855, 1993.
14. Kwong YL, Wong KF, Chan LC, et al: Large granular lymphocyte leukemia: A study of nine cases in a Chinese population. *Am J Clin Pathol* 103:76–81, 1995.
15. Ho FCS, Srivastava G, Loke SL, et al: Presence of Epstein–Barr virus DNA in nasal lymphomas of B and T-cell type. *Hematol Oncol* 8:271–281, 1990.
16. Pandolfi F, Pezzuto A, DeRossi G, et al: Characterization of two patients with lymphomas of large granular lymphocytes. *Cancer* 53:445–452, 1984.
17. Swerdlow SH, Habeshaw JA, Richards MA, et al: T-lymphoblastic lymphoma with Leu 7 positive phenotype and unusual clinical course: A multiparameter study. *Leuk Res* 9:167–173, 1985.

18. Wantanabe S, Sato Y, Shimoyama M, et al: Immunoblastic lymphadenopathy, angioimmunoblastic lymphadenopathy and IBL-like T-cell lymphoma: A spectrum of T-cell neoplasia. *Cancer* 58:2224–2232, 1986.
19. Sheibani K, Nathwani BN, Winberg CD, et al: Antigenically defined subgroups of lymphoblastic lymphoma: Relationship to clinical presentation and biologic behavior. *Cancer* 60:183–190, 1987.
20. Sheibani K, Winberg CD, Burke JS, et al: Lymphoblastic lymphoma expressing natural killer cell-associated antigens: A clinicopathologic study of six cases. *Leuk Res* 11:371–377, 1987.
21. Ng CS, Chan JKC, Lo STH: Expression of natural killer cell markers in non-Hodgkin's lymphomas. *Hum Pathol* 18:1257–1262, 1987.
22. Kanavaros P, Lavergne A, Galian A, et al: A primary immunoblastic T malignant lymphoma of the small bowel with azurophilic intracytoplasmic granules. *Am J Surg Pathol* 12:641–647, 1988.
23. Berceanu S, Roman S, Butoianu E, et al: A particular case of large granular lymphocytic lymphoma. *Haematologia* 22:43–53, 1989.
24. Longacre TA, Listrom MB, Spigel JH, et al: Aggressive jejunal lymphoma of large granular lymphocytes. *Am J Clin Pathol* 93:124–132, 1990.
25. Wong KF, Chan JKC, Ng CS, et al: CD56 (NKH-1) positive hematolymphoid malignancies. *Hum Pathol* 23:798–804, 1992.
26. Kern WF, Spier CM, Hanneman EH, et al: Neural cell adhesion molecule-positive peripheral T-cell lymphomas: A rare variant with a propensity for unusual sites of involvement. *Blood* 79:2432–2437.
27. Prasthofer EF, Barton JC, Zarcone D, et al: Ultrastructural morphology of granular lymphocytes (GL) from patients with immunophenotypically homogeneous expansions of GC populations (GLE). *J Submicrosc Cytol* 19:345–354, 1987.
28. Bassan R, Introna M, Rambaldi A, et al: Large granular lymphocyte/natural killer cell proliferative disease: Clinical and laboratory heterogeneity. *Scand J Haematol* 37:91–96, 1986.
29. Suzumiya J, Takeshit M, Kimura N, et al: Expression of adult and fetal natural killer cell markers in sinonasal lymphomas. *Blood* 83:2255–2260, 1994.
30. Gentile TC, Uner AH, Hutchinson RE, et al: CD3+, CD56+ aggressive variant of large granular lymphocyte leukemia. *Blood* 84:2315–2321, 1994.
31. McDaniel HL, MacPheron BR, Tindle BH, et al: Lymphoproliferative disorder of granular lymphocytes. *Arch Pathol Lab Med* 116:242–248, 1992.
32. Chan WC, Gu LB, Masih A, et al: Large granular lymphocyte proliferation with the natural killer cell phenotype. *Am J Clin Pathol* 97:353–358, 1992.
33. Sun T, Cohen NS, Marino J, et al: CD3+ CD4− CD8− large granular T-cell lymphoproliferative disorder. *Am J Hematol* 37:173–178, 1991.
34. Vie H, Chevalier S, Garand R, et al: Clonal expansion of lymphocytes bearing the γδ T-cell receptor in a patient with large granular lymphocyte disorder. *Blood* 74:285–290, 1989.
35. Tefferi A, Greipp PR, Thibodeau S: Demonstration of clonality by X-linked DNA analysis in chronic natural killer cell lymphocytosis and successful therapy with oral cyclophosphamide. *Leukemia* 6:477–480, 1992.

19
Mycosis Fungoides/Sézary Syndrome vs. Adult T-Cell Leukemia/Lymphoma

Cutaneous lymphoid tumors are often secondary to an extracutaneous primary lymphoma, and rarely, primary skin tumors. When mycosis fungoides/Sézary syndrome (MF/SS) is excluded, the frequency of primary cutaneous lymphomas represents about 5% of all cutaneous lymphomas.[1] There is great variation in the histologic patterns of cutaneous lymphomas.[1,2] A study of 52 cases of primary cutaneous lymphomas, excluding MF/SS, showed that 21% of cases were high-grade lymphomas, 58% intermediate-grade, and 21% low-grade, as classified by the Working Formulation.[1] In the same study, 73% were of B-cell lineage, 25% T-cell, and 2% non-T non-B cell origin. In a combined study of both primary and secondary cutaneous lymphomas, however, the majority of cases belong to the T-cell lineage.[2] Among the cutaneous T-cell lymphomas, there are two distinct groups: MF/SS and adult T-cell leukemia/lymphoma (ATCL). The remaining cases are other types of peripheral T-cell lymphomas and very rarely, lymphoblastic lymphomas.

CLINICAL FEATURES

MF/SS

MF is a special type of peripheral T-cell lymphoma presenting with an orderly progression from stages of patch, plaque, and tumor formation. SS is characterized by the presence of erythroderma, lymphadenopathy, and atypical lymphocytes (Sézary cells) in the peripheral blood. However, MF may have an erythrodermatous variant, lymphadenopathy, and small numbers of circulating tumor cells, which are indistinguishable from Sézary cells.[2] Therefore, the distinction between MF and SS is sometimes blurred, and these two entities will be discussed together.

The incidence of MF/SS has increased in recent years and up to 1000 new cases are seen in the United States annually.[3] The average age of patients at presentation is about 50 years, and the male:female ratio is 2.2:1. Although the etiology of MF/SS is still unknown, a retroviral cause has been suggested. HTLV-1 is usually associated with adult T-cell leukemia/lymphoma, but its antibodies have also been detected in a few cases of MF/SS.[4,5] HTLV-1-like retroviral particles have been detected by electron microscopy in cultured lymphocytes from 18 HTLV-1 seronegative patients with MF/SS.[6] Partially deleted HTLV-1 DNA sequences have been found integrated in cell lines from MF patients.[7] A more recent study discovered deleted viral sequences of both HTLV-I and HTLV-II in the mononuclear leukocytes from patients with MF.[8] In addition, a new human retrovirus, HTLV-V, has been isolated from an MF/SS case.[9]

The clinical course of SS/MF is insidious. Cutaneous lesion is the earliest clinical manifestation, progressing from patch to plaque and finally tumor stage. Nodal and visceral involvement are usually present in the later stages. However, lymphadenopathy is found in about 60% of patients at presentation.[10] In autopsy series, extracutaneous involvement by MF/SS can be as high as 71–100%.[11] The leukemic phase appears in 12% of patients in the plaque stage, 16% in the tumor stage, and 100% in patients with generalized erythroderma.[12] When peripheral blood is involved, about 50% of patients have lymphadenopathy.[12] Infection is still the major cause of death.

A study of the National Cancer Institute identified three prognostic groups.[12] The low-risk group has a median survival exceeding 12 years, including patients with plaque-only skin disease but no lymph node, blood, or visceral involvement. The intermediate group has a median survival of about 5 years, including those with skin plaque, tumor, or erythroderma disease and lymph node or blood involvement but no visceral disease. The high-risk group has a median survival of only 2.5 years, including those with visceral involvement or complete effacement of lymph node by tumor cells. Alternatively, a TNM (tumor, lymph node, and metastases) staging system can be used to evaluate the patient's prognosis (Table 19.1).[2,10,12]

ATCL

The first cases of ATCL were reported from southwestern Japan.[13] Subsequently, patients with similar symptoms were reported from the Caribbean Basin, western Africa, and the southeastern United States.

TABLE 19.1
TNM Staging System for Cutaneous T-Cell Lymphomas

T (tumor)
  T_0: clinically or histopathologically suspicious lesions
  T_1: cutaneous patches and/or plaques covering <10% of body surface
  T_2: generalized patches and/or plaques covering >10% of body surface
  T_3: one or more cutaneous tumor nodules
  T_4: generalized erythroderma
N (lymph node)
  N_0: lymph nodes clinically normal and histologically negative for tumor cells
  N_1: lymph nodes clinically enlarged but histologically negative
  N_2: lymph nodes clinically normal but histologically positive
  N_3: lymph nodes clinically enlarged and histologically positive
M (metastases, visceral organs)
  M_0: no visceral organ involvement
  M_1: visceral involvement present
PB (peripheral blood)
  PB_0: atypical circulating cells not present (≤5%)
  PB_1: atypical circulating cells present (>5%)
Staging
  Ia: T_1, N_0, M_0, PB_0
  Ib: T_2, N_0, M_0, PB_0
  IIa: T_{1-2}, N_1, M_0, PB_0
  IIb: T_3, N_{0-1}, M_0, PB_0
  IIIa: T_4, N_0, M_0, PB_0
  IIIb: T_4, N_1, M_0, PB_0
  IVa: $T_{1-4}, N_{2-3}, M_0, PB_0$
  IVb: $T_{1-4}, N_{0-3}, M_1, PB_1$

Modified from references 2, 9, and 11.

Currently, ATCL has been found in the European continent, Hawaii, and Taiwan.[14,15] The circumscribed geographic distribution of the Japanese patients in southwestern Japan raised the question of a viral cause, which was later proved to be a retrovirus, human T-cell leukemia/lymphoma virus 1 (HTLV-1) by seroepidemiologic study and molecular biologic techniques. The viral genome of HLTV-1 is integrated into the nuclear DNA sequence of the host cells, which can be detected by the Southern blotting technique.[16]

The clinical course of ATCL may evolve through several stages: preleukemic, smoldering, chronic, and subacute/acute.[14] In the preleukemic stage, patients are asymptomatic with no organ involvement except for occasional bone marrow infiltrate. A diagnosis is usually made by the incidental finding of peripheral atypical lymphocytosis, which is further confirmed by serologic or genotypic evidence of HTLV-1 infection. About half of the preleukemic patients recovered spontaneously and the remaining half progressed to other stages.

When ATCL becomes clinically evident, it can be divided into four clinical subtypes. In addition to the three temporally related stages (smoldering, chronic, and acute), an independent lymphoma subtype is recognized. The differential criteria include multiple clinical and laboratory parameters (Table 19.2).[15,17,18] The characteristic clinical features in ATCL, such as peripheral lymphocytosis with atypical lymphocytes, skin lesions, lymphadenopathy, and hepatosplenomegaly, are usually demonstrated in the acute subtype. Hypercalcemia, one of the pathognomonic features of ATCL, is also seen only in the acute stage because of osteolytic bone lesions. The polylobated lymphocytes (flower cells) are frequently demonstrated in the acute stage, but are seldom seen in other subtypes. However, atypical T-lymphocytes with various morphology can be demonstrated in other subtypes. The lymphoma subtype generally shows only a few ATCL features, and a leukemic phase is demonstrated only in a later stage.[13] The smoldering subtype may manifest as long-lasting cutaneous lesions, pulmonary infiltration of small lymphocytes, or peripheral lymphocytosis with low percentage of atypical lymphocytes.[13] Disseminated lesions are most frequently seen in the lungs, the CNS, and the GI tract. However, dissemination is seldom found in the smoldering and chronic subtypes.

PATHOLOGY

MF/SS

As mentioned above, the skin lesions in MF/SS may show patch, plaque, tumor, or erythroderma forms; the last form is most frequently seen in SS. A patch lesion may reveal scanty to patchy lymphocytic infiltration in the upper dermis. It is usually perivascular rather than band-like. Intraepidermal lymphoid infiltrates or Pautrier abscesses are rare or absent. Cytologic atypia, if present, is minimal. The plaque lesion is characterized by a dense band-like infiltrate of atypical lymphoid cells in the upper dermis (Fig. 19.1). Pautrier microabscesses are often present (Figs. 19.2, 19.3). The atypical lymphoid cells show hyper-

TABLE 19.2
Clinical and Laboratory Findings in Various Clinical Subtypes of ATCL

	Smoldering	Chronic	Lymphoma	Acute
Anti-HTLV antibody	+	+	+	+
Peripheral lymphocytosis (× 10/L)	<4	≥4	<	≥4
Abnormal T-lymphocytes (%)	≥5	≥5	≤1	≥5
Polylobated lymphocytes	Rare	Rare	None	Frequent
Bone marrow infiltrate	−	+	−	+
Lymphadenopathy	−	+	+	+
Skin lesions	+	+	+	+
Hepatomegaly	−	+	±	+
Splenomegaly	−	+	±	−
Lytic bone lesions	−	−	−	+
Pulmonary lesions	−	−	±	+
CNS lesions	−	−	±	±
GI-tract lesions	−	−	±	±
Hypercalcemia	−	−	−	+
Elevated lactate dehydrogenase	±	+	+	+
Elevated alkaline phosphatase	−	−	−	+
Hypoproteinemia	−	−	±	±
Hyperbilirubinemia	−	−	−	±
Anemia	−	±	±	−
Thrombocytopenia	−	−	−	±
Eosinophilia	−	±	−	±

From Sun T: *Color Atlas/Text of Flow Cytometric Analysis of Hematologic Neoplasms*, New York, Igaku-Shoin, 1993.

chromatic and convoluted nuclei and scant cytoplasm. The deep dermis and subcutis are seldom involved. The tumor lesion, on the other hand, shows a dense infiltrate of atypical lymphoid cells that may extend into the lower dermis and subcutis. The erythrodermatous lesions seen in SS reveal a dense infiltrate of Sézary cells, mixed with normal lymphocytes, eosinophils, plasma cells, and fibroblasts, in the upper dermis. Pautrier microabscesses may be present. The Sézary cells are characterized by their highly convoluted (cerebriform) nuclei (Figs. 19.4, 19.5). In equivocal cases, ultrastructural morphometric measurement

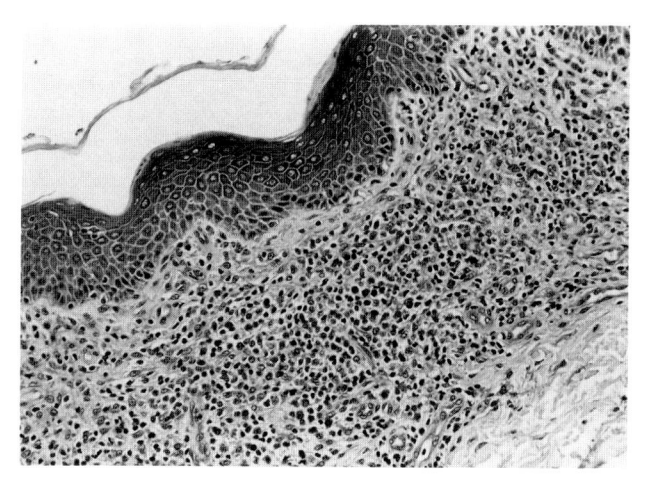

Fig. 19.1. The plaque lesion in mycosis fungoides showing a dense band-like infiltration of atypical lymphoid cells in the upper dermis. H&E, ×250.

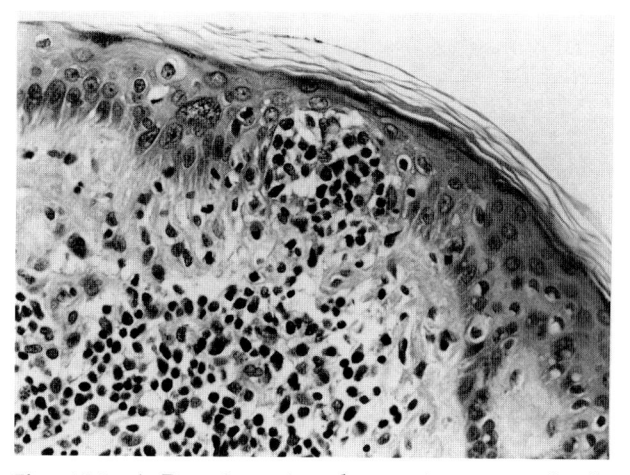

Fig. 19.2. A Pautrier microabscess is present in the epidermis from a case of mycosis fungoides. H&E, ×500.

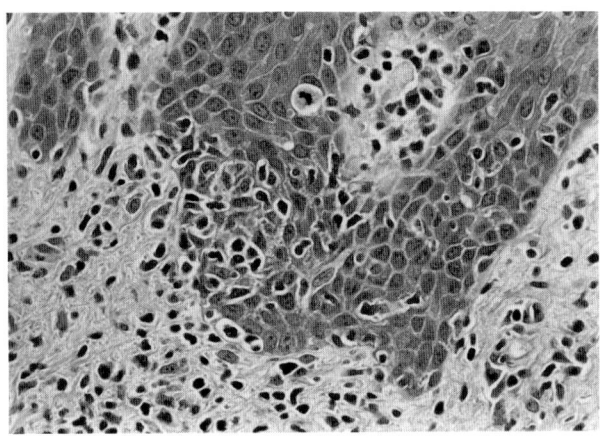

Fig. 19.3. Neoplastic infiltration of the epidermis from a case of B-cell lymphoma mimicking Pautrier microabscess. H&E, ×500.

of the nuclear size and shape (Fig. 19.6), chromatin distribution, and nuclear/cytoplasmic ratio are helpful in differential diagnosis.[19]

After studying 222 cases of MF/SS, Shapiro and Pinto found that there was a broad histologic spectrum of MF/SS, covering practically all patterns described for inflammatory skin disease.[20] These authors suggest that the most helpful diagnostic clues are "Pautrier's microabscesses, epidermotropism with slight or no spongiosis, lining up of lymphocytes along the basal layer, a lichenoid infiltrate that spares the dermal–epidermal junction and the clear presence of lymphocytes that are slightly large and hyperconvoluted."[20]

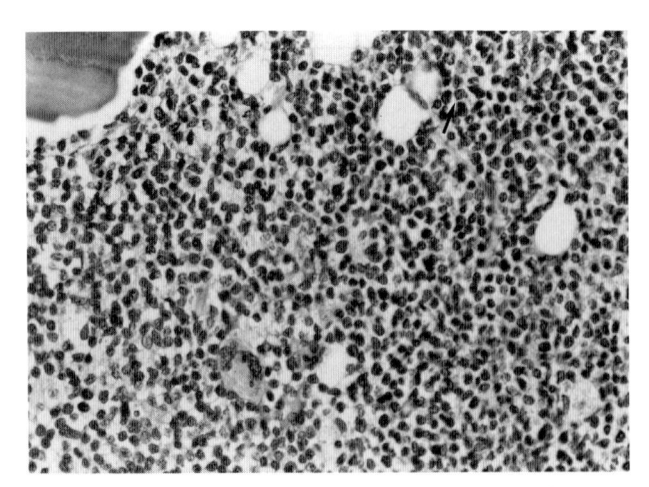

Fig. 19.4. Bone marrow biopsy from a case of Sézary syndrome showing cerebriform nuclei in many Sézary cells (arrow). H&E, ×500.

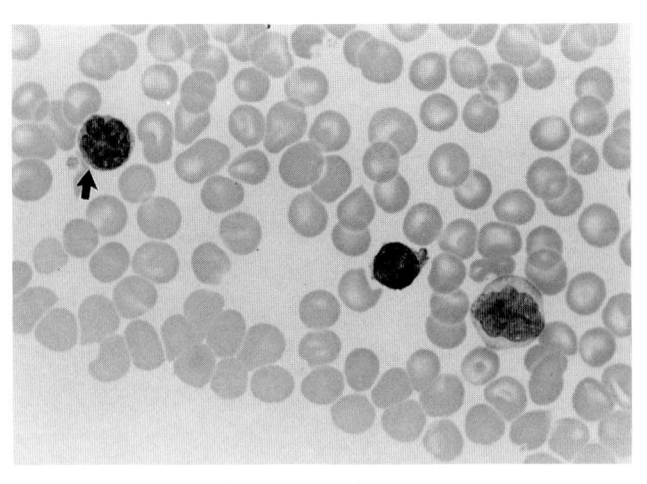

Fig. 19.5. A peripheral blood smear from a case of Sézary syndrome showing a Sézary cell with a cerebriform nucleus at the upper left corner (arrow). A lymphocyte and a monocyte are at right. Wright–Giemsa, ×1250.

The histologic features in the lymph node of an MF/SS patient are most commonly those of dermatopathic lymphadenopathy (Figs. 19.7–19.9). In a later stage, the lymph nodes may be involved by the tumor cells to various degrees. A grading system divides the lymph node (LN) changes into four categories.[21] LN1 shows dermatopathic lymphadenopathy with occasional atypical lymphocytes. LN2 is designated when fewer than 6 atypical lymphoid cells are demonstrated. When more than 15 atypical cells are seen, it is graded as LN3. When the normal architecture of the lymph node is partially or completely effaced, it becomes LN4

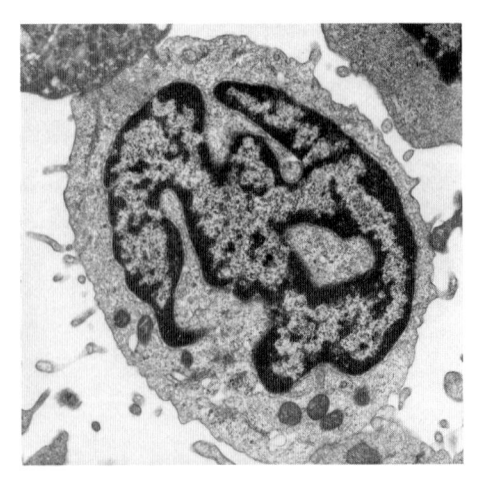

Fig. 19.6. A Sézary cell in a peripheral blood smear showing a folded cerebriform nucleus. ×17,600.

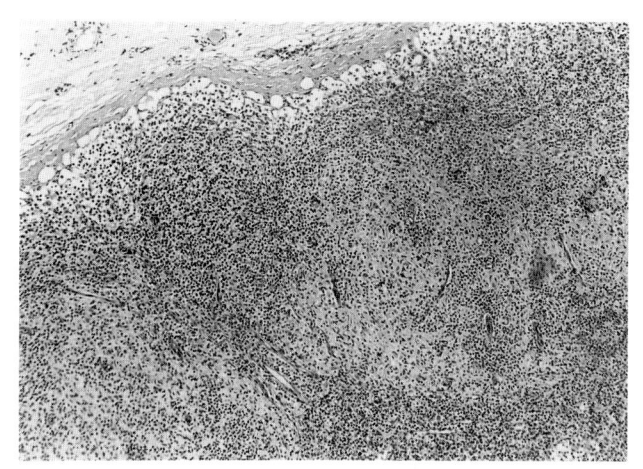

Fig. 19.7. Dermatopathic lymphadenitis showing expansion of the paracortical zone by the pale-stained histiocytes and darkly stained lymphocytes. H&E, ×125.

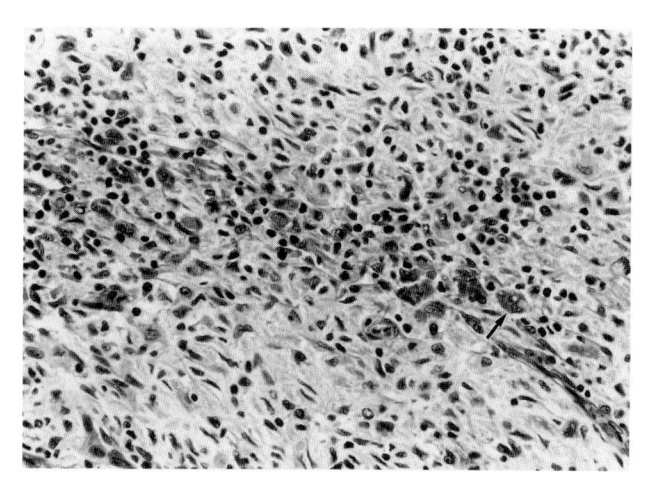

Fig. 19.9. A higher-power view of the same lymph node as showing in Figs. 19.7 and 19.8, revealing melanin-laden macrophages (arrow) among the pale-stained histiocytes. H&E, ×500.

(Fig. 19.10). A recent study of 251 lymph nodes from 200 patients with MF/SS revealed that 89 specimens or 35% belonged to the LN4 category. Among these 89 cases, 16 showed small-cell lymphoma; 16, poorly differentiated lymphocytic lymphoma; 22, mixed small- and large-cell lymphoma; 32, large cell lymphoma; and 3, pleomorphic lymphoma.[22] The large-cell or mixed-cell lymphomas may represent transformation from the small-cell components of MF/SS. A transformation to higher-grade lymphomas occurs in about 10% of MF cases and is associated with a shorter survival time (< 20 months).[23,24]

In a review of 29 autopsies of MF patients, lymph nodes were involved in 37.9%; spleen, 34.5%; liver, 31.0%; lungs, 27.6%; bone marrow, 24.1%; and pleura, stomach, and kidneys, 17.2% each.[11] Hepatic involvement by MF/SS usually manifests as nodular aggregates of tumor cells in the portal zones or lobules, and bone marrow involvement also shows nodular aggregates of tumor cells.[2]

ATCL

A morphologic diagnosis of ATCL usually depends on the identification of the characteristic tumor cells with

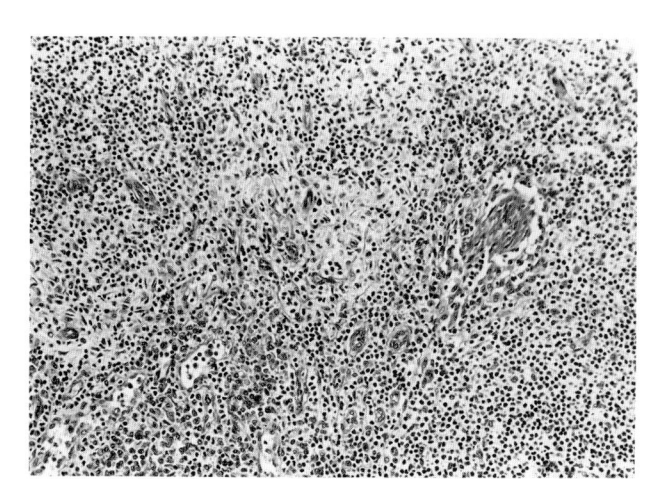

Fig. 19.8. A higher magnification of Fig. 19.7 demonstrating the lymphohistiocytic cells. H&E, ×250.

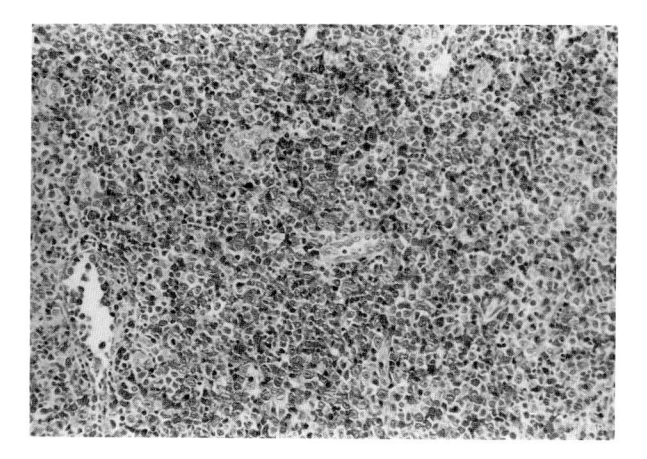

Fig. 19.10. Dermatopathic lymphadenitis (LN4) with lymphoma showing complete effacement of normal nodal architecture by lymphoma cells stained with UCHL-1. Immunoperoxidase, ×500.

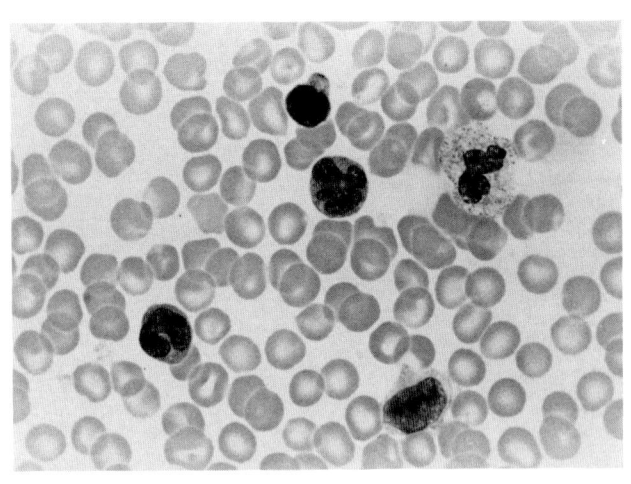

Fig. 19.11. A peripheral blood smear from a case of adult T-cell leukemia/lymphoma showing a polylobated (flower) cell in the center. Wright–Giemsa, ×1250.

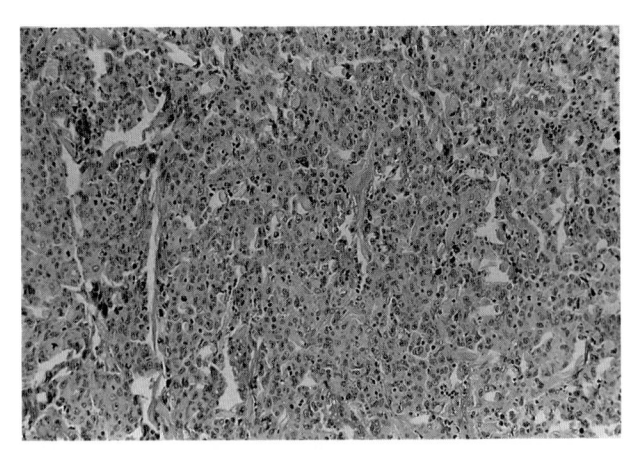

Fig. 19.13. Another view of the same case as in Fig. 19.12 showing large pleomorphic tumor cells. H&E, ×250.

polylobated nuclei (flower cells) (Fig. 19.11). In the chronic subtype, the tumor cells show less atypism. In the smoldering subtype, minimal atypism and lower percentage of tumor cells are seen in the peripheral blood.

Skin lesions are a constant feature of ATCL and may mimic MF/SS by showing plaque, tumor and erythroderma forms (Figs. 19.12–19.14).[13] Only the papular form is specific for ATCL. Pautrier microabscesses are present in more than 50% of the ATCL cases and thus do not constitute an absolute index for distinguishing ATCL from MF/SS.[13] When the lymph nodes are involved, the normal architecture is completely replaced by pleomorphic tumor cells of varying sizes (Figs. 19.15, 19.16).[13] Reed–Sternberg-like cells may be present in some cases.[13]

LABORATORY FINDINGS

Identification of HTLV-1 infection by various means was previously a major criterion for distinguishing ATCL from MF/SS (Table 19.2). However, since HTLV-1 antibody and partially deleted HTLV-1 genome have been found in some patients with MF/SS, evidence of HTLV-1 infection is no longer an absolute criterion for differential diagnosis. On the

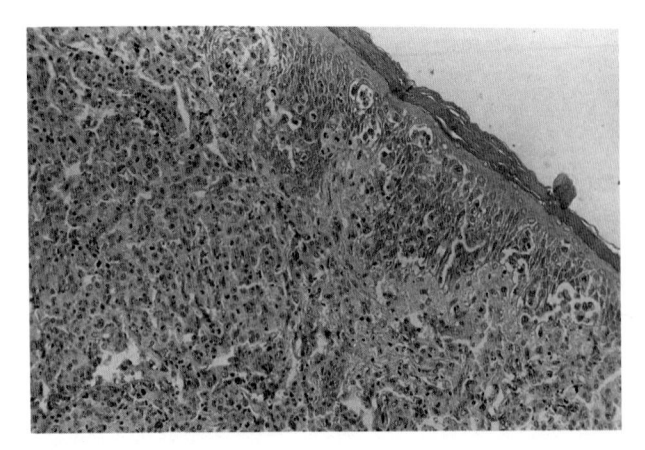

Fig. 19.12. Skin lesion in adult T-cell leukemia/lymphoma showing diffuse dermal infiltration by pleomorphic large tumor cells and multiple Pautrier microabscesses in the epidermis. H&E, ×125. (Case contributed by Dr. I. J. Su.)

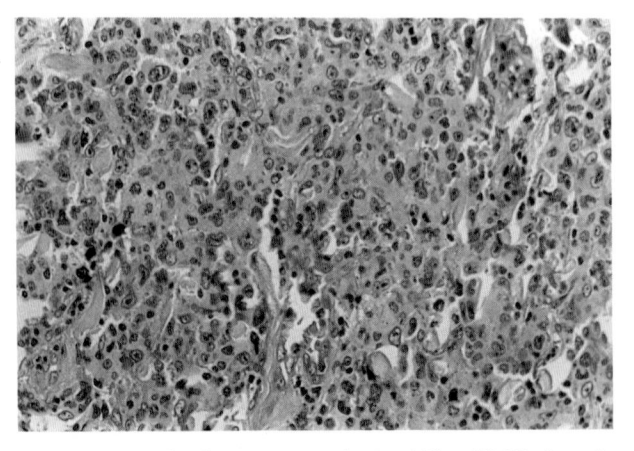

Fig. 19.14. A higher-power view of Fig. 19.12 showing a few polylobated cells. H&E, ×500.

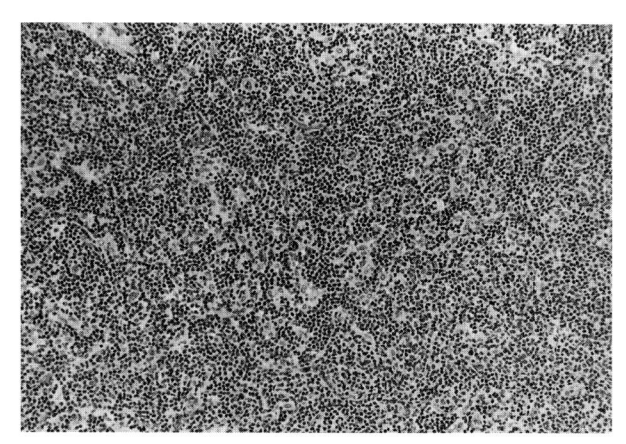

Fig. 19.15. Lymph node biopsy of adult T-cell leukemia/lymphoma showing pale-stained pleomorphic small tumor cells intermingled with small lymphocytes. H&E, ×250. (Case contributed by Dr. I. J. Su.)

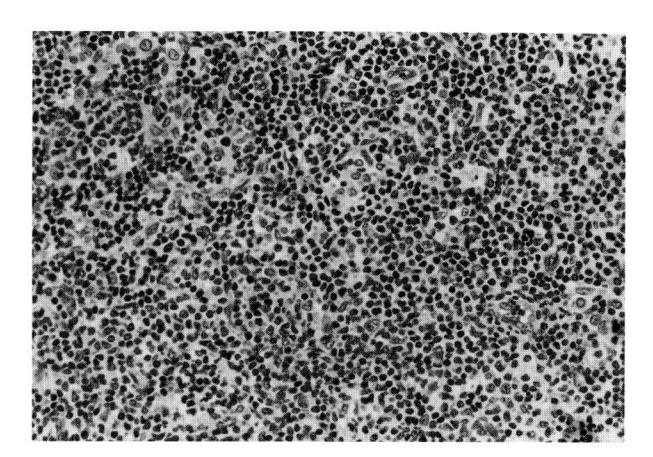

Fig. 19.16. A higher-power view of Fig. 19.15 showing the small polymorphic tumor cells (arrow). H&E, ×500.

other hand, a rare form of HTLV-1-negative ATCL has been reported.[25] Notwithstanding the situations mentioned above, the etiologic role of HTLV-1 in ATCL remains clinically important, because patients may transmit the virus to other people through sexual contact, blood transfusion, or the transplacental route, leading to ATCL development. A current theory, however, emphasizes that only carriers infected at birth ultimately develop leukemia, as age-dependent accumulation of somatic mutations may be required in leukemogenesis.[13] In addition to serologic and the Southern blotting technique, HTLV-1 can also be detected by the polymerase chain reaction using a probe specific for the HTLV-1 *pol* sequences.[26]

Phenotypically, MF/SS and ATCL share many similar features, but a few important markers can be used to distinguish these two entities (Table 19.3).[2,11,13,14] They both share the helper T-cell type, and have selective loss of one pan-T antigen, CD7. Activation antigens, such as CD38 and CD71, are present, while thymic antigens (CD1 and terminal deoxynucleotidyl transferase) are absent in both. HLA-DR is absent in circulating Sézary cells but is present in lymphocytic infiltrates of the skin.[27] However, HLA-DR is persistently demonstrated in ATCL cases.[28] CD25, the low-affinity IL-2 receptor, is present on ATCL cells and is enhanced by the Px protein, a gene product of HTLV-1.[29] The response of IL-2 receptor to the T-cell growth factor with resultant excessive proliferation may be part of the mechanism of leukemogenesis.[27,28] The soluble IL-2R levels are also elevated in the serum of ATCL cases. However, CD25 may also be present on MF/SS tumor cells in some cases; thus, its presence is not an absolute distinguishing feature for these two entities.[2] The most useful marker appears to be Leu8, the lymph node homing receptor, which is absent on MF/SS cells but is present on ATCL cells.[2,13]

The current interest in adhesion receptor molecules may also be applied to distinguish MF/SS from ATCL as well as to explain the mechanisms of tumoregenesis. MF/SS cells carry an adhesion molecule, LFA-1, which may bind to another adhesion receptor molecule, ICAM-1, on keratinocytes in the skin. This may explain the epidermiotropic phenomenon of the MF/SS cells.[11] However, the expression of ICAM-1 on keratinocytes depends on α-interferon (α-IFN) stimulation. When the patients' MF cells fail to produce α-IFN, ICAM-1 is no longer expressed on keratinocytes, and the tumor cells may not be attracted to the skin and may become disseminated.[11]

TCR gene rearrangement as demonstrated by Southern blotting or polymerase chain reaction has been used for the confirmation of diagnosis in MF/SS, especially when no typical tumor cells are identified in a lymph node. In one comparison study of 8 histopathologically negative lymph nodes for MF/SS, 6 were found to be immunogenetically positive and 3 were immunophenotypically positive.[2] However, some benign lesions that mimic MF/SS, such as follicular mucinosis, lymphomatoid papulosis, and pagetoid reticulosis, may also show T-cell receptor gene rearrangement.[11]

Another approach is to use a series of monoclonal

TABLE 19.3
Comparison Between Mycosis Fungoides/Sézary Syndrome and Adult T-Cell Leukemia/Lymphoma

	Mycosis fungoides/Sézary syndrome	*Adult T-cell leukemia/lymphoma*
Geographic distribution	Universal	Limited to HTLV-1 endemic areas
Clinical course	Generally insidious	Generally aggressive
Nuclear morphology	Cerebriform (convoluted)	Polylobated (flower-like)
Lymphocytosis	Moderate	Moderate
Hepatosplenomegaly	Late stage	Acute stage
Lymphadenopathy	Late stage	Acute stage
Skin lesion	Patch, plaque, tumor, or erythroderma	Papules
Pautrier microabscesses	Frequently present	Present in 50% of cases
Pan-T antigens	CD2+, CD3+, CD5+, CD7−	CD2+, CD3+, CD5+, CD7−
T-cell subset	CD4+, CD8−	CD4+, CD8−
CD25 (IL-2R)	Occasionally positive	Positive
Leu8	Negative	Positive
Activation antigens	CD38+, CD71+	CD38+, CD71+
TdT, CD1	Negative	Negative
LFA1	Positive	Negative
TCR gene rearrangement	Positive	Positive
HTLV-1 antibody	Occasionally positive	Positive
HTLV-1 proviral DNA	Partially deleted genome identified	Complete geome identified
Hypercalcemia	Absent	Present

antibodies specific for the variable region of T-cell receptor β-chain gene (V_β) to test the tumor cells. There are only 20–30 genes in this region, so not many antisera are required. In a neoplastic population, all cells will react to the same V_β antibody, while cells in a polyclonal population may react to several V_β antibodies in a low percentage (3–5%).[30]

The most common cytogenetic abnormalities in ATCL are trisomy 3, trisomy 7, and the absence of the X chromosomes.[14] Cytogenetic abnormalities have also been demonstrated in cases of MF/SS. However, none of them are specific for MF/SS.[2]

Finally, cytochemical reaction may also help in differential diagnosis. Sézary cells are positive for tartrate-resistant acid phosphatase, β-glucuronidase, and periodic-acid Schiff (PAS) stain, which can be used to distinguish reactive T-lymphocytes.[31]

REFERENCES

1. Joly P, Charlotte F, Leibowitch M, et al: Cutaneous lymphomas other than mycosis fungoides: Follow-up study of 52 patients. *J Clin Oncol* 9:1994–2001, 1991.
2. Wood GS: Benign and malignant cutaneous lymphoproliferative disorders including mycosis fungoides. In Knowles DM (ed): *Neoplastic Hematopathology*, Baltimore, Williams & Wilkins, 1992, pp 917–952.
3. Weinstock MA, Horm JW: Mycosis fungoides in the United States—increasing incidence and descriptive epidemiology. *JAMA* 260:42–46, 1988.
4. Knobler RM, Rehle T, Grossman M, et al: Clinical evolution of cutaneous T-cell lymphoma in a patient with antibodies to human T-lymphotropic virus type I. *J Am Acad Dermatol* 17:903–909, 1987.
5. Wantzin GL, Thomsen K, Nissen NI, et al: Occurrence of human T-cell lymphotropic virus (type I) antibodies in cutaneous T-cell lymphoma. *J Am Acad Dermatol* 15:598–602, 1986.
6. Zucker-Franklin D, Coutavas EE, Rush MG, et al: Detection of human T-lymphotropic virus-like particles in cultures of peripheral blood lymphocytes from patients with mycosis fungoides. *Proc Natl Acad Sci* (USA) 88:7630–7634, 1991.
7. Hall WW, Liu CR, Schneewing O, et al: Deleted HTLV-1 provirus in blood and cutaneous lesions of patients with mycosis fungoides. *Science* 253:317–320, 1991.
8. Zucker-Franklin D, Hooper WC, Evatt BL: Human lymphotropic retroviruses associated with mycosis fungoides: Evidence that human T-cell lymphotropic virus type II (HTLV-11) as well as HTLV-I may play a role in the disease. *Blood* 80:1537–1545, 1992.
9. Manzari V, Gismondi A, Barillari G, et al: A new human retrovirus isolated in a tac-negative T-cell lymphoma/leukemia. *Science* 1581–1583, 1987.
10. Bunn PA, Lamberg SI: Report of the committee on staging and classification of cutaneous T-cell lymphomas. *Cancer Treat Rep* 63:725–728, 1979.

11. Barcos M: Mycosis fungoides: Diagnosis and pathogenesis. *Am J Clin Pathol* 99:452–458, 1993.
12. Sausville EA, Eddy JL, Malsuch RW, et al: Histopathologic staging at initial diagnosis of mycosis fungoides and the Sézary syndrome: Definition of three distinctive prognostic groups. *Ann Intern Med* 109:372–382, 1988.
13. Watanabe S, Mukai K, Shimoyama M: Adult T-cell leukemia/lymphoma. In Knowles D (ed): *Neoplastic Hematopathology*, Baltimore, Williams & Wilkins, 1992, pp 1281–1294.
14. Wachsman W, Golde DW, Chen ISY: HTLV and human leukemia: Perspective 1986. *Semin Hematol* 23:245–256, 1986.
15. Shih LY, Kuo TT, Dunn P, et al: Human T-cell lymphotropic virus type I associated adult T-cell leukemia/lymphoma in Taiwan Chinese. *Br J Haematol* 79:156–161, 1991.
16. Yoshiba M, Seiki M, Yamaguchi K, et al: Monoclonal integration of HTLV in all primary tumors of adult T-cell leukemia suggests causative role of HTLV in the disease. *Proc Natl Acad Sci* (USA) 81:2534–2537, 1984.
17. Shimoyama M: Diagnostic criteria and classification of clinical subtypes of adult T-cell leukemia/lymphoma: A report from the lymphoma study group (1984–87). *Br J Haematol* 79:428–437, 1991.
18. Sun T: *Color Atlas/Text of Flow Cytometric Analysis of Hematologic Neoplasms*, New York; Igaku-Shoin, 1993, pp 138–142.
19. Payne CM, Glasser L: Ultrastructural morphometry in the diagnosis of Sézary syndrome. *Arch Pathol Lab Med* 114:661–671, 1990.
20. Shapiro PE, Pinto FJ: The histologic spectrum of mycosis fungoides/Sézary syndrome (cutaneous T-cell lymphoma). *Am J Surg Pathol* 18:645–667, 1994.
21. Matthews MJ: Surgical pathology of mycosis fungoides and Sézary syndrome. In Jaffe ES (ed): *Surgical Pathology of the Lymph Nodes and Related Organs*, Philadelphia, Saunders, 1985, pp 329–356.
22. Vonderheid EC, Diamond LW, Lai SM, et al: Lymph node histopathologic findings in cutaneous T-cell lymphoma: A prognostic classification system based on morphology assessment. *Am J Clin Pathol* 97:121–129, 1992.
23. Dmitrovsky E, Matthews MJ, Bunn PA, et al: Cytologic transformation in cutaneous T-cell lymphoma: A clinicopathologic entity associated with poor prognosis. *J Clin Oncol* 5:208–215, 1987.
24. Salhany KE, Cousar JB, Greer JP, et al: Transformation of cutaneous T-cell lymphoma to large cell lymphoma. *Am J Pathol* 132:265–277, 1988.
25. Shimoyama M, Kagami Y, Shimotomo K, et al: Adult T-cell leukemia/lymphoma not associated with human T-cell leukemia virus type I. *Proc Natl Acad Sci* (USA) 83:4524–4528, 1986.
26. Gessain A, Caumes E, Feyeux C, et al: The cutaneous form of adult T-cell leukemia/lymphoma in a woman from Ivory Coast. *Cancer* 69:1362–1367, 1992.
27. Haynes BF, Hensley LL, Jegasothy BV: Differentiation of human T-lymphocytes: 2. Phenotypic difference in skin and blood of malignant T-cells in cutaneous T-cell lymphoma. *J Invest Dermatol* 78:323–326, 1982.
28. Shirono K, Haltori T, Hata H, et al: Profiles of expression of activated cell antigens on peripheral blood and lymph node cells from different clinical stages of adult T-cell leukemia. *Blood* 73:1664–1671, 1989.
29. Yodoi J, Uchiyama T: IL-2 receptor dysfunction and adult T-cell leukemia. *Immunol Rev* 92:135–156, 1986.
30. Clark DM, Boylston AW, Hall PA, et al: Antibodies to T-cell antigen receptor beta chain families detect monoclonal T-cell proliferation. *Lancet* 2:835–836, 1986.
31. Naeim F, Capostagno VJ, Johnson CE Jr, et al: Sézary syndrome: Tartrate-resistant acid phosphatase in the neoplastic cells. *Am J Clin Pathol* 71:528–533, 1979.

20
Cutaneous Lymphomas vs. Carcinomas

Besides mycosis fungoides/Sézary syndrome and adult T-cell leukemia/lymphoma, there are other lymphomas, such as peripheral T-cell lymphoma, lymphoblastic lymphoma, and B-cell lymphoma, which may involve the skin. In addition, nonlymphomatous tumors, including cutaneous neuroendocrine (Merkel-cell) carcinoma, undifferentiated carcinoma, small-cell carcinoma, and amelanotic melanoma, should be considered in the differential diagnosis. In typical cases, these tumors can be readily distinguished by their clinical or pathologic features. However, immunohistochemical studies are frequently needed in difficult cases.

CLINICAL FEATURES

Cutaneous Lymphoma

The cutaneous lesions in lymphomas include papules, plaques, nodules, erythroderma, and exfoliative dermatitis.[1,2] In localized lesions, patients do not have constitutional symptoms, lymphadenopathy, bone marrow and/or blood involvement, or hypercalcemia. However, a few patients may have peripheral eosinophilia.[1] In a later stage (stage IV), most patients have lymphadenopathy and bone marrow involvement and some patients may have B symptoms, such as fever, night sweats, or weight loss. These patients also have high serum levels of lactate dehydrogenase, and a few patients may show atypical lymphocytes in the peripheral blood or eosinophilia.[1] The clinical course depends on the histologic type and stage. Patients with low-grade lymphomas may have a long period of complete remission, and the tumor may show spontaneous regression.[1,2] Patients with intermediate-grade or high-grade lymphoma detected at an early stage usually have a high frequency of recurrence, while those detected at a later stage often fail to respond to chemotherapy and may show a shorter survival.[1] The presence of multifocal skin lesions usually predicts a poor prognosis.[3]

Cutaneous Neuroendocrine (Merkel-Cell) Carcinoma

This tumor is most frequently seen in the head and neck region and less frequently in the lower extremity.[4] Half of the patients may have recurrence or metastasis. In a study of 19 patients, 9 cases had recurrent and/or metastatic disease, and among these 9 cases, 4 survived, and 5 died in a follow-up over 5–80 months.[4]

Other Carcinomas

Carcinomas that may mimic cutaneous lymphomas are mainly undifferentiated or poorly differentiated carcinoma and small-cell carcinoma. The poorly differentiated carcinoma is usually of skin adnexal origin. The small-cell carcinoma, on the other hand, is generally metastatic, with the oat-cell carcinoma from the lung most frequently mentioned.[5] The clinical manifestation of these tumors depends on the primary carcinoma.

Amelanotic Melanoma

Melanoma is usually a pigmented skin cancer, but nonpigmented melanoma may occur and cause confusion with lymphoma. This tumor may produce rapid visceral metastasis and cause a high mortality, worse than most of the other skin cancers. Change in size, color, or texture of a preexisting nevus should suggest the possibility of a melanoma.

PATHOLOGY

When mycosis fungoides and Sézary syndrome are excluded, most cutaneous lymphomas are of B-cell origin (Figs. 20.1–20.4).[1,3] Among B-cell lymphomas, most are of follicular center cell origin,[3,6] but immunoblastic lymphoma and immunocytoma (lymphoplasmacytic lymphoma) have also been reported.[3,6,7] Among T-cell lymphomas, most are peripheral T-cell lymphoma (Figs. 20.5, 20.6) and seldom T-cell lymphoblastic lymphoma.[8] In Hong Kong, cutaneous T-cell lymphomas, even after exclusion of mycosis fungoides, are more frequently encountered than cutaneous B-cell lymphomas, and 51% of a series of 37 cutaneous lymphomas were angiocentric T-cell lymphoma[6] (see Chapter 21). When classified by histopathologic patterns in a study of 52 cases, 21% were high-grade lymphomas, 58% intermediate-

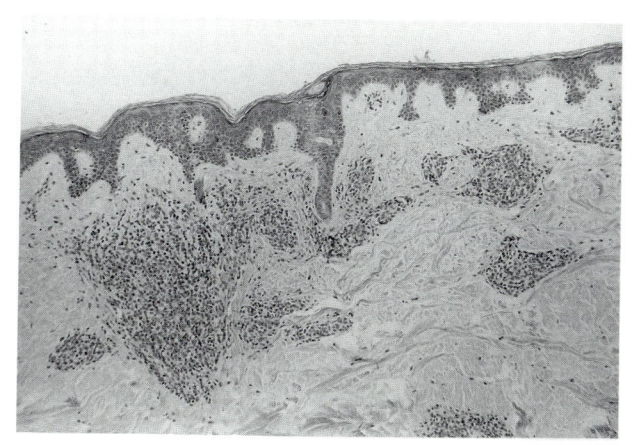

Fig. 20.1. Cutaneous B-cell lymphoma showing several patches of lymphoma cells in the dermis. The epidermis is not involved. H&E, ×125.

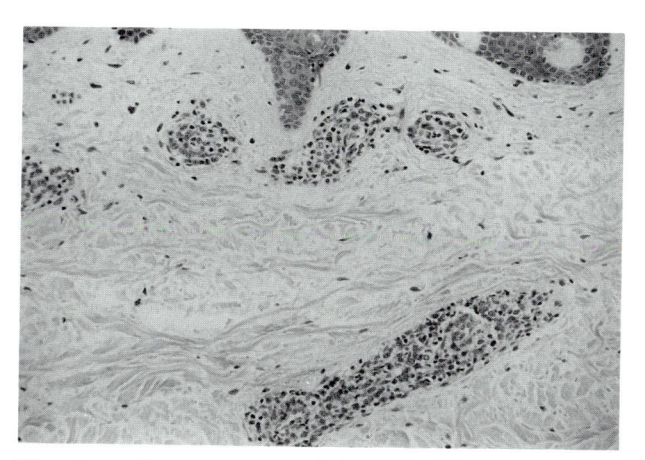

Fig. 20.2. Cutaneous B-cell lymphoma showing focal perivascular infiltration of the dermis. H&E, ×250.

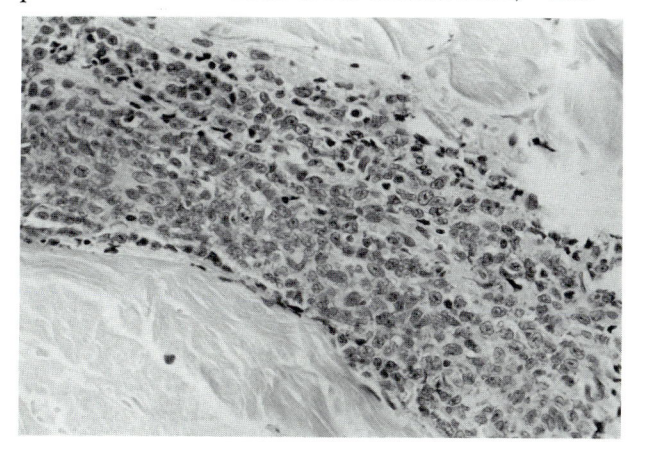

Fig. 20.3. Cutaneous B-cell lymphoma showing medium-sized lymphoma cells with prominent nucleoli. H&E, ×500.

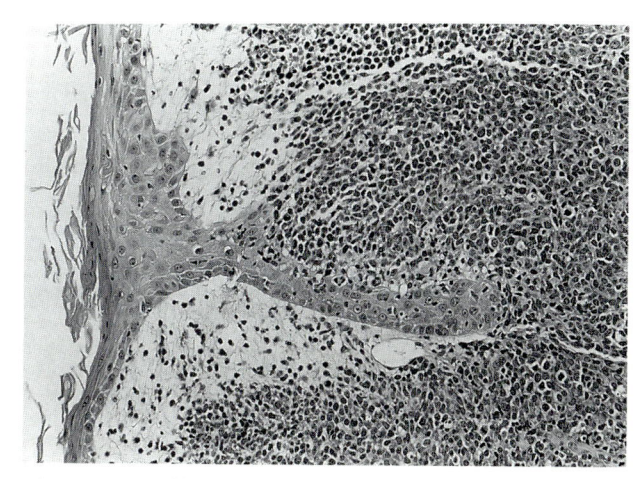

Fig. 20.4. Diffuse large-cell lymphoma infiltrating the papillary dermis with invasion of epidermis. H&E, ×250.

grade, and 21% low grade.[1] Nodal involvement is usually seen in diffuse large-cell or immunoblastic lymphomas.

Lymphoma cells mainly infiltrate the dermis. In B-cell lymphomas, perivascular and periappendageal infiltration is the most common pattern.[6,7] When atypical lymphoid cells with cerebriform or noncerebriform nuclei infiltrate mainly the epidermis, it is either mycosis fungoides or an unusual condition called *pagetoid reticulosis* or *Woringer–Kolopp disease*.[9] The lymphoid component in pagetoid reticulosis is usually of T-cell origin, either predominantly CD4+ or CD8+. T-cell receptor gene rearrangement has been

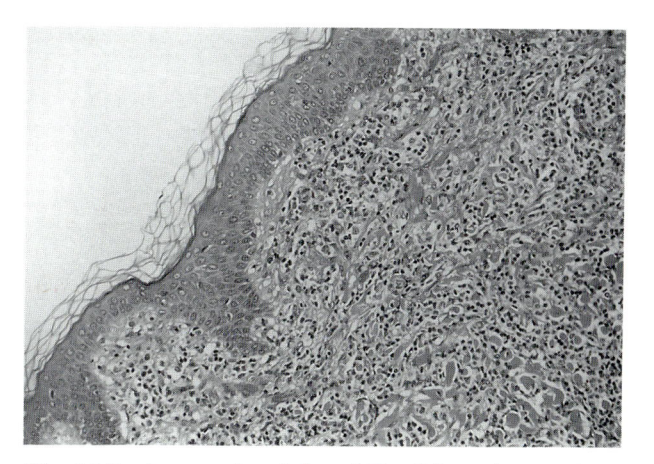

Fig. 20.5. A case of peripheral T-cell lymphoma showing extensive infiltration of dermis without involving the epidermis. H&E, ×250.

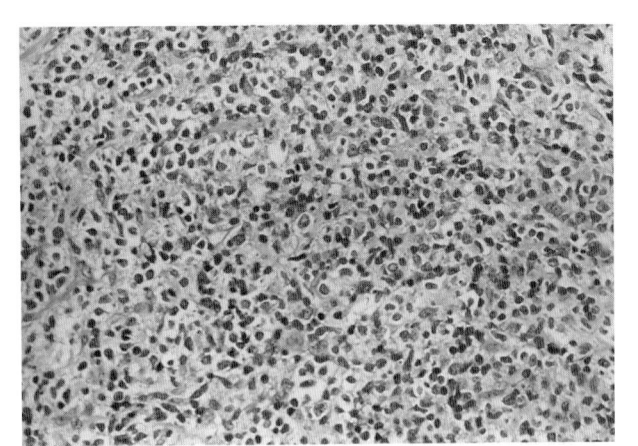

Fig. 20.6. A case of peripheral T-cell lymphoma with mixed small and large cells showing extensive pleomorphic infiltration. H&E, ×500.

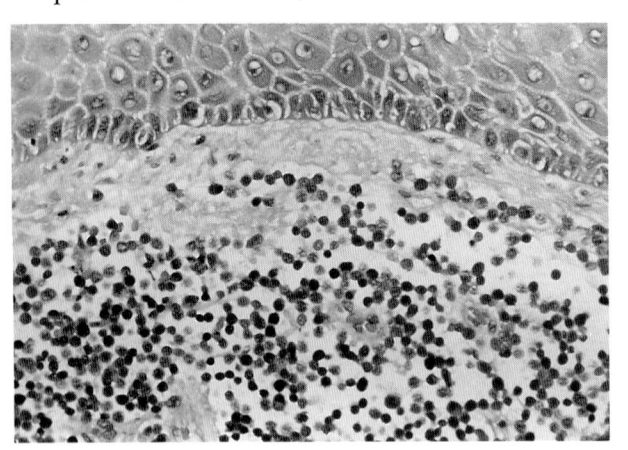

Fig. 20.7. A case of Merkel-cell carcinoma of small-cell type with dermal infiltration simulating cutaneous lymphoma. H&E, ×500.

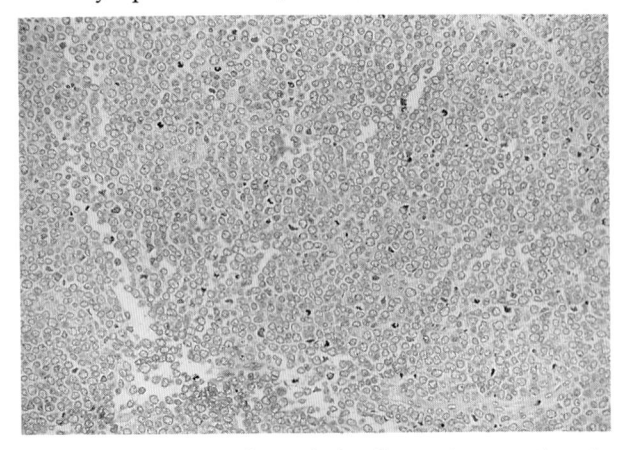

Fig. 20.8. A case of Merkel-cell carcinoma showing monotonous round nuclei, scant cytoplasm, and multiple mitotic figures. H&E, ×250.

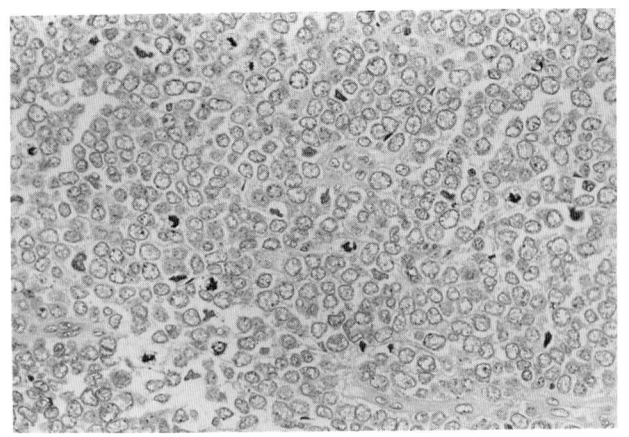

Fig. 20.9. A higher-power view of Fig. 20.8 showing vesicular nuclei and inconspicuous nucleoli. H&E, ×500.

demonstrated in this disorder.[8] Pagetoid reticulosis and mycosis fungoides can be distinguished only on clinical grounds.

Another condition that must be distinguished from cutaneous lymphoma is pseudolymphoma. *Pseudolymphoma* refers to a heterogenous group of diseases, including lymphomatoid papulosis, pseudo-Hodgkin's disease, actinic reticuloid, angioimmunoblastic lymphadenopathy, lymphomatoid granulomatosis, Jessner's lymphocytic infiltration, and drug-induced skin lesions. For differential diagnosis of cutaneous pseudolymphomas, the reader is referred to Wood's review.[8]

Although not a common tumor, neuroendocrine (Merkel-cell) carcinoma is frequently mentioned in

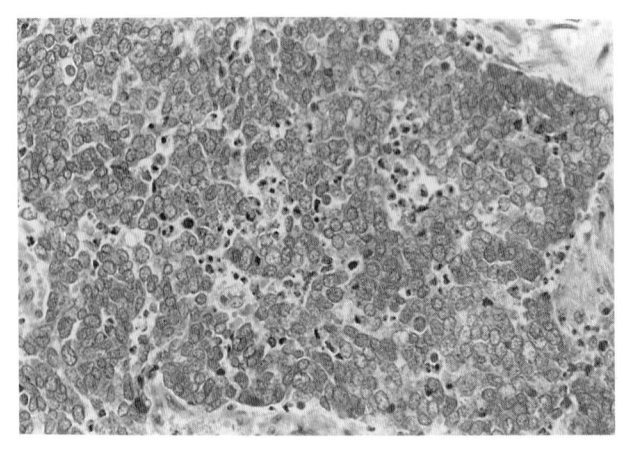

Fig. 20.10. A case of Merkel-cell carcinoma showing the trabecular pattern. H&E, ×500.

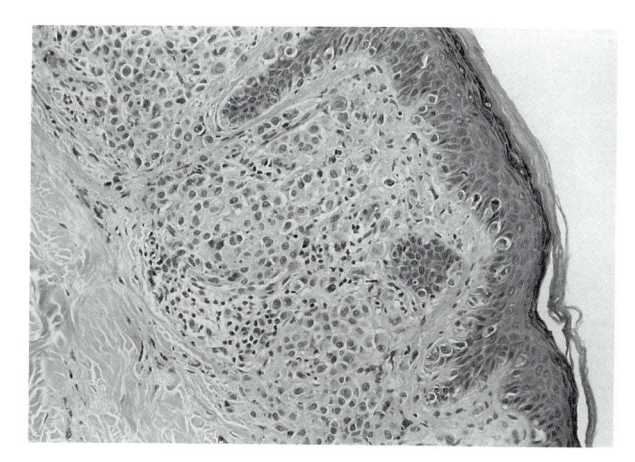

Fig. 20.11. A case of malignant melanoma showing nests of tumor cells at the dermoepidermal junction and the papillary dermis with invasion of epidermis. H&E, ×250.

the differential diagnosis of lymphomas. These carcinoma cells have monotonous reniform round nuclei with scant cytoplasm, mimicking lymphoma cells (Figs. 20.7–20.10).[10] Their vesicular nuclei often contain one or more inconspicuous nucleoli. The neoplasm usually infiltrates the dermis without involvement of the epidermis. However, a special form of Merkel-cell carcinoma shows pagetoid intraepidermal spread.[11] The major distinction of Merkel-cell carcinoma from lymphoma is the arrangement of the tumor cells in ill-defined nodules or trabeculae, but they may also show a diffuse lymphoma-like pattern.[10] Gould and DeLellis have divided Merkel-cell carcinoma into three histologic patterns: trabecular, intermediate-, and small-cell types.[12] Electron microscopy may reveal small dense-core secretory granules, perinuclear intermediate filaments, and desmosomes. These ultrastructures can help distinguish Merkel-cell carcinoma from lymphoma but not from metastatic small-cell neuroendocrine carcinoma, such as oat-cell carcinoma.

Oat-cell carcinoma and undifferentiated or poorly differentiated carcinoma may also be confused with lymphomas. The cohesiveness of carcinoma cells and their cluster formation are useful features in distinguishing carcinoma from lymphoma. The demonstration of desmosomes and tonofilaments in carcinoma cells by electron microscopy can help exclude lymphoma.

Malignant melanoma forms nests at the dermoepidermal junction, protrudes into the papillary dermis, and invades the epidermis (Figs. 20.11, 20.12). The demonstration of melanin may substantiate the diagnosis.[10]

LABORATORY FINDINGS

When the distinction between cutaneous lymphoma and carcinoma cannot be made morphologically, phenotyping becomes necessary. Flow cytometric analysis can demonstrate the lymphoid nature of the lymphoma cells by cell-lineage-specific antibodies (Fig. 20.13); and the clonality of B-lymphocytes, by surface immunoglobulin studies. Thus, a B-cell lymphoma can be diagnosed on the basis of light-chain

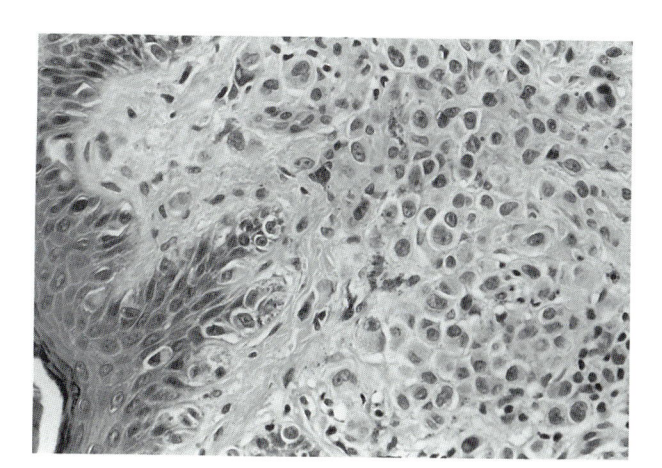

Fig. 20.12. A higher-power view of Fig. 10.11 showing intracellular pigment in tumor cells and epidermal invasion. H&E, ×500.

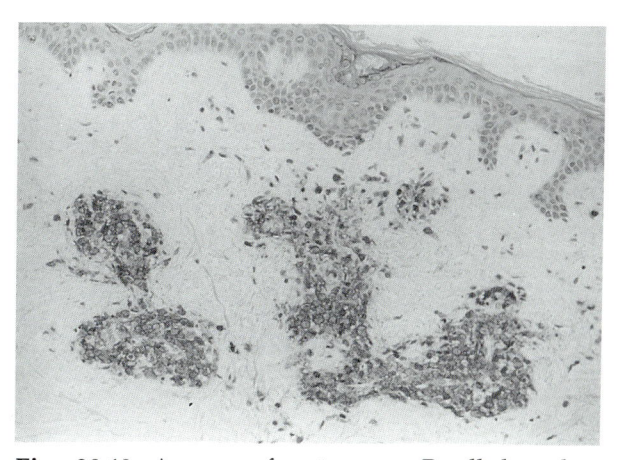

Fig. 20.13. A case of cutaneous B-cell lymphoma showing positive CD20 staining. Immunoperoxidase, ×250.

194 DIFFERENTIAL DIAGNOSIS OF LYMPHOID DISORDERS

TABLE 20.1
Differences in Markers Between Lymphoma and Nonlymphomatous Tumors

	Lymphoma	Neuroendocrine CA	Other CA	Melanoma
LCA (CD45)	+++	−	−	−
T- or B-cell antigen	+++	−	−	−
Keratin	−	+++	+++	−
Neurofilament	−	++	−	−
Chromogranin	−	++	−	−
NSE	−	++	−	−
Synaptophysin	−	++	−	−
Bombesin	−	++	−	−
EMA	−	NA	+++	−
S100 protein	−	−	−	+++
HMB-45	−	−	−	+++
Calcitonin	−	+	−	−
Somatostatin	−	+	−	−
VIP	−	+	−	−

Key: +, ++, and +++ represent low, intermediate, or high positive rate, respectively; Ca = carcinoma, EMA = epithelial membrane antigen, HMB-45 = melanoma-associated antigen, LCA = leukocyte common antigen, NSE = neuron-specific enolase, VIP = vasoactive intestinal polypeptide, NA = no information available.

restriction, whereas a T-cell lymphoma cannot be diagnosed unless there is selective loss of pan-T antigens, such as CD2, CD3, CD5, or CD7.[8] In peripheral T-cell lymphoma, CD7 is frequently absent, whereas T-cell lymphoblastic lymphoma usually expresses CD7 but loses CD3.[13,14] The diagnosis of lymphoblastic lymphoma can also be made when a majority of the cell population shows positive terminal deoxynucleotidyl transferase. Concerning T-cell subsets, most of peripheral T-cell lymphomas have a CD4+, CD8-phenotype,[8] and about 50% of the lymphoblastic lymphoma shows a CD4+, CD8+ (common thymocyte) phenotype.[15] The presence of surface CD30 antigen, regardless of the morphology (whether anaplastic or not), often confers a favorable prognosis.[3] Epithelial markers are not routinely used in flow cytometric studies, but the scattergram may show a widely dispersed dot plot, providing a clue for the diagnosis of carcinoma.[16]

For the differential diagnosis of various types of carcinomas, immunohistochemistry is most helpful.

Fig. 20.14. A case of Merkel-cell carcinoma showing the characteristic cytoplasmic inclusion-like pattern of cytokeratin staining. Immunoperoxidase with hematoxylin counterstain, ×250.

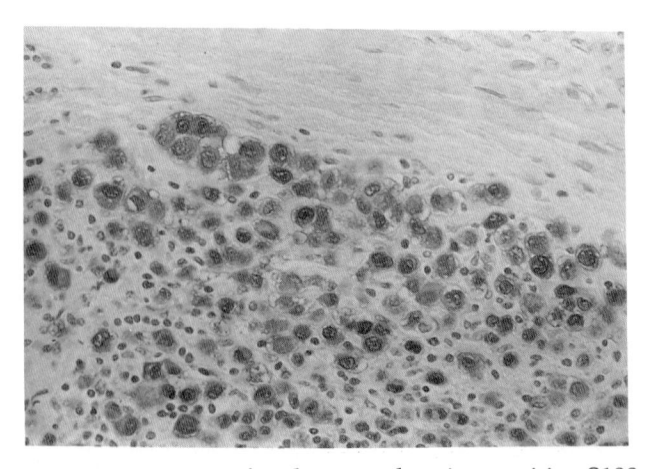

Fig. 20.15. A case of melanoma showing positive S100 staining in both cytoplasm and nuclei. Immunoperoxidase, ×500.

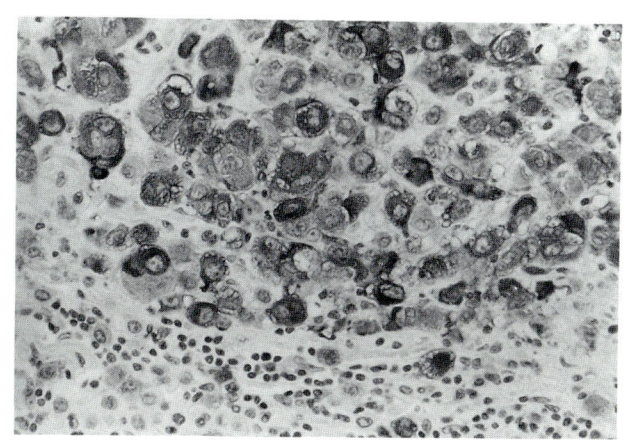

Fig. 20.16. A case of melanoma showing positive cytoplasmic staining of HMB-45. Immunoperoxidase, ×500.

Generally speaking, carcinomas should stain positive by cytokeratin and epithelial membrane antigen (EMA), and are negative for leukocyte common antigen (LCA or CD45) (Table 20.1). In Merkel-cell carcinoma, the keratin stain shows a dense, inclusion-like, cytoplasmic globule pattern (Fig. 20.14), which is characteristic for this tumor, although the same pattern may be demonstrated in pulmonary and intestinal carcinoids.[4,5] Neurofilament antigen, and neuroendocrine markers (chromogranin, neuron-specific enolase, synaptophysin, and bombesin) are demonstrated in a lower percentage of cases with Merkel-cell carcinoma.[4,5,12] A variety of polypeptide hormones have been identified in neuroendocrine carcinomas, most frequently calcitonin, vasoactive intestinal polypeptide (VIP), and somatostatin and occasionally, gastrin and adenocorticotropic hormone (ACTH).[4,5] However, because of the low positive rates in demonstrating these polypeptides, their detection is seldom used for diagnostic purposes.

Staining for neuroendocrine markers in formalin-fixed tissues is usually weak and focal, but the staining can be enhanced in frozen unfixed tissues.[4] It has been found that prolonged protease digestion of fixed tissues may compensate for the detrimental effect of fixation.[5]

For the diagnosis of amelanotic melanoma, S-100 protein and melanoma-associated antigen (HMB-45) should be used (Figs. 20.15, 20.16).[17]

Finally, gene rearrangement analysis and cytogenetic studies may be useful in distinguishing lymphoma from carcinoma.

REFERENCES

1. Joly P, Charlotte F, Leibowitch M, et al: Cutaneous lymphomas other than mycosis fungoides: Follow-up study of 52 patients. *J Clin Oncol* 9:1994–2001, 1991.
2. Maeda K, Takahashi M, Takatsuka N, et al: Cutaneous T-cell lymphoma differing from classical mycosis fungoides and Sézary syndrome: Clinical, histological and immunohistochemical studies of six cases. *J Dermatol* 17:226–234, 1990.
3. Kurtin PJ, DiCaudo DJ, Haberman TH, et al: Primary cutaneous large cell lymphomas: Morphologic, immunophenotypic and clinical features of 20 cases. *Am J Surg Pathol* 18:1183–1191, 1994.
4. Visscher D, Cooper PH, Zarbo RJ, et al: Cutaneous neuroendocrine (Merkel cell) carcinoma: An immunophenotypic, clinicopathologic and flow cytometric study. *Modern Pathol* 2:331–338, 1989.
5. Battifora H, Silva EG: The use of antikeratin antibodies in the immunohistochemical distinction between neuroendocrine (Merkel cell) carcinoma of the skin, lymphoma, and oat cell carcinoma. *Cancer* 58:1040–1046, 1986.
6. Chan JKC, Ng CS, Ngan KC, et al: Angiocentric T-cell lymphoma of the skin: An aggressive lymphoma distinct from mycosis fungoides. *Am J Surg Pathol* 12:861–876, 1988.
7. LeBoit PE, McNutt NS, Reed JA, et al: Primary cutaneous immunocytoma: A B-cell lymphoma that can easily be mistaken for cutaneous lymphoid hyperplasia. *Am J Surg Pathol* 18:969–978, 1994.
8. Wood GS: Benign and malignant cutaneous lymphoproliferative disorder including mycosis fungoides. In Knowles D (ed): *Neoplastic Hematopathology*, Baltimore, Williams & Wilkins, 1992, pp 917–952.
9. Deneau DG, Wood GS, Beckstead JH, et al: Woringer–Kolopp disease (pagetoid reticulosis): Four cases with histologic, ultrastructural, and immunohistologic observations. *Arch Dermatol* 120:1045–1051, 1984.
10. Cruz DJS, Leyva WH: Neoplasm of skin. In Sternberg SS (ed): *Diagnostic Surgical Pathology*, New York, Raven Press, 1989, pp 59–102.
11. LeBoit PE, Crutcher WA, Shapiro PE: Pagetoid intraepidermal spread in Merkel cell (primary neuroendocrine) carcinoma of the skin. *Am J Surg Pathol* 16:585–592, 1992.
12. Gould VE, DeLellis RA: The neuroendocrine system. In Silverberg SG (ed): *Principles and Practice of Surgical Pathology*, 2nd ed, New York, Churchill Livingston, 1990, pp 1981–1995.
13. Sun T, Ngu M, Henshall J, et al: Marker discrepancy as a diagnostic criterion for lymphoid neoplasms. *Diagn Clin Immunol* 5:393–399, 1988.
14. Sheibani K, Nathwani BN, Winberg CD, et al: Antigenically defined subgroup of lymphoblastic lymphoma:

Relationship to clinical presentation and biologic behavior. *Cancer* 60:183–190, 1987.
15. Hollema H, Poppema S: T-lymphoblastic and peripheral T-cell lymphomas in the northern part of Netherlands. An immunologic study of 29 cases. *Cancer* 64:1620–1628, 1989.
16. Sun T: *Color Atlas/Text of Flow Cytometric Analysis of Hematologic Neoplasms*, New York, Igaku-Shoin, 1993, p 12.
17. Ioachim HL: *Lymph Node Pathology*, 2nd ed, Philadelphia, Lippincott, pp 674–681, 1994.

21
Differential Diagnosis of Angiocentric Immunoproliferative Lesions

There is a group of extranodal lymphoproliferative disorders that show angiocentric and angiodestructive lesions. Depending on the site of involvement, they are termed differently.[1] *Lymphomatoid granulomatosis* (LG or Stewart's granuloma) involves the lungs, upper respiratory tract, central nervous system (CNS), skin, kidneys, and gastrointestinal (GI) tract. *Lymphomatoid vasculitis* is seen in the skin and lungs. *Polymorphic reticulosis*, which is also known as *midline malignant reticulosis* and *lethal midline granuloma*, is found in the nose, paranasal sinuses, nasopharynx (Fig. 21.1), and palate. DeRemee et al. first suggested that these disorders represented the same pathologic process at different anatomic sites.[2] Jaffe subsequently proposed a unifying concept of angiocentric immunoproliferative lesions (AIL) to encompass all the above-mentioned lesions as well as the angiocentric T-cell lymphoma.[3] Lipford et al. further divided AIL into three histologic grades.[4] Although there have been some reports showing low-grade lesions of AIL transforming to high-grade lesions, whether these low-grade lesions are malignant at their inception is still a controversial issue. In fact, Pisani and DeRemee have postulated that AIL may represent a host immune response to many different diseases and not a distinct clinicopathologic entity.[5]

CLINICAL FEATURES

Clinically, AILs is included in the midline granuloma syndrome (MGS). This is a localized relentlessly progressive, destructive disease of the upper aerodigestive tract, including nasal cavity, paranasal sinuses, hard palate, trachea, soft tissue of the orbit, and the face.[6,7] MGS can be divided into three categories: infectious diseases, neoplastic diseases, and inflammatory diseases of unknown etiology.[7,8] AIL is classified as neoplastic diseases together with conventional lymphoma, carcinoma, and sarcoma.[7] The inflammatory diseases of unknown etiology category include Wegener's granulomatosis and idiopathic midline destructive disease.

LG is a better-defined clinical entity than other AILs, frequently seen in the middle age (mean 48) with a male:female ratio of 1.7:1.[9] It is usually presented as a primary lesion in lungs; therefore, the most common clinical presentation is the finding of pulmonary nodules on chest roentgenograms.[10] The most common radiographic findings is bilateral multiple rounded mass densities.[9] Unilateral involvement is seen in about one fifth of the cases, and these cases may eventually show involvement of another lung. Although a few patients may be asymptomatic at presentation, most have pulmonary symptoms, such as deep-chest discomfort, pleuritic chest pain, cough, shortness of breath, and dyspnea on exertion.[9,10] Constitutional symptoms such as fever, malaise, and weight loss are also common. Skin and CNS are the most frequently involved sites of secondary lesions, and neurologic symptoms are seen in about one third of the patients. Uncommon clinical manifestations include arthralgias, myalgias, and GI symptoms.

Physical examination may demonstrate skin rash and/or nodules, splenomegaly, hepatomegaly, and, less frequently, lymphadenopathy. The enlarged lymph nodes, however, seldom show LG lesions, unless lymphomatous transformation has taken place.[9,10] Extranodal involvement is typical for LG.

In a study of 152 cases, 12% evolved into lymphoma.[9] This incidence is obviously an underestimation of the actual rate, as only lymph node—but not pulmonary—malignancy was included in that study because of difficulty in diagnosing pulmonary lymphoma. In the same study, about two-thirds of patients died with a median survival of 14 months.[9]

PATHOLOGY

Histologically, AIL encompasses a spectrum of disorders, ranging from benign to malignant. Its salient feature is polymorphous cellular infiltration around blood vessels (angiocentric) with destruction of vessel walls (angiodestructive) and necrosis.[3,4] The grade of malignancy depends heavily on the number of large atypical cells within the infiltrate.[10] As the grade of malignancy increases, the inflammatory background becomes less conspicuous and necrosis becomes more prominent (Table 21.1).

On the basis of these three variants (cytologic atypia, inflammatory background, and necrosis), Lipford et al. have divided AIL into three grades.[4] On the basis of an angiocentric and angiodestructive back-

197

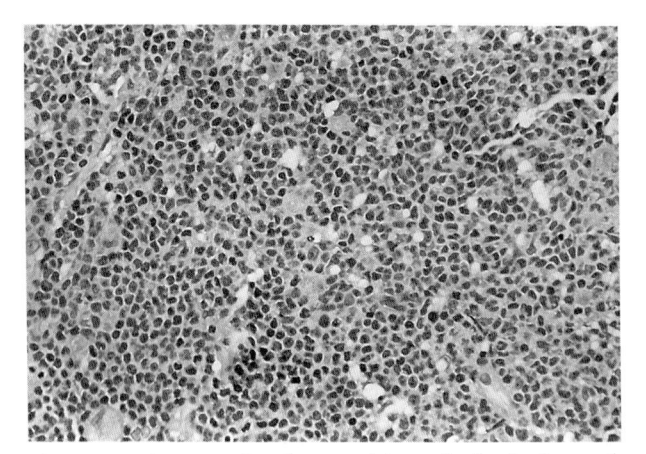

Fig. 21.1. A case of polymorphic reticulosis from the nasopharynx showing small cleaved lymphoma cells. H&E, ×500. (Case contributed by I. J. Su.)

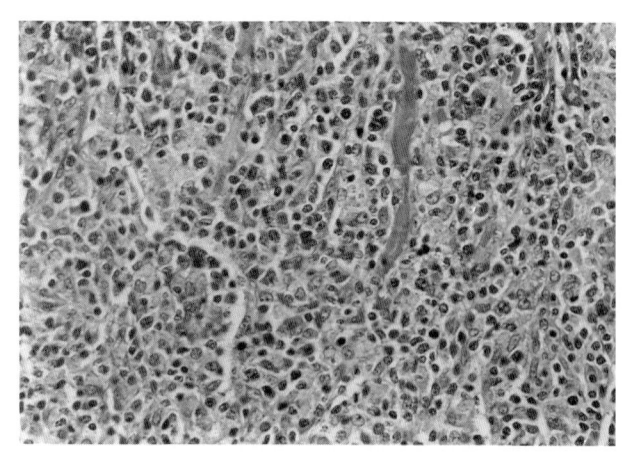

Fig. 21.2. A case of low-grade lymphomatoid granulomatosis showing polymorphic infiltrate of atypical lymphocytes, histiocytes, and plasma cells in the lung (angiocentric immunoproliferative lesion, grade II). H&E, ×500. (Case contributed by Dr. A-L. A. Katzenstein.)

ground, grade I is characterized by a polymorphous infiltrate of lymphocytes, plasma cells, and histiocytes, with or without eosinophils (Fig. 21.2). Large lymphoid cells and immunoblasts are rare and do not show cytologic atypia. Necrosis is absent. Grade II is similar to grade I in cellular composition. However, some cytologic atypia is present in small lymphoid cells, and necrosis is more common (Fig. 21.3). Grade III shows marked cytologic atypia in both small and large lymphoid cells. Polymorphous inflammatory background becomes inconspicuous, while necrosis is usually prominent. Although the composition of atypical lymphoid cells may vary from case to case, leading to different classification (e.g., diffuse, mixed small- and large-cell type, and diffuse, large-cell type), the grade III lesions are collectively called *angiocentric lymphoma* (Figs. 21.4–21.7). It should be emphasized that clearcut distinctions between these grades are not always achievable.

These lesions can evolve from low-grade to high-grade. For instance, a benign lymphocytic angiitis and granulomatosis can transform into LG. The latter lesion, in turn, may transform into angiocentric lymphoma.[9] In a study with sequential biopsies of 8 cases of polymorphic reticulosis, 6 cases showed progression to a higher grade.[13] It is still unclear whether the low-grade lesions are a neoplastic process at onset and gradually express their malignant nature or they are a benign process and gradually evolve into lymphoma. Medeiros et al. have hypothesized that patients with AILs may have an underlying immunodeficiency similar to that in transplant recipients who develop lymphomas secondary to immunosuppression.[11] Indeed, the histology in posttransplant lymphoma is very similar to that of AIL.[11,12] In addition, EB virus genomes are identified in both diseases, and they also share the variable presence of gene rearrangements.[11] The immunodeficient status in patients with AIL may contribute to the frequent association between AIL and other malignancies, such as acute and chronic myelogeneous leukemia, Hodgkin's disease, and non-Hodgkin's lymphoma.[10,14–16]

TABLE 21.1
Grading of Angiocentric Immunoproliferative Lesions

Grade	Angiocentric lesion	Angiodestructive lesion	Polymorphous infiltration	Necrosis	Cytologic atypia
I	++	++	+++	−	−
II	++	++	++	+	+
III	++	++	+	++	++

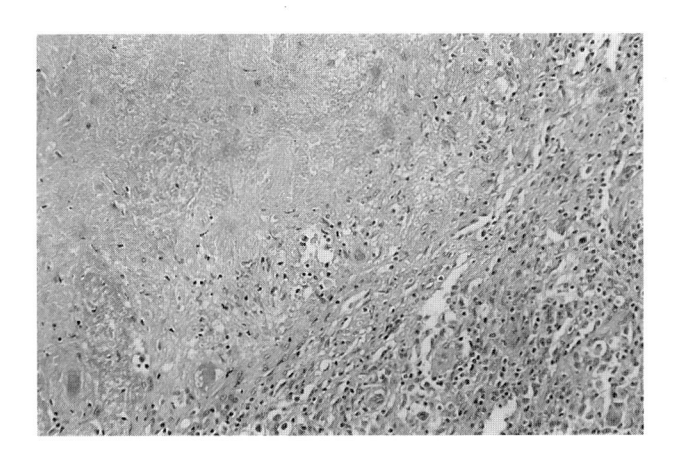

Fig. 21.3. A case of pulmonary lymphomatoid granulomatosis showing a large area of necrosis (angiocentric immunoproliferative lesion, grade II). H&E, ×250. (Case contributed by Dr. A-L. A. Katzenstein.)

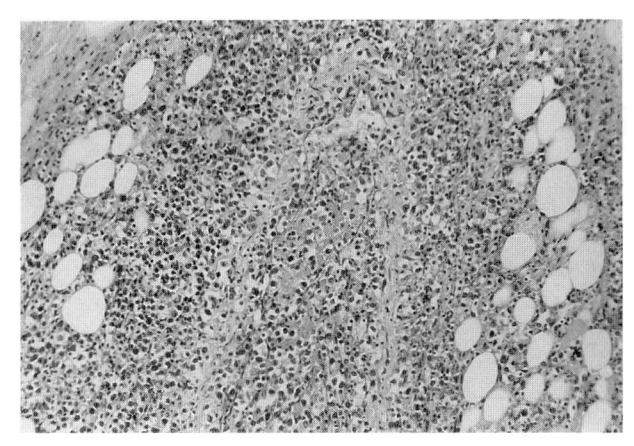

Fig. 21.5. A higher-power view of Fig. 21.4 showing angiocentric infiltration and angiodestructive lesion. H&E, ×250.

Angiocentric T-cell lymphomas are occasionally associated with hemophagocytic syndrome.[17,18] The phagocytic cells are benign histiocytes presumably responding to a lymphokine produced by neoplastic T-cells.

The cutaneous lesion of AIL is usually manifested as skin nodules involving one or multiple sites, with or without ulceration.[19,20] The patch and plaque stages, as seen in mycosis fungoides, are not present in AIL. AIL is characterized by infiltration of mid- and deep dermis with sparing of epidermis and papillary dermis. The infiltration pattern is perivascular and periadnexal. These features of AIL are distinguished from those of mycosis fungoides and other cutaneous lymphomas.

The clinical behavior of AIL appears analogous to the follicular center-cell lymphomas of B-cell origin in that the low-grade lesions may have an indolent clinical course for many years but do not respond to chemotherapy as well as high-grade lesions do.[4] When grade I or grade II AIL progresses to grade III in spite of chemotherapy, the prognosis is especially ominous. Therefore, the single most important prognostic indicator for ultimate survival is achievement of an initial complete remission.[4]

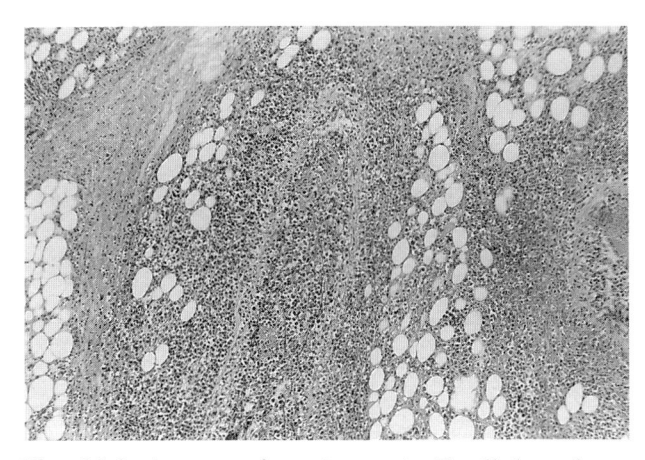

Fig. 21.4. A case of angiocentric T-cell lymphoma showing polymorphic cellular infiltration around blood vessels with destruction of blood vessel walls and necrosis (angiocentric immunoproliferative lesion, grade III). H&E, ×125. (Case contributed by Dr. I. J. Su.)

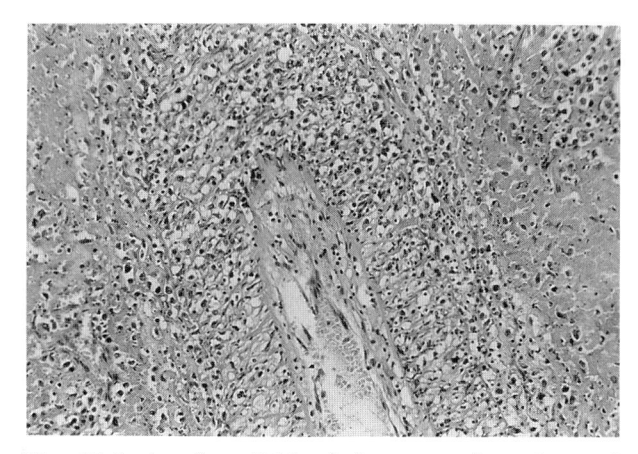

Fig. 21.6. Another field of the case of angiocentric T-cell lymphoma showing marked necrosis in the area of polymorphic infiltration. H&E, ×250.

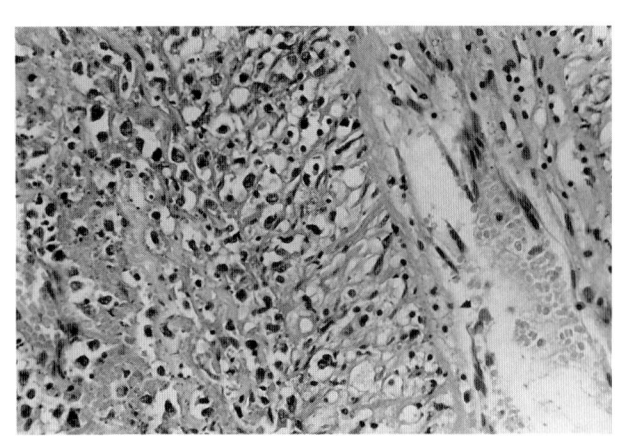

Fig. 21.7. A higher-power view of Fig. 21.6 showing malignant infiltration of the blood vessel wall. H&E, ×500.

LABORATORY FINDINGS

Immunophenotyping is sometimes difficult to perform in AILs because of the presence of polymorphous cellular components. The recent consensus is that AIL is a T-cell lesion with a helper T-cell phenotype (CD4+), as has been demonstrated in most studies.[4,13–16,19–25] Aberrant T-cell phenotype (loss of certain pan-T-cell antigens) is also a frequent finding. In other words, all major T-cell markers (CD2, CD3, CD4, CD5, CD7, CD8, and T-cell receptor protein) except for CD1 have been demonstrated in varying percentages in AIL cases, but for an individual case, one or more pan-T-cell markers can be negative. Activated T-cell markers (HLA-DR and CD25) are frequently found.[19,21] B-cell and myelomonocytic markers are seldom expressed on the neoplastic lymphoid cells in AIL.

By using combined immunohistochemistry and *in situ* hybridization, Guinee et al. found Epstein–Barr virus within CD20+ B-lymphocytes in cases of pulmonary lymphomatoid granulomatosis and considered pulmonary lesions distinguished from angiocentric T-cell lymphoma in other sites, such as the head and neck.[26]

Molecular studies have demonstrated T-cell receptor (TCR) gene rearrangement in a small number of cases, but immunoglobulin gene rearrangement was not observed in AIL cases[4,11,14,16,22,25] until a recent study showing immunoglobulin heavy-chain gene rearrangement in 6 of 9 cases of pulmonary lymphomatoid granulomatosis.[26] A comprehensive study for TCR β-, γ-, and δ-chain genes in 8 cases of AIL revealed TCR gene rearrangement in only 1 case.[11] The unexpectedly low frequency of TCR gene rearrangement can be explained by several hypotheses.[11] First, the low-grade AILs may be polyclonal and may transform into monoclonal only when a genuine lymphoma develops. Alternatively, the number of the malignant cells may be insufficient for detection by Southern blot analysis in most cases, or the tumor cells of AILs might be arrested before gene rearrangement has taken place. However, the most plausible explanation is that most cases of AIL are derived from natural-killer (NK) cells that do not show TCR gene rearrangement.[11,13,15,25] Indeed, NK-cell markers, especially CD56, have been detected in angiocentric lymphomas in several studies.[13,25,27,28]

One of the most interesting findings in recent years is the association of AIL with Epstein–Barr virus (EBV).[11,29–33] Katzenstein and Peiper used the polymerase chain reaction (PCR) technique to identify EBV DNA sequences in 21 of 29 cases of LG.[29] The Southern blotting technique may provide evidence of clonality of the EBV genomes.[30] However, only the EBV-encoded latent membrane protein (LMP) demonstrated by immunohistochemical technique[32,33] or the EBV mRNA identified by the RNA *in situ* hybridization (RISH)[30,32,33] can provide direct evidence of the association of EBV with the tumor cells and not the reactive cellular components. All the abovementioned tests demonstrated EBV genomes or LMP in high percentages of AIL cases. However, the frequency varies in relation to site. The study conducted by deBruin et al. identified EBV at the DNA, RNA, and protein levels in 5 of 5 nasal T-cell lymphomas, 2 of 6 pulmonary T-cell lymphomas, 1 of 12 GI T-cell lymphomas, and none (0) of 17 primary cutaneous T-cell lymphomas.[33] That EBV is more closely associated with the angiocentric T-cell lymphoma than other non-Hodgkin's lymphomas is illustrated by the study of Borisch et al., in which EBV was demonstrated in 6 of 6 angiocentric T-cell lymphomas but in none of the other 6 lymphomas studied.[31]

AIL has also been found related to other viruses, such as human T-cell lymphotropic virus type I (HTLV-I) by polymerase chain reaction and human immunodeficiency virus (HIV) by serologic assays.[15,24] However, their role in the etiology of AIL is not clear.

DIFFERENTIAL DIAGNOSIS

The major differential diagnosis for LG is Wegener's granulomatosis (WG), as both lesions are present

TABLE 21.2
Comparison of Wegener's Granulomatosis and Lymphomatoid Granulomatosis

	Wegener's granulomatosis	Lymphamatoid granulomatosis
Granuloma with multinucleated giant cells	Common	Absent
Palisading histiocytes	Present	Absent
Lymphocytic infiltrate	Rare	Common
Neutrophilic infiltrate	Common	Rare
Atypical lymphocytes	Absent	Present
Necrosis	Cellular and nuclear debris	Coagulative
Lymphoma transformation	Never occurs	Frequently occurs
Immunophenotype	Nonspecific	Frequently T-helper cell
TCR gene rearrangement	Absent	Occasionally present
EB virus	Unrelated	Frequently associated

mainly in the lungs with systemic involvement (Table 21.2).[4,6,7] Histologically, they share some common features such as polymorphic infiltration, vasculitis, and necrosis (Figs. 21.8, 21.9). However, WG is characterized by the presence of well-formed granulomas with multinucleated giant cells and palisading histiocytes, whereas a characteristic granuloma is not seen in LG. Although both lesions show polymorphous infiltration, the major cellular component in LG is lymphoid cells with varying percentages of atypical lymphocytes, whereas neutrophils are prevalent and atypical lymphoid cells are never seen in WG. While cellular infiltrate of the blood vessel walls is seen in both LG and WG, angiodestructive lesion is not present in WG. Necrosis is also present in both lesions, but necrosis in LG is coagulative and perivascular, like infarction, and that in WG contains cellular and nuclear debris due to disintegration of neutrophils. The most important reason for the distinction between LG and WG is that LG frequently transforms into angiocentric lymphoma, but WG never evolves into malignancy. The immunophenotype of LG is frequently that of helper T-cell, but TCR gene is not demonstrable in most cases. EBV genomes are frequently demonstrated in LG. WG has neither specific immunophenotype, nor gene rearrangement and EB genomes identified.

Angiocentric T-cell lymphoma or grade III AIL should be distinguished from pseudolymphoma and other lymphomas. Katzenstein and Peiper emphasized the difficulty in distinguishing AIL from pseudolymphoma in the lungs.[29] Pinkus and Said indicated that cytologic pleomorphism, the presence of

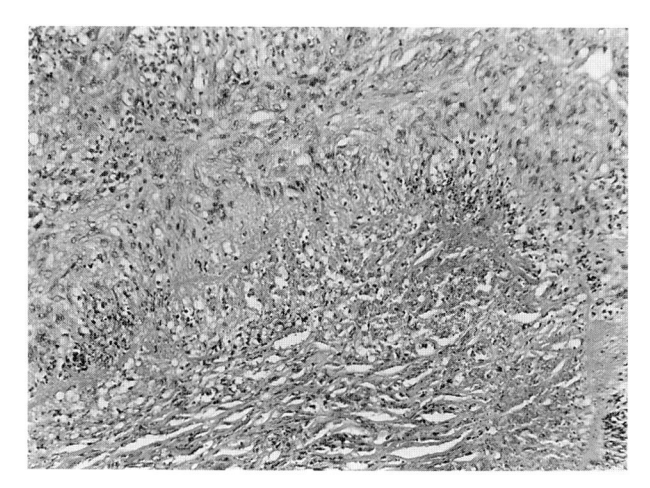

Fig. 21.8. A case of Wegener's granulomatosis in the lung showing extensive necrosis and palisading epithelioid histiocytes mimicking lymphomatoid granulomatosis. H&E, ×250. (Courtesy of Dr. A-L. A. Katzenstein.)

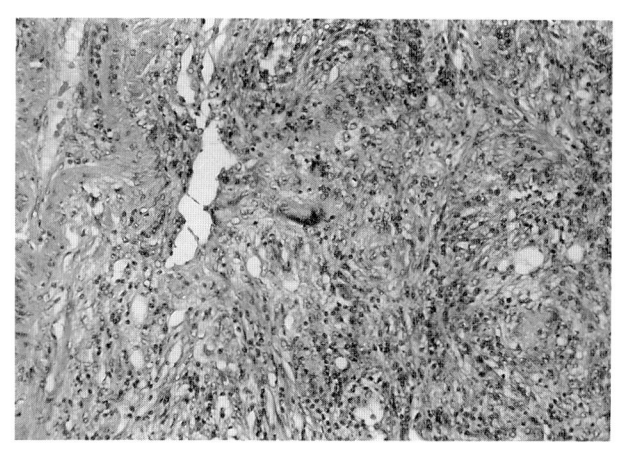

Fig. 21.9. The same case as in Fig. 21.8 showing polymorphic infiltration and a multinucleated giant cell in the center. H&E, ×250.

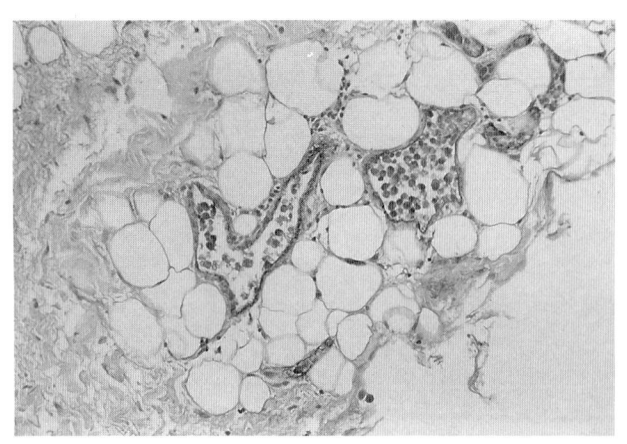

Fig. 21.10. A case of malignant angioendotheliomatosis (intravascular lymphoma) in subcutaneous tissue showing lymphoma cells inside the lumen of blood vessels, but the blood vessel wall is not involved. H&E, ×250.

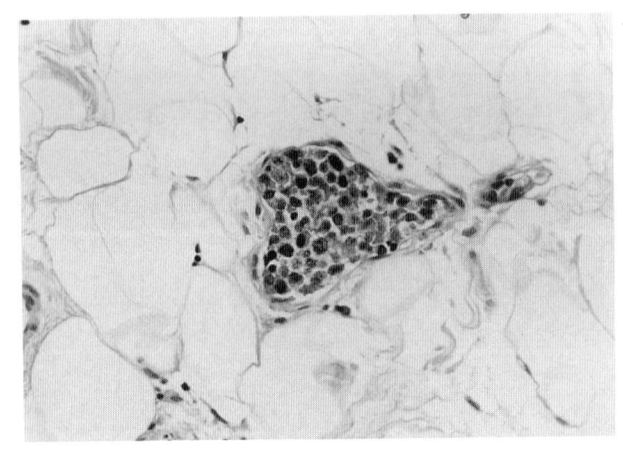

Fig. 21.11. A higher-power view of the case of intravascular lymphoma (Fig. 21.10) showing polymorphic lymphoma cells and intact blood vessel wall. H&E, ×500.

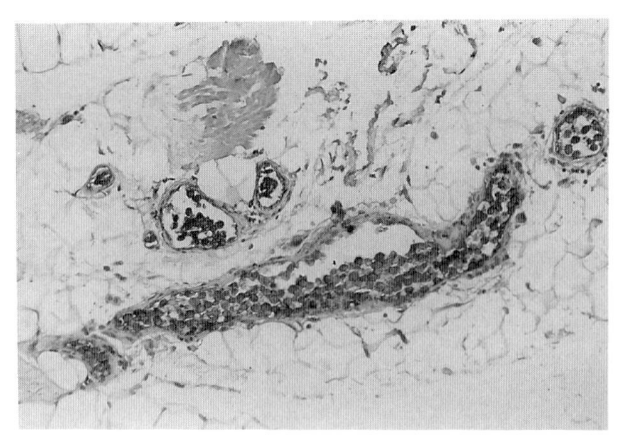

Fig. 21.12. The same case of Fig. 21.11 showing CD20 staining of lymphoma cells. Immunoperoxidase, ×250.

large lymphoid cells, and the angiodestructive character of angiocentric lymphoma are in marked contrast to the reactive process.[1] Pseudolymphoma is usually composed of small lymphocytes and is sometimes associated with germinal centers, but angiocentric and angiodestructive lesions are inconspicuous. A dominant helper-T-cell phenotype or TCR gene rearrangement is helpful to substantiate the diagnosis of lymphoma.

Other lymphomas may also involve the blood vessels and show necrosis. However, vascular infiltration is usually restricted to veins[1] and necrosis is seldom associated with vascular distribution.[4] In addition, angiocentric lymphoma shows more cellular and nuclear pleomorphism than large-cell and small non-cleaved-cell lymphomas.[4] When the skin is involved, angiocentric lymphoma is confined to the mid and deep dermis, in contrast to mycosis fungoides, which shows a predilection for the papillary dermis and epidermis.[19,20] Some T-cell lymphomas may occasionally involve subcutaneous fat manifested as panniculitis. These T-cell lymphomas usually show atypical mixed-cell or large-cell infiltration in the connective tissue septa between adipocytes with fat necrosis, histiocytic infiltrate, and karyorrhexis.[1] Angiocentric and angiodestructive features are inconspicious, and hemophagocytic syndrome is frequently observed in these T-cell lymphomas.[1] Finally, malignant angioendotheliomatosis (intravascular lymphoma) may be present in the skin and CNS, mimicking angiocentric lymphoma (Figs. 21.10–21.12). However, the tumor cells of this lymphoma are in the lumina of small blood vessels and do not infiltrate the blood vessel walls or cause tissue infarction.[1]

REFERENCES

1. Pinkus GS, Said JW: Peripheral T-cell lymphomas. In Knowles DM (ed): *Neoplastic Hematopathology*, Baltimore, Williams & Wilkins, 1992, pp 837–867.
2. DeRemee RA, Weiland LH, McDonald TJ: Polymorphic reticulosis, lymphomatoid granulomatosis: Two diseases or one? *Mayo Clin Proc* 53:634–640, 1978.

3. Jaffe ES: Pathologic and clinical spectrum of post-thymic T-cell malignancies. *Cancer Invest* 2:413–426, 1984.
4. Lipford EH Jr, Margolick JB, Longo DL, et al: Angiocentric immunoproliferative lesions: A clinicopathologic spectrum of post-thymic T-cell proliferations. *Blood* 72:1674–1681, 1988.
5. Pisani RJ, DeRemee RA: Clinical implications of the histopathologic diagnosis of pulmonary lymphomatoid granulomatosis. *Mayo Clin Proc* 65:151–163, 1990.
6. Crissman JD, Weiss MA, Gluckman J: Midline granuloma syndrome: A clinicopathologic study of 13 patients. *Am J Surg Pathol* 6:335–346, 1982.
7. Costa J, Delacretaz F: The midline granuloma syndrome. *Pathol Annu* 21:159–171, 1986.
8. Tsokos M, Fauci AS, Costa J: Idiopathic midline destructive disease (IMDD): A subgroup of patients with the "midline granuloma" syndrome. *Am J Clin Pathol* 77:162–168, 1982.
9. Fauci AS, Haynes GF, Costa J, et al: Lymphomatoid granulomatosis: Prospective clinical and therapeutic experience over 10 years. *N Engl J Med* 306:68–74, 1982.
10. Katzenstein A-LA, Carrington CB, Liebow AA: Lymphomatoid granulomatosis: A clinicopathologic study of 152 cases. *Cancer* 43:360–373, 1979.
11. Medeiros LJ, Peiper SC, Elwood L, et al: Angiocentric immunoproliferative lesions: A molecular analysis of eight cases. *Hum Pathol* 22:1150–1157, 1991.
12. Shimokawa I, Ushijima N, Moriuchi R, et al: A case of angiocentric immunoproliferative lesions (angiocentric lymphoma) associated with human T-cell lymphotropic virus type 1. *Hum Pathol* 24:921–923, 1993.
13. Ho FCS, Choy D, Loke SL, et al: Polymorphic reticulosis and conventional lymphomas of the nose and upper aerodigestive tract: A clinicopathologic study of 70 cases and immunophenotypic studies of 16 cases. *Hum Pathol* 21:1041–1050, 1990.
14. Vergier B, Capron F, Trojani M, et al: Benign lymphocytic angiitis and granulomatosis: A T-cell lymphoma? *Hum Pathol* 23:1191–1194, 1992.
15. Hseuh C, Gonzalez-Crussi F, Murphy SB: Testicular angiocentric lymphoma of post-thymic T-cell type in a child with T-cell acute lymphoblastic leukemia in remission. *Cancer* 72:1801–1805, 1993.
16. Troussard X, Galateau F, Gaulard P, et al: Lymphomatoid granulomatosis in a patient with acute myeloblastic leukemia in remission. *Cancer* 65:107–111, 1990.
17. Jaffe ES, Costa J, Fauci AS, et al: Malignant lymphoma and erythrophagocytosis simulating malignant histiocytosis. *Am J Med* 75:741–749, 1983.
18. Falini B, Pileri S, DeSolas I, et al: Peripheral T-cell lymphomas associated with hemophagocytic syndrome. *Blood* 75:434–444, 1990.
19. Chan JKC, Ng CS, Ngan KC, et al: Angiocentric-T-cell lymphoma of the skin: An aggressive lymphoma distinct from mycosis fungoides. *Am J Surg Pathol* 12:861–876, 1988.
20. Carlson KC, Gibson LE: Cutaneous signs of lymphomatoid granulomatosis. *Arch Dermatol* 127:1693–1698, 1991.
21. Chan JKC, Ng CS, Lau WH, et al: Most nasal/nasopharyngeal lymphomas are peripheral T-cell neoplasms. *Am J Surg Pathol* 11:418–429, 1987.
22. Gaulard P, Henni T, Marolleau JP, et al: Lethal midline granuloma (polymorphic reticulosis) and lymphomatoid granulomatosis: Evidence for a monoclonal T-cell lymphoproliferative disorder. *Cancer* 62:705–710, 1988.
23. Aviles A, Rodriquez L, Guzman R, et al: Angiocentric T-cell lymphoma of the nose, paranasal sinuses and hard palate. *Hematol Oncol* 10:141–147, 1992.
24. Shimokawa I, Ushijima N, Moriuchi R, et al: A case of angiocentric immunoproliferative lesions (angiocentric lymphoma) associated with human T-cell lymphotropic virus type 1. *Hum Pathol* 24:921–923, 1993.
25. Nakamura S, Suchi T, Koshikawa T, et al: Aggressive rectal lymphoma of large granular lymphocytes with the histologic feature of an angiocentric grown pattern. *Cancer* 71:249–256, 1993.
26. Guinee D, Jr., Jaffe E., Kingma D, et al: Pulmonary lymphomatoid granulomatosis. Evidence of a proliferation of Epstein-Barr virus infected B-lymphocytes with a prominent T-cell component and vasculitis. *Am J Surg Pathol* 1994; 18:753–764.
27. Wong KF, Chan JKC, Ng CS, et al: CD56 (NKH-1)-positive hematolymphoid malignancies: An aggressive neoplasm featuring frequent cutaneous/mucosal involvement, cytoplasmic azurophilic granules and angiocentricity. *Hum Pathol* 23:798–804, 1992.
28. Suzumiya J, Takeshita M, Kimura N, et al: Expression of adult and fetal natural killer cell markers in sinonasal lymphomas. *Blood* 83:2255–2260, 1994.
29. Katzenstein A-LA, Peiper SC: Detection of Epstein–Barr virus genomes in lymphomatoid granulomatosis: Analysis of 29 cases by the polymerase chain reaction technique. *Mod Pathol* 3:435–441, 1990.
30. Medeiros LJ, Jaffe ES, Chen YY, et al: Localization of Epstein–Barr viral genomes in angiocentric immunoproliferative lesions. *Am J Surg Pathol* 16:439–447, 1992.
31. Borisch B, Hennig I, Laeng RH, et al: Association of the subtype 2 of the Epstein–Barr virus with T-cell non-Hodgkin's lymphoma of the midline granuloma type. *Blood* 82:858–864, 1993.
32. Sabourin JC, Kanavaros P, Briere J, et al: Epstein–Barr virus (EBV) genomes and EBV-encoded latent membrane protein (LMP) in pulmonary lymphomas occurring in non-immunocompromised patients. *Am J Surg Pathol* 17:995–1002, 1993.
33. deBruin PC, Jiwa M, Oudejans JJ, et al: Presence of Epstein–Barr virus in extranodal T-cell lymphomas: Differences in relation to site. *Blood* 83:1612–1618, 1994.

22
Lymphoplasmacytic Lymphoma vs. Plasmacytoma vs. Plasmacytoid T-Cell Lymphoma (Plasmacytoid Monocytoid Sarcoma)

Many lymphoproliferative disorders may contain significant numbers of plasma cells. In some lymphomas, the presence of plasma cells may be a constant feature but not the integral component of malignancy, such as splenic lymphoma with villous lymphocytes, lymphoma of mucosa-associated lymphoid tissue, immunoblastic lymphadenopathy-like T-cell lymphoma, and Hodgkin's disease. Another group of lymphomas, such as lymphoplasmacytic lymphoma, plasmacytoma, and myeloma, the plasma cells or plasmacytoid cells are monoclonal and are thus an integral part of the tumor. In Castleman's disease, plasma-cell subtype, the plasma cells may occasionally be monoclonal but are not considered to be neoplastic. The plasmacytoid T-cell lymphoma is a newly described entity, but it turns out to be a misnomer; the origin of the neoplastic cells is, in fact, monocyte/macrophage.

CLINICAL MANIFESTATION

Lymphoplasmacytic Lymphoma

Lymphoplasmacytic lymphoma is designated *lymphoplasmacytic/lymphoplasmacytoid lymphoma* (immunocytoma) in the updated Kiel classification. It is also equivalent to malignant lymphoma, small lymphocytic, plasmacytoid subtype in the Working Formulation. This lymphoma is associated mainly with Waldenstrom's macroglobulinemia (WM), but not chronic lymphocytic leukemia.[1] The median age of WM patients is 63 years, with a 55% male predominance.[2] In the so-called splenomegalic immunocytoma, the patients usually have splenomegaly but not lymphadenopathy.[3] These cases are now classified as splenic lymphoma with villous lymphocytes.[4] Besides the splenomegalic subtype, most patients have slow-developing, multiregional lymphadenopathy. Immunocytoma may also develop primarily at an extranodal site.

Monoclonal gammopathy is encountered in at least 36% of patients with immunocytoma.[1] Most cases show monoclonal IgM, but some patients may have monoclonal IgG, and rarely IgA or IgE.[1] Approximately 60% of patients have lymphocytosis (>4 × 10^9/L), which can be small lymphocytes or lymphoplasmacytoid cells.

Cases with symptomatic monoclonal IgM gammopathy are referred to as WM. The IgM level required for distinction between WM and monoclonal gammopathy of unknown significance (MGVS) varies from 10 to 30 g per liter.[5,6] However, it is more reliable to use a multifactorial criterion, such as clinical symptoms, bone marrow, and/or lymph node involvement, serum-β microglobulin levels, to make the diagnosis.

Major clinical symptoms in WM include hyperviscosity syndrome, bleeding diathesis, cryoglobulinemia, cold agglutinin hemolytic anemia, peripheral neuropathy, renal disease, and amyloidosis.[2] The most important, independent, prognostic factors for WM in a recent study are age, hemoglobin concentration, weight loss, and cryoglobulinemia.[5] In patients who are refractory to treatment, the median survival is 2.5 years. For those who respond to adequate treatment, the median survival is about 5–7 years.[2]

Plasmacytoma

Plasmacytoma is also called *plasmacytic lymphoma*. It may be presented as solitary plasmacytoma of bone (SPB) or extramedullary plasmacytoma (EP). In bone, the spine, pelvis, and femurs are the most common sites of involvement.[7] EP most commonly involves the upper air passageway, including the nasopharynx, paranasal sinuses, nasal cavity, tonsils, epiglottis, and floor of the mouth.[8] Lymph nodes of the head and neck are frequently involved. Involvement of lymph nodes in the axillary, mesenteric, and pelvic regions is also not rare.[9] Because of the partial neoplastic replacement of the lymph node that is ipsilateral to the primary lesion, the lymph node lesion is usually secondary. However, primary plasmacytoma in lymph nodes also exists. Recently, several cases of plasmacytoma of the gastrointestinal (GI) tract have been reported.[10–13] Cases of cutaneous, pulmonary, pancreatic, renal, and bladder plasmacytoma have also been reported.[14–18]

Serum paraprotein and Bence–Jones protein are seldom seen in EP probably because of the low tumor mass. However, in four recently reported cases of GI plasmacytoma, all were associated with paraprotein production, including one to three classes of heavy chains (although the presence of different heavy chains was proved to be due to heavy-chain switching and not different clonal origin).[10-13] In any event, 36% of EPs may finally develop osteolytic bone lesion or convert into myeloma when monoclonal gammopathy appears.[8,9] SPB produces paraprotein in the serum and urine in less than half of the patients.[7] Of these cases, 53% may also evolve into multiple myeloma.[8] In addition, SPB may also develop into multiple EP lesions.[19]

Patients with SPB are 50–55 years old and 70% of patients are male.[7] The average age of patients with EP is 52 years, and the male:female ratio is 2:1.[8] The median survival period for patients with either disease exceeds 10 years.[7,8]

Plasmacytoid T-Cell Lymphoma

The term *plasmacytoid T-cell lymphoma* was originally designated because the lymphoma cells are morphologically plasmacytoid and yet they are located in the T-zone of lymph nodes and are positive for several T-cell markers. As will be discussed later, this tumor is now recognized as of monocyte/macrophage origin on the basis of marker studies and the association with myelomonocytic leukemias. This is a rare clinicopathologic entity, as less than 10 cases have been reported.[20-27]

In the 8 reported cases, the male:female ratio is 3:1 and the median age is 73 years. Most are elderly patients over 58 years, except one 6-year-old girl. This lymphoma is associated with myeloproliferative disorders (acute myelogenous leukemia, chronic myelogenous leukemia, or myelodysplastic syndrome), which occur before, after, or at the same time as the lymphoma develops. The clinical symptoms are usually nonspecific constitutional symptoms, such as fatigue, weight loss, night sweats, asthma, anorexia, and abdominal discomfort. Generalized lymphadenopathy has been encountered in all cases and hepatosplenomegaly in 5 of 8 cases.[20-27] Five patients died of leukemia at 3 weeks to 28 months after diagnosis. Three patients were lost to follow-up, but one of the three expired of leukemia-related complications.

PATHOLOGY

Lymphoplasmacytic Lymphoma

In the Working Formulation, small lymphocytic lymphoma (SLL) is divided into two subtypes: chronic lymphocytic leukemia (CLL) and plasmacytoid. The current thinking is that SLL, CLL, and lymphoplasmacytic lymphoma should be considered as similar but separate entities.[28] For instance, patients with SLL usually have no lymphocytosis. Therefore, it is inappropriate to make a diagnosis of SLL consistent with CLL when there is no leukemic phase detected (Fig. 22.1). On the other hand, lymphoplasmacytic lymphoma should not be considered equivalent to WM because the major diagnostic criterion of WM is the presence of monoclonal IgM gammopathy,[2,6] so the presence of lymphoplasmacytic lymphoma may or may not be associated with WM and vice versa.

In the Kiel classification, lymphoplasmacytic lymphoma is called *immunocytoma* with the subtypes of lymphoplasmacytoid and lymphoplasmacytic lymphomas. In this chapter, we use the term *lymphoplasmacytic lymphoma* to include both subtypes. The lymphoplasmacytoid subtype is usually CD5-positive, more often leukemic but less often paraproteinemic.[1] The lymphoplasmacytic subtypes is just the opposite. The polymorphic subtype, which contains large numbers of immunoblasts, is no longer included in the updated Kiel classification.

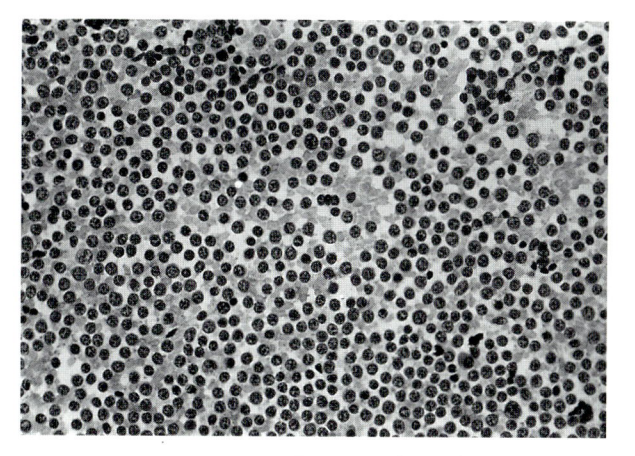

Fig. 22.1. An imprint of a lymph node of a case of small lymphocytic lymphoma consistent with chronic lymphocytic leukemia showing uniform, small, mature-looking lymphoid cells. H&E, ×500.

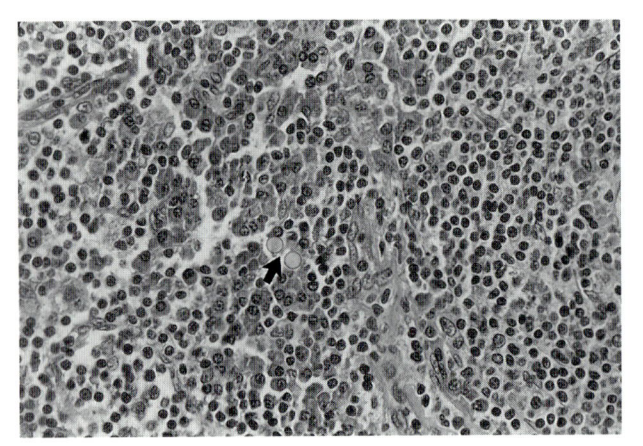

206 DIFFERENTIAL DIAGNOSIS OF LYMPHOID DISORDERS

Fig. 22.2. A case of lymphoplasmacytic lymphoma showing predominantly lymphoid cells at right and plasma cells at left. Note two Russell bodies (arrow) in the center. H&E, ×500.

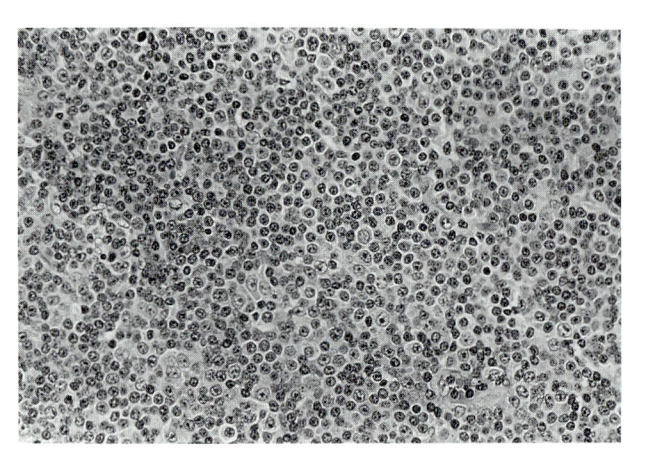

Fig. 22.4. A case of small lymphocytic lymphoma showing predominantly small, uniform, lymphoid cells with a few prolymphocytes. H&E, ×500.

The basic pattern of lymphoplasmacytic lymphoma is the diffuse infiltration of well-differentiated small lymphoid cells with the normal architecture of the lymph node partially or completely effaced. The small lymphocytes make up 50–90% of the tumor cells, and the plasma cells or plasmacytoid cells usually make up less than 10% of the population (Fig. 22.2).[1] these plasma/plasmacytoid cells may contain intracytoplasmic (Russell bodies) (Fig. 22.3) and/or intranuclear inclusions (Dutcher bodies). They bear a monoclonal cytoplasmic immunoglobulin pattern, as in contrast to the reactive plasma cells, which are polyclonal. In addition, varying numbers of immunoblasts are often present (Fig. 22.4). Similar to small lymphocytic lymphoma, proliferation centers may be found (Figs. 22.5–22.7).[1] In some cases of lymphoplasmacytic lymphoma, there are numerous epithelioid cells; those cases should be distinguished from lymphoepithelioid T-cell lymphoma (Lennert's lymphoma) (Fig. 22.8).[29]

In lymphoplasmacytic lymphoma the bone marrow is frequently involved and the infiltrating pattern can be nodular, interstitial, mixed, or diffuse (Figs. 22.9–22.15).[28] The presence of a lymphoplasmacytic population in the bone marrow may help establish the diagnosis.

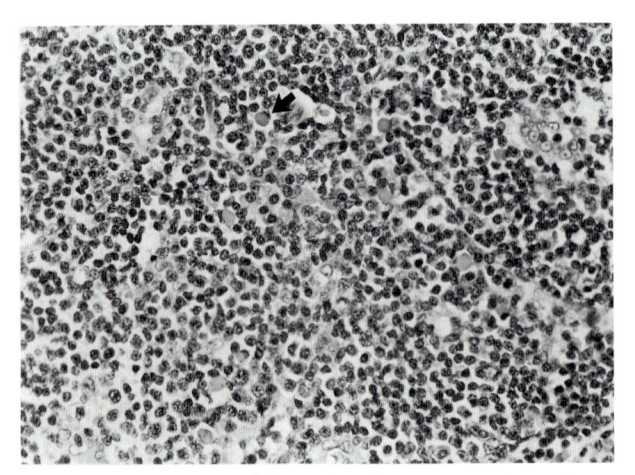

Fig. 22.3. A case of lymphoplasmacytic lymphoma showing Russell bodies in a few cells (arrow). H&E, ×500.

Fig. 22.5. A case of small lymphocytic lymphoma showing proliferation centers. H&E, ×125.

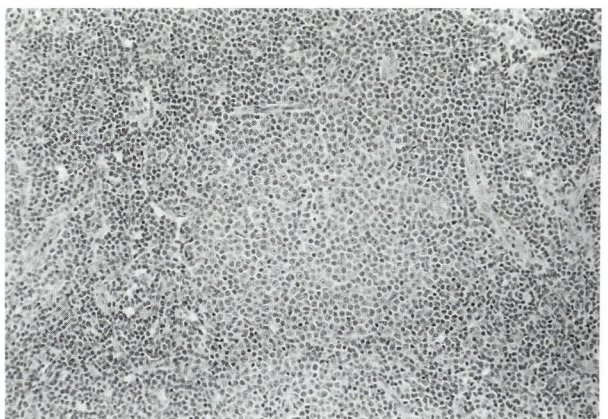

Fig. 22.6. The higher-power view of a proliferation center with pale-staining activated lymphocytes or prolymphocytes, imparting a pseudofollicular appearance. H&E, ×250.

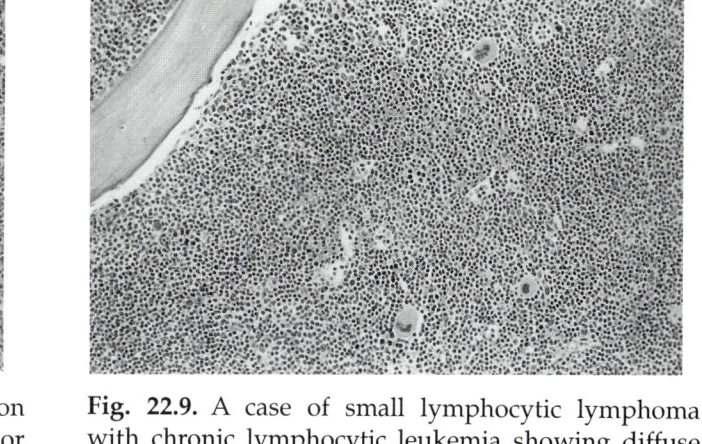

Fig. 22.9. A case of small lymphocytic lymphoma with chronic lymphocytic leukemia showing diffuse small-lymphoid-cell infiltration in the bone marrow. H&E, ×250.

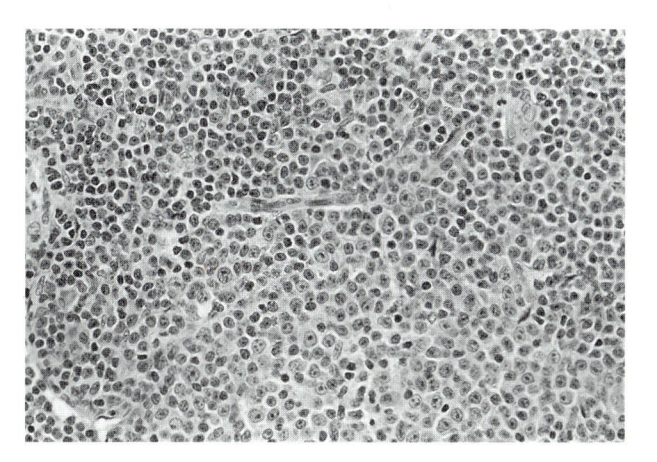

Fig. 22.7. A high-power view of the proliferation center showing the morphology of the prolymphocytes. H&E, ×500.

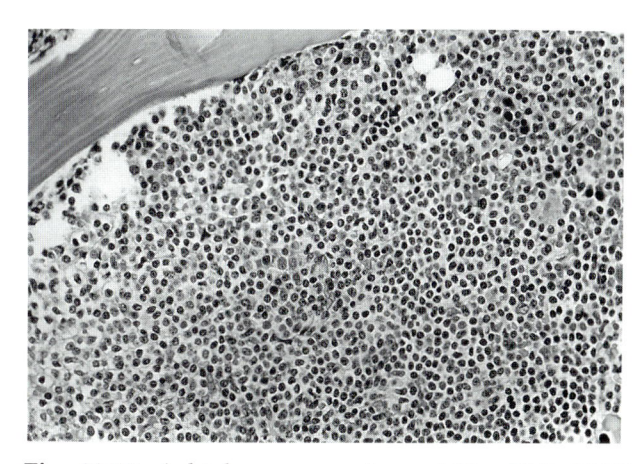

Fig. 22.10. A higher-power view of Fig. 22.9. H&E, ×500.

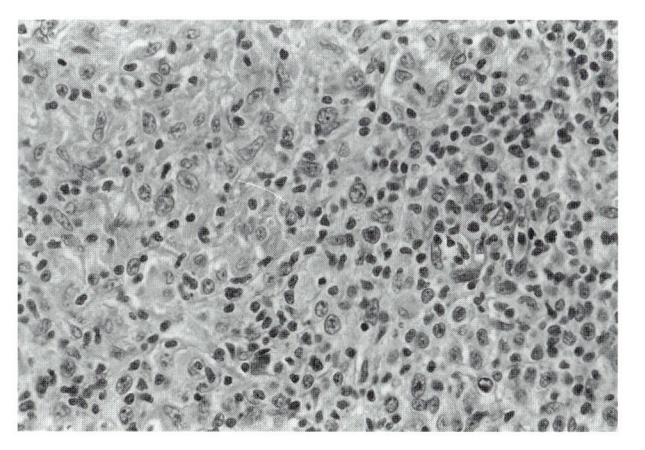

Fig. 22.8. Lymph node biopsy of Lennert's lymphoma showing epithelioid histiocytes at left and mixed small and large lymphoid cells at right. H&E, ×500.

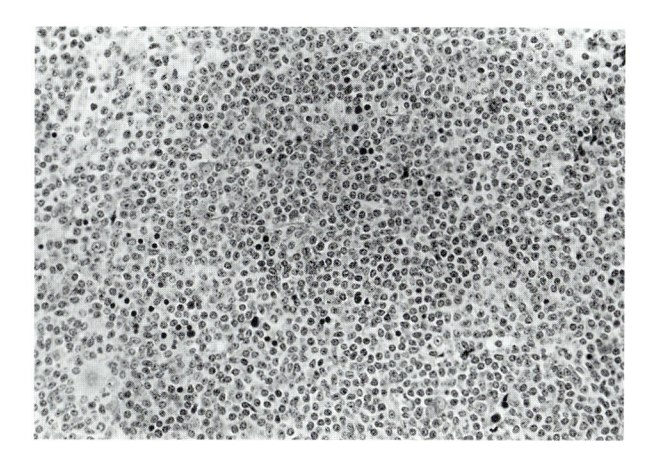

Fig. 22.11. Bone marrow biopsy of a case of small lymphocytic lymphoma with chronic lymphocytic leukemia showing a delicate chromatin pattern with the Giemsa stain. ×500.

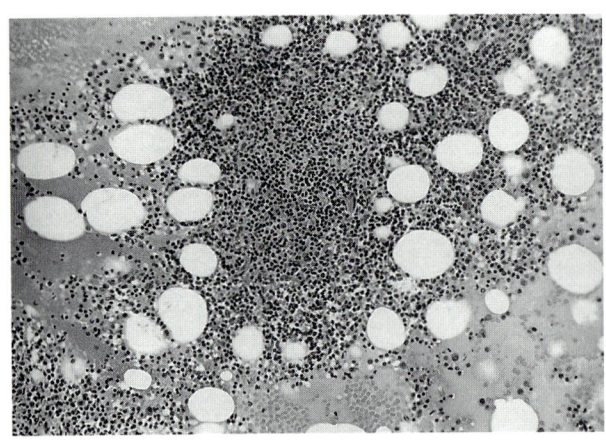

208 DIFFERENTIAL DIAGNOSIS OF LYMPHOID DISORDERS

Fig. 22.12. A case of lymphoplasmacytic lymphoma with Waldenström's macroglobulinemia showing a nodular pattern in the bone marrow. H&E, ×250.

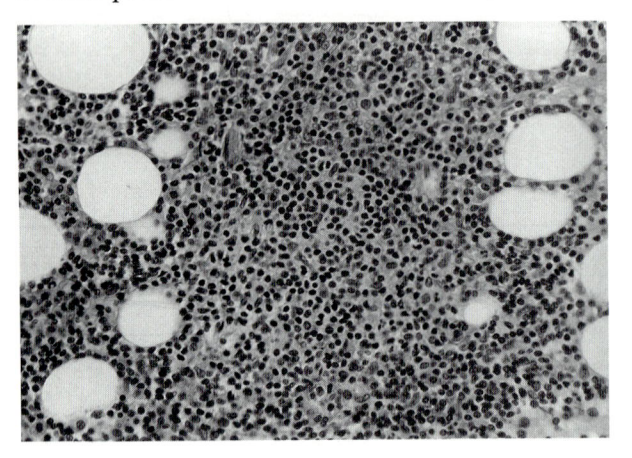

Fig. 22.13. A higher magnification of Fig. 22.12 showing lymphoplasmacytic infiltrate. H&E, ×500.

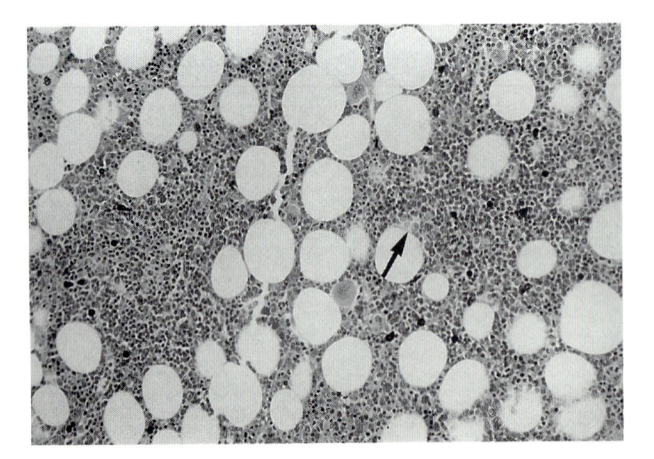

Fig. 22.14. A case of lymphoplasmacytic lymphoma with Waldenström's macroglobulinemia showing clusters of plasma cells (arrow) that are easily recognized in this Giemsa-stained preparation, ×250.

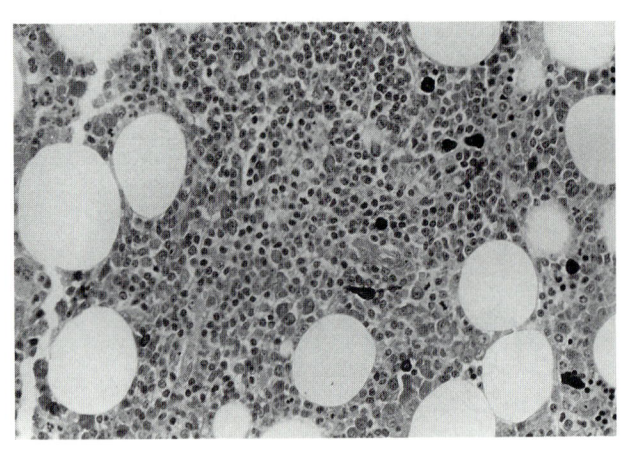

Fig. 22.15. A higher-power view of Fig. 22.14 showing lymphoplasmacytic infiltrate. A few darkly stained mast cells are also present. Giemsa, ×500.

Plasmacytoma

Plasmacytoma includes EP and SPB; both are solitary plasmacytic tumor located in soft tissue or bone, respectively. They are distinguished from multiple myeloma (Figs. 22.16–22.23) by the absence of a plasma cell infiltration in random bone marrow biopsies, no evidence of other bone lesions (besides the SPB lesion) by radiographic examination and absence of renal failure, hypercalcemia, and anemia that are possibly caused by myeloma.[7] EP and SPB differ from lymphoplasmacytic lymphoma by their exclusive composition of mature and/or immature plasma cells. However, in secondary lesions, such as in the lymph

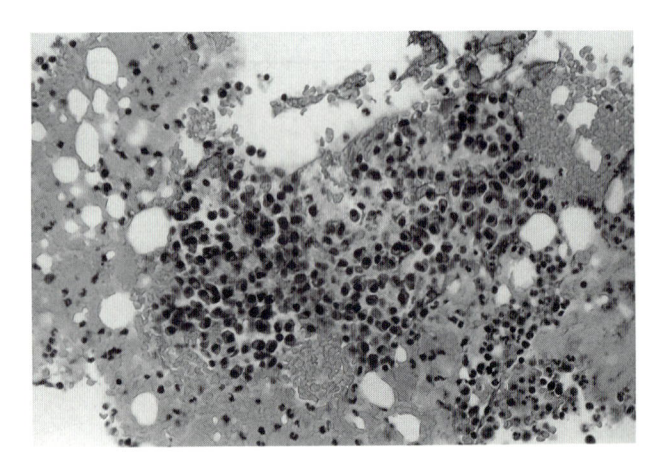

Fig. 22.16. A case of solitary plasmacytoma of bone composed exclusively of mature plasma cells. H&E, ×500.

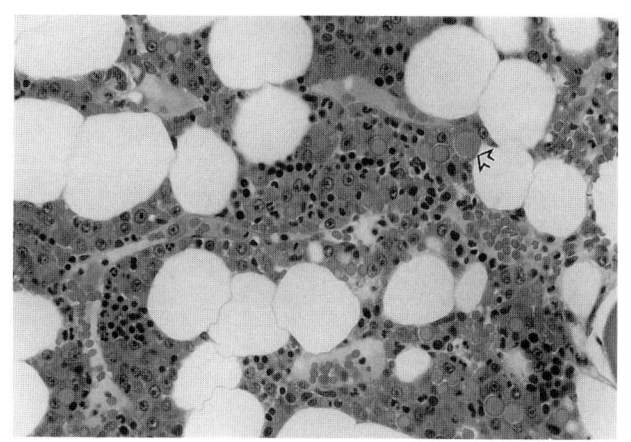

Fig. 22.17. A case of multiple myeloma showing that the normal bone marrow components are partially replaced by immature plasmacytoid cells with prominent nucleoli. Note the presence of multiple Russell bodies (arrow). H&E, ×500.

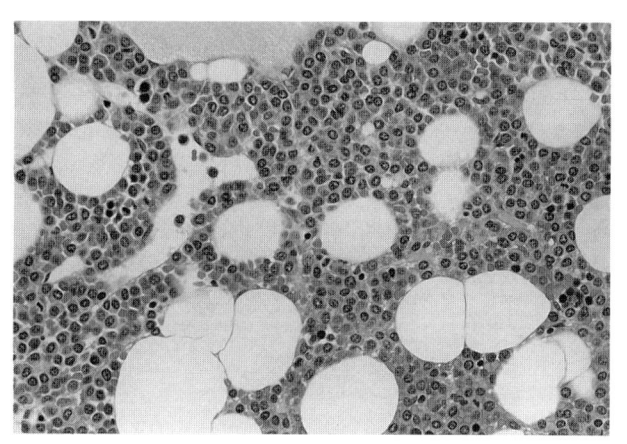

Fig. 22.18. A case of multiple myeloma showing complete bone marrow replacement by uniform plasma cells. H&E, ×500.

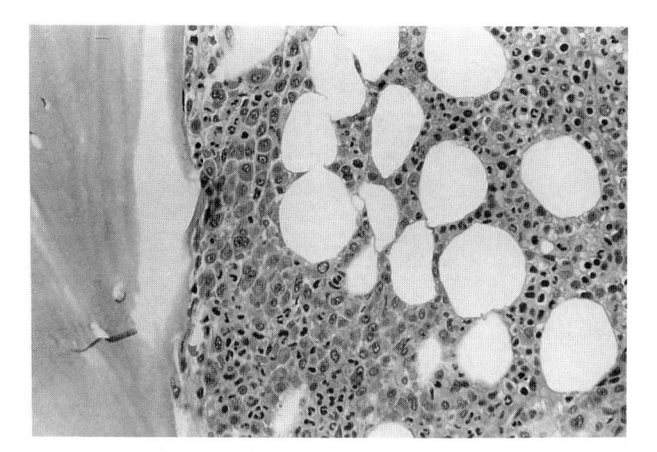

Fig. 22.19. A case of multiple myeloma showing paratrabecular infiltration by pleomorphic plasma cells. H&E, ×500.

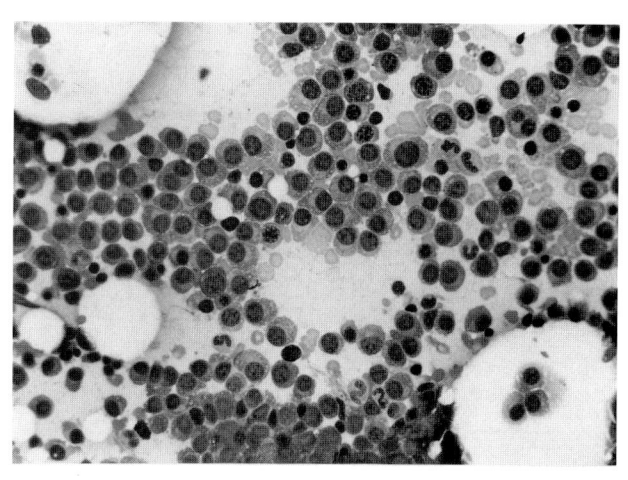

Fig. 22.20. A bone marrow aspirate in a case of multiple myeloma showing a sheet of plasma cells. Wright–Giemsa, ×125.

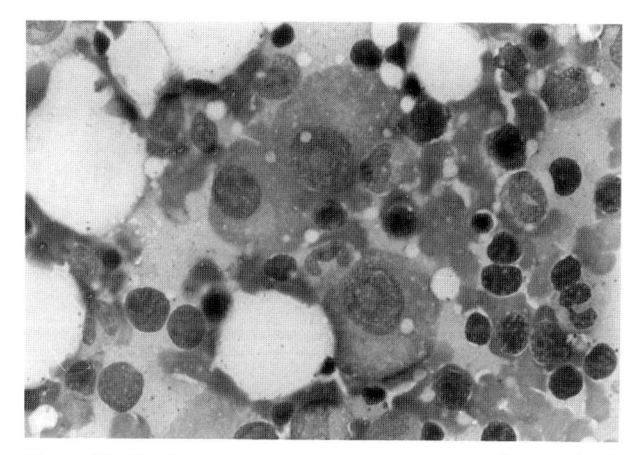

Fig. 22.21. Bone marrow aspirate of multiple myeloma showing two plasmoblasts with prominent nucleoli and a plasma cell in the center. Wright–Giemsa, ×1250.

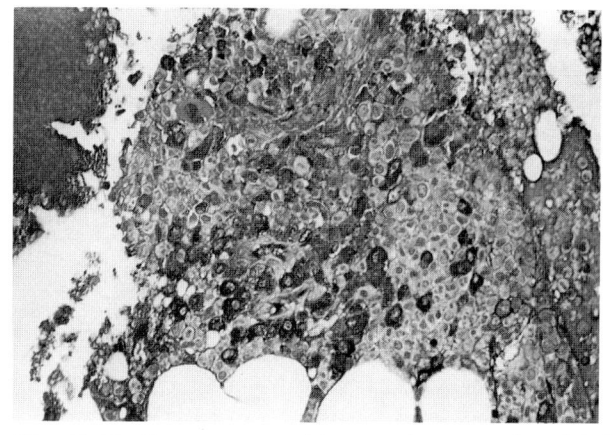

Fig. 22.22. Bone marrow biopsy of a case of multiple myeloma showing cytoplasmic κ light-chain stain in most tumor cells. Immunoperoxidase, ×500.

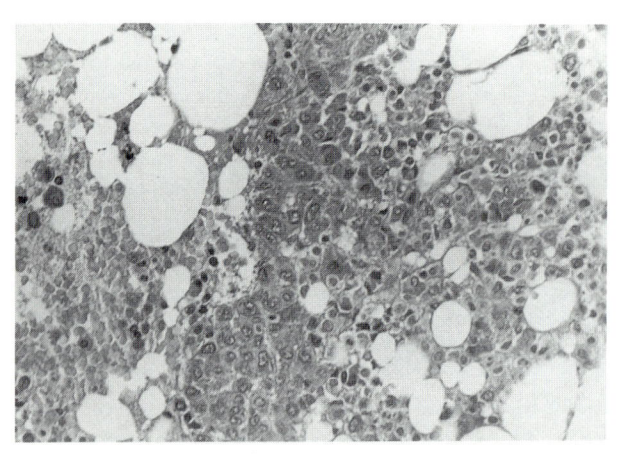

Fig. 22.23. The same specimen as in Fig. 22.22 showing negative stain for λ light chain. Immunoperoxidase, ×500.

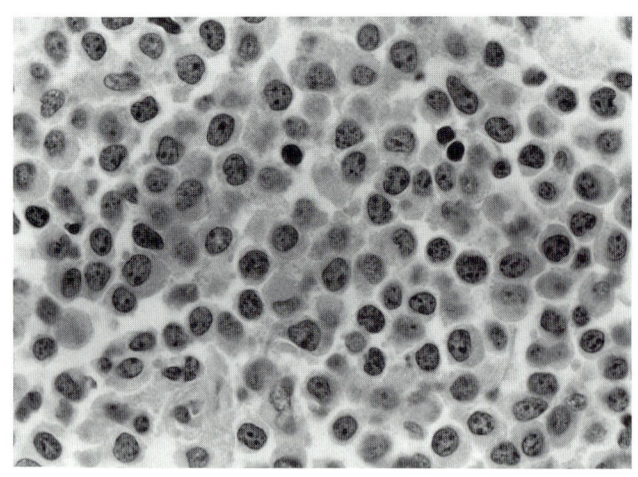

Fig. 22.24. Plasmacytoid T-cell lymphoma in lymph node showing eccentrically located nuclei and a plasmacytoid cytoplasm. H&E, ×1,250. (Case contributed by Dr. C. H. Koo, Kaiser Foundation Hospital.)

nodes, the tumor cells can be intermingled with the remaining normal cellular components.

The mature plasma cells are easily recognizable by their oval configuration, eccentric nucleus, paranuclear halo (hof), and the typical "cartwheel" chromatin pattern. In the immature plasma cells, the only recognized feature may be an eccentric nucleus with or without a hof. These immature cells may have finely dispersed chromatin and prominent nucleoli.[30] The tumor cells can be pleomorphic with varying size and shape and may show binucleation, irregular nuclei, and mitoses. Intracytoplasmic inclusions of immunoglobulin (Russell bodies) are frequently present. They are usually homogeneously stained, but can also be crystalline.[12] The crystals may also appear in intercellular space or inside macrophages.[31] Amyloid deposition may be found in the interstitium and blood vessel walls.[30]

Several factors may be used to predict the conversion of plasmacytoma to multiple myeloma: nuclear immaturity, presence of prominent nucleoli, high serum protein level, presence of monoclonal gammopathy, and large size of primary lesions.[9,30]

Plasmacytoid T-Cell Lymphoma

As mentioned above, *plasmacytoid T-cell lymphoma* is a misnomer. Plasmacytoid T-cell has been renamed by Beiske et al. as *plasmacytoid T-zone cells*[22] and by Facchetti et al. as *plasmacytoid monocytes*.[23] Accordingly, Baddoura et al. have suggested to designate this tumor as *plasmacytoid T-zone lymphoma* or *plasmacytoid monocyte proliferation*,[27] and Thomas et al. have suggested the term *plasmacytoid monocyte sarcoma*.[26]

As indicated by these terms, the tumor cells are plasmacytoid. In other words, they have eccentric nuclei, coarsely stippled chromatin with marginal condensation or cartwheel-like chromatin, and a moderate amount of basophilic cytoplasm, which is evident in Giemsa stained preparations (Figs. 22.24, 22.25). The tumor cells are of intermediate size. The nuclei are round to oval and occasionally indented. A small

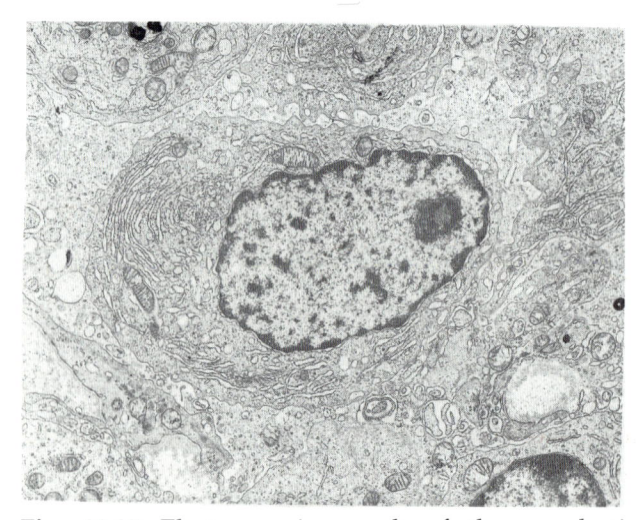

Fig. 22.25. Electron micrograph of the neoplastic "plasmacytoid T-cell" showing parallel strands of rough endoplasmic reticulum resembling those seen in plasma cells. ×11,000. (Same source as Fig. 22.24.)

distinct nucleolus is frequently present. The mitotic rate is low. A paranuclear halo (hof) as seen in true plasma cells is sometimes present. However, secretory products (immunoglobulins) have never been identified in these cells.

Characteristically, these plasmacytoid cells infiltrate the paracortical or T-zone area, and may expand to the deep cortex and medulla.[20-27] The tumor cells are topographically close to interdigitating reticulum cells and high endothelial venules. The infiltration pattern is nodular and diffuse, causing partial or complete effacement of the normal architecture of the lymph node. Scattered tingible-body macrophages are seen, giving the starry-sky appearance. When myelogenous leukemia coexists, myelomonocytic cells may be intermingled with the plasmacytoid cells. Scattered true plasma cells are seen in a few cases.[22]

In the bone marrow, the infiltrating cells are usually those of myeloid or monocytoid leukemic cells or those with myelodysplastic changes. Plasmacytoid tumor cells are seen in the marrow only occasionally.[27] Tumor cells have not been found in the peripheral blood in any of the cases reported.

LABORATORY FINDINGS

Lymphoplasmacytic Lymphoma

The major diagnostic feature for lymphoplasmacytic lymphoma is a well-differentiated small lymphocytic lymphoma with a monoclonal population of plasma/plasmacytoid cells. Lennert and Feller have recommended the use of Giemsa stain to facilitate the recognition of the plasmacytoid cells, which may be inconspicuous in H&E-stained preparations.[1] They have also advocated the use of PAS stain to demonstrate the Russell and Dutcher bodies.[1] Dutcher bodies are found in only one-quarter of the cases, but their presence is valuable in ruling out reactive plasmacytosis. The Goldner or Ladewig stain can stain IgM green or grayish-blue but stain other immunoglobulins red.[1]

The immunophenotype of the neoplastic cells show a monoclonal surface immunoglobulin pattern (mostly IgM) with positive B-cell surface antigens, CD19, CD20, and CD22. The lymphoplasmacytoid subtype expresses, in addition, CD5 and CD23, but the lymphoplasmacytic subtype is always CD5-negative and CD23-positive in 50% of the cases.[1] The plasma/plasmacytoid cell population may show FMC7 and several activation antigens: CD25, CD38, and CD71.[28] This population seldom expresses B-cell surface antigen, such as CD19, CD20, and CD22. However, CD5, CD19, CD22, and Leu8 have been demonstrated in the Russell bodies of a case of lymphoplasmacytic lymphoma.[32] Surface immunoglobulin pattern is particularly useful in diagnosing Waldenström's macroglobulinemia in the bone marrow. In 16 morphologically normal or nondiagnostic bone marrow biopsies, 13 cases were diagnosed by demonstrating a monoclonal immunoglobulin pattern.[33]

Cytogenetic abnormalities, such as t(11;14) (q13;32) and trisomy 12, have been demonstrated in CLL, SLL, and lymphoplasmacytic lymphoma.[28] Recently, t(9;14) (p13;q32) has been found to be more specific for small-cell lymphoma with plasmacytoid differentiation.[34] In this study, 8 cases with t(9;14) were found among 426 consecutive specimens on non-Hodgkin's lymphoma, and 6 of them were small-cell lymphoma with plasmacytoid features.[34]

Plasmacytoma

The tumor cells in plasmacytoma characteristically show monoclonal cytoplasmic immunoglobulin, but not surface immunoglobulin. Among the immunoglobulins, IgA is most frequently expressed; IgG is less often and IgM is rarely demonstrated.[1,30] Surface B-cell antigens, such as CD19 and CD20, are usually negative. Plasma-cell antigens, PCA-1 and CD38, are always positive.[1,8] Some cases also express CD45R (Ki-B3+).[1]

As normal plasma cells, the tumor cells also show positive PAS and pyronine staining. Electron microscopy may demonstrate an elaborate endoplasmic reticulum and help identify the plasma cell nature.

The differences in adhesion molecules between the tumor cells of a subcutaneous plasmacytoma and those of the secondary plasma-cell leukemia in the same patient are interesting.[35] The subcutaneous plasmacytoma showed the adhesion molecules LFA-1 α (CD11a) and LFA-1 β (CD18), but was negative for ICAM-1 (ligand for LFA-1), while the phenotype of the leukemic cells was the reverse. ICAM-1 was also present in the capillary cells in this case. This situation is similar to that seen in the SLL and CLL. The former bears LFA-1 molecules and remains in the lymph node, while the latter carries no LFA-1 molecules and spreads to the blood.[28]

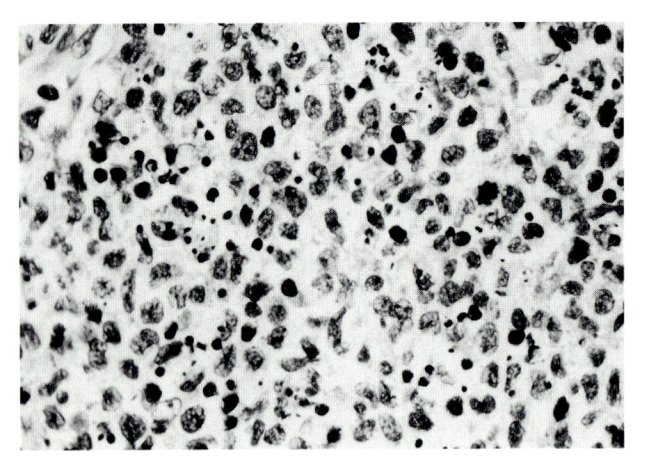

Fig. 22.26. Neoplastic "plasmacytoid T-cells" are stained with a macrophage marker KP1 (CD68). APAAP stain, ×1,250. (Same source as Fig. 22.24.)

Plasmacytoid T-Cell Lymphoma

The common phenotype of plasmacytoid T-cell lymphoma is the expression of CD2 (2 of 4 cases), CD4 (7 of 7 cases), CD5 (4 of 6 cases), CD71 (5 of 6 cases), and HLA-DR (5 of 6 cases), and the absence of CD3 and CD8 (in all cases tested).[20-27] Further study has demonstrated positivity in two more T-cell markers (CD7 and CD43).[27] All B-cell markers (CD19, CD20, CD22, and CDw75 or LN1), except for CD74 (LN2), are negative. CD10 was positive in 2 of 3 cases tested.[20,22,27] Because of this phenotype, the tumor was first considered to be T-cell in origin. Later studies, however, have revealed that two monocytic antigens (CD14 and CD68) are consistently positive (Fig. 22.26).[22-24,27] In spite of the negative results in other myelomonocyte markers, such as CD11b, CD13, CD15, and CD33, the current consensus is that the so-called plasmacytoid T-cell lymphoma is most likely derived from the monocyte/macrophage lineage, not only because of the markers but also because of the frequent association with myelomonocytic leukemias.

Cytochemical studies on lymph node imprints show that the tumor cells are positive for α-naphthyl butyrate esterase lysozyme, α$_1$-antichymotrypsin, cathepsin B, and acid phosphatase, but negative for myeloperoxidase, Sudan black and chloroacetate esterase.[27] These findings further suggest the monocytic origin of the tumor cells.

The absence of both immunoglobulin and T-cell receptor gene rearrangement further excludes the possibility of this tumor being of T-cell origin.[24,27] The positivity of T-cell antigens including CD2, CD4, CD7, and CD43 do not negate the monocytic origin of this tumor, as these antigens have been demonstrated in myelomonocytic cells.[24,27] The demonstration of CD5 in individual cases is difficult to explain and may represent aberrant expression by tumor cells.[23] The case reported by Caldwell et al. shows positive reactions to almost all T-cell markers (CD1, CD2, CD3, CD4, CD5, and CD7); thus it is a true T-cell lymphoma and differs from other reported cases.[25]

DIFFERENTIAL DIAGNOSIS

For lymphoplasmacytic lymphoma, the major differential diagnosis is to distinguish it from SLL and CLL. The most important element for their distinction is the presence of a monoclonal population of plasma cells in lymphoplasmacytic lymphoma. Plasma cells can also be seen in the other two conditions, but they are polyclonal.[1,28] SLL and CLL are characteristically positive for CD5, but lymphoplasmacytic lymphoma is CD5 positive only in its lymphoplasmacytoid subtype.[1]

TABLE 22.1
Comparison of Lymphoplasmacytic Lymphoma, Plasmacytoma, and Plasmacytoid T-Cell Lymphoma

	Lymphoplasmacytic lymphoma	Plasmacytoma	Plasmacytoid T-cell lymphoma
Plasma-cell component	<10%	100%	0%
Lymphocytosis	Present in 60% cases	Absent	Absent
Paraproteinemia	~36%	Rare	None
Prevalent Ig[a]	IgM	IgA	None
Major markers	Cytoplasmic Ig for plasma cells Surface Ig and B-cell markers for lymphoid cells	Cytoplasmic Ig, CD38, PCA-1	Monocyte markers—CD14, CD68; T-cell markers—CD4
Ig gene rearrangement	Present	May be present	Absent

[a]Ig = immunoglobulin.

For plasmacytoma, the major differential diagnosis is from myeloma. Plasmacytoma is a solitary tumor seen mainly in extramedullary and extranodal tissues (EP) and occasionally in bone (SPB). Paraproteinemia is seldom seen in either EP or SPB. Multiple myeloma, on the other hand, involves multiple foci of the bone marrow with prominent paraproteinemia and frequent Bence–Jones proteinuria. Plasmacytoma should contain exclusively plasma or plasmacytoid cells, except for secondary plasmacytoma in the lymph node. The presence of even small clusters of lymphocytes in a predominant plasmacytic population is considered to be lymphoplasmacytic lymphoma rather than plasmacytoma (Table 22.1).[1]

Plasmacytoid T-cell lymphoma may resemble a plasmacytic tumor or T-zone lymphoma, but the absence of cytoplasmic and surface immunoglobulin and the presence of monocytic markers readily exclude other diagnosis.

REFERENCES

1. Lennert K, Feller AC: *Histopathology of non-Hodgkin's Lymphomas* (based on the updated Kiel classification), Berlin, Springer-Verlag, pp 64–76, 1992.
2. Dimopoulos MA, Alexanian R: Waldenstrom's macroglobulinemia. *Blood* 83:1452–1459, 1994.
3. Theml H, Burger A, Keiditsch E, et al: Klinische Beobachtungen zur charakteriaierung des splenomegalen Immunozytoms. *Med Klin* 72:1019–1032, 1977.
4. Melo JV, Hegde V, Parreira A, et al: Splenic B-cell lymphoma with circulating villous lymphocytes: Differential diagnosis of B-cell leukemia with large spleens. *J Clin Pathol* 40:642–651, 1987.
5. Gobbi PG, Bettini R, Montecucco C, et al: Study of prognosis in Waldenström's macroglobulinemia: A proposal for a simple binary classification with clinical and investigational utility. *Blood* 83:2939–2945, 1994.
6. Kyle RA, Garton JP: The spectrum of IgM monoclonal gammopathy in 430 cases. *Mayo Clin Proc* 62:719–731, 1987.
7. Brunning RD, McKenna RW: *Atlas of Tumor Pathology: Tumors of the Bone Marrow*, Washington DC, Armed Forces Institute of Pathology, 1994, p 348.
8. Ioachim HL: *Lymph Node Pathology*, 2nd ed, Philadelphia, Lippincott, 1994, pp 431–438.
9. Holland J, Trenkner DA, Wasserman TH, et al: Plasmacytoma. Treatment results and conversion to myeloma. *Cancer* 69:1513–1517, 1992.
10. Yatabe Y, Mori N, Oka K, et al: A case with primary gastric lymphoma producing IgM and IgG immunoglobulins. *Arch Pathol Lab Med* 118:655–658, 1994.
11. Murata T, Fujita H, Harano H, et al: Triclonal gammopathy (IgAκ, IgGκ, and IgMκ) in a patient with plasmacytoid lymphoma derived from a monoclonal origin. *Am J Hematol* 42:212–216, 1993.
12. Kornstein MJ, de Blois GG, Williams ME: Unusual biclonal plasma cell dyscrasia with crystal-like inclusions producing colonic tumors (plasma cell polyposis) and terminating in T-cell lymphoma. *Arch Pathol Lab Med* 116:168–172, 1992.
13. Ishido T, Mori N: Primary gastric plasmacytoma: A morphological and immunohistochemical study of five cases. *Am J Gastroenterol* 87:875–878, 1992.
14. Schmitz L, Simrell CR, Thorning D: Multiple plasmacytomas in skin. Harbinger of aggressive B-immunocytic malignancy. *Arch Pathol Lab Med* 117:214–216, 1993.
15. Joseph G, Pandit M, Korfhage L: Primary pulmonary plasmacytoma. *Cancer* 71:721–724, 1993.
16. Davidson BS, Lee JE, Dodd LG, et al: Extramedullary plasmacytoma of the pancreas. *Am J Clin Oncol* 16:363–368, 1993.
17. Kanoh T, Katoh H, Izuni T, et al: Renal plasmacytoma. *Rinsho Ketsueki* 34:1470–1473, 1993 (in Japanese with English abstract).
18. Ho DS, Patterson AL, Orozco RE, et al: Extramedullary plasmacytoma of the bladder; case report and review of the literature. *J Urol* 150:473–474, 1993.
19. Matsumoto A, Negata K, Hamaguchi H, et al: Solitary bone plasmacytoma terminally develop myeloma with multiple extramedullary lesions and myelomatous effusion and ascites. *Int J Hematol* 59:59–65, 1993.
20. Muller-Hermelink HK, Steinmann G, Stein H, et al: Malignant lymphoma of plasmacytoid T-cells: Morphologic and immunologic studies characterizing a special type of T-cell. *Am J Surg Pathol* 7:849–862, 1983.
21. Prasthofer EF, Prchal JT, Grizzle WE, et al: Plasmacytoid T-cell lymphoma associated with chronic myeloproliferative disorder. *Am J Surg Pathol* 9:380–387, 1985.
22. Beiske K, Langholm R, Godal T, et al: T-zone lymphoma with predominance of "Plasmacytoid T-cells" associated with myelomonocytic leukemia—a distinct clinicopathologic entity. *J Pathol* 150:247–255, 1986.
23. Facchetti F, DeWolf-Peeters C, Kennes C, et al: Leukemia-associated lymph node infiltrates of plasmacytoid monocytes (so-called plasmacytoid T-cells): Evidence for two distinct histological and immunophenotypical patterns. *Am J Surg Pathol* 14:101–112, 1990.
24. Koo CH, Mason DY, Miller R, et al: Additional evidence that "plasmacytoid T-cell lymphoma" associated with chronic myeloproliferative disorders is of macrophage/monocyte origin. *Am J Clin Pathol* 93:822–827, 1990.
25. Caldwell CW, Yesus YW, Loy TS, et al: Acute leukemia/lymphoma of plasmacytoid T-cell type. *Am J Clin Pathol* 94:778–786, 1990.
26. Thomas JO, Beiske K, Hann I, et al: Immunohistological diagnosis of plasmacytoid T-cell lymphoma in paraffin wax sections. *J Clin Pathol* 44:632–635, 1991.

27. Baddoura FK, Hanson C, Chan WC: Plasmacytoid monocyte proliferation associated with myeloproliferative disorders. *Cancer* 69:1457–1467, 1992.
28. Pangalis GA, Boussiotis VA, Kittas C: Malignant disorders of small lymphocytes: Small lymphocytic lymphoma, lymphoplasmacytic lymphoma and chronic lymphocytic leukemia: Their clinical and laboratory relationship. *Am J Clin Pathol* 99:402–408, 1993.
29. Patsouris E, Noel H, Lennert K: Lymphoplasmacytic/lymphoplasmacytoid immunocytoma with a high content of epithelioid cells: Histologic and immunocytochemical findings. *Am J Surg Pathol* 14:660–670, 1990.
30. Meis JM, Butler JJ, Osborne BM, et al: Solitary plasmacytomas of bone and extramedullary plasmacytomas. A clinicopathologic and immunohistochemical study. *Cancer* 59:1475–1485, 1987.
31. Addis BJ, Isaacson P, Billings JA: Plasmacytoma of lymph nodes. *Cancer* 46:340–346, 1980.
32. El-Okda M, Hyeh Y, Xie SS, et al: Russell bodies consist of heterogeneous glycoproteins in B-cell lymphoma cells. *Am J Clin Pathol* 97:866–871, 1992.
33. Feiner HD, Rizk CC, Finfer MD, et al: IgM monoclonal gammopathy/Waldenström's macroglobulinemia: A morphological and immunophenotypic study of the bone marrow. *Mod Pathol* 3:348–356, 1990.
34. Offit K, Parsa NZ, Filippa D, et al: t(9;14) (p13;q32) denotes a subset of low-grade non-Hodgkin's lymphoma with plasmacytoid differentiation. *Blood* 80:2594–2599, 1992.
35. Tsutani H, Sugiyama T, Shimizu S, et al: Discordant LFA-1/ICAM-1 expression in a case of secondary plasma cell leukemia associated with subcutaneous plasmacytoma. *Am J Hematol* 42:299–304, 1993.

23
Granulocytic Sarcoma vs. Large-Cell Lymphoma vs. True Histiocytic Lymphoma

Granulocytic sarcoma (GS) was initially defined by Rappaport as tumor masses composed of immature cells of the granulocytic series.[1] Nieman et al. further expanded the definition to include leukemic infiltrate by myeloid cells.[2] Recently, Davey et al. adopted a new term, *extramedullary myeloid-cell tumor*, to include both tumor masses and leukemic infiltration.[3] However, in the early literature, GS was known as *chloroma* because of its green color, which fades on exposure to air. It was subsequently found that this color is due to the presence of myeloperoxidase in the tumor cells and that the faded color can be restored by the application of peroxide. Other terms used in the literature include *myeloid sarcoma*,[2] *myelosarcoma*,[4] and *myeloblastoma*.[5] When the tumor mass is composed mainly of a monocytic component, the tumor is also referred to as *monocytic sarcoma*.[5] For all practical purposes, monocytic sarcoma should also be included under the same title (GS or extramedullary myeloid-cell tumor) in spite of the clinical differences sometimes demonstrated between these two tumors. By morphology alone, it is very difficult to distinguish a granulocytic sarcoma from a large-cell lymphoma, and rarely, a true histiocytic lymphoma. When a blastic form of GS is encountered, one must distinguish it from lymphoblastic lymphoma or Burkitt's lymphoma. Fortunately, large panels of cytochemical stains and monoclonal antibodies are now available to help in the differential diagnosis.

CLINICAL FEATURES

GS is a rare tumor when compared with other myeloid neoplasms. Its incidence is about 3%, but, in a study in Hiroshima and Nagasaki (Japan) after atomic bomb explosions, the incidence of granulocytic sarcoma was 7% in patients with myeloid leukemia.[6] In most studies, patients were predominantly children or young adults, with a slight male predominance,[6] but in one series of 61 biopsies, the mean age of the patients was 48 years.[2]

GS may occur in three different clinical settings: (a) antecedent to acute myelogenous leukemia in nonleukemic patients, (b) in association with myelodysplastic syndrome with leukemic transformation or chronic myelogenous leukemia with impending blast crisis, or (c) in association with acute myelogenous leukemia. In a study of 478 patients with myeloid leukemias, GS occurs twice as frequently with chronic myelogenous leukemia than with acute myelogenous leukemia.[6] In a series of 50 patients of GS, 15 were without known leukemia, 24 with myeloproliferative disorders, and 13 with acute myelogenous leukemia.[2] Most nonleukemic patients with GS finally developed leukemia several months (mean, 10 months) after the diagnosis of GS.[2] However, GS patients may survive for 3.5–16 years without development of acute myelogenous leukemia.[7–9] A possible explanation for these long-term survivals may be due to the aggressive anti-acute-myelogenous-leukemia treatment, which prevented the development of leukemia.[7–9] In some early studies, patients with GS usually survived for less than 5 months.[1] So far, no prognostic factor (such as differentiation of tumor cells or mitotic rate) has been identified for the prediction of eventual development of leukemia.[7]

GS may involve multiple anatomic sites. In children and young adults, the orbit is most frequently involved.[6] Other organs, and tissues, such as paranasal sinuses, nasopharynx, lymph nodes, bone, soft tissue, skin, breast, central and peripheral nervous systems, gastrointestinal, respiratory, and genitourinary tracts, have also been involved in varying series.[2,3,4,6,7]

The clinical manifestation of GS depends on its location and the accompanying myeloproliferative disorder or leukemia. The symptoms of acute monocytic leukemia, for instance, may differ from those of acute myeloblastic leukemia. Monocytic leukemia has a propensity for tissue and organ infiltration; the gingiva, skin, liver, spleen, lymph nodes, kidney, and central nervous system (CNS) are frequently involved.[5,10,11] Renal failure in monocytic leukemia may be caused by leukemic infiltration of the kidney and nephrotoxicity of the lysozyme, which is markedly elevated in this condition. Disseminated intravascular coagulation is also seen more frequently in acute monocytic leukemia than in myeloblastic leukemia.[5]

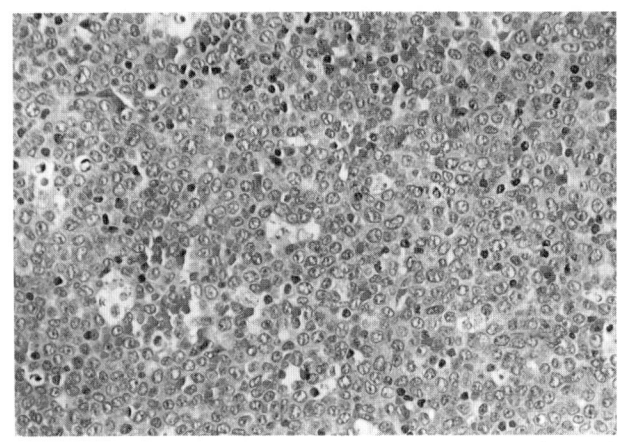

216 DIFFERENTIAL DIAGNOSIS OF LYMPHOID DISORDERS

Fig. 23.1. Granulocytic sarcoma in a lymph node showing total replacement of the normal architecture by myeloblasts with vesicular nuclei and conspicuous nucleoli. Myelocytes are not recognizable. H&E, ×500.

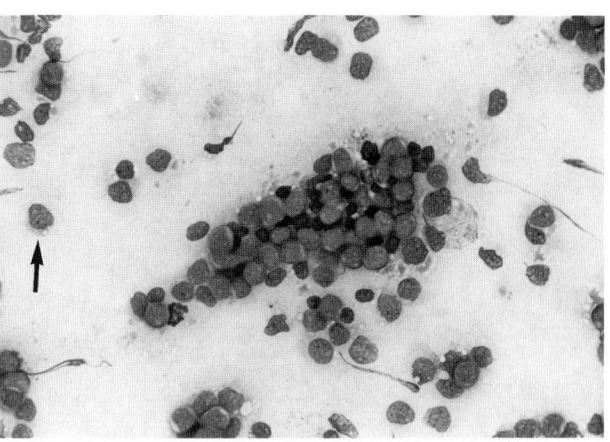

Fig. 23.2. An imprint of lymph node from a case of granulocytic sarcoma showing myeloblasts with delicate chromatin pattern, prominent nucleoli, and cytoplasmic granules (arrow). H&E, ×500.

PATHOLOGY

Morphologically, it may be difficult to distinguish GS from lymphoma. The only clue that may be demonstrated in a routine histologic section stained with hematoxylin and eosin is the presence of eosinophilic myelocytes (Fig. 23.1).[2,7] The presence of the more mature granulocytes does not help, as this may be considered as leukocytic infiltration of lymphoma cells. Unfortunately, about 50% of GS contains no myelocytes.[2,3,12] In those cases, a tissue imprint is most helpful for the distinction between lymphoma cells and myeloblasts/monoblasts (Fig. 23.2). Pure monocytic sarcoma is rare, but most GS contain a certain percentage of monoblasts.[7] A myeloblast is usually larger and with more cytoplasm than a lymphoblast (Table 23.1).[13] The presence of cytoplasmic granules and/or Auer rods is particularly helpful in identifying myeloblasts. Myeloblasts usually have delicate and dispersed chromatin pattern with 1–4 prominent nucleoli. Cytochemical stain of tissue imprints may

TABLE 23.1
Differentiating Features between Acute Lymphoblastic and Acute Myeloblastic Leukemias

	Lymphoblastic	Myeloblastic
Size of blasts	Variable, depending on subtype	Usually large and uniform
Cytoplasm	Scant	Moderate amount
Cytoplasmic granules	Absent	Frequently present
Auer rods	Absent	Seen in ~21% of cases
Nuclear chromatin	Coarse to fine	Delicate and dispersed
Nucleoli	0–2, less prominent	1–4, often prominent
Myelodysplastic changes	Absent	May be present
Myeloperoxidase/Sudan black	Negative	Often positive
Chloroacetate esterase	Negative	Often positive
Nonspecific esterase	Negative	May be positive
Periodic-acid Schiff	Positive in ~ 80–90% of cases	Positive in ~ 10–15% of cases
Terminal deoxynucleotidyl transferase	Positive	Positive in small percentage
Common ALL antigen (CD10)	Positive in most cases	Negative
Myeloid antigens	Negative	Positive
Gene rearrangement	Frequently positive	Occasionally positive

From Sun T: *Color Atlas/Text of Flow Cytometric Analysis of Hematologic Neoplasms*, Igaku-Shoin, New York, 1993.

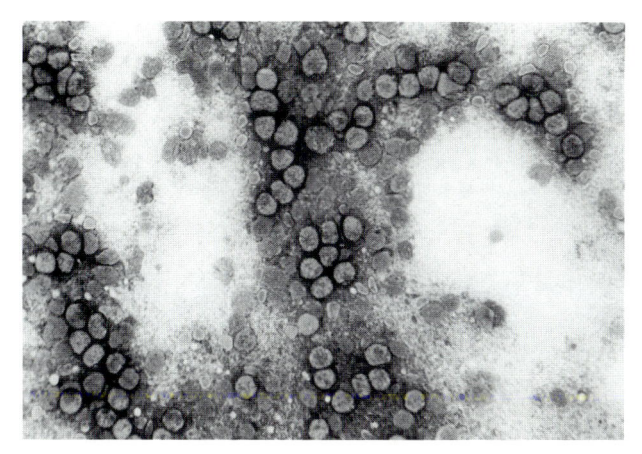

Fig. 23.3. Myeloperoxidase stain of the imprint from the same case as shown in Fig. 23.2 reveals positive cytoplasmic stain in myeloblasts. ×500.

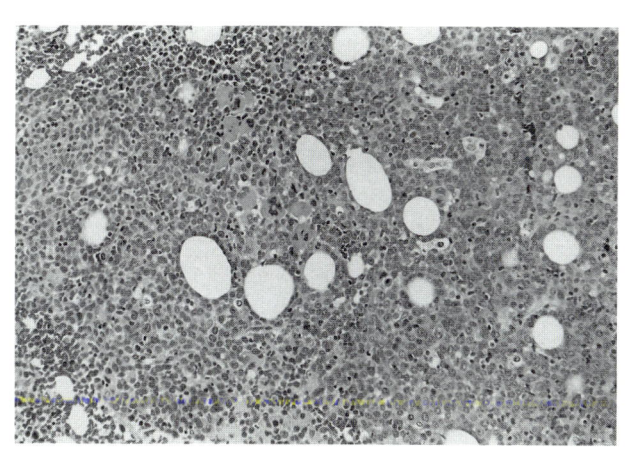

Fig. 23.5. Acute myelogenous leukemia in bone marrow showing diffuse myeloblastic infiltration. H&E, ×250.

show positive myeloperoxidase/Sudan black (Fig. 23.3), chloroacetate esterase (Fig. 23.4) and/or nonspecific esterase staining in myeloblasts and monoblasts and positive periodic-acid Schiff (PAS) stain in some lymphoblasts. Immunofluorescence stain of the imprints for terminal deoxynucleotidyl transferase (TdT) may show positive reaction with lymphoblasts but negative reaction with myeloblasts; although TdT was demonstrated in one case of GS in a very immature form.[14]

On the basis of tumor-cell differentiation, GS can be classified into three groups: well-differentiated, poorly differentiated, and blastic.[2,15] The well-differentiated group is composed primarily of promyelocytes, but nearly all stages of granulocyte may be present. The poorly differentiated group consists of myeloblasts and promyelocytes. In tissue sections, the tumor cells have vesicular nuclei with conspicuous nucleoli (Figs. 23.5–23.7). The nuclei may be variable in size and show nuclear grooves, creases, or convolutions (Figs. 23.8, 23.9).[15] The cytoplasm is moderate to abundant, and a small number of tumor cells may show cytoplasmic granules consistent with myeloid differentiation. The blastic group is formed predominantly of myeloblasts. In tissue sections, the nuclei of the tumor cells are uniform and relatively round. The nuclear chromatin is dispersed, and small inconspicuous nucleoli are seen only occasionally. The cytoplasm varies in amount and contains no granules.

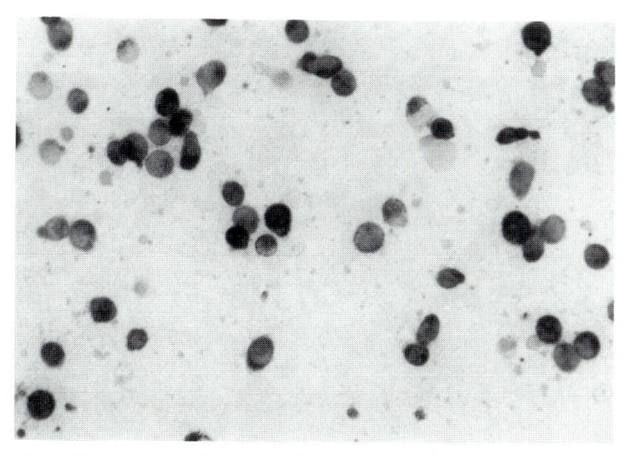

Fig. 23.4. Combined chloroacetate esterase and α-naphthyl butyrate esterase stain of the imprint from the same case as shown in Fig. 23.2 reveals positive chloroacetate esterase staining in myeloblasts. ×500.

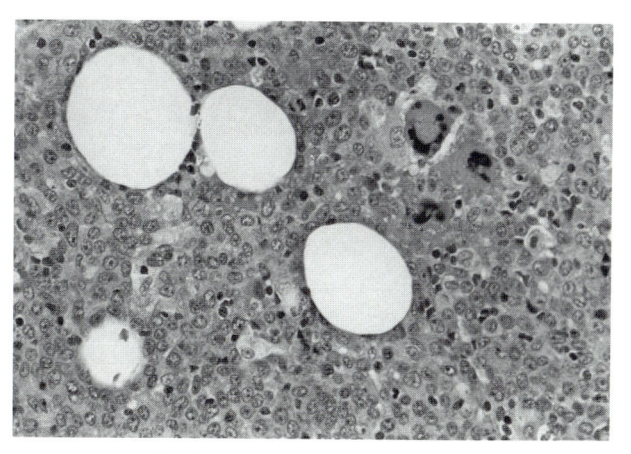

Fig. 23.6. A higher-power view of Fig. 23.5 showing myeloblasts with vesicular nuclei and prominent nucleoli. H&E, ×500.

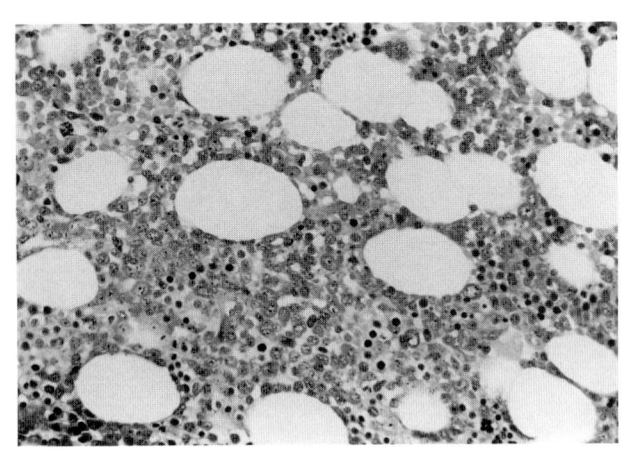

Fig. 23.7. A Giemsa-stained bone marrow biopsy from a case of relapsed acute myelogenous leukemia showing focal myeloblastic infiltrate. The delicate chromatin and vesicular nuclei of the tumor cells readily distinguish them from other marrow components. ×500.

GS usually manifests as sheets of tumor cells invading the adjacent tissues. In the periphery of the tumor mass, tumor cells may form strands and cords (Figs. 23.10, 23.11), and sometimes, a targetoid pattern vaguely reminiscent of invasive lobular breast carcinoma is formed.[7] The tumor infiltrates by expansion, so that normal tissues, such as the glandular and tubular structures, may be separated but the overall architecture is preserved (Fig. 23.12). In lymph nodes, the sinuses and occasionally the paracortex and medulla are infiltrated by leukemic cells, but the germinal centers are preserved.[7] A reported case of monocytic sarcoma showed a myxoid stroma with cording of tumor cells in the lymph node (Figs. 23.13–23.16).[16] In another case of GS, the tumor cells assumed plasmacytoid features, simulating nonsecretory multiple myeloma.[17]

When the tumor cells appear to be monocytes or histiocytes, the differential diagnosis is between a monocytic sarcoma and a true histiocytic lymphoma. Some authors consider these two entities identical,[11] while others feel that they can be separated on a morphologic basis.[18] A soft-tissue mass presentation occurs more frequently in acute monocytic leukemia (Figs. 23.17, 23.18) than in acute myeloblastic leukemia.[11] However, because acute monocytic leukemia is rare, the absolute number of monocytic sarcoma cases is lower than that

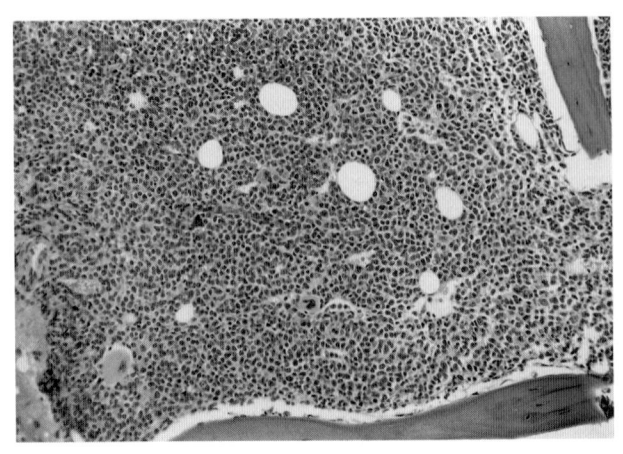

Fig. 23.8. A bone marrow biopsy showing diffuse myeloblast infiltration. H&E, ×250.

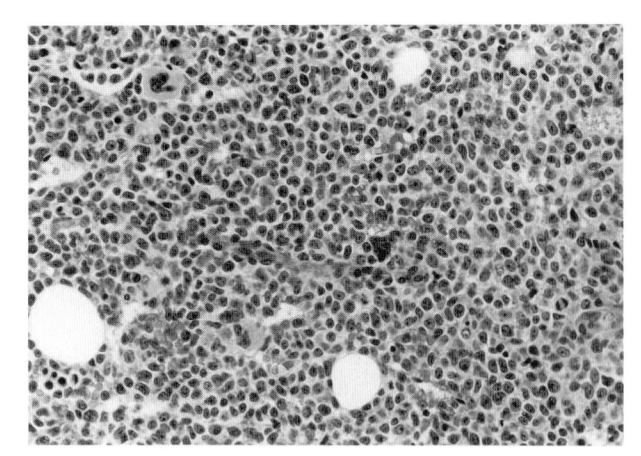

Fig. 23.9. A higher-power view of Fig 23.8 showing the pleomorphic configuration of myeloblasts with nuclear grooves, creases, and convolutions. H&E, ×500.

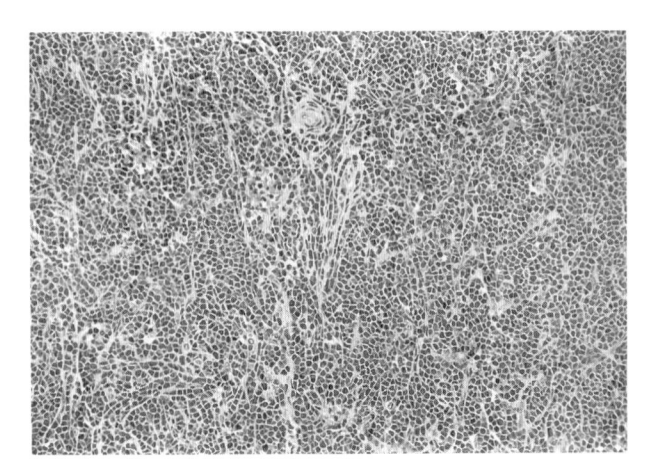

Fig. 23.10. Granulocytic sarcoma in a lymph node showing total replacement of normal architecture by myeloblasts that form strands and cords. H&E, ×250.

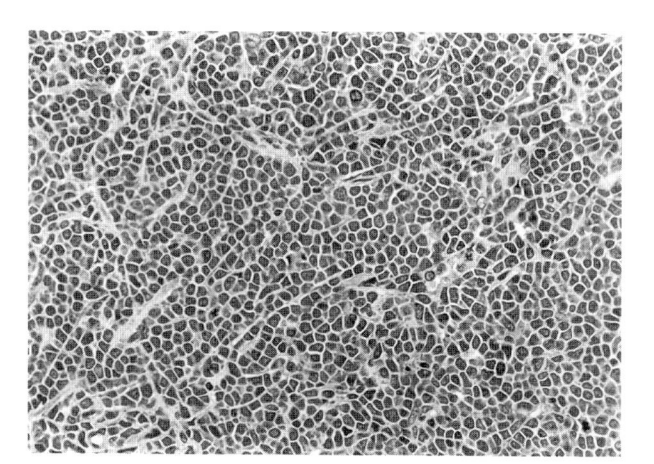

Fig. 23.11. A higher-power view of Fig. 23.10 showing cording or myeloblasts. The morphology of tumor cells is not as typical as the case shown in Fig. 23.1. H&E, ×500.

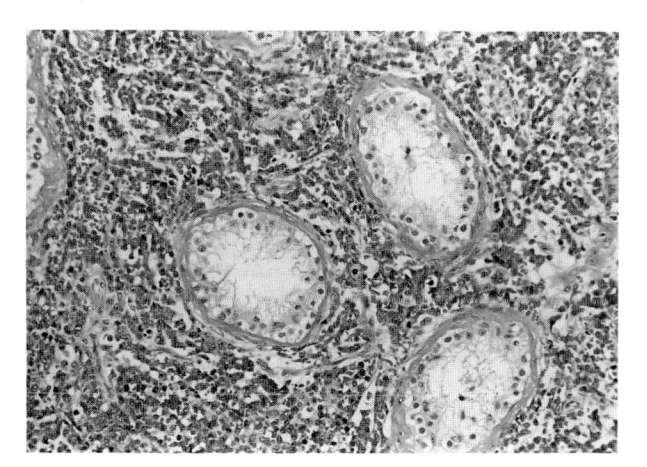

Fig. 23.12. Monocytic sarcoma infiltrating the testis. Note the preservation of seminiferous tubules. H&E, ×250.

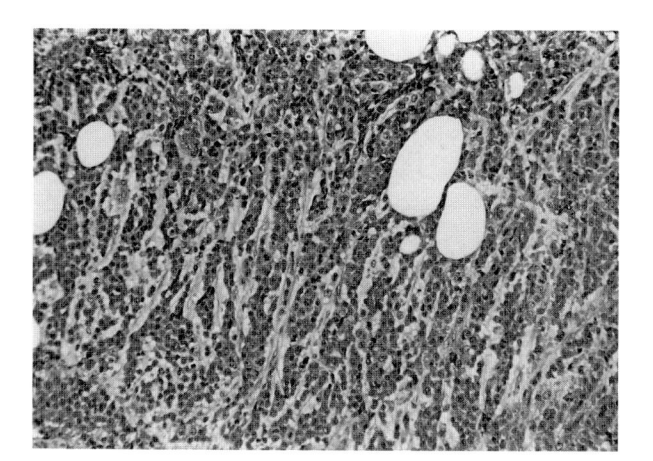

Fig. 23.13. A lymph node biopsy of monocytic sarcoma showing cording pattern of tumor cells. H&E, ×2,500.

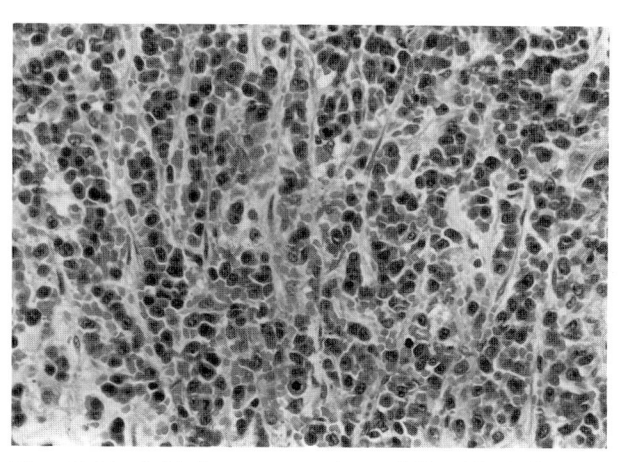

Fig. 23.14. A higher-power view of Fig. 23.13 showing tumor cells with moderate amount of cytoplasm. H&E, ×500.

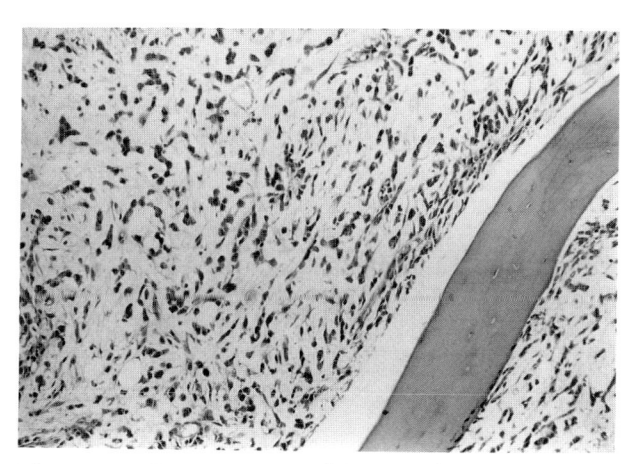

Fig. 23.15. Bone marrow biopsy of monocytic sarcoma showing a myxoid stroma. H&E, ×250.

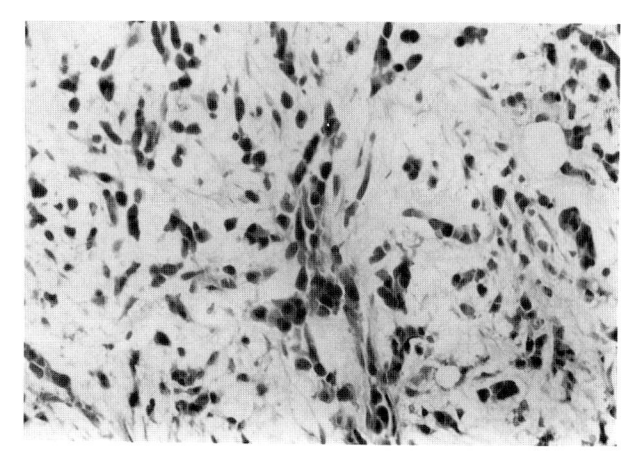

Fig. 23.16. A higher-power view of Fig. 23.15 showing stellate-shaped tumor cells in a myxoid stroma. H&E, ×500.

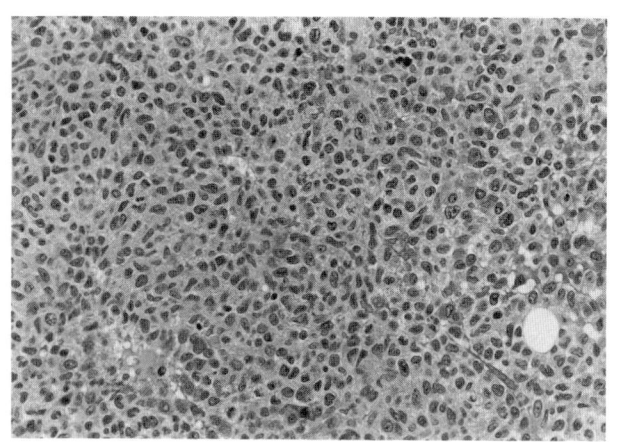

Fig. 23.17. A bone marrow biopsy of acute monoblastic leukemia showing folded nuclei in many tumor cells, characteristic of monoblasts. H&E, ×500.

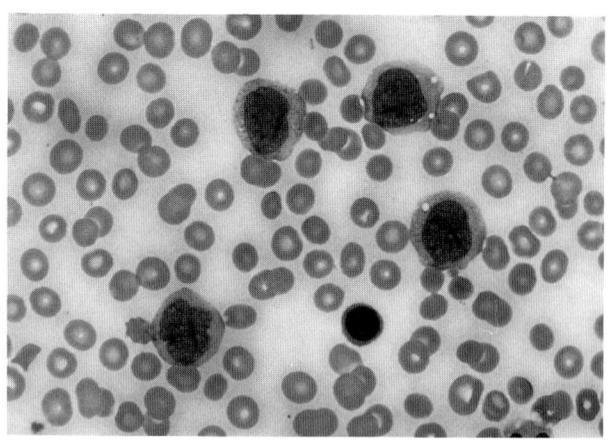

Fig. 23.18b. A higher-power view of Fig. 23.18a showing the characteristic folded nuclei in monocytes and monoblasts. Wright-Giemsa, ×1,250.

of myelocytic sarcoma. On the other hand, true histiocytic lymphoma is extremely low; in one study its incidence was 4 cases among more than 900 lymphomas studied.[18] The morphologic differences between monocytic sarcoma and true histiocytic lymphoma are listed in Table 23.2. The cells in histiocytic lymphoma are more pleomorphic with irregular nucleus, one or more inconspicuous nucleoli, and vacuolated basophilic cytoplasm.[10,18] The nuclear/cytoplasmic ratio is higher in histiocytic lymphoma than in monocytic sarcoma. The latter shows monotonous cell size and shape, with regular nucleus and a single prominent nucleolus and eosinophilic cytoplasm. Phagocytosis is more frequently seen in histiocytic lymphoma than monocytic sarcoma. In the lymph node, both tumors show sinusoidal infiltration, but the tumor cells are noncohesive in histiocytic lymphoma, while those of monocytic sarcoma are closely packed.[10,18]

In two study series, 66% and 75% of GS cases, respectively, were initially diagnosed as large-cell lymphoma (Figs. 23.19, 23.20).[2,7] GS may also show a starry-sky pattern with a high mitotic rate, mimicking lymphoblastic and Burkitt's lymphomas.[2,7] Leder (chloroacetate esterase) stain (Fig. 23.21) used to be the gold standard for the differential diagnosis, but a negative Leder stain has been found in one quarter to one third of GS cases.[2,3,15] Furthermore, a strongly positive Leder stain may also be demonstrated in mast cell tumors.[7] Occasionally, GS may also simulate embryonal rhabdomyosarcoma, amelanotic melanoma, or undifferentiated carcinomas.[3] Electron microscopy may help in the differential diagnosis by demonstrating specific cytoplasmic granules and/or Auer rods, but the most useful techniques for this purpose are immunohistochemistry and immunocytochemistry.

LABORATORY FINDINGS

In addition to the time-honored Leder stain for chloroacetate esterase, several polyclonal/monoclonal antibodies specific for myeloperoxidase (Fig. 23.22), lysozyme, elastase, α_1-antitrypsin, α_1-antichymotrypsin, lactoferrin, and cathepsin are now available for immunohistochemical staining (Table 23.3). These enzymes are positive in variable percentages of GS.[2,3,4,14,15,19–21] In one comparative study, lysozyme was more sensitive in diagnosing GS than was chloroacetate esterase.[2] Elastase is present in the pri-

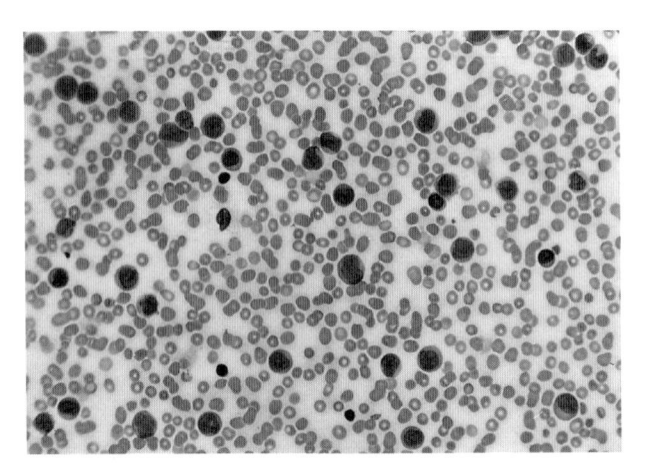

Fig. 23.18a. A peripheral blood smear of acute monocytic leukemia showing many monocytes and monoblasts. Wright-Giemsa, ×500.

TABLE 23.2
Comparison of Monocytic Sarcoma and True Histiocytic Lymphoma

	Monocytic sarcoma	True histiocytic lymphoma
Cell size and shape	Monotonous, large	Pleomorphic, large
Cytoplasm	Abundant, eosinophilic	Abundant, basophilic, vacuolated
Nucleus	Round to oval	Oval, convoluted or multilobulated
Nucleolus	Single, prominent	One or more, less prominent
Nuclear:cytoplasmic ratio	Lower	Higher
Phagocytosis	Rare	More common
Mitoses	Fairly frequent	Numerous
Lymph node involvement	Sinuses	Sinuses
Infiltrating pattern	Compact	Noncohesive

mary granules of granulocytes and monocytes, but it appears later than myeloperoxidase; therefore elastase is not demonstrated in acute myeloblastic leukemia without maturation (M1). Lysozyme appears in primary granules of both myeloblasts and monoblasts, while lactoferrin appears at a stage of secondary granule formation. α_1-Antitrypsin and α_1-antichymotrypsin are strongly positive for myeloblasts and weakly positive or negative for monoblasts.[3]

There are many monoclonal antibodies specific for myelomonocytic series.[3,4,10,14,19,21] In the series conducted by Furebring-Freden et al., a large panel of myelomonocytic antibodies were used.[4] Three of them (CD11c, CD13, CD33) were positive in GS, but the results of CD11b and CD14 were equivocal.[4] CD15 was positive in 50% of the cases in this series, similar to the results reported by Davey et al.[3] In the study by Traweek et al., CD15 (LeuM1) and CD68 (KP-1) were positive for all well-differentiated GS, and 76% of poorly differentiated GS.[15] However, for the blastic groups, CD68 was positive in only 3 of 5 cases, and CD15 was negative in all 5 cases.[15] The insensitivity of these two markers in least differentiated GS was confirmed by Hudock et al.[22] CD68, a lysozyme-associated antigen, is also consistently demonstrated in the monocyte–histiocyte–phagocyte system, and multiple monoclonal antibodies are now available for the detection of this antigen (KP-1 and KiM6 for paraffin sections and EBM 11 for frozen sections).[18] Another antigen that is consistently positive in GS is CD43 (Leu22), which was positive in all 28 cases in the study series of Traweek et al.[15] and in 26 of 29 GS cases in the report of Hudock et al.[22] CD43 is a multilineage marker reactive to myelomonocytic leukemias, T-cell lymphomas, B-cell lymphomas, and plasmacytomas.[23]

With cytochemical and monoclonal antibody stains,

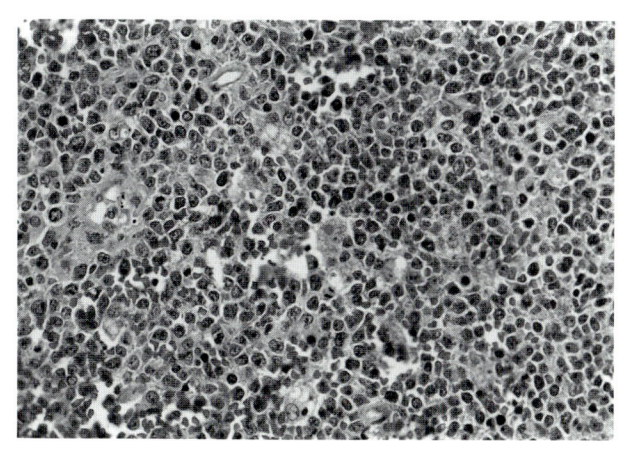

Fig. 23.19. Lymph node biopsy showing large-cell lymphoma that should be distinguished from granulocytic sarcoma. H&E, ×500.

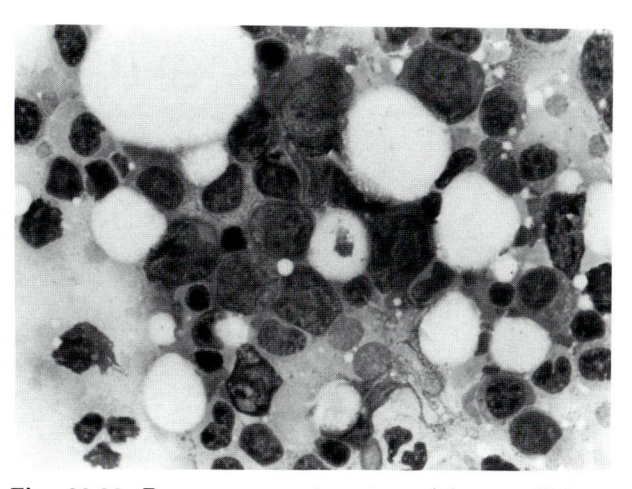

Fig. 23.20. Bone marrow imprint of large-cell lymphoma showing a cluster of large neoplastic cells with clumped chromatin in the center of the field. Wright–Giemsa, ×1,250.

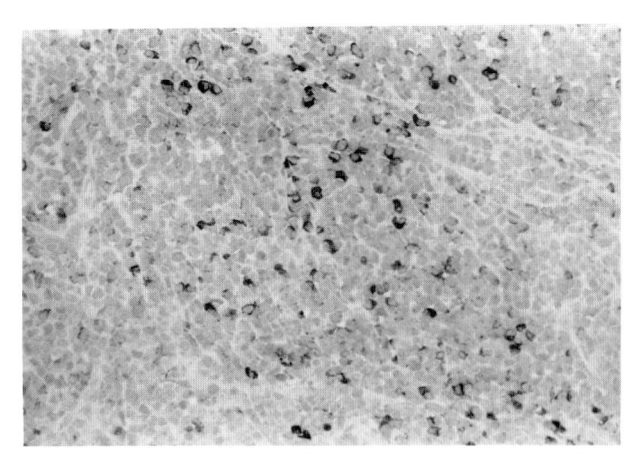

Fig. 23.21. Lymph node biopsy of granulocytic sarcoma, showing positive Leder stain (chloroacetate esterase) in some tumor cells. ×500.

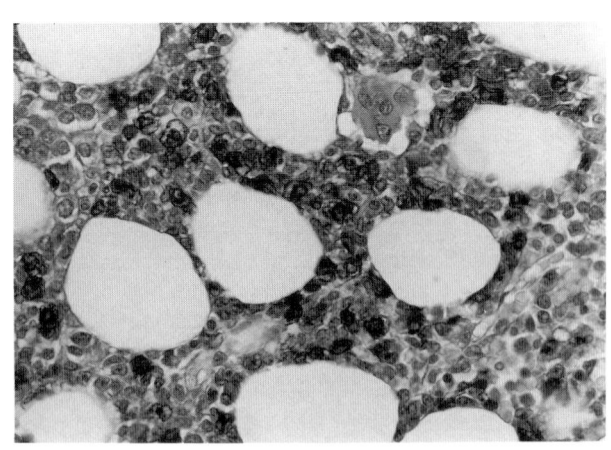

Fig. 23.22. Bone marrow biopsy of acute myeloblastic leukemia showing positive myeloperoxidase antibody staining in blast cells. ×500.

GS can be diagnosed with confidence by most pathologists. However, many other antigens can also be demonstrated in GS cases, thus causing some confusion. For instance, S-100 and MT1 (another CD43 antibody) may be present in cases of GS.[19,24] Other T-cell antigens, such as CD45RO (UCHL1), CD3, and CD7, have also been demonstrated in some cases.[3,4,19,21] The B-cell antigens are less frequently detected in GS cases than T-cell antigens.[4,15] However, in some studies, 20–30% of cases of GS or acute myeloid leukemia showed B-cell antigens (L26, Ki-B3, 4kB5, MB1, LN2).[3,19] Besides nonspecific cross-reactivity, the reaction to T- or B-cell antibodies may, in some cases, represent a mixed lymphoid–myeloid phenotype.[4,19]

TABLE 23.3
Comparison of Marker Studies in Granulocytic Sarcoma, True Histiocytic Lymphoma, and Lymphocytic Lymphoma

	Granulocytic sarcoma	True histiocytic lymphoma	Lymphocytic lymphoma
CD11c	+	±	−
CD13	+	+	−
CD14	±	+	−
CD15	±	+	−
CD25	NT[a]	+	−
CD30	−	+	−
CD33	+	+	−
CD43	+	+	+
CD45	+	±	+
CD68	+	+	−
HLA-DR	+	+	+
Myeloperoxidase	+	±	−
Lysozyme	+	+	−
Chloroacetate esterase	+	−	−
Nonspecific esterase	−	+	−
α_1-antitrypsin	+	+	−
α_1-antichymotrypsin	+	+	−
Acid phosphatase	+	+	+
Neutrophil elastase	+	−	−
Cathepsin B	−	+	−
Cathepsin G	+	−	−

[a]NT = not tested.

Since histiocytes and monocytes are derived from the same stem cells, monocytic sarcoma, true histiocytic lymphoma, and malignant histiocytosis represent a spectrum of related disorders.[18,26] The difference in markers between malignant histiocytosis and true histiocytic sarcoma is that the former expresses more frequently monocytic markers (CD11b, CD11c, and CD14), while the latter more frequently expresses Reed–Sternberg cell markers (CD25, CD30).[25] The major differences between GS and the group of monocytic/histiocytic disorders is in their enzymes (Table 23.3). GS shows consistent positivity in myeloperoxidase, chloroacetate esterase, neutrophil elastase, and cathepsin G but absence of nonspecific esterase and cathepsin B.[3,4,15,19,20] The monocyte/histiocyte entities, on the other hand, are positive for nonspecific esterase and cathepsin B, but are negative for chloroacetate esterase, neutrophil elastase, and cathepsin G.[18,20] Myeloperoxidase is also negative in most cases of monocyte/histiocyte disorders. The results of monoclonal antibody staining are similar between these two groups of diseases, but CD30 is negative in GS but positive in true histiocytic lymphoma.[15,24] In addition, CD14 and CD15 are more frequently negative in GS than in monocyte/histiocyte disorders.[3,4,21]

All non-Hodgkin's lymphomas are negative for myelomonocytic antigens and for all the enzymes discussed above except for acid phosphatase, which appears as punctate staining in T-lymphocytes. HLA-DR and CD45 (LCA) are positive in GS, monocyte/histiocyte disorders, and lymphoma, but CD45 stains weaker in GS and monocyte/histiocyte cases than in lymphoma cases.[4,14,16] As mentioned before, CD43 is a multilineage antigen; therefore, it is present in GS as well as in lymphomas.

In summary, there is a large panel of enzymes and monoclonal antibodies that may help in distinguishing GS from similar diseases. The selection of a few of them should be sufficient to serve the purpose; for instance, chloroacetate esterase, CD13, CD33, CD43, and CD68 are able to successfully identify the vast majority of GS cases.

REFERENCES

1. Rappaport H: *Atlas of Tumor Pathology: Tumors of the Hematopoietic System*, Washington DC, Armed Forces Institute of Pathology, pp 241–243; 1966.
2. Neiman RS, Barcos M, Berard C, et al: Granulocytic sarcoma: A clinicopathologic study of 61 biopsied cases. *Cancer* 48:1426–1437, 1981.
3. Davey FR, Olsen S, Kurec AS, et al: The immunophenotyping of extramedullary myeloid cell tumors in paraffin-embedded tissue sections. *Am J Surg Pathol* 12:699–707, 1988.
4. Furebring-Freden M, Martinsson U, Sundstrom C: Myelosarcoma without acute leukemia. Immunohistochemical and clinicopathologic characterization of eight cases. *Histopathology* 16:243–250, 1990.
5. Case records of the Massachusetts General Hospital: Case 50-1990. *N Engl J Med* 323:1689–1697, 1990.
6. Ioachim HL: *Lymph Node Biopsy*, Philadelphia, Lippincott, 1994, pp 560–565.
7. Meiss JM, Butler JJ, Osborne BM, et al: Granulocytic sarcoma in nonleukemic patients. *Cancer* 58:2697–2709, 1986.
8. Beck TM, Day JC, Smith CE, et al: Granulocytic sarcoma treated as an acute leukemia: Report of a case. *Cancer* 53:1764–1766, 1984.
9. Eshghabadi M, Shojama AM, Carr I: Isolated granulocytic sarcoma: Report of a case and review of the literature. *J Clin Oncol* 4:912–917, 1986.
10. Peterson L, Dehner LP, Brunning RD: Extramedullary masses as presenting features of acute monoblastic leukemia. *Am J Clin Pathol* 75:140–148, 1981.
11. Bain B, Manoharan A, Lampert I, et al: Lymphoma-like presentation of acute monocytic leukemia. *J Clin Pathol* 36:559–565, 1983.
12. Kurec AS, Cruz VE, Barrett D, et al: Immunophenotyping of acute leukemia using paraffin embedded tissue sections. *Am J Clin Pathol* 93:502–509, 1990.
13. Sun T: *Color Atlas/Text of Flow Cytometric Analysis of Hematologic Neoplasms*, New York, Igaku-Shoin, 1993, p 158.
14. van Veen S, Kluin PM, de Keizer RJW, et al: Granulocytic sarcoma (chloroma): Presentation of an unusual case. *Am J Clin Pathol* 95:567–571, 1991.
15. Traweek ST, Arber DA, Rappaport H, et al: Extramedullary myeloid cell tumors: An immunohistochemical and morphologic study of 28 cases. *Am J Surg Pathol* 17:1011–1019, 1993.
16. Strauchen JA: Sarcomatoid neoplasm of monocytic lineage. *Am J Surg Pathol* 15:1206–1208 (letter), 1991.
17. Carmichael GP, Lee YT: Granulocytic sarcoma simulating "non-secretory" multiple myeloma. *Hum Pathol* 8:697–700, 1977.
18. Malone M: The histiocytoses of childhood. *Histopathology* 19:105–119, 1991.
19. Horny HP, Campbell M, Steinke B, et al: Acute myeloid leukemia: Immunohistologic findings in paraffin-embedded bone marrow biopsy specimens. *Hum Pathol* 21:648–655, 1990.
20. Muller S, Sangster G, Crocker G, et al: An immunohistochemical and clinicopathological study of granulocytic sarcoma (chloroma). *Hematol Oncol* 4:101–112, 1986.
21. Fellbaum C, Hansmann ML: Immunohistochemical differential diagnosis of granulocytic sarcomas and malig-

nant lymphomas on formalin-fixed material. *Virchows Archiv A Pathol Anat* 416:351–355, 1990.
22. Hudock J, Chatten J, Miettinen M: Immunohistochemical evaluation of myeloid leukemia infiltrates (granulocytic sarcomas) in formaldehyde-fixed, paraffin-embedded tissue. *Am J Clin Pathol* 102:55–60, 1994.
23. Segal GH, Stoler MH, Tubbs R: The "CD43 only" phenotype: An aberrant, nonspecific immunophenotype requiring comprehensive analysis for lineage resolution. *Am J Clin Pathol* 97:861–865, 1992.
24. Elliot CJ, McCarthy KP, Carter RL, et al: Granulocytic sarcoma: Misleading immunological staining with MT1 and S100 protein antibodies. *J Clin Pathol* 42:188–190, 1989.
25. Hsu SM, Ho YS, Hsu PL: Lymphomas of true histiocytic origin: Expression of different phenotypes in so-called true histiocytic lymphoma and malignant histiocytosis. *Am J Pathol* 138:1389–1404, 1991.
26. Lauritzen AF, Delsol G, Hansen NE, et al: Histiocytic sarcomas and monoblastic leukemias: A clinical, histiologic and immunophenotypical study. *Am J Clin Pathol* 102:45–54, 1994.

INDEX

A

Acquired immunodeficiency syndrome (AIDS), *see* AIDS
Adipose tissue, perinodal, follicular lymphoma infiltrating, 93
AIDS,
    reactive lymphoid hyperplasias, 25–26, 27t, *27–28*
    lymph node biopsy, 27
AIDS-related lymphadenopathy, Castleman's disease, 87–88
Ancillary studies, lymphoid disorders, 13–24
    chromosomal translocation, in lymphoid neoplasms, 23
    contourgram, 16
    cytogenetics, oncogenes and, 21–23, *22*, 23t
    flow cytometry, 15–16, *15–17*
        basic structure of, 15
    hematologic neoplasms, criteria for diagnosis of, 14
    histogram, with prominent K light-chain-positive population, 16
    immunoglobulin
        heavy chain gene rearrangement, 18
    immunohistochemistry, 14, *14*
    immunophenotyping, 13–16, 14t
        immunogenotyping, comparison, 17
    isometric plot, composite, 17
    karyotype, lymph node cells, 22
    molecular genetics, 16–21, 17t
    natural-killer-cell lymphoma, spleen, 21
    polymerase chain reaction, *20*, 20–21
    receptor genes, characteristics of, 18
    scattergram, with side scatter, 16
    in situ hybridization, 21, *21*
    Southern blotting, *19*, 19–20
    T-cell receptor β-chain gene, Southern blot hybridization analysis, 19
Angiocentric immunoproliferative lesions, 197–203, *198*
    clinical features, 198
    differential diagnosis, 200–202, 201t, *201–202*
    laboratory findings, 200
    pathology, 198t, *198–199*, *198–200*
Angiofollicular hyperplasia, 82–89
    AIDS-related lymphadenopathy, 87–88
    angioimmunoblastic lymphadenopathy, 88
    autoimmune disorders, 88
    clinical features, 82–83
    differential diagnosis, 87–88
    Hodgkin's disease coexistent with, 86
    hyaline-vascular type, 82–84, *83–84*
    intermediate type, 82, 85
        showing hyperplastic, vascular follicular center, 85
    laboratory findings, 87
    lymphoplasmacytic lymphoma, 88
    mantle-cell lymphoma, 88
    multicentric type, 82–83, 85, *85–86*
        burned-out phase, 85
    neoplasms associated with, 86, *86*
    pathogenesis, 87
    pathology, 83–87
    plasma-cell type, 82, 84, *84–85*
        extensive plasma-cell, 84
    plasmacytoma, 88
    Reed-Sternberg cell, in case of Hodgkin's disease, 86
    rheumatoid arthritis, 88
    syphilis, 88
    systemic lupus erythematosus, 88
Angioimmunoblastic lymphadenopathy
    Castleman's disease, 88
    vs. immunoblastic lymphadenopathy-like T-cell lymphoma, 158–163
        clinical features, 158
        laboratory findings, 162
        pathology, 158–162, *159–161*
Angiolymphoid hyperplasia, reactive lymphoid hyperplasias, skin biopsy in, 31
Antibodies, monoclonal
    cell specificity, clinical applications of, 8–9
    used in paraffin-embedded sections, 9
Antigens
    lymphoid, 6–9, 7–9t
    surface, categories of, 7
Autoimmune disorders, Castleman's disease, 88

B

Bacillary angiomatosis, reative lymphoid hyperplasias, 41, *41*
B-cell differentiation, intranodal, 7
B-cell lymphoma, monocytoid, vs. splenic lymphoma with villous lymphocytes vs. hairy-cell leukemia, 120–131
    B-cell neoplasms, low-grade, comparison, 126
    blood lakes, pseudosinuses, 122
    bone marrow biopsy, hairy-cell leukemia, 121
    clinical features, 120–121
    cytochemistry, 129, *129*
    cytopreparation, from peripheral blood, 129
    fried-egg pattern, 121
    hairy cell, 120–122, *121–122*, 127–128, *128*
    immunophenotyping, 127–129
    laboratory findings, 125–130
    lymphocytic leukemia, chronic, 129
    mast cells, 125
        with dark cytoplasmic staining, 125
        showing spindle tumor cells, 125
        systemic, 124, *125*
    molecular-genetic studies, 129–130
    monocytoid B-cell lymphoma, 120, 122–124, *123–124*, 128
    pathology, 121–124
    peripheral blood, 125–127, 126t, *126–127*
    prolymphocytic leukemia, 129
    splenectomy specimen, 128
    splenic lymphoma, with villous lymphocytes, 120–121, 124, *124–125*, 128
    T-cell phenotype, 129
    toxoplasmic lymphadenopathy, 123
    variants, hybrid forms, 129
    villous lymphocyte(s), 126
        showing polar distribution, 127
B-cell neoplasms, low-grade, 126
Blood lakes, pseudosinuses, 122
Bone marrow
    aspirate, sea-blue histiocyte, storage histiocyte disorder, 65
    biopsy, granuloma, 58
Brucellosis, 52, *53*
    kidney, 53
Burkitt's lymphoma vs. acute lymphoblastic leukemia vs. lymphoblastic lymphoma, 132–142, 133t, *135–141*, *137–138*, 139t
    acute lymphoblastic leukemia, 135, 135t, *136*
    clinical features, 132–133
    laboratory findings, 139–141
    lymphoblastic lymphoma, 132–135, *133–134*, 134t, 139–140, *140*, 140t
    pathology, 133–139

C

Carcinoma vs. lymphoma
  cutaneous, 190–196
    amelanotic melanoma, 190
    clinical features, 190
    cutaneous lymphoma, 190
    laboratory findings, 193–195, *193–195*, 194t
    pathology, 190–193, *191–193*
  neuroendocrine carcinoma, cutaneous, 190
Castleman's disease, 82–89, *83–86*
  AIDS-related lymphadenopathy, 87–88
  angioimmunoblastic lymphadenopathy, 88
  autoimmune disorders, 88
  clinical features, 82–83
  differential diagnosis, 87–88
  Hodgkin's disease coexistent with, 86
  hyaline-vascular type, 82–84, *83–84*
  intermediate type, 82, 85
    showing hyperplastic, vascular follicular center, 85
  laboratory findings, 87
  lymphoplasmacytic lymphoma, 88
  mantle-cell lymphoma, 88
  multicentric type, 82–83, 85, *85–86*
    burned-out phase, 85
  neoplasms associated with, 86, *86*
  pathogenesis, 87
  pathology, 83–87
  plasma-cell type, 82, 84, *84–85*
    extensive plasma-cell, 84
  plasmacytoma, 88
  Reed-Sternberg cell, in case of Hodgkin's disease, 86
  rheumatoid arthritis, 88
  syphilis, 88
  systemic lupus erythematosus, 88
Cat-scratch disease, 50–51, *50–51*
Cell markers, lymphoid neoplasms, 3–12, 4t
  antibodies, monoclonal
    cell specificity, clinical applications of, 8–9
    used in paraffin-embedded sections, 9
  antigens
    lymphoid, 6–9, *7–9t*
    nuclear, categories of, 7
    surface, categories of, 7
  B-cell differentiation, intranodal, 7
  B-lymphocytes, immunophenotypes, of different developmental stages of, 4
  cortex, of normal lymph node, 4
  European-American classification, revised, 11–12
  follicle dendritic cells, in germinal center, meshwork, 6
  Kiel classification, updated, of non-Hodgkin's lymphomas, 11
  lymph follicle
    B-cell, positive, 5
    germinal center, 5
  lymph node, normal
    with capsule, 4
    with cortex containing lymph follicles with germinal centers, 4
    with subscapular sinus, cortex containing lymph follicles with germinal centers, 4
  lymphocytes
    development of, 3–6, *4–7*
    intranodal distribution, 3–6, *4–7*
  lymphomas, classification of, 9–12, 10–12t
  medulla, of normal lymph node, 5
  non-Hodgkin's lymphoma, 10
  paracortex, of normal lymph node, 4
  T-cell, positive, lymph node, 6
  T-lymphocytes, immunophenotype, different developmental stages of, 4
Chromosomal translocation, in lymphoid neoplasms, 23

Classification, lymphoid neoplasms, 3–12, 4t
  antibodies, monoclonal
    cell specificity, clinical applications of, 8–9
    used in paraffin-embedded sections, 9
  antigens
    lymphoid, 6–9, *7–9t*
    surface, categories of, 7
  B-cell differentiation, intranodal, 7
  B-lymphocytes, immunophenotypes, of different developmental stages of, 4
  cortex, of normal lymph node, 4
  European-American classification, revised, 11–12
  follicle dendritic cells, in germinal center, meshwork, 6
  Kiel classification, updated, of non-Hodgkin's lymphomas, 11
  lymph follicle
    B-cell, positive, 5
    germinal center, 5
  lymph node, normal
    with capsule, 4
    with cortex containing lymph follicles with germinal center, 4
    with subcapsular sinus, 4
  lymphocytes
    development of, 3–6, *4–7*
    intranodal distribution, 3–6, *4–7*
  lymphomas, classification of, 9–12, 10–12t
  medulla, of normal lymph node, 5
  non-Hodgkin's lymphoma, 10
  paracortex, of normal lymph node, 4
  T-cell, positive, lymph node, 6
  T-lymphocytes, immunophenotype, different developmental stages of, 4
Coccidioides lymphadenitis, 59–60, *59–60*
Composite lymphoma, 102–104, *103–105*, 106
  vs. Richter's syndrome vs. mixed small- and large-cell lymphoma, 102–109, *106–107*
  clinical features, 102
  composite lymphoma, 102–104, *103–105*
  differential diagnosis, 106–107
  immunoperoxidase stain, of composite lymphoma, 103
  laboratory finding, 105–106
  mycosis fungoides, 103
  pathology, 102–105
  Reed-Sternberg cell, 105
  Richter's syndrome, 102, 104–105, *105*
  small lymphocytic lymphoma, with proliferation centers, 107, *107*
Cortex, of normal lymph node, 4
Cryptococcus lymphadenitis, 55–57, *56–57*
  with yeast cells, 56
Cutaneous lymphomas vs. carcinomas, 190–196
  amelanotic melanoma, 190
  clinical features, 190
  cutaneous neuroendocrine carcinoma, 190
  laboratory findings, 193–195, *193–195*, 194t
  pathology, 190–193, *191–193*
Cytogenetics, oncogenes and, 21–23, *22*, 23t
Cytomegalovirus lymphadenitis, reactive lymphoid hyperplasias, 37, *37*

D

Dermatopathic lymphadenopathy, reactive lymphoid hyperplasias, 43, *185*

E

European-American classification, revised, 11–12

F

Flow cytometer, 15–16, *15–17*
  basic structure of, 15
Follicle dendritic cells, in germinal center, meshwork, 6
Follicular hyperplasia, 90–92, 91t, *92*
  atypical, 92
  and follicular lymphoma, differentiation between, 91
  germinal center, 92
  lymph node biopsy, 92
  vs. mantle-cell lymphoma vs. follicular lymphoma, 90–101, 91t, *92*
    atypical follicular hyperplasia, 92
    blastic variant, of mantle-cell lymphoma, 98
    clinical manifestation, 90–91
    floral variant, follicular lymphoma, 96
    follicular lymphoma, 90, 92–96, *93–96*
      infiltrating perinodal adipose tissue, 93
      lymph node biopsy, 93
    germinal center, follicular hyperplasia, 92
    laboratory findings, 98–100, 99t
    liver, in mantle-cell lymphoma, 99
    lymph node biopsy, 92
    lymph node imprint, 98
    mantle cell lymphoma, 90–91, 96–98, *97–99*
      involving tonsil, 97
    paratrabecular infiltration, follicular lymphoma with, 96
    pathology, 91–98
    signet-ring-cell variant, follicular lymphoma, 95
    small-cleaved-cell follicular lymphoma, 96
    spleen, in mantle-cell lymphoma, 98
Follicular lymphoma, 90, 92–96, *93–96*
  floral variant, 96
  vs. follicular hyperplasia vs. mantle-cell lymphoma, 90–101, *93–96*
    atypical follicular hyperplasia, 92
    blastic variant, of mantle-cell lymphoma, 98
    clinical manifestation, 90–91
    floral variant, follicular lymphoma, 96
    follicular hyperplasia, 90–92, 91t, *92*
      and follicular lymphoma, differentiation between, 91
      lymph node biopsy, 92
    follicular lymphoma infiltrating perinodal adipose tissue, 93
    germinal center, follicular hyperplasia, 92
    laboratory findings, 98–100, 99t
    liver, in mantle-cell lymphoma, 99
    lymph node biopsy, 93
    lymph node imprint, 98
    mantle-cell lymphoma, 90–91, 96–98, *97–99*
      involving tonsil, 97
    paratrabecular infiltration, follicular lymphoma with, 96
    pathology, 91–98
    signet-ring-cell variant, follicular lymphoma, 95
    small-cleaved-cell follicular lymphoma, 96
    spleen, in mantle-cell lymphoma, 98
  lymph node biopsy, 93
  paratrabecular infiltration, 96
  signet-ring-cell variant, 95
  small-cleaved-cell, 96
Follicular pattern, reactive lymphoid hyperplasias, 25–31

G

Gaucher cell
  in bone marrow, positive PAS staining, 64
  electron micrograph of, 64
Gaucher disease, 62–64, *63–64*, 67
Germinal centers, reactive lymphoid hyperplasias, progressive transformation of, 27–28, *29*
Granulocytic sarcoma vs. large-cell lymphoma vs. true histiocytic lymphoma, 215–224
  clinical features, 215
  laboratory findings, 220–223, *222*, 222t
  pathology, 216t, 216–220, *216–222*, 221t
Granulomatous lymphadenitis, 49–61
  asteroid body, 50
  bone marrow biopsy, granuloma, 58
  brucellosis, 52, *53*
    kidney, 53
  cat-scratch disease, 50–51, *50–51*
  coccidioides lymphadenitis, 59–60, *59–60*
  cryptococcus lymphadenitis, 55–57, *56–57*
    with yeast cells, 56
  histoplasma lymphadenitis, 57–59, 58t, *58–59*
  lepromatous leprosy, 55
  lymphogranuloma venereum, 51–52, *51–52*
  McCoy cells, 52
  mycobacterial lymphadenitis, 53–54, *53–54*
    caused by Mycobacterium tuberculosis, 53
  mycobacterium avium-intracellularae, spleen, 54
  mycobacterium leprae lymphadenitis, 54–55, *55*
  pneumocystis carinii, cysts of, 57
  pneumocystis lymphadenitis, 57
  pulmonary blastomycosis, 57
  pulmonary hilar lymph node, coccidiodomycosis in, 59
  pulmonary histoplasmosis
    with caseous necrosis, 58
    GMS-positive organisms, 59
  sarcoidosis, 49, *50*
  tularemia, 52
Gene rearrangements
  immunoglobulin, 18
  T-cell receptor, 17–19, *18*, 18t

H

Hairy cell leukemia, 120–122, *121–122*, 127–128, *128*
  bone marrow biopsy, 121
Hematologic neoplasms, criteria for diagnosis of, 14
Hemophagocytic syndrome, infection-associated, 164–167, *166*
Herpes simplex esophagitis, reactive lymphoid hyperplasias, *38*
Herpes zoster/herpes simplex lymphadenitis, reactive lymphoid hyperplasias, 38, *38*
Histiocytic lymphoma vs. large-cell lymphoma, vs. granulocytic sarcoma, 215–224
  clinical features, 215
  laboratory findings, 220–223, *222*, 222t
  pathology, 216t, 216–220, *216–222*, 221t
Histiocytosis, malignant, 164, 166, *166*
  and benign vs. T-cell lymphoma, 164–174, 165t
    clinical features, 164–166
    familial, gene-related diseases, 165
    hemophagocytic syndrome, infection-associated, 164–167, *166*
    histiocytosis malignant, 166, *166*
    Langerhans' cell histiocytosis, 165, 167, *167–168*
    lymphohistiocytosis, familial erythrophagocytic, 167–168
    lymphoproliferative syndrome, X-linked, 168
    malignant histiocytosis, 164
    pathology, 166–170
    Rosai-Dorfman disease, 165, *168*, 168–169
    T-cell lymphomas, with sinusoidal infiltration and/or hemophagocytosis, 165–166
  metastatic carcinoma, Hodgkin's disease, vs. Ki-1 lymphoma, anaplastic large-cell, 143–149
    clinical features, 143
    laboratory findings, 146, 146–147
    pathology, 143–146, *144–146*
Histogram, with prominent K light-chain-positive population, 16

Histoplasma lymphadenitis, 57–59, 58t, *58–59*
Hodgkin's disease, 153, *153*
   coexistent with Castleman's disease, 86
   vs. lymphomas with Reed-Sternberg-like cells, 69–81, 70t
     Ann Arbor staging system, Hodgkin's disease, 70
     B-cell lymphoma
       mediastinal large, with sclerosis, 80
       T-cell rich, 79
     clinical features, 69–70, 70t
     comparison of four types of, 71
     cytogenetics, 78
     differential diagnosis, 78–80
     Epstein-Barr virus, and Hodgkin's disease, relationship between, 78
     extranodal Hodgkin's disease, 76
     immunoblastic proliferations, benign, 80
     immunogenotyping, 78
     immunophenotyping, 77t, 77–78
     Ki-1 positive anaplastic large cell lymphoma, 79
     laboratory findings, 77–78
     lacunar cells, nodular sclerosis, 72
     large-cell immunoblastic lymphoma, 79
     Lennert's lymphoma, 79
     lymphocyte depletion, 70, 75–76, *76*
       positive CD15, 76
     lymphocyte predominance, 69–72, 71t, *71–72*
     lymphocytic lymphoma, small, 80
     mixed cellularity, 69–70, 73–75, *74–75*
       interfollicular variant, 75
       with mummified cells, 74
     nodular sclerosis, 69, 72–73, *72–74*
       lacunar cells, 72
       obliterative sclerosis variant of, 74
       syncytial variant of, 73
     oncogene alterations, 78
     pathology, 70–76, *71–72*
     phenotypes, four types of, 77
     Richter's syndrome, 79
     T-cell lymphomas, peripheral, 79
   metastatic carcinoma, and malignant histiocytosis, vs. Ki-1 lymphoma, anaplastic large-cell, 143–149
     clinical features, 143
     laboratory findings, *146*, 146–147
     pathology, 143–146, *144–146*
   vs. thymoma vs. malignant lymphoma, 150–157
     clinical features, 150
     Hodgkin's disease, 153, *153*
     laboratory findings, 154–156, *155*, 155t
     non-Hodgkin's lymphoma, 150, 153–154, *154*
     pathology, 150–154
     thymoma, 150–153, *151–152*
Hunter syndrome, 66
Hyaline-vascular type, Castleman's disease, 82
Hyperplasias, lymphoid, reactive, 25–48, 26t
   AIDS, 25–26, 27t, *27–28*
     lymph node biopsy, 27
   angiolymphoid hyperplasia, skin biopsy in, 31
   bacillary angiomatosis, 41, *41*
   cytomegalovirus lymphadenitis, 37, *37*
   dermatopathic lymphadenopathy, 43, *185*
   follicular pattern, 25–31
   germinal centers, progressive transformation of, 27–28, *29*
   herpes simplex esophagitis, 38
   herpes zoster/herpes simplex lymphadenitis, 38, *38*
   Kaposi's sarcoma, 34–35, *34–35*
     lymph node, 34, 35
   Kawasaki disease, 46
   Kikuchi-Fujimoto disease, 44–46, *44–45*
   Kirmura disease, 29–31, *30–32*, 31t
     angiolymphoid hyperplasia, comparison of, 31
     subcutaneous lesion in, 30
   leishmaniasis, spleen, 43
   lipogranuloma, after lymphangiography, lymph node biopsy, 33
   lymphadenitis, luetic, with florid follicular hyperplasia, 29
   lymphadenopathy
     AIDS-related, histologic patterns in, 27
     drug-induced, 40–41
   lymphangiographic effect, 32–33, *33*
   measles lymphadenitis, 38–39, *39*
   mononucleosis, infectious, 35–37, *36*
   mucocutaneous lymph node syndrome, 46
   polykaryocytes of Warthin and Finkeldey, 38, *39*
   posttransplantation lymphoproliferative disorders, 39–40, *39–40*
   postvaccinial lymphadenitis, 38
   rheumatoid arthritis, 26, *28–29*
     lymph node biopsy, 28
   sinus
     pattern, 31–35, *32*
     vascular transformation of, 33–34, *34*
   syphilis, 26–27, *29*
   systemic lupus lymphadenopathy, 43–44
   toxoplasma
     pseudocyst, 42
   toxoplasmic lymphadenitis, 41–43, *42*
   transformation of germinal centers, progressive, lymph node biopsy of, 29
   Whipple's disease, 32, *33*
     lymph node, 33

I
Immunogenotyping, immunophenotyping, comparison, 17
Immunoglobulin
   heavy chain gene rearrangement, 18
Immunohistochemistry, 14, *14*
Immunoperoxidase stain, of composite lymphoma, 103
Immunophenotyping, 13–16, 14t
   immunogenotyping, comparison, 17
Immunoproliferative lesions, angiocentric, 197–203, *198*
   clinical features, 198
   differential diagnosis, 200–202, 201t, *201–202*
   laboratory findings, 200
   pathology, 198t, 198–199, *198–200*
In situ hybridization, 21, *21*
Isometric plot, composite, 17

K
Kaposi's sarcoma, reactive lymphoid hyperplasias, 34–35, *34–35*
   lymph node, 34, 35
Karyotype, lymph node cells, 22
Kawasaki disease, reactive lymphoid hyperplasias, 46
Ki-1 lymphoma, anaplastic large-cell vs. Hodgkin's disease, metastatic carcinoma, and malignant histiocytosis, 143–149
   clinical features, 143
   laboratory findings, *146*, 146–147
   pathology, 143–146, *144–146*
Kiel classification, updated, of non-Hodgkin's lymphomas, 11
Kikuchi-Fujimoto disease, reactive lymphoid hyperplasias, 44–46, *44–45*
Kirmura disease, reactive lymphoid hyperplasias, 29–31, *30–32*, 31t
   angiolymphoid hyperplasia, comparison of, 31
   subcutaneous lesion in, 30

L
Langerhans' cell histiocytosis, 165, 167, *167–168*
Leishmaniasis, reactive lymphoid hyperplasias, spleen, 43

Lepromatous leprosy, 55
Leukemia
    acute lymphoblastic vs. lymphoblastic lymphoma vs. Burkitt's lymphoma vs., 132–142, 135t, *136*
        Burkitt's lymphoma, 132–133, 133t, 135–141, *137–138*, 139t
        clinical features, 132–133
        laboratory findings, 139–141
        lymphoblastic lymphoma, *133–134*, 133–135, 134t
            and acute lymphoblastic leukemia, 132, 139–140, *140*, 140t
        pathology, 133–139
    hairy-cell vs. monocytoid B-cell lymphoma vs. splenic lymphoma with villous lymphocytes, 120–131, *121–122*, *128*
        B-cell neoplasms, low-grade, comparison, 126
        blood lakes, pseudosinuses, 122
        bone marrow biopsy, hairy-cell leukemia, 121
        clinical features, 120–121
        cytochemistry, 129, *129*
        cytopreparation, from peripheral blood, 129
        fried-egg pattern, 121
        immunophenotyping, 127–129
        laboratory findings, 125–130
        lymphocytic leukemia, chronic, 129
        mast cell, 125
            showing spindle tumor cells, 125
            systematic, 124, *125*
        molecular-genetic studies, 129–130
        monocytoid B-cell lymphoma, 120, 122–124, *123–124*, 128
        pathology, 121–124
        peripheral blood, 125–127, 126t, *126–127*
        prolymphocytic leukemia, 129
        splenectomy specimen, 128
        splenic lymphoma, with villous lymphocytes, 120–121, 124, *124–125*, 128
        T-cell phenotype, 129
        toxoplasmic lymphadenopathy, 123
        variants, hybrid forms, 129
        villous lymphocyte, 126
            showing polar distribution, 127
    lymphocytic, chronic, 129
    prolymphocytic, 129
Lipogranuloma, reactive lymphoid hyperplasias, after lymphangiography, lymph node biopsy, 33
Liver
    in mantle-cell lymphoma, 99
    mycopolysaccharidosis, 66
Lymph follicle
    B-cell, positive, 5
    germinal center, 5
Lymphadenitis
    asteroid body, 50
    granulomatous, 49–61
        bone marrow biopsy, granuloma, 58
        brucellosis, 52, *53*
            kidney, 53
        cat-scratch disease, 50–51, *50–51*
        coccidioides lymphadenitis, 59–60, *59–60*
        cryptococcus lymphadenitis, 55–57, *56–57*
            with yeast cells, 56
        histoplasma lymphadenitis, 57–59, 58t, *58–59*
        lepromatous leprosy, 55
        lymphogranuloma venereum, 51–52, *51–52*
        McCoy cells, 52
        mycobacterial lymphadenitis, 53–54, *53–54*
            caused by Mycobacterium tuberculosis, 53
        mycobacterium avium-intracellulare, spleen, 54
        mycobacterium leprae lymphadenitis, 54–55, *55*
        pneumocystis carinii, cysts of, 57
        pneumocystis lymphadenitis, 57
        pulmonary blastomycosis, 57
        pulmonary hilar lymph node, coccidiodomycosis in, 59
        pulmonary histoplasmosis
            with caseous necrosis, 58
            GMS-positive organisms, 59
        sarcoidosis, 49, *50*
        tularemia, 52
    reactive lymphoid hyperplasias, luetic, with florid follicular hyperplasia, 29
Lymphadenopathy, reactive lymphoid hyperplasias
    AIDS-related, histologic patterns in, 27
    drug-induced, 40–41
Lymphangiographic effect, reactive lymphoid hyperplasias, 32–33, *33*
Lymphoblastic lymphoma vs. Burkitt's lymphoma vs. acute lymphoblastic leukemia, 132–142
    acute lymphoblastic leukemia, 135, 135t, *136*
    Burkitt's lymphoma, 132–133, 133t, 135–141, *137–138*, 139t
    clinical features, 132–133
    laboratory findings, 139–141
    lymphoblastic lymphoma, *133–134*, 133–135, 134t
        and acute lymphoblastic leukemia, 132, 139–140, *140*, 140t
    pathology, 133–139
Lymphocytes, intranodal distribution, 3–6, *4–7*
Lymphocytic lymphoma, small, with proliferation centers, 107, *107*
Lymphogranuloma venereum, 51–52, *51–52*
Lymphohistiocytosis, familial erythrophagocytic, 167–168
Lymphoid disorders, *see also* specific disorder
    ancillary studies for, 13–24
        chromosomal translocation, in lymphoid neoplasms, 23
        contourgram, 16
        cytogenetics, oncogenes and, 21–23, *22*, 23t
        flow cytometer, 15–16, *15–17*
            basic structure of, 15
        hematologic neoplasms, criteria for diagnosis of, 14
        histogram, with prominent K light-chain-positive population, 16
        immunoglobulin
            heavy chain gene rearrangement, 18
        immunohistochemistry, 14, *14*
        immunophenotyping, 13–16, 14t
            immunogenotyping, comparison, 17
        isometric plot, composite, 17
        karyotype, lymph node cells, 22
        molecular genetics, 16–21, 17t
        natural-killer-cell lymphoma, spleen, 21
        polymerase chain reaction, *20*, 20–21
            with stages of denaturation, 20
        in situ hybridization, 21, *21*
        receptor genes, characteristics of, 18
        scattergram, with side scatter, 16
        Southern blotting, *19*, 19–20
        T-cell receptor ß-chain gene, Southern blot hybridization analysis, 19
Lymphoid hyperplasias, reactive, 25–48, 26t; *see also* Reactive lymphoid hyperplasias
Lymphoid neoplasms, 3–12, 4t
    antibodies, monoclonal
        cell specificity, clinical applications of, 8–9
        used in paraffin-embedded sections, 9
    antigens
        lymphoid, 6–9, 7–9t
        surface, categories of, 7
    associated with Castleman's disease, 86, *86*
    B-cell differentiation, intranodal, 7
    B-lymphocytes, immunophenotypes, of different developmental stages of, 4
    cell markers and classification of, 3–12, 4t
        lymph node, normal

230 INDEX

Lymphoid neoplasms (*cont.*)
    with cortex containing lymph follicles with germinal centers, 4
    with subcapsular sinus, 4
    lymphocytes, development of, 3–6, *4–7*
    paracortex, of normal lymph node, 4
  cortex, of normal lymph node, 4
  European-American classification, revised, 11–12
  follicle dendritic cells, in germinal center, meshwork, 6
  Kiel classification, updated, of non-Hodgkin's lymphomas, 11
  lymph follicle
    B-cell, positive, 5
    germinal center, 5
  lymph node, normal, with capsule, 4
  lymphocytes, intranodal distribution, 3–6, *4–7*
  lymphomas, classification of, 9–12, 10–12t
  medulla, of normal lymph node, 5
  non-Hodgkin's lymphoma, 10
  T-cell, positive, lymph node, 5
  T-lymphocytes, immunophenotype, different developmental stages of, 4
Lymphoma
  classification of, 9–12, 10–12t
  large-cell vs. true histiocytic lymphoma
    vs. granulocytic sarcoma, 215–224, *220*
      clinical features, 215
      laboratory findings, 220–223, *222*, 222t
      pathology, 216t, 216–220, *216–222*, 221t
  malignant vs. thymoma vs. Hodgkin's disease, 150–157
    clinical features, 150
    Hodgkin's disease, 153, *153*
    laboratory findings, 154–156, *155*, 155t
    non-Hodgkin's lymphoma, 150, 153–154, *154*
    pathology, 150–154
    thymoma, 150–153, *151–152*
  small- and large-cell vs. composite lymphoma vs. Richter's syndrome, 102–109, *106–107*
    clinical features, 102
    composite lymphoma, 102–104, *103–105*
      and Richter's syndrome, 106
    differential diagnosis, 106–107
    immunoperoxidase stain, of composite lymphoma, 103
    laboratory findings, 105–106
    mycosis fungoides, 103
    pathology, 102–105
    Reed-Sternberg cell, 105
    Richter's syndrome, 102, 104–105, *105*
    small lymphocytic lymphoma, with proliferation centers, 107, *107*
Lymphoplasmacytic lymphoma
  Castleman's disease, 88
  vs. plasmacytoma vs. plasmacytoid T-cell lymphoma, 204–214
    clincial manifestation, 204–205
    differential diagnosis, 212t, 212–213
    laboratory findings, 211–212
    lymphoplasmacytic lymphoma, 204–207, *205–208*, 211
    pathology, 205–211
    plasmacytoid T-cell lymphoma, 205, 210, 210–212, *212*
    plasmacytoma, 204–205, 208–211, *208–210*
Lymphoproliferative syndrome, X-linked, 168

M
Mantle-cell lymphoma, 90–91, 96–98, *97–99*
  blastic variant, 98
  Castleman's disease, 88
  vs. follicular lymphoma vs. follicular hyperplasia, 90–101
    atypical follicular hyperplasia, 92
    clinical manifestation, 90–91

    floral variant, follicular lymphoma, 96
    follicular hyperplasia, 90–92, 91t, *92*
      and follicular lymphoma, differentiation between, 91
      lymph node biopsy, 92
    follicular lymphoma, 90, 92–96, *93–96*
      infiltrating perinodal adipose tissue, 93
      lymph node biopsy, 93
    germinal center, follicular hyperplasia, 92
    involving tonsil, 97
    laboratory findings, 98–100, 99t
    liver, in mantle-cell lymphoma, 99
    lymph node imprint, 98
    mantle-cell lymphoma, 90–91, 96–98, *97–99*
    paratrabecular infiltration, follicular lymphoma with, 96
    pathology, 91–98
    signet-ring-cell variant, follicular-lymphoma, 95
    small-cleaved-cell follicular lymphoma, 96
    spleen, in mantle-cell lymphoma, 98
    involving tonsil, 97
Mast cell disease, 125
  with dark cytoplasmic staining, 125
  showing spindle tumor cells, 125
  systemic, 124, *125*
McCoy cells, 52
Measles lymphadenitis, reactive lymphoid hyperplasias, 38–39, *39*
Medulla, of normal lymph node, 5
Melanoma, amelanotic, 190
Merkel-cell carcinoma, 190
Molecular genetics, 16–21, 17t
Monocytoid B-cell lymphoma, 120, 122–124, *123–124*, 128
Monocytoid sarcoma, plasmacytoid, T-cell lymphoma, vs. lymphoplasmacytic lymphoma, 204–214
  clinical manifestation, 204–205
  differential diagnosis, 212t, 212–213
  laboratory findings, 211–212
  lymphoplasmacytic lymphoma, 204–207, *205–208*, 211
  pathology, 205–211
  plasmacytoid T-cell lymphoma, 205, 210, 210–212, *212*
  plasmacytoma, 204–205, 208–210, *208–210*, 211
Mononucleosis, reactive lymphoid hyperplasias, infectious, 35–37, *36*
Mucocutaneous lymph node syndrome, reactive lymphoid hyperplasias, 46
Mucopolysaccharidoses, 63, 67, 67t
  enzyme deficiency in, 67
Mucopolysaccharidosis, 65–67, *66*
Mucosa-associated lymphoid tissue vs. T-cell-rich-B-cell lymphoma vs. pseudolymphoma
  clinical manifestation, 110–111
  gastric lymphoma, 113
    of MALT type, 112
  Hashimoto's thyroiditis, 113
  Helicobacter pylori gastritis, 113
  MALT-type lymphoma, 110–114, *111–114*
  monocytoid B-cells, 114
  pathology, 111–115
  pulmonary lymphoma, 111, 113
    MALT type, 112
  salivary gland, 116
    with MALT-type lymphoma, 112
  T-cell-rich-B-cell lymphoma, 111, 114–115, *115*
Mycobacterial lymphadenitis, 53–54, *53–54*
  caused by Mycobacterium tuberculosis, 53
Mycobacterium avium-intracellularae, spleen, 54
Mycobacterium leprae lymphadenitis, 54–55, *55*
Mycosis fungoides, 103
  Sézary syndrome vs. adult T-cell leukemia/lymphoma, 181–189, 182t, 183t, *183–187*

clinical features, 181–182
laboratory findings, 183t, 186–188, 188t
pathology, 182–186

N

Natural-killer-cell lymphoma
vs. natural-killer-like T-cell lymphoma, 175–180, *176*
clinical features, 175–176, 176t
laboratory findings, 176t, 177–179, 179t
pathology, 176–177, *176–178*
spleen, 21
Niemann-Pick disease, 62–64, *65*, 67
cells, from spleen, showing positive stain, 65
foamy cells in spleen, 65
type C cell, from bone marrow, 65
Non-Hodgkin's lymphoma, 10

P

Plasmacytoid T-cell lymphoma vs. lymphoplasmacytic lymphoma vs. plasmacytoma, 204–214
clinical manifestation, 204–205
differential diagnosis, 212t, 212–213
laboratory findings, 211–212
lymphoplasmacytic lymphoma, 204–207, *205–208*, 211
pathology, 205–211
plasmacytoid T-cell lymphoma, 205, *210*, 210–212, *212*
plasmacytoma, 204–205, 208–211, *208–210*
Plasmacytoma
Castleman's disease, 88
vs. plasmacytoid T-cell lymphoma vs. lymphoplasmacytic lymphoma, 204–214
differential diagnosis, 212t, 212–213
laboratory findings, 211–212
lymphoplasmacytic lymphoma, 211
plasmacytoid T-cell lymphoma, *210*, 210–212, *212*
plasmacytoma, 211
Pneumocystis carinii, cysts of, 57
Pneumocystis lymphadenitis, 57
Polykaryocytes of Warthin and Finkeldey, reactive lymphoid hyperplasias, 38
Polymerase chain reaction, *20*, 20–21
Posttransplantation lymphoproliferative disorders, reactive lymphoid hyperplasias, 39–40, *39–40*
Postvaccinial lymphadenitis, reactive lymphoid hyperplasias, 38
Prolymphocytic leukemia, 129
Pseudolymphoma vs. lymphoma of mucosa-associated lymphoid tissue vs. T-cell-rich-B-cell lymphoma, 110–119
clinical manifestation, 110–111
gastric lymphoma, 113
of MALT type, 112
Hashimoto's thyroiditis, 113
Helicobacter pylori gastritis, 113
MALT-type lymphoma, 110–114, *111–114*
monocytoid B-cells, 114
pathology, 111–115
pulmonary lymphoma, 111, 113
MALT type, 112
salivary gland, with MALT-type lymphoma, 112
T-cell-rich-B-cell lymphoma, 111, 114–115, *115*
Pulmonary blastomycosis, 57
Pulmonary hilar lymph node, coccidiodomycosis in, 59
Pulmonary histoplasmosis
with caseous necrosis, 58
GMS-positive organisms, 59

R

Reactive lymphoid hyperplasias, 25–48, 26t
AIDS, 25–26, 27t, *27–28*
lymph node biopsy, 27
angiolymphoid hyperplasia, skin biopsy in, 31
bacillary angiomatosis, 41, *41*
cytomegalovirus lymphadenitis, 37, *37*
dermatopathic lymphadenopathy, 43, *185*
follicular pattern, 25–31
germinal centers, progressive transformation of, 27–28, *29*
herpes simplex esophagitis, 38, *38*
herpes zoster/herpes simplex lymphadenitis, 38, *38*
Kaposi's sarcoma, 34–35, *34–35*
lymph node, 34, 35
Kawasaki disease, 46
Kikuchi-Fujimoto disease, 44–46, *44–45*
Kirmura disease, 29–31, *30–32*, 31t
angiolymphoid hyperplasia, comparison of, 31
subcutaneous lesion in, 30
leishmaniasis, spleen, 43
lipogranuloma, after lymphangiography, lymph node biopsy, 33
lymphadenitis, luetic, with florid follicular hyperplasia, 29
lymphadenopathy
AIDS-related, histologic patterns in, 27
drug-induced, 40–41
lymphangiographic effect, 32–33, *33*
measles lymphadenitis, 38–39, *39*
mononucleosis, infectious, 35–37, *36*
mucocutaneous lymph node syndrome, 46
polykaryocytes of Warthin and Finkeldey, 38, *39*
posttransplantation lymphoproliferative disorders, 39–40, *39–40*
postvaccinial lymphadenitis, 38
rheumatoid arthritis, 26, *28–29*
lymph node biopsy, 28
sinus
pattern, 31–35, *32*
vascular transformation of, 33–34, *34*
syphilis, 26–27, *29*
systemic lupus lymphadenopathy, 43–44
toxoplasma
lymphadenitis, 41–43, *42–43*
pseudocyst, 42
transformation of germinal centers, progressive, lymph node biopsy of, 29
Whipple's disease, 32, *33*
lymph node, 33
Receptor genes, characteristics of, 18
Reed-Sternberg-like cells, lymphomas with, Hodgkin's disease vs., 69–81, 70t
Ann Arbor staging system, Hodgkin's disease, 70
B-cell lymphoma
mediastinal large, with sclerosis, 80
T-cell rich, 79
clinical features, 69–70, 70t
cytogenetics, 78
differential diagnosis, 78–80
Epstein-Barr virus, and Hodgkin's disease, relationship between, 78
extranodal Hodgkin's disease, 76
Hodgkin's disease
comparison of four types of, 71
phenotypes, four types of, 77
immunoblastic proliferations, benign, 80
immunogenotyping, 78
immunophenotyping, 77t, 77–78
Ki-1 positive anaplastic large cell lymphoma, 79
laboratory findings, 77–78
lacunar cells, nodular sclerosis, 72
large-cell immunoblastic lymphoma, 79

Reed-Sternberg-like cells (*cont.*)
　Lennert's lymphoma, 79
　lymphocyte
　　depletion, 70, 75–76, *76*
　　　positive CD15, 76
　　predominance, 69–72, 71t, *71–72*
　lymphocytic lymphoma, small, 80
　mixed cellularity, 69–70, 73–75, *74–75*
　　interfollicular variant, 75
　　mummified cells, 74
　nodular sclerosis, 69, 72–73, *72–74*
　　lacunar cells, 72
　　obliterative sclerosis variant of, 74
　　syncytial variant of, 73
　oncogene alterations, 78
　pathology, 70–76, *71–72*
　Richter's syndrome, 79
　T-cell lymphomas, peripheral, 79
Rheumatoid arthritis
　Castleman's disease, 88
　reactive lymphoid hyperplasias, 26, *28–29*
　　lymph node biopsy, 28
Richter's syndrome, 102, 104–105, *105*
　vs. mixed small- and large-cell lymphoma vs composite
　　　lymphoma, 102–109
　　clinical features, 102
　　composite lymphoma, 102–104, *103–105*
　　　and Richter's syndrome, 106
　　differential diagnosis, 106–107
　　immunoperoxidase stain, of composite lymphoma, 103
　　laboratory findings, 105–106
　　mixed small and large cell lymphoma, 106, *106–107*
　　mycosis fungoides, 103
　　pathology, 102–105
　　Reed-Sternberg cell, 105
　　Richter's syndrome, 102, 104–105, *105*
　　small lymphocytic lymphoma, with proliferation centers, 107, *107*
Rosai-Dorfman disease, 165, *168*, 168–169

S

Sézary syndrome, mycosis fungoides, vs. adult T-cell
　　　leukemia/lymphoma, 103, 181–189, 182t, 183t, *183–187*
　　clinical features, 181–182
　　laboratory findings, 183t, 186–188, 188t
　　pathology, 182–186
Sarcoidosis, 49, *50*
Scattergram, with side scatter, 16
Sinus
　pattern, reactive lymphoid hyperplasias, 31–35, *32*
　reactive lymphoid hyperplasias, vascular transformation of, 33–34, *34*
Southern blotting, *19*, 19–20
Spleen
　lymphoma, with villous lymphocytes, 120–121, 124, *124–125*, 128
　　vs. hairy-cell leukemia vs. monocytoid B-cell lymphoma,
　　　120–131, *121–122*, *124–125*, *128*
　　　B-cell neoplasms, low-grade, comparison, 126
　　　blood lakes, pseudosinuses, 122
　　　bone marrow biopsy, hairy-cell leukemia, 121
　　　clinical features, 120–121
　　　cytochemistry, 129, *129*
　　　cytopreparation, from peripheral blood, 129
　　　fried-egg pattern, 121
　　　hairy cell, 127
　　　immunophenotyping, 127–129
　　　laboratory findings, 125–130
　　　lymphocytic leukemia, chronic, 129

　　　mast cell, 125
　　　　showing spindle tumor cells, 125
　　　systematic, 124, *125*
　　　molecular-genetic studies, 129–130
　　　monocytoid B-cell lymphoma, 120, 122–124, *123–124*, 128
　　　pathology, 121–124
　　　peripheral blood, 125–127, 126t, *126–127*
　　　prolymphocytic leukemia, 129
　　　splenectomy specimen, 128
　　　T-cell phenotype, 129
　　　toxoplasmic lymphadenopathy, 123
　　　variants, hybrid forms, 129
　　　villous lymphocyte, 126
　in mantle-cell lymphoma, 98
Storage histiocyte disorders, 62–68, 63t
　bone marrow aspirate, sea-blue histiocyte, 65
　clinical manifestation, 62–67
　comparison of, 63
　Gaucher cell, 62–64, *63–64*, 67
　　in bone marrow, positive PAS staining, 64
　　showing, electron micrograph of, 64
　laboratory findings, 67
　liver, mycopolysaccharidosis, 66
　mucopolysaccharidoses, 63, 67, 67t
　　enzyme deficiency in, 67
　mucopolysaccharidosis, 65–67, *66*
　Niemann-Pick disease, 62–64, 65, 67
　　foamy cells in spleen, 65
　　from spleen, showing positive stain, 65
　　type C cell, from bone marrow, 65
　pathology, 63–67
　"zebra body" membrane-delimited inclusion, electron micrograph, 66
Syphilis
　Castleman's disease, 88
　reactive lymphoid hyperplasias, 26–27, *29*
Systemic lupus erythematosus, Castleman's disease, 88
Systemic lupus lymphadenopathy, reactive lymphoid hyperplasias, 43–44

T

T-cell
　B-cell lymphoma
　　vs. pseudolymphoma vs. lymphoma of mucosa-associated
　　　lymphoid tissue, 110–119
　　vs. pseudolymphoma vs. mucosa-associated lymphoid tissue
　　　vs., 114
　　clinical manifestation, 110–111
　　comparison of immunophenotype and immunogenotype
　　　among low-grade B-cell lymphomas, 117
　　gastric lymphoma, 113
　　　of MALT type, 112
　　Hashimoto's thyroiditis, 113
　　Helicobacter pylori gastritis, 113
　　MALT-type lymphoma, 110–114, *111–114*
　　monocytoid B-cells, 114
　　pathology, 111–115
　　pulmonary lymphoma, 111, 113
　　　MALT type, 112
　　salivary gland, with MALT-type lymphoma, 112
　　T-cell-rich B-cell lymphoma, 111, 114–115, *115*
　leukemia/lymphoma, adult
　　Sézary syndrome, mycosis fungoides, 103, 181–189, 182t, 183t, *183–187*
　　　clinical features, 181–182
　　　laboratory findings, 183t, 186–188, 188t
　　　pathology, 182–186
　　vs. Sézary syndrome, mycosis fungoides, 181–189

lymphoma
    immunoblastic lymphadenopathy-like, vs. angioimmunoblastic
        lymphadenopathy, 158–163
        clinical features, 158
        laboratory findings, 162
        pathology, 158–162, *159–161*
    natural-killer-cell lymphoma, vs. natural-killer-like, 175–180, *176*
        clinical features, 175–176, 176t
        laboratory findings, 176t, 177–179, 179t
        pathology, 176–177, *176–178*
    plasmacytoid, vs. lymphoplasmacytic lymphoma vs.
        plasmacytoma, 204–214
        clinical manifestation, 204–205
        differential diagnosis, 212t, 212–213
        laboratory findings, 211–212
        lymphoplasmacytic lymphoma, 204–207, *205–208*, 211
        pathology, 205–211
        plasmacytoid T-cell lymphoma, 205, *210*, 210–212, *212*
        plasmacytoma, 204–205, 208–210, *208–210*, 211
    with sinusoidal infiltration and/or hemophagocytosis, 165–166
    vs. histiocytosis, malignant and benign, 164–174, 165t
        clinical features, 164–166
        familial, gene-related diseases, 165
        hemophagocytic syndrome, infection-associated, 164–167, *166*
        histiocytosis, malignant, 166, *166*
        laboratory findings, 170–173, 171t, *172*
        Langerhans' cell histiocytosis, 165, 167, *167–168*
        lymphohistiocytosis, familial erythrophagocytic, 167–168
        lymphomas, 169–170, *169–170*
        lymphoproliferative syndrome, X-linked, 168
        malignant histiocytosis, 164
        pathology, 166–170
        Rosai-Dorfman disease, 165, *168*, 168–169
        T-cell lymphomas, with sinusoidal infiltration and/or
            hemophagocytosis, 165–166
T-cell receptor β-chain gene, Southern blot hybridization analysis, 19

Thymoma vs. malignant lymphoma vs. Hodgkin's disease, 150–157
    clinical features, 150
    Hodgkin's disease, 153, *153*
    laboratory findings, 154–156, *155*, 155t
    non-Hodgkin's lymphoma, 153–154, *154*
    pathology, 150–154
    thymoma, 150–153, *151–152*
Toxoplasma, reactive lymphoid hyperplasias, pseudocyst, 42
Toxoplasmic lymphadenitis, reactive lymphoid hyperplasias, 41–43, *42–43*
Toxoplasmic lymphadenopathy, 123
Transformation of germinal centers, reactive lymphoid hyperplasias, progressive, lymph node biopsy of, 29
Tularemia, 52

V
Villous lymphocyte, 126
    polar distribution, 127

W
Whipple's disease, reactive lymphoid hyperplasias, 32, *33*
    lymph node, 33

X
X-linked lymphoproliferative syndrome, 168

Z
"Zebra body" membrane-delimited inclusion, electron micrograph, storage histiocyte disorders, 66